Karl Neno
Gunter Carloff

Einsatz für den Rettungshubschrauber
Mission for the Rescue Helicopter

FORTES FORTUNA ADIUVAT.
Den Mutigen hilft das Glück.
Fortune assists the brave.

TERENZ, *Phormio,* 203

KISTERKALL VERLAG GMBH

Impressum / Imprint

Die Deutsche Bibliothek - CIP – Standard Einheitsaufnahme (Standard Bibliographic Entry)
Karl Neno / Gunter Carloff
Einsatz für den Rettungshubschrauber – Mission for the Rescue Helicopter
Köln/Cologne 2001
ISBN 3-935604-00-9

Postfach 90 60 81
D-51127 Köln
Fax: +49 (0) 22 03 / 96 50 01
E-Mail: info@kisterkall.de
Internet: www.kisterkall.de.

Die Fotos, auf denen ich im Einsatz zu sehen bin, verdanke ich freundlichen Helfern, denen ich meine vorher eingestellte Kamera in die Hand drücken konnte und sie bat, bei eingeschaltetem Kameramotor in meine Richtung auszulösen.
Das Studioportrait von Karl Neno verdanke ich Photographie Göbel's Kunst.
Das Portrait von Herrn Genscher machte Helmut R. Schulze.

Die Bildunterschriften wurden teilweise zum Schutz von Patienten verfremdet, damit Vorgänge zu deren Nachteil nicht nachvollzogen werden können.
Die Fotos sind, außer mit einer Säuberungsretusche, nicht bearbeitet oder verfremdet worden.

Karl Neno

The credit for the photos showing me in action goes to friendly helpers who obligingly accepted the camera I shoved into their hands and who then pressed the release button (which activated the motor) with the camera pointed in my direction. The studio portrait of Karl Neno was made by Göbel's Art Photography Studio.
The portrait of Mr. Genscher was made by Helmut R. Schulze.

In some cases the information in the photo captions has been altered to protect the privacy of the patients.
Except for slight cosmetic retouching, the photos have not been tampered with in any way.

Karl Neno

Layout und Lithographie: Becker Satz GmbH, Köln
Druck: Rasch Druckerei und Verlag GmbH & Co. KG, Bramsche
Printed in Germany

ISBN 3-935604-00-9

Einsatz für den Rettungshubschrauber

Mission for the Rescue Helicopter

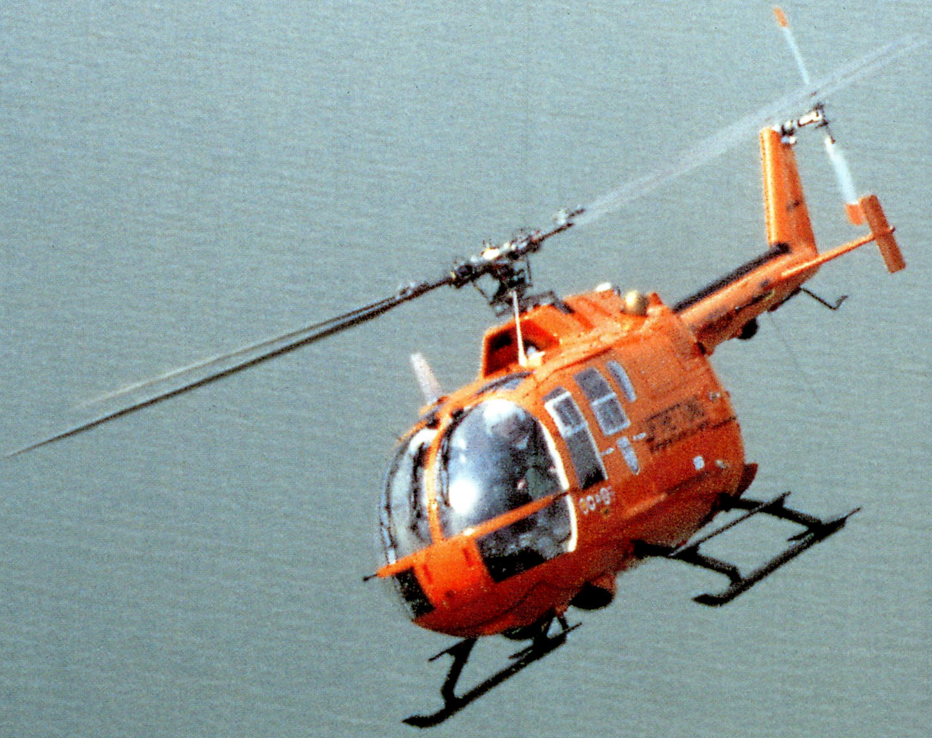

Karl Neno
Gunter Carloff

KISTERKALL VERLAG GMBH

Inhaltsverzeichnis der Textbeiträge
Table of Contents for the Rescue Helicopter Texts

Mit Indienststellung des ersten Rettungshubschraubers „Christoph 1“ wurde Ende 1970 in München der Grundstein für den Aufbau des öffentlich-rechtlichen Luftrettungsnetzes in Deutschland gelegt.

Dieser Luftrettungsstation folgten bis heute bundesweit 51 Stationen. Damit besteht in Deutschland ein flächendeckendes und dichtes Luftrettungsnetz zur schnellen Notfallversorgung wie in keinem anderen Land. Es verdankt seinen hohen Standard dem Zusammenwirken verschiedener Einrichtungen – Bund, Ländern, Bundeswehr und nicht zuletzt dem ADAC und der Deutschen Rettungsflugwacht. Auch der Bundesgrenzschutz ist in besonderer Weise eingebunden und hat die Entwicklung der Flugrettung in Deutschland durch die Bereitstellung einer leistungsfähigen Flugdienstorganisation maßgeblich voran gebracht. Die mit den Rettungshubschraubern geflogenen Einsätze, die als luftgestützte Notarztwagen fungieren, werden im ersten Halbjahr 2001 die Millionenmarke erreichen. Unzähligen Menschen konnte hierdurch das Leben gerettet und die Gesundheit erhalten werden.

Mit der nun vorliegenden Veröffentlichung haben Gunter Carloff und Karl Neno – beide sind seit vielen Jahren aktiv in der Luftrettung tätig – eine Dokumentation vorgelegt, die ihresgleichen sucht. Ausführlich wir hier in Bild und Wort die Arbeit des Rettungshubschrauberdienstes am Beispiel der Station „Christoph 3“ in Köln-Merheim nachgezeichnet. Dieses Buch lebt von den Erfahrungen aus erster Hand, die erstmals so umfangreich dokumentiert werden, dass sie nicht nur für die von Berufs wegen Interessierten eine erstklassige Informationsquelle bieten.

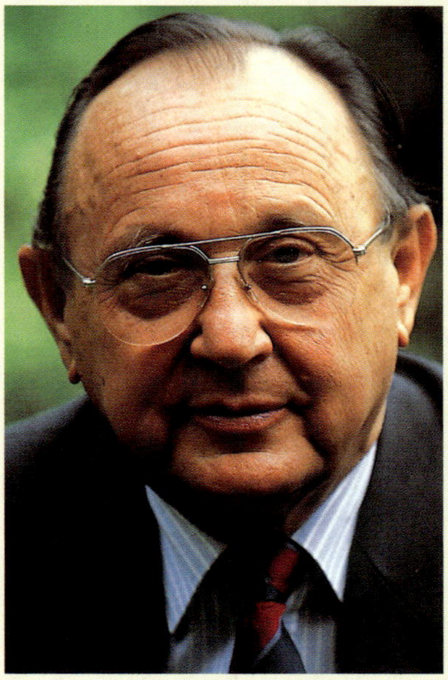

Bundesminister a. D.
Former German Minister
HANS-DIETRICH GENSCHER

When the first rescue helicopter, "Christoph 1", was put into service in Munich in 1970, the cornerstone was laid for the establishment of an helicopter emergency medical service (HEMS) under public law in Germany.

This first station has spawned 50 others to date; today the 51 HEMS stations in Germany form a tightly meshed network covering the entire territory of Germany and providing rapid emergency medical care as part of an emergency medical system that is unique in the world. The high standard of this system is the result of cooperation between various organizations – the federal and state governments, the German Air Force and, not least, the German Automobile Club (ADAC) and the German Air Rescue Service (DRF). The German Federal Border Police is also involved in this system and plays a very special role: its contribution, an efficient flight operations organization, has been instrumental in moving the HEMS forward. The number of missions flown by the rescue helicopters, each of which serves as a flying rescue ambulance carrying a physician with emergency & rescue certification, will reach the one million mark during the first six months of 2001. Since its inception this system has saved the life and health of countless individuals.

With their book "Mission for the Rescue Helicopter", co-authors Gunter Carloff and Karl Neno – both active in the helicopter emergency medical service for many years – have put together an unparalleled documentation on the rescue helicopter system. The book paints a detailed picture, in both photos and texts, of the work of the helicopter emergency medical service, with the "Christoph 3" HEMS station in Cologne-Merheim serving as a representative example. This book lives from the first-hand experience – and experiences – of the authors; both have now been documented so comprehensively, for the first time, that the book will surely serve as a first-class source of information for everyone interested in rescue helicopters – regardless of whether this interest is private or professional.

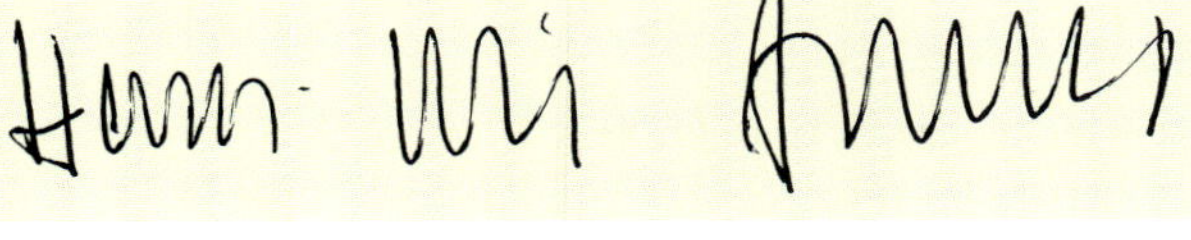

Vorwort / Foreword

von/by Karl Neno

Meine Aufgabe als Luftrettungsassistent war vom 7.8.1978 bis zum 1.1.2000 die gleiche, wie für jeden anderen Luftrettungsassistenten auch. Die Kamera begleitete mich von Beginn an, zunächst als mein eigenes fotografisches Notizbuch, dann wurden meine Fotos recht schnell für Fortbildungsveranstaltungen genutzt. Dort tauchten immer wieder die gleichen Fragen auf, die auch dieses Buch beantworten will. Und immer wieder war es auch die Frage, wie denn eine Einsatzstelle aus der Luft, also aus der Sicht der RTH-Crew aussieht.

Nachdem der Pilot an der Einsatzstelle den Rotor abgebremst hatte, wurde er nach anfänglicher Scheu dann mit Fragen bombardiert. Wir, der Notarzt und ich, waren unterwegs zum Notfallort, und wenn wir zum RTH zurückkamen, war unser Pilot umringt von fragenden und interessierten Menschen. Kinder hatten dabei die wenigste Scheu. In den „meistgestellten Fragen an der Einsatzstelle" hat Thomas Helbig diese Fragen aufgegriffen und in leicht verständlicher Form beantwortet. Piloten und RTH-Besatzungen haben täglich die Möglichkeit, untereinander zu fragen, sie haben die Cockpitsicht auf Einsatzstellen und kennen natürlich alle das, was in diesem Buch steht. Die überwiegende Zahl des bodengebundenen Rettungspersonals hat dieses Privileg nicht und versteht oft erst nach einem Einsatz mit dem RTH, warum eine RTH-Besatzung mit möglichst genauen Informationen versorgt werden muss, damit eine Einsatzstelle schnellstmöglich erreicht werden kann. Dies hat Gunter Carloff in den „Einsatzmöglichkeiten von Rettungshubschraubern" aufgegriffen und für den Rettungsassistenten vor Ort nachvollziehbar erklärt. Sein Artikel kann als Information zur Zusammenarbeit mit RTH für alle gelten, die diese noch vor sich haben. Wenn man seine Anregungen aufgreift, wird der erste Einsatz nicht zum Stress, der vernünftiges Handeln blockiert. PD Dr. Bertil Bouillon und die anderen Autoren auch haben es auf den Punkt gebracht: (Nur) Gemeinsam sind wir stark.

Der RTH ist nur ein Glied in der Rettungskette. Die Bilder dieses Buch belegen dies in allen Facetten. Die Fortsetzung dieses Gedankens ist eine Maxime des Buches: Menschen sind es, die Rettung entscheidend gestalten. Deshalb sind überall dort, wo Personen einen Vorgang verdeutlichen können, Personen abgebildet. Und wieder waren es Menschen, Pioniere beseelt von der Idee, mit Christoph 3, einer der ersten Luft-

During the 22 years I worked as an air rescue paramedic – from 7 August 1978 to 1 January 2000 – I performed the same duties as any other air rescue paramedic. My camera was my constant companion from the start. At first these photos served as a personal journal; before long, however, the crew numbers asked if they could use them at their continued education seminars.

At these seminars, the same questions were posed time and again – questions this book has tried to answer. One question raised on numerous occasions was: what does an operating site look like from the air, i.e. from the point of view of a rescue helicopter crew member? The book contains numerous photos which answer this question. At the operating site, after the rotors had stopped turning, we were first greeted with shyness and then curiosity. We – the physician with emergency & rescue certification and myself – headed quickly to the scene of the emergency. When we returned to the helicopter, we were often circled by people bombarding us with questions. Children displayed the least hesitancy in this respect. In the chapter Frequently Asked Questions, the pilot Thomas Helbig answers many of these questions in a manner even a layperson can understand. Pilots and rescue helicopter crews have a daily opportunity to ask each other any questions that are on their minds. From the cockpit, moreover, they have a clear view of the operating site and are naturally already familiar with most of the information in this book. However, the vast majority of the rescue workers on the ground have not yet had this privilege; as a result, they frequently do not understand why the rescue helicopter crew has to be given such extremely precise information to help them locate the emergency site at top speed.

Gunter Carloff has taken up this subject in Possibilities for Employing Rescue Helicopters. Carloff's explanation of the possibilities for rescue helicopters is written in an understandable style aimed mainly at the paramedic at the emergency site. This chapter can also serve as a guide to cooperating with rescue helicopter crews for all rescue workers who have not yet had this experience. By following his recommendations, rescue personnel can assist the rescue helicopter crew – or go on their own first rescue helicopter mission – without the kind of stress which precludes level-headed action. In his chapter on The Rescue Helicopter: An Important Link in the Rescue Chain, PD Dr. Bertil Bouillion drives home a point made by other authors as well: rescue work is by definition a team effort. The rescue helicopter is only one link in the rescue chain. The photos in this book document all aspects of this powerful cooperation.

The authors have taken this idea and developed it further to formulate one of the main messages of the book: individuals play a decisive role in rescue activities. This

rettungsstationen, einen erfolgreichen Modellversuch zur Rettung anderer Menschen zu starten. In den Beiträgen dieser Pioniere werden die ersten Tage beschrieben, der Modellversuch Rettungshubschrauber und die Bauwagenzeit. Eine spannende Hubschraubergeschichte am Beispiel eines Hubschraubers. Und hier findet sich ein weiterer Grundgedanke des Buches: Was auf einer Hubschrauberstation geschieht, ist in Deutschland ähnlich nach dem pars - pro - toto Prinzip. 365 Tage jedes Jahr! Die auch in den Medien geführte Diskussion über die Qualität von Landeplätzen wird durch den Beitrag von Gunter Carloff auf den Stand des Jahres 2001 gebracht. Gunter Carloff bringt auch die von vielen Rettungsassistenten erwünschten Informationen zu den HEMS-Crew-Membern. Christoph-Luftrettungsstationen im Internet zeigen Präsentations- und Kommunikationsformen des 21.Jahrhunderts. Nichts ist vorhersehbar und alles ist jederzeit möglich, das ist Rettungsdienst. So soll auch die Abfolge der Einsatzsequenzen nur Rettungsalltag widerspiegeln.

Diese Widerspiegelung von Rettungshubschrauberalltag bestimmt auch die Abfolge der Fotosequenzen. Mit wenigen Ausnahmen wird nur die Sicht aus dem Cockpit und an der Einsatzstelle, meistens nach der Patientenversorgung, gezeigt. Die Skalpierungsverletzung eines Kleinkindes durch den eigenen Schäferhund und die Schussverletzung sollen zeigen, dass Rettungshubschrauberbesatzungen auch mit sehr tragischen und brutalen Einsätzen konfrontiert werden. In wenigen Bildbeispielen muss dies anklingen, in einem Bildband, der den Leser eher mit schönen Bildern verwöhnt.

Die Übersetzung der deutschen Texte ins Englische bedarf in vielen Fällen weiterer Umschreibungen, da die Rettungskonzepte weltweit unterschiedlich sind. Das deutsche Konzept schreibt vor, dass der Notarzt schnell zum Patienten gebracht werden soll, das amerikanische Konzept sieht vor, dass der Arzt im Krankenhaus bleibt und der Patient von Paramedics versorgt und ins Krankenhaus gebracht werden soll. Das ist sicher auch durch die deutlich größeren Entfernungen in Amerika bedingt. Die Übersetzung beschreibt deshalb so anschaulich, dass der deutsche Text nachvollziehbar wird.

Die vielen Fotos gewähren über Landesgrenzen und Sprachbarrieren hinaus einen anschaulichen Einblick in den Alltag der Rettungshubschrauberbesatzungen, jeden Tag, 365 Tage im Jahr.

is the reason we have included photographs of individuals wherever possible to illustrate rescue procedures.

It was individuals, furthermore, who were first inspired by the idea of starting a model project centered on Christoph 3, one of the first air rescue stations. Since then this program has met with enormous success and benefited countless individuals. The early days of the rescue helicopter service provided material for The Early Days, the Rescue Helicopter Model Program and the Construction-Site Trailer Days.

These chapters make exciting reading: an action-packed helicopter story starring a rescue helicopter! Here we find another central idea of the book: the events taking place aboard one helicopter on a typical operational day are – in keeping with the principle pars pro toto – happening at numerous other locations throughout Germany 365 days a year!

In his chapter on Hospital Heliports, Gunter Carloff has brought the discussion on heliports and rooftop heliports up to date as of 2001. Carloff is also the author of Information on HEMS Crew Members.

It was several crew members, moreover, who hit upon the idea of using the presentation and communication forms of the 21st century to provide information on the Christoph rescue helicopters. The result is the Christoph website.

In the rescue business, nothing is predictable and everything is possible. The photos of individual missions have been arranged in an order that reflects the sequence of events during a rescue operation.

It was the sequence of events during a day in the life a rescue helicopter crew, moreover, that determined the order in which the various photo sequences are presented in the book. With few exceptions, the photos show the view from the cockpit or depict the provision of emergency medical care at the emergency site. The photos of the little girl scalped by the family's German shepherd and of the man with gunshot wounds were included to show that rescue helicopter crews are often confronted with tragic and brutal incidents. This message has to be brought across, with only a few photos, in a photo book which generally tends to spoils the reader with esthetic pictures.

In many cases, the English text has had to explain or describe – rather than translate word for word – to do justice to the differences between the national rescue systems. In the German system, for example, the physician with emergency & rescue certification goes out to the patient. In the American system, in contrast, the emergency physician remains in the hospital; the patient is given emergency medical care by paramedics and then transported by ambulance to the hospital.

The photos, however, convey a vivid impression of the work carried out at a rescue helicopter base day in, day out – 365 days a year – which can be understood across all national boundaries or language barriers.

Einleitung / Introduction

von/by Gunter Carloff

Der Anfang

„Christoph 1", der erste Rettungshubschrauber Deutschlands, benannt nach dem Heiligen Christophorus, dem Schutzpatron der Fahrenden und Reisenden, nimmt in München am 1. November 1970 seinen Dienst auf.

Bereits in den 1960er Jahren war eine Vielzahl von zumeist privaten Versuchen vorausgegangen, den Rettungsdienst mit Hilfe von Hubschraubern effektiver zu gestalten. Neue Ideen waren notwendig, denn aufgrund der zunehmenden Motorisierung war die Zahl der Verkehrstoten auf nahezu 20.000 im Jahr gewachsen. Das Projekt, nicht den Patienten so schnell wie möglich ins Krankenhaus zu transportieren, sondern das therapiefreie Intervall dadurch zu verkürzen, dass der Notarzt zum Patienten fliegt, war zunächst nur als Großversuch auf Zeit gedacht.

Den Betrieb des ersten zivilen Rettungshubschraubers, einer BO 105 von Messerschmitt-Bölkow-Blohm, ausgerüstet nach dem neuesten Stand der Notfallmedizin und ausschließlich für Notfalleinsätze bereitgehalten, übernahm der Allgemeine Deutsche Automobil Club (ADAC), der dieses Konzept federführend vorangetrieben hatte. An der Finanzierung beteiligten sich der Bund, der Freistaat Bayern und die Allianz-Versicherungsgruppe.

Die Konzeption

Wesentlich für das deutsche Modell der Luftrettung waren die Grundsätze, die noch heute Geltung besitzen: Der speziell ausgestattete Hubschrauber wird ausschließlich für die Notfallrettung bereitgehalten, er ist grundsätzlich innerhalb von zwei Minuten nach der Alarmierung startbereit. Die medizinische Besatzung besteht aus einem erfahrenen Notarzt und einem Sanitäter, heute Luftrettungsassistenten (HEMS-Crew-Member).

Die medizinische Ausrüstung entspricht der eines bodengebundenen Notarztwagens. Die Luftrettung und der bodengebundene Rettungsdienst werden durch regionale Leitstellen koordiniert. Die Hubschrauber werden grundsätzlich an leistungsfähigen Krankenhäusern stationiert.

How It All Began

The first rescue helicopter in Germany, "Christoph 1" (named after the patron saint of travelers), was put into service on 1 November 1970. In the 1960s a large number of attempts were already mounted, mainly by private individuals and organizations, to use rescue helicopters to raise the effectiveness of emergency medical services. New ideas were in high demand: owing to Germany's increasing motorization, the number of deaths on the nation's highways had risen to almost 20,000 per year. The rescue helicopter project – which was based on the idea of shortening the time between the call for help and the provision of emergency medical care by sending the physician with emergency & rescue certification out to the patient instead of bringing the patient as quickly as possible to the hospital – was initially designed as a large-scale trial of limited duration. The first civilian rescue helicopter, the BO 105 made by Messerschmitt-Bölkow-Blohm, was operated by the German Automobile Club (ADAC), which had played a leading role in promoting this concept from the start. This helicopter was equipped with state-of-the-art emergency medical equipment and reserved for emergency missions. Financing was provided by the German government, the German state of Bavaria and the Allianz Insurance Group.

Concept

The German air rescue model embodied basic principles which are still valid today: the specially equipped rescue helicopter is used exclusively for emergency medical care and is ready to take off within two minutes of receiving an emergency call. The original medical crews consisted of an experienced physician with emergency & rescue certification and an emergency medical technician; today the EMT has been supplanted by an air rescue paramedic (HEMS Crew Member). The helicopter carries the same medical equipment as a road-bound rescue ambulance. Both HEMS and emergency medical services on the ground are coordinated by regional Coordination Centers. The helicopters are normally stationed at efficient hospitals with a broad spectrum of capabilities.

Die Funktion der Luftrettung umfasst folgende Aufgaben:

1. Schnelle Heranführung des qualifizierten Rettungsteams bestehend aus Notarzt und Rettungsassistent,
2. optimale präklinische Versorgung des Patienten am Notfallort,
3. schonender und schneller Transport des Patienten in das für die definitive Behandlung geeignete Krankenhaus,
4. Transport von Patienten zwischen Kliniken (Interhospitaltransfer),
5. Transport von lebenswichtigen Organen für Transplantationen, Blutkonserven, Arzneimitteln, etc.,
6. Transport von Spezialisten, z.B. für technische Rettungsmaßnahmen bei Großschadensereignissen und
7. Suchflüge nach vermissten Personen.

Die Einsatzbereitschaft beginnt bei Sonnenaufgang, in der Regel nicht vor 7.00 Uhr, und endet bei Sonnenuntergang.

Das deutsche Modell

Nach der föderativen Staatsverfassung der Bundesrepublik Deutschland sind für den Rettungsdienst ausschließlich die Bundesländer zuständig. Diese sahen sich jedoch nicht in der Lage, die Finanzierung und den Betrieb der Luftrettung zu übernehmen.

Für den erweiterten Katastrophenschutz bzw. Zivilschutz im Verteidigungsfall ist wiederum das Bundesinnenministerium zuständig. Der damalige Bundesinnenminister Hans-Dietrich Genscher schuf über die Erweiterung des Gesetzes für den Katastrophenschutz die Voraussetzung, Luftrettungsmittel für diesen Zweck zu beschaffen. Diese Zivilschutzhubschrauber sollten als Führungs-, Lenkungs- und Erkundungsmittel sowie zum Transport von Einsatzpersonal und Einsatzausstattung eingesetzt werden. Da diese Hubschrauber in Friedenszeiten nicht ungenutzt bleiben sollten, wurden sie auf der Basis von Zuweisungsverfügungen den Ländern für die Verwendung im friedensmäßigen Katastrophenschutz und Rettungsdienst im Wege der Doppelnutzung zur Verfügung gestellt.

Air rescue comprises the following activities:

1. rapid transport of a qualified rescue team, consisting of a physician with emergency & rescue certification and an air rescue paramedic, to the emergency site
2. provision of optimal emergency medical care to the patient at the emergency site
3. quick and gentle transport of the patient to a hospital equipped to provide the type of treatment the patient needs
4. transport of patients between hospitals (inter-hospital transfer)
5. transport of vital organs for transplantations, banked blood, pharmaceuticals, etc.
6. transport of rescue specialists, e.g. for technical rescue measures at major disasters
7. search flights for missing persons.

The on-call duty of the rescue helicopter starts at sunrise – not before 7.00 a.m. as a rule – and ends at sunset.

The German model

In accordance with the federative constitution of the Federal Republic of Germany, emergency medical services fall exclusively within the jurisdiction of the German states. However, the states declared that they were in no financial position to support the operation of the air rescue service.

The German Minister of the Interior is, in turn, responsible for disaster services and civil defense in the event of a military attack. Hans-Dietrich Genscher, Minister of the Interior at that time, was instrumental in broadening the Law on Disaster Services, thus creating the prerequisite for purchasing air rescue resources for this purpose.

The civil defense helicopters were originally intended for management, control and surveillance activities as well as for the transport of operating personnel and operating equipment. To prevent these helicopters from lying idle in peacetime, they were made available to the states for use in peacetime disaster and emergency medical services – within the scope of a "dual utilization" concept – by means of Allocation Orders issued by the German government.

Während der Bund die Kosten für die Beschaffung der Hubschrauber und das Personal des BGS trägt, das den Flugbetrieb gewährleistet, werden die Betriebskosten von den Bundesländern zu 100% übernommen. Ein Grossteil der Kosten wird ihnen von Kranken- und Sozialversicherungen erstattet. Wesentlich ist auch, dass der Anfordernde oder der Patient den Flug nicht persönlich zu zahlen hat. Die Krankenkassen zahlen die Flüge mit versicherten Patienten. Nicht abrechenbare Flüge zahlen die Trägergemeinschaften.

Die Bundesländer übernehmen auch die Standortbestimmung der Luftrettungs-Stationen, die Regelungen zur Durchführung des Luftrettungsdienstes und die Finanzierung der Standortanlagen wie Hangar, Betankungsanlage und Rettungswache beim Standortkrankenhaus.

Den Kommunen obliegt die unternehmerische Funktion in Gestalt der öffentlich-rechtlichen Trägerschaft des Luftrettungsdienstes. Die Absicherung ungedeckter Kosten ist dabei der wichtigste Punkt in dieser Aufgabenstellung. In vielen Fällen haben sich mehrere kommunale Gebietskörperschaften zu Trägergemeinschaften zusammengeschlossen, um durch Lastenteilung das finanzielle Risiko für den einzelnen überschaubar zu halten.

Die Hilfsorganisationen und Berufsfeuerwehren stellen die mitfliegenden Sanitäter, heute Luftrettungsassistenten: Arbeiter-Samariter-Bund (ASB), Deutsches Rotes Kreuz (DRK), Johanniter-Unfall-Hilfe (JUH) und Malteser-Hilfsdienst (MHD). Der ADAC betreibt eigene Rettungshubschrauber als Ergänzung der staatlichen Hubschrauber und führt organisatorische Aufgaben als Treuhänder für die Zivilschutzhubschrauber des Bundes durch.

Bei so vielen beteiligten Organisationen erscheint der Rettungshubschrauber als „Verwaltungswunder". Es ist ein Wunder, dass er bei so vielen unterschiedlichen Kompetenzen aufsteigen kann. Andererseits ist diese Vielfalt die Stärke dieser Konstruktion: Eine leistungsstarke Flugdienstorganisation, der Bundesgrenzschutz (BGS), der diese Aufgabe mit hoher Motivation übernommen hat und ein breites Fundament, das ausgewogen alle Zuständigkeiten in einem föderalen Staat berücksichtigt.

Whereas the federal government carries the costs for purchasing helicopters and obtaining personnel from the Federal Border Police, which is responsible for keeping flight operations going, 100% of the operating costs are covered by the German states. The majority of these costs are reimbursed by the health insurance schemes and social security system.

The states are also responsible for determining the locations of HEMS stations, for setting down regulations for the HEMS, and for financing base station facilities such as hangars, fuelling facilities and rescue helicopter bases at selected hospitals. The municipalities play an entrepreneurial role by serving as the public authority supporting the HEMS. Securing the financing of the non-covered costs is the most important item on this list of responsibilities. In many cases, several municipal bodies have banded together to establish cooperative supporting organizations, the idea being to limit the financial risk for the individual municipality by sharing the burdens.

The emergency medical organizations and professional fire services provided the emergency medical technicians, and later the air rescue paramedics, who fly with the rescue helicopter: Arbeiter Samariter Bund (ASB), German Red Cross (DRK), Johanniter Unfall Hilfe (JUH) and Malteser-Hilfsdienst (MHD). The ADAC operates its own rescue helicopters as a supplement to the state-owned helicopters and carries out certain organizational tasks in the role of trustee for the cicil defense helicopters owned by the German government.

With so many organizations involved, the rescue helicopter appears to be an "administrative wonder". With all the different regulations, standards, jurisdictions, etc. to which it is subject, it is a miracle that it can fly at all. However, this diversity is also a source of strength: the efficient aviation organization provided by the German Federal Border Police, which has taken up this task with a high degree of motivation, can be seen as a sound superstructure resting on a solid administrative foundation that takes account of the complicated balance of responsibilities characteristic of a federative state.

Expansion Phase

Taking "Christoph 1" as his model, the German Minister of the Interior set up three additional

Der Aufbau

Nach dem Vorbild des „Christoph 1" hatte der Bundesinnenminister seit 1971 drei weitere Rettungshubschrauber-Stationen in Köln, Frankfurt und Hannover in einem Modellversuch eingerichtet. Schon 1974 wurde die Phase der Modellversuche beendet und aufgrund der überzeugenden Ergebnisse mit dem planmäßigen Ausbau begonnen. Zur Unterstützung der staatlichen Bestrebungen hat der ADAC 1973 seinen Münchener Rettungshubschrauber in den Pool der Zivilschutzhubschrauber eingebracht und 1974 noch eine weitere BO 105 dem Bundesinnenminister übergeben. Die Björn-Steiger-Stiftung und eine Benefizschallplatte helfen 1972, den Rettungshubschrauber in Frankfurt zu finanzieren. Die von Siegfried Steiger gegründete Deutsche Rettungsflugwacht (DRF;German Air Rescue) stellt 1973-1975 drei Rettungshubschrauber in Dienst. Auch die Bundeswehr beteiligte sich mit SAR - (Search and Rescue) Hubschraubern in Ulm, Koblenz und Hamburg nachdem nachgewiesen wurde, dass Notfallrettung dual über bodengebundene Rettungsmittel sowie gleichzeitig mit Rettungshubschraubern zu betreiben sei. Bis 1980 konnte so ein Netz von 18 Zivilschutz-Stationen ergänzt durch die bereits erwähnten Betreiber über die Bundesrepublik gelegt werden. Mitte der 1980er Jahre waren es dann bereits 35 Stationen. Den heutigen Stand zeigt die Übersicht auf Seite 299 des Buches.

Das Konzept hat sich trotz vieler Schwierigkeiten überzeugend durchgesetzt.

Die Rückschläge

Am 17.August 1971 kam es beim Landeanflug des „Christoph 1", weniger als zehn Monate nach seiner Indienststellung, zu einem tödlichen Unfall mit Totalschaden des Hubschraubers. Nur durch die nahtlose Übernahme der Luftrettung durch den BGS konnte eine Beendigung des Modellversuchs verhindert werden. Anfang der 1980er Jahre kam es neben Unfällen durch Einflug in Schlechtwetter oder Berührung mit Hindernissen zu einer Serie von technisch bedingten Triebwerkausfällen beim Hubschrauber BO 105. Zwei Fälle seien beispielhaft dargestellt: Am 21. Mai 1980 fielen beim Landeanflug zu einem Schulhof in etwa 10 Metern Höhe beide Triebwerke aus. Durch die schnelle Reaktion des Piloten konnte erreicht werden, dass die beteiligten Personen unverletzt blieben.

rescue helicopter stations – in Cologne, Frankfurt/Main and Hannover – after 1971 as part of a model program. On the basis of the excellent results achieved by this model program, which was terminated in 1974, the expansion of the rescue helicopter system commenced on schedule. To support the efforts of the German government, the ADAC placed its rescue helicopters in the pool of civil defense helicopters in 1973; in 1974 it handed over an additional BO 105 to the Minister of the Interior. The Björn Steiger Foundation and a benefit LP produced in 1972 also did their part to finance the rescue helicopter in Frankfurt/Main. The organization "German Air Rescue" founded by Siegfried Steiger put three rescue helicopters into service in the years 1973-1975. The German Air force also contributed three search-and-rescue (SAR) helicopters earmarked for the cities of Ulm, Koblenz and Hamburg, respectively, after studies showed that emergency medical care could be provided by a "dual system" including both rescue ambulances on the ground and rescue helicopters. On this basis a network consisting of 18 civil defense stations – supplemented by the above-mentioned rescue helicopter operators – was established in the Federal Republic of Germany by 1980. By the mid-1980s this network had grown to 35 stations. The present figures are shown in the overview provided on page 299.

This dual system is now firmly established despite the numerous hurdles it has had to overcome.

Setbacks

On 17 August 1971, less than 10 months after its commissioning, "Christoph 1" was involved in a fatal accident, with the helicopter written off as a total loss, during an approach to landing. It was only thanks to the seamless transfer of HEMS activities to the German Federal Border Police that termination of the model program could be averted. In the early 1980s the rescue helicopter service suffered a number of accidents after flying into bad weather or coming into contact with obstacles in addition to a series of engine failures caused by technical problems affecting the BO 105. Two incidents are provided by way of illustration. On 21 May 1980 both engines of a BO 105 kicked out at about 10 m above the ground during the approach to a landing site at a school.

Ursache war der Bruch eines Turbinenrades. Ein grösseres Bruchstück dieses Rades drang in die Brennkammer des zweiten Triebwerks ein, und der gleichzeitige Ausfall beider Triebwerke war die Folge. Am 31.12.82 fiel in einer Höhe von 150 Metern über Grund auf dem Weg zum Krankenhaus mit einem Patienten an Bord ein Triebwerk aus. Unmittelbar darauf brach im Triebwerkraum Feuer aus und drang in die Kabine ein. Der Pilot führte ohne Triebwerkleistung eine sofortige Notlandung (Autorotation) aus. Die Besatzung konnte den Hubschrauber unverletzt verlassen und anschließend den bei einem Verkehrsunfall verletzten Patienten sicher evakuieren. Der Hubschrauber brannte aus. In weiteren Fällen konnten Piloten durch umsichtiges Verhalten Unfälle verhindern.

Ohne eine leistungsfähige Flugdienstorganisation – hier der BGS – wäre die Luftrettung ohne Zweifel in eine Sackgasse geraten. So wurden die Unfallursachen sorgfältig analysiert, die Schulung der Piloten weiter optimiert und die Triebwerke durch den Hersteller einem langwierigen Verbesserungsprozess unterzogen. Nirgendwo ist die Belastung für einen Hubschrauber so hoch wie in der Luftrettung: Schnelles Anlassen, extrem kurze Flugzeiten mit maximaler Dauerleistung und sehr viele Landungen kennzeichnen diesen Flugbetrieb.

Die Wiedervereinigung

Kurz nach Öffnung der Grenzen der ehemaligen Deutschen Demokratischen Republik (DDR) im November 1989 begannen auf verschiedenen Ebenen intensive Gespräche um den Aufbau eines Luftrettungssystems. Bereits im April 1990 wurden in Zusammenarbeit mit der Nationalen Volksarmee (NVA) und der sogenannten Schnellen Medizinischen Hilfe (SMH) fünf Luftrettungsstützpunkte errichtet und bis Juli 1990 auf neun erweitert. Durch die schnelle Vereinigung am 3.10.1990 wurde der Aufbau der Luftrettung in den neuen Bundesländern wiederum beschleunigt. Die Bundeswehr führte mit Hubschraubern MI-2 der ehemaligen NVA die Luftrettung solange fort, wie die logistischen Ressourcen es erlaubten. ADAC und DRF engagierten sich mit „Know how" und eigenen Hubschraubern. Der BGS übernahm von der Bundeswehr leichte Transporthubschrauber Bell UH-1D, um insgesamt fünf neue Stationen im Beitrittsgebiet aufbauen zu können. Tarnfarbene

Fortunately, none of the persons involved in the accident was injured, thanks to the quick reaction of the pilot. This accident was caused by a broken turbine wheel. A large fragment of this wheel flew into the combustion chamber of the second turbine engine, resulting in the simultaneous failure of both engines. During the second accident, which occurred on 31 December 1982, one engine failed at about 150 m above ground while the helicopter was en route to a hospital with a patient on board. Fire broke out in the engine space and spread to the helicopter's cabin. The pilot made an emergency landing (autorotation) without engine power. The crew emerged from the helicopter uninjured and safely evacuated the patient, who had sustained injuries during an automobile accident. The helicopter was totally destroyed by the fire. In numerous other cases, accidents were prevented by judicious action on the part of the pilots.

Without an efficient aviation service organization – in this case the German Federal Border Police – the air rescue system would undoubtedly have run into a dead end. As it was, the causes of the accidents were meticulously analyzed, the training of the pilots further optimized, and the helicopter engines subjected to an extensive improvement process by the manufacturer. Nowhere are the stresses and strains of helicopter flight as high as in air rescue: quick takeoffs, extremely short flight times at maximum power, and a large number of landings are characteristic of this kind of flight operation.

German Reunification

Shortly after the opening of the borders of the former German Democratic Republic (DDR) in November 1989, intensive discussions were mounted on various levels concerning the establishment of an helicopter emergency medical system in the DDR. In April 1990 five air rescue stations were set up in cooperation with the Nationale Volksarmee (NVA) and the so-called Rapid Medical Assistance Program (SMH); by July 1990 this number had risen to nine.

The speed of German reunification accelerated the establishment of air rescue systems in what were now the new German states. The German Air Force initially carried out air rescue activities in this part of Germany with MI-2 helicopters

militärische Hubschrauber erhielten die Farbe orange des Katastrophenschutzes. Ehemalige Kampfhubschrauber-Piloten der NVA, die die MI-24 geflogen hatten, wurden nach Übernahme in den BGS und intensiver Schulung zu hochmotivierten Rettungsfliegern. Bis Jahresmitte 1994 nahmen 12 Rettungshubschrauberstationen auf dem gleichen Niveau wie in den alten Bundesländern den Betrieb auf.

Durch die Auflösung des Warschauer Paktes und die damit einhergehende weltpolitische Entspannung wurden jedoch neue Gefahren für den Bestand der Luftrettung sichtbar. In geheimen Papieren des Bundesministeriums des Innern (BMI) wurde nicht nur eine drastische Reduzierung der Katastrophenschutzeinrichtungen und -einheiten, sondern auch der Totalausstieg aus der Luftrettung erwogen, da für den zivilen Verteidigungsfall nun nicht mehr so viele Einsatzmittel für erforderlich gehalten wurden. Alle nunmehr 22 Stationen des Zivilschutzes sollten vom BGS an zivile Betreiber übergeben werden. Als diese Papiere öffentlich wurden, wurde das BMI in den Medien von leitenden Rettungsmedizinern und von vielen Landesministerien bedrängt, diese Pläne nicht umzusetzen. In Bielefeld, am Standort des Christoph 13, gründete sich sogar eine Bürgerinitiative, die für den Verbleib des BGS in der Luftrettung kämpfte. Auch die BGS-Fliegergruppe begründete, dass ohne die fliegerischen Fortbildungen der Piloten in der Luftrettung erhebliche Haushaltsmittel für diese Fortbildungen bereitgestellt werden müssten. Die hohe Qualität des BGS-Flugdienstes gründet nicht zuletzt auf dem in der Luftrettung erworbenen Erfahrungsschatz und könnte ohne seine angemessene Beteiligung in der Luftrettung nicht aufrechterhalten werden.

Hinsichtlich der Beteiligung in der Luftrettung änderte das BMI schließlich seine Auffassung, es wurde mit dem neuen Konzept für den Zivilschutz die Beteiligung von Zivilschutzhubschraubern in verringertem Umfang festgeschrieben. Von 22 Stationen übergab der BGS 6 an ADAC und DRF. Der damals im BMI federführende Abteilungsleiter, Dr. Rüdiger Kass, erklärte sinngemäß, er sei vom Saulus zum Paulus geworden. Gute und zahlreiche Argumente von vielen Seiten hatten ihn von der Richtigkeit der Beteiligung des BGS in der Luftrettung überzeugt.

formerly owned by the NVA as long as the necessary logistic resources were available. The German Automobile Club (ADAC) and the German Air Rescue Service (DRF) took an active role by contributing needed know-how and rotary aircraft. With lightweight transport helicopters, type Bell UH-1D, it had obtained from the Federal Armed Forces, the Federal Border Police set up a total of five new stations in the new German states. Camouflage-colored helicopters were painted orange – the international color of disaster relief. Former combat helicopter pilots who had flown the MI-24 for the NVA became highly-motivated rescue helicopter pilots after being admitted to the FBP and undergoing intensive training. By mid 1994 12 rescue helicopter stations – of the same quality as their Western German counterparts – had been commissioned in the new German states.

With the dissolution of the Warsaw Pact and the resulting global political thaw, however, new dangers emerged for the continued existence of air rescue. In a confidential paper drawn up by the Federal Ministry of the Interior (BMI), consideration was given to a drastic reduction of disaster relief facilities and units – and even a total withdrawal from air rescue – since a smaller amount of resources now had to be kept operational for civil defense. The paper envisaged turning all 22 civil defense stations now run by the Federal Border Police over to private operators. After this paper was published, the BMI was urged, in the media, by physicians high in the rescue hierarchy and by many departments on the state level not to act on the recommendations it contained.

The proposals also came under fire from another direction. The Aviation Group of the Federal Border Police pointed out that the air rescue activities of the FBP made a contribution to the continued training of FBP pilots. If the air rescue programs were terminated, the government would have to earmark substantial budgetary funds top to such training. They went on to argue that the high quality of the FBP Aviation Service was based to a signitican texttent on the experience gained by FBP pilots turing air rescue activities and could not be maintained without a commensurate participation in HEMS.

In Bielefeld, the base of Christoph 13, a Citizens' Group was founded to keep the Federal Border Police in air rescue.

Die Organisationen

Die Luftrettung in Deutschland wird heute von vier Organisationen geprägt. Die Bundeswehr, die für den Such- und Rettungsdienst (SAR – Search and Rescue) nach vermissten oder abgestürzten Flugzeugen zuständig ist, hat ihre SAR-Hubschrauber von Anfang an in die Luftrettung integriert. Mit der Ausphasung des leichten Transporthubschraubers Bell UH-1D, die bereits begonnen hat, zieht sich das Bundesministerium der Verteidigung aus der Luftrettung zurück. Das Nachfolgemodell, der NH 90, ist mit seiner Flugmasse von rund 9000 kg nicht für die Luftrettung in dicht besiedelten Gebieten geeignet. Daher hat die Bundeswehr bereits mehrere Stationen an zivile Betreiber übergeben. Die ADAC-Luftrettung GmbH engagiert sich unverändert stark in der Luftrettung und betreibt heute in Deutschland die meisten RTH-Stationen. Eine weitere große Organisation ist die Deutsche Rettungsflugwacht e.V. (DRF; German Air Rescue). (siehe Seite 299).

Die Zivilschutzhubschrauber, die vom BGS betrieben werden, stellen heute mit 16 Stationen unverändert das Rückgrat der deutschen Luftrettung. Der Ausschuss Rettungswesen, in dem alle Bundesländer vertreten sind, hat im Jahr 2000 festgestellt, dass sich das System der organisierten Luftrettung in Deutschland in der Vergangenheit bewährt hat. Dies schließt die Durchführung der Luftrettung seitens der beteiligten Leistungserbringer und hier nicht zuletzt des Bundes, insbesondere des BGS, ein. Die BGS-Hubschrauberbesatzungen können sich durch ihre Erfahrungen aus der Luftrettung aus dem Stand bei Katastrophen und beim Massenanfall von Verletzten effektiv in den Rettungsdienst eingliedern. Bei all diesen Ereignissen der letzten Jahrzehnte, Waldbrand-, Schnee- und Hochwasserkatastrophen, Flugzeugabstürzen, Eisenbahn-, Seilbahn- und Lawinenunglücken waren nicht nur Zivilschutzhubschrauber, sondern auch Führungs- und Transporthubschrauber des BGS, sowie eine leistungsfähige Flugdienstorganisation mit Spezialkraftfahrzeugen vor Ort, die sich in die örtlich zuständigen Katastrophenschutzstäbe integriert hat.

Daher kann der o.g. Ausschuss Rettungswesen feststellen, dass die Bundesrepublik Deutschland über ein insgesamt bewährtes, leistungsfähiges und international anerkanntes Rettungswesen verfügt. Hierbei kommt neben den bodengebundenen Organisationen des Rettungsdienstes

The BMI finally changed its position concerning the participation in air rescue: the new civil defense concept assigned a lesser role to civil defense helicopters. The FBP turned six of its 22 helicopter stations over to the German Automobile Club (ADAC) and the German Air Rescue Service (DRF). Dr. Rüdiger Kass, the BMI department head concerned with air rescue at that time, admitted that he had made a radical about-face. The numerous sound arguments put forth had convinced him that the FBP should keep its present role in air rescue.

The Organizations

Today air rescue in Germany bears the stamp of four organizations. The German Air Force, which is responsible for search and rescue (SAR) missions to locate missing or crashed aircraft, had integrated its SAR helicopters into air rescue from the beginning. With the phasing-out of the lightweight Bell UH-1D transport helicopters which is already underway, the Federal Ministry of Defense is pulling out of air rescue. The successor to the Bell UH-1D, the NH 90, is not suitable for air rescue in congested areas by virtue of maximum take-off weight (MTOW) of about 9,000 kg. For this reason, the German Air Force has already turned several stations over to civilian operators. ADAC-Luftrettung GmbH has retained its high commitment to air rescue; today this organization operates the largest group of rescue helicopter stations of any operator in Germany. The German Air Rescue Service (DRF) (Cf. page 299) also plays a major role.

The civil defense helicopters operated by the FBP and stationed at 16 rescue helicopter bases are still the backbone of the German air rescue system. The Rescue System Committee, which contains representatives of all the German states, stated in 2000 that the system of organized air rescue in service in Germany has proved its worth in the past. This vote of approval also extended to the services provided by the various organizations involved in air rescue, including most importantly the German government and the German Federal Border Police.

With the experience they have gained in air rescue, the FBP helicopter crews would be able to join the ranks of rescue workers and work effectively immediately at disasters or

insbesondere der Luftrettung eine erhebliche Bedeutung zu.

Die Motivation

Die Motivation der beteiligten fliegerischen Besatzungen ist in der Luftrettung außergewöhnlich hoch. Die Gründe hierfür liegen im humanitären Sinngehalt der Luftrettung, in dem ihr innewohnenden besonderen Zuverlässigkeitsansprüchen, in konkreten Einsatzerfolgen auf der Grundlage hochqualifizierter Teamarbeit (Pilot-Notarzt-Rettungsassistent) und in der Anerkennung des sozialen Stellenwertes der Tätigkeit durch die Öffentlichkeit, die Medien und das private Umfeld.

Dafür werden die Herausforderungen der Luftrettung gerne angenommen:

- Flugführung ausnahmslos in Alarmsituationen ohne den normalerweise üblichen zeitlichen Vorlauf, dabei Inanspruchnahme von Sonderrechten nach dem Luftrecht unter erheblicher physischer und psychischer Belastung,
- außergewöhnliche fliegerische Anforderungen unter Einsatzbedingungen und
- stressintensive Mehrfachfunktionsbelastungen.

Die Ergebnisse

Die Luftrettung in Deutschland hat 30 Jahre nach ihrem Beginn ein nahezu flächendeckendes Netz mit heute 51 Stationen erreicht. Es wird ergänzt durch weitere Hubschrauber für den Interhospitaltransfer (Intensivtransporte) bei Tag und Nacht. Im ersten Halbjahr 2001 wird der einmillionste Rettungseinsatz geflogen. Jährlich kommen mehr als 63.000 Einsätze hinzu. Dabei ist es unerheblich, welche Farbe die Luftrettung trägt, ob das Natooliv der Bundeswehr, das Gelb des ADAC, das Rot der DRF oder das Orange des Zivilschutzes/BGS: Selbst bei konservativer Bewertung gelten mindestens 10% der Einsätze als lebensrettend. Allein in Deutschland verdanken ca. 100.000 Notfallpatienten ihr Leben dem Einsatz eines Rettungshubschraubers.

large-scale accidents with numerous casualties. At all of the disasters and related incidents which have taken place in recent years – forest fires, severe snows and floods, airplane crashes, train and cable car accidents, avalanches, etc.– control & guidance and transport helicopters from the German FBP – and an efficient flight service organization with special vehicles – were on the scene quickly and were fully integrated into efforts mounted by the local disaster relief coordinators.

As a result, the above-mentioned committee concluded that the Federal Republic of Germany possesses an efficient and internationally recognized rescue system. In this context an important role is played by both the rescue service organizations on the ground and the air rescue system.

The Motivation

Aviation crews involved in air rescue display an exceptionally high motivation. The reasons for this high motivation include the humanitarian ideals of air rescue, the inherent high demands for dependability, and the concrete "success stories" achieved via a qualified teamwork between the pilot, physician with emergency & rescue certification and air rescue paramedic. Another important factor is the recognition of the social value of these activities by the public, the media and the rescue worker's immediate environment.

This motivation enables the crew members to gladly take on the particular challenges of air rescue, i.e.:

- Rescue flights are by definition exceptional flights carried out in emergency situations, without the normal sequence of flight guidance events, with pilots taking advantage of special privileges under aviation law, and with considerable physical and emotional stress.
- They are always flown under mission conditions and thus place unusual demands on the crew.
- They require all crew members to perform several functions and are thus stress-intensive.

Die Zukunft

Der Luftrettung wird auch zukünftig vornehmlich die Funktion einer Ergänzung und Unterstützung des bodengebundenen Rettungsdienstes zugewiesen. Mit der Verfügbarkeit von Nachtsehhilfen (Bildverstärkerbrillen), Wärmebildgeräten und Hinderniswarnsystemen sind die technischen Voraussetzungen für einen Flugbetrieb rund um die Uhr gegeben. GPS-Satellitennavigation, digitale Kartensysteme und automatisierte Flugführungssysteme erlauben bereits den Instrumentenflug zu Flugplätzen. Ob und wann diese Technologien in der Luftrettung in größerem Umfang genutzt werden, hängt vom politischen Gestaltungswillen der Gesellschaft bzw. des Staates ab, da die erheblichen Mehrkosten finanziert werden müssen.

Ein Schwerpunkt der nächsten Jahre wird sicherlich die Qualitätssicherung und das Qualitätsmanagement in der Luftrettung darstellen. Die Leistungen der Luftrettung sind bundesweit nach einheitlichen Kriterien zu dokumentieren, zusammenzuführen und auszuwerten. Die sachgerechte Kostenbewertung wird die Voraussetzung für ein stabiles Luftrettungssystem der Zukunft darstellen. Trotz des äußeren Drucks auf dem Rettungswesen zur Kostenreduzierung wird meiner Meinung nach die optimale Versorgung von Notfallpatienten – der Mensch steht im Mittelpunkt – auch zukünftig gewährleistet werden.

The Results

Thirty years after its inception, the air rescue system in Germany consists of a network of 51 stations covering nearly the entire country. This network is supplemented by additional helicopters used for inter-hospital transfer (intensive-care transports) 24 hours a day. During the first six months of 2001, the one-millionth rescue mission was flown. More than 63,000 missions are flown each year. The color of the rescue helicopter – NATO olive green for the German Air Force, yellow for the ADAC, red for the DRF, and orange for civil defense or the Federal Border Police – does not matter since, even according to conservative estimates, at least 10% of the missions are life-saving. In Germany alone approx. 100,000 former emergency patients owe their lives to emergency medical care which arrived by rescue helicopter.

The Future

In the future air rescue will continue to play mainly a supporting role supplementing the work of rescue services on the ground. With the advent of night vision goggles, thermal imaging units and obstacle-recognition systems, the technical prerequisites for round-the-clock operation will be met. GPS satellite navigation, digital cartographic systems and automatic flight guidance already allow pilots to fly by instrument to airfields. Whether and when these technologies will be used on a large scale in air rescue depends on the political will of society and of the government since their use would entail substantial additional costs.

During the next few years, quality assurance and quality management will surely be an area of focus in air rescue. The services provided by air rescue are to be documented, compiled and analyzed nation-wide according to uniform criteria. The establishment of an effective system of cost evaluation will be one of the prerequisites for a stable air rescue system in the future. Despite the external pressures on the rescue system to cut costs, the provision of optimal emergency medical care to patients – a concept focused on the human being who is ill or injured –will, in my opinion, be assured in the future as well.

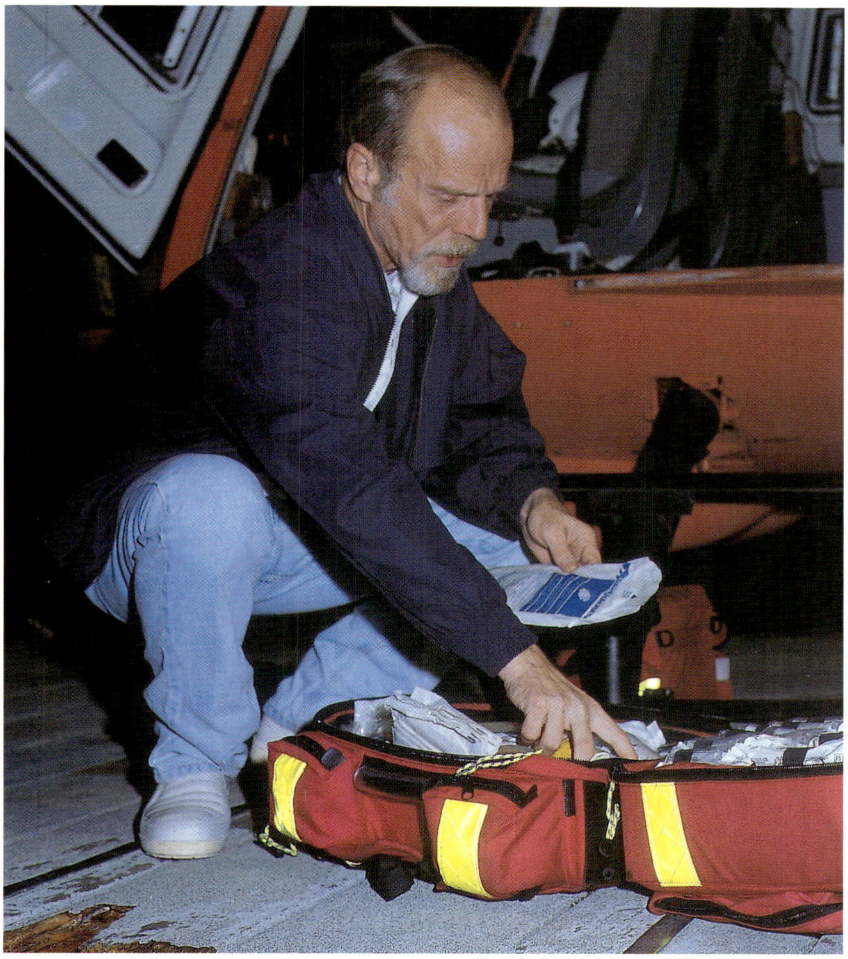

Die Rettungsassistenten überprüfen vor Dienstbeginn Geräte und Material auf Vollständigkeit und Funktionsfähigkeit.

The paramedic who has just come on duty inspects the medical equipment and supplies to make sure they are complete and functional.

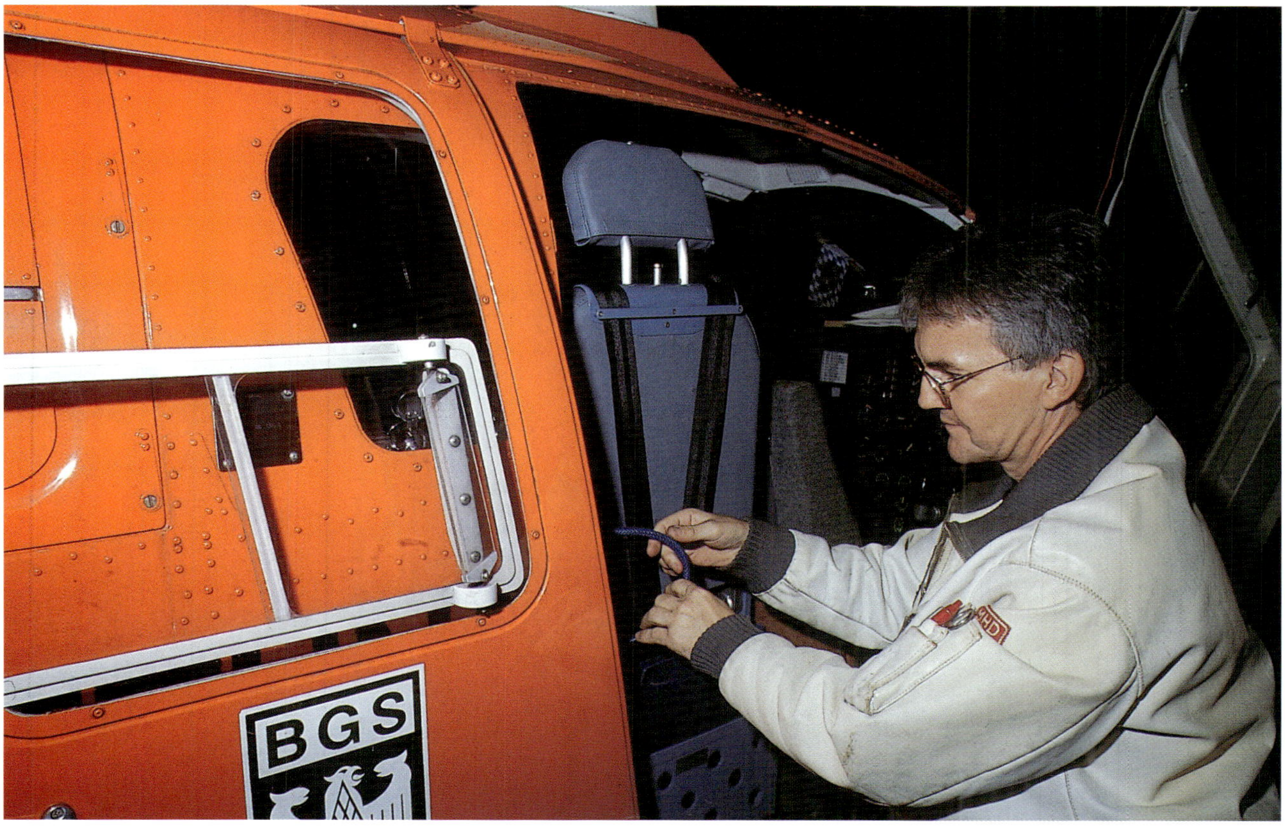

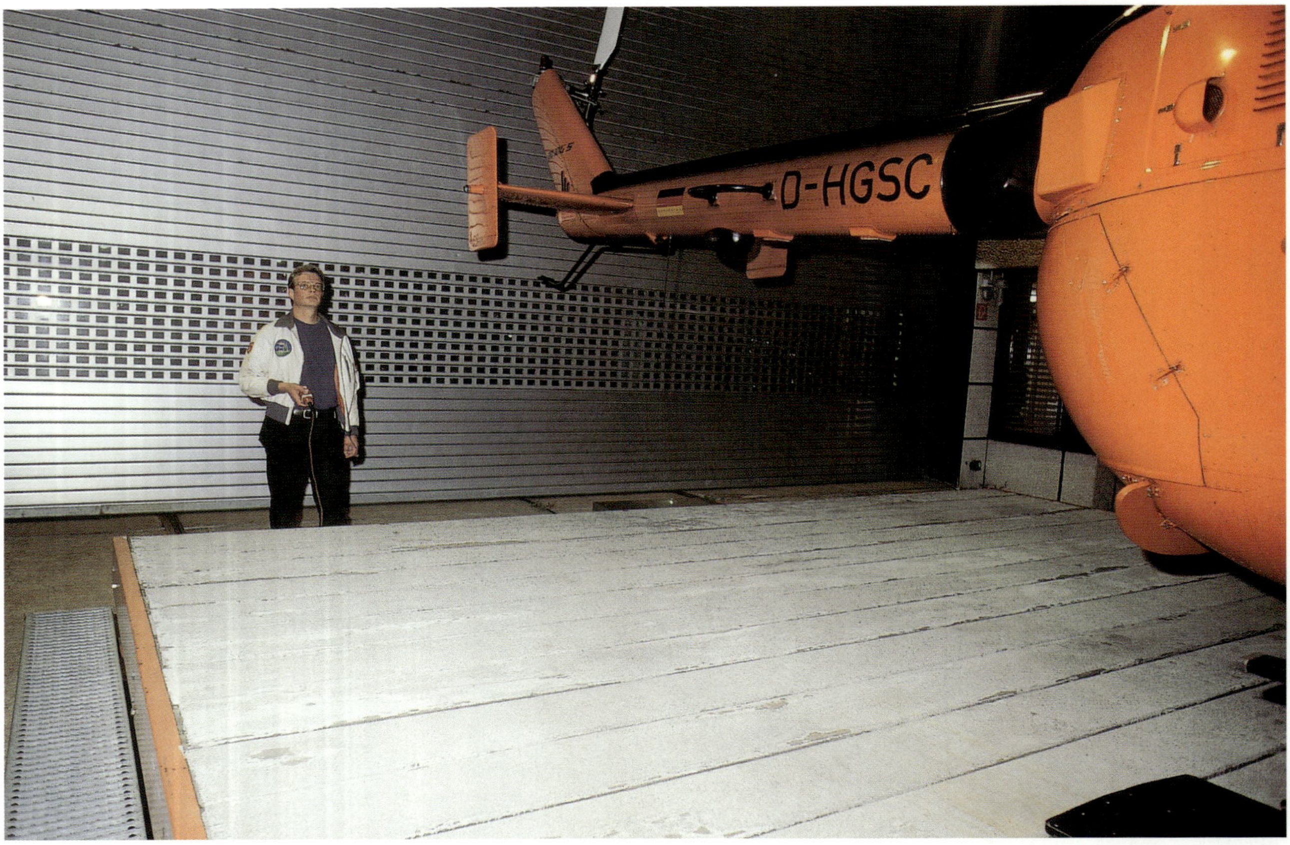

Der Rettungshubschrauber wird mit einer elektrisch angetriebenen Plattform aus dem Hangar auf seine Startposition gefahren.

The rescue helicopter is pushed out of the hangar to its starting position with an electric platform.

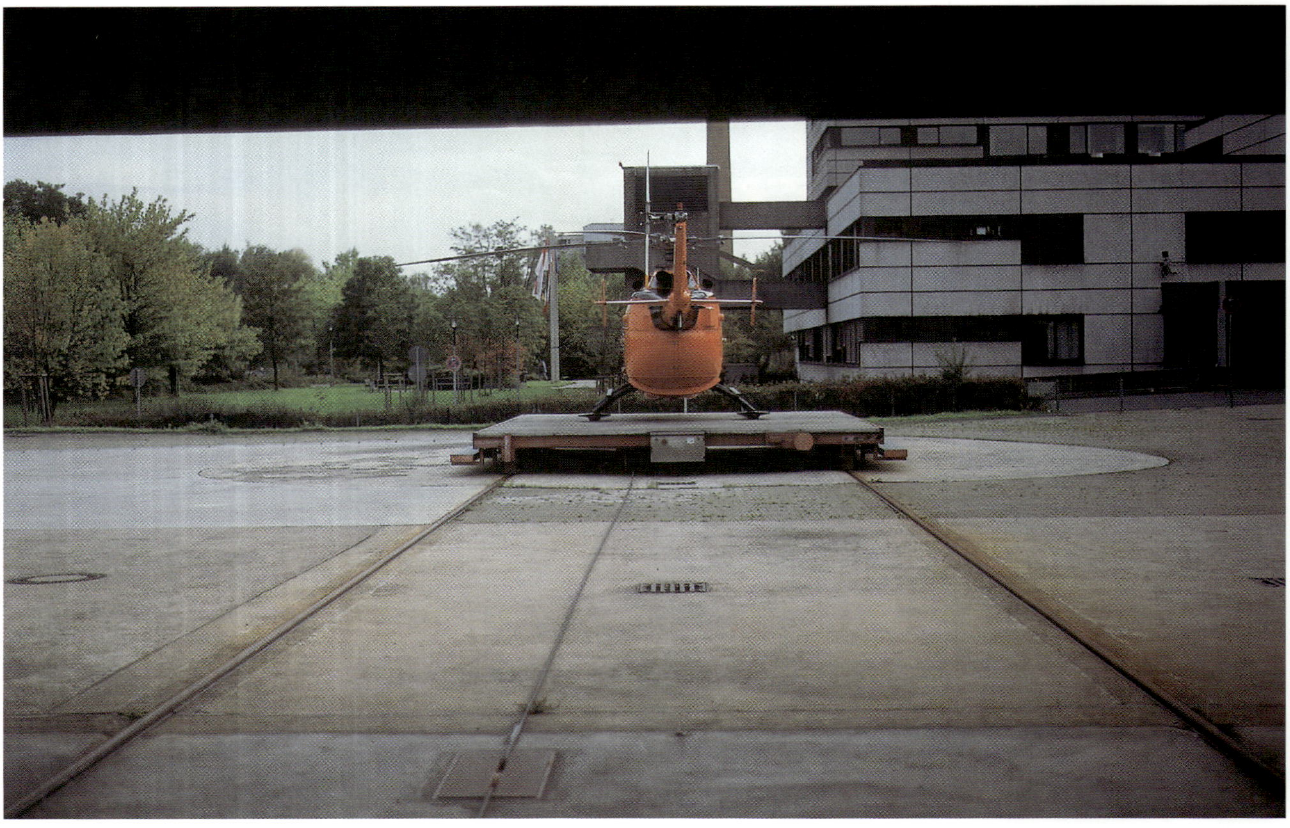

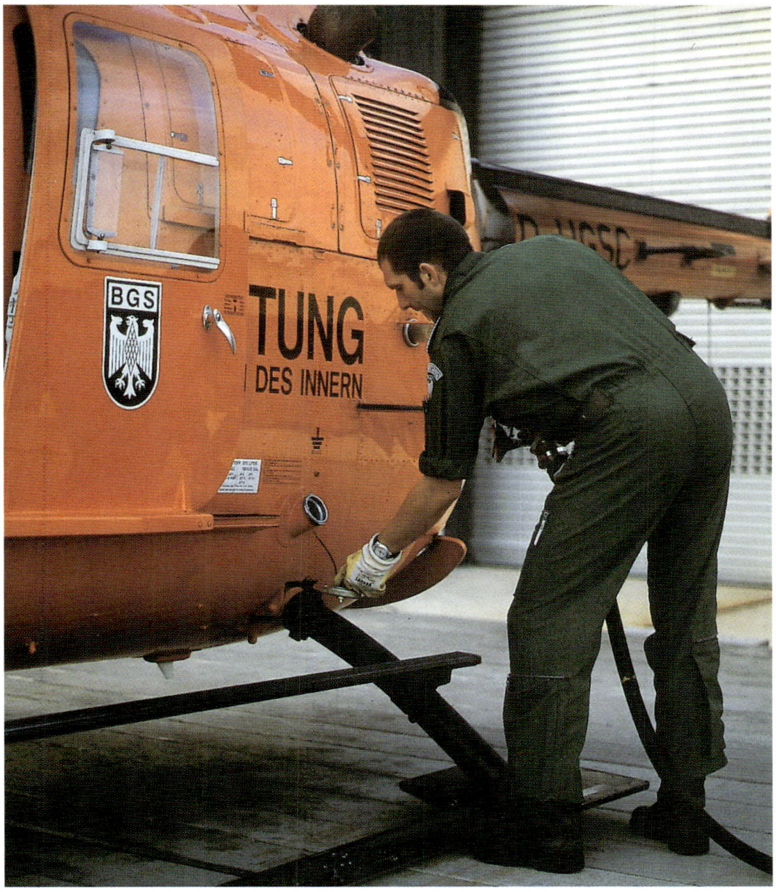

Der Pilot betankt den Rettungshubschrauber (RTH).

The pilot refuels the rescue helicopter (RH).

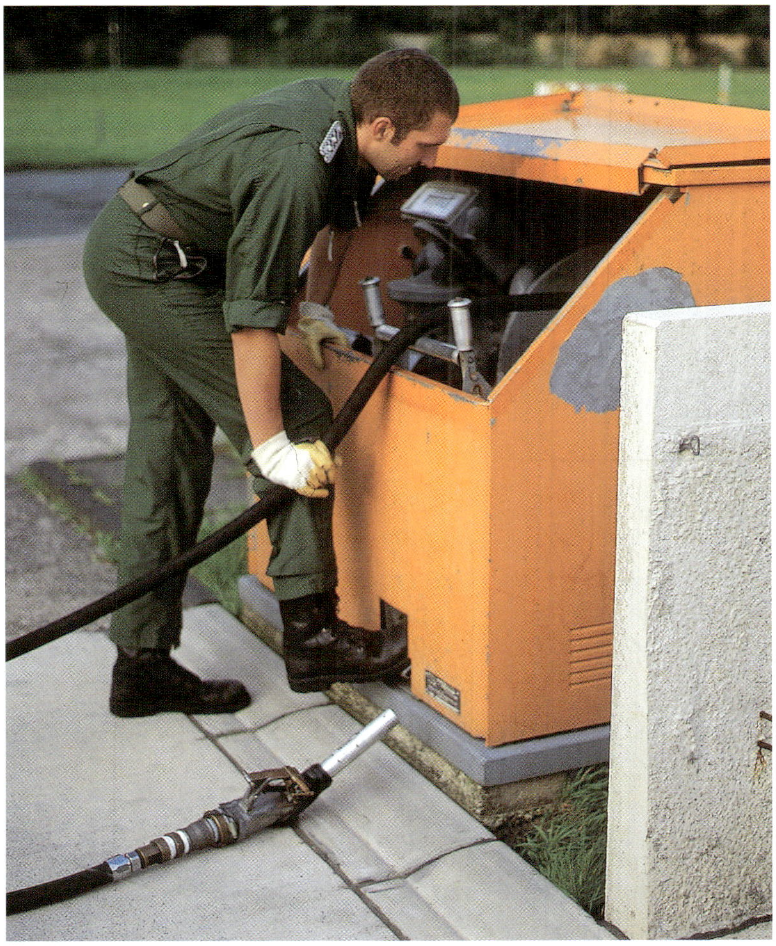

Einsatzmöglichkeiten von Rettungshubschraubern
Possibilities for Employing Rescue Helicopters

von/by Gunter Carloff

Im folgenden soll, ähnlich wie in den Fortbildungsveranstaltungen des Kölner Rettungshubschraubers, aufgezeigt werden, welche Möglichkeiten aber auch Grenzen mit dem Einsatz von Rettungshubschraubern verbunden sind.

Medizinische Aspekte werden bewusst nicht erwähnt, es werden ausschließlich fliegerische Belange angesprochen.

Bereitschaft am Krankenhaus

Der Rettungshubschrauber (RTH) steht täglich startbereit an seinem Standortkrankenhaus. Der Pilot versieht seinen Dienst in einem Bereitschaftsraum, maximal 50 Meter vom Hubschrauber entfernt, zusammen mit dem Luftrettungsassistenten. Der Einsatzradius ist grundsätzlich begrenzt auf etwa 50 bis 70 Kilometer, um jeden Notfallort sicher innerhalb von 15 Minuten erreichen zu können.

An Verwaltungsgrenzen ist der RTH nicht gebunden. Einsätze über die deutschen Grenzen hinweg sind möglich. Ein Start ist auch im Winter innerhalb von zwei Minuten ohne Vorwärmzeit möglich. Nur bei vereisendem Regen, bei Hagel, starkem Schneefall, Gewitterschauern oder stark böigen Winden wird der RTH zurück in den Hangar gefahren. In diesem Fall verzögert sich der Start um 1 bis 2 Minuten.

Die Einsatzbereitschaft beginnt in der Regel um 7 Uhr und endet mit dem Sonnenuntergang.

Alarmierung

Durch die Rettungsleitstelle wird die RTH-Besatzung über einen Funkmeldeempfänger alarmiert. Der Pilot läuft zum Hubschrauber und startet die Triebwerke. In der Zwischenzeit nimmt der Luftrettungsassistent vom Leitstellendisponenten Ort und Umstände des Einsatzes auf. Der Notarzt, der in der Regel seinen Dienst im Krankenhaus versieht, wird zeitgleich alarmiert.

Die Genauigkeit und Eindeutigkeit der Ortsangabe bestimmen wesentlich die Flugzeit des RTH zum Notfallort. In jedem Einsatzbereich eines RTH gibt es Orte gleichen Namens. Es ist bei der Beschreibung des Einsatzortes daher zu

Like the Continuing Education Seminars held by the Cologne Rescue Helicopter Station, this chapter intends to outline the various possibilities for using the rescue helicopter – and the limitations on the use of this rescue resource. This chapter focuses exclusively on the aviation aspects of the rescue helicopter; medical considerations have been deliberately left out.

Operational readiness at the hospital

Every day the rescue helicopter (RH) is on duty, in a state of operational readiness, at the hospital where it is based. When they are not in the air, the pilot and the air rescue paramedic are working in the Rescue Helicopter Staff Room located no more than 50 m from the helicopter. The action of radius of the helicopter is basically limited to around 50 to 70 kilometers so that the helicopter can safely reach the scene of any emergency within 15 minutes.

The RH is not limited by administrative boundaries. It can fly missions taking it beyond Germany's borders. The helicopter can take off, even in winter, within two minutes. It is rolled into its hangar only under extreme weather conditions, e.g. icy rain, hail, heavy snowstorms, thunderstorms or strong winds. In this case take-off is delayed by one to two minutes.

The helicopter's operational day usually starts at 7 a.m. and ends at sunset.

Emergency calls

The rescue helicopter crews receive emergency calls from the Coordination Center via a pager system. When a call comes in, the pilot runs over to the helicopter and starts up the engines. At the same time, the air rescue paramedic records the location and details of the emergency provided by the dispatcher at the Coordination Center. The physician with emergency & rescue certification, who is usually on duty in the hospital, is notified at the same time.

The rescue helicopter's flight time to the scene of the emergency depends mainly on the exactness and non-ambiguity with which the location is described. In every area serviced by

empfehlen, sich zunächst auf einen größeren Ort in der Nähe zu beziehen, z.B.: „(Name der größeren Ortschaft), von dort aus 5 Kilometer im Westen (Name des kleineren Ortes)", dann eine weitergehende Detailbeschreibung der genauen Einsatzstelle durch Zusätze wie etwa: „An der Landstraße, am südlichen Ortsrand, Richtung B-Dorf" zu geben.

Die Piloten navigieren nach der Generalkarte im Maßstab 1:200 000, nach Spezialkarten in anderen Maßstäben oder Stadtplänen. Bei Einsätzen in Innenstädten sind Straßenname und Hausnummer dann wichtig, wenn der Rettungshubschrauber nicht unmittelbar an der Einsatzstelle landen kann und deshalb die Besatzung durch ein Zubringerfahrzeug der Polizei oder der Feuerwehr an die Einsatzstelle gefahren wird.

Wenn der Notfallort eindeutig auf der Karte oder im Stadtplan markiert ist, läuft der Luftrettungsassistent zum startbereiten RTH. Sobald die Crew mit dem Notarzt komplett ist, startet der RTH zum Rettungseinsatz.

Flug zum Notfallort

Der Flug zum Notfallort erfolgt grundsätzlich auf direktem Weg. Der Pilot nimmt, so weit erforderlich oder sinnvoll, Sprechfunkverbindung zur Flugsicherung auf, um erforderliche Genehmigungen für den Flugweg einzuholen oder Informationen über sonstigen Flugverkehr zu erhalten. Die Flughöhe beträgt – abhängig von Entfernung, Gelände, Wetter und sonstigem Luftverkehr – zwischen 100 und 600 Meter über Grund. Der Flug wird nach Sichtflugregeln durchgeführt, der Instrumentenflug zum nicht erkundeten Notfallort kommt für Rettungsflieger bisher nicht in Betracht.

Das Orientieren erfolgt mit Karte, Kompass und Uhr, Anzeigen zu Funkfeuern für die Luftfahrt werden unterstützend ausgewertet. Zahlreiche RTH verfügen bereits über GPS - Satellitennavigation und digitale Kartengeräte, die elektronisch den genauen Standort darstellen. Für den Sichtflug sind grundsätzlich mindestens 800 Meter Flugsicht, d.h. Sicht aus dem Cockpit in Flugrichtung, und die Wolkenuntergrenze von nicht weniger als 150 Meter über Grund vorgeschrieben. Diese Werte werden zur Rettung von Menschenleben im Einzelfall auch unterschritten.

In Grenzwetterlagen sind Informationen über die Wetterverhältnisse an der Einsatzstelle für den

a rescue helicopter there are towns with the same name. When describing the scene of an emergency, therefore, it is advisable to first name a larger city or town nearby, e.g. (name of the larger town), 5 km west of the town (name of the smaller town), followed by a more detailed description of the exakt location of the emergency scene containing details such: on the rural road, on the southern edge of the town, in the direction of B-Village. For navigation the pilots refer to a general map on the scale of 1:200 000, special maps on other scales, and street atlases. During missions in downtown areas, street addresses are especially important in situations where the rescue helicopter cannot land directly at the scene of the emergency and the crew has to be brought to the scene in police or fire service vehicles.

Once the emergency site has been clearly marked on the map or street atlas, the air rescue paramedic runs over to the rescue helicopter, which is now ready to start. As soon as the entire crew and physician with emergency & rescue certification are aboard, the rescue helicopter takes off on its emergency mission.

Flight to the emergency site

The pilot always flies to the emergency site by the shortest route. He takes up contact to the air traffic controllers, if he or she deems such contact necessary or advisable, to obtain any necessary clearance for the planned flight path and information about other air traffic. The flight altitude is – depending on the distance to the destination, the terrain, the weather and the other air traffic – between 100 and 600 m. The rescue helicopter pilots fly according to the visual flight rules; so far rescue helicopters have not had to make any flights according to instrument flight rules to unfamiliar landing spots.

The crew member responsible for navigation works with a map, a compass and a watch; additional information is provided by radio navigational aids used for aviation purposes. Numerous rescue helicopters are already equipped with GPS – satellite navigation and digital moving maps which display the precise location. The visual flight rules stipulate a minimum flight visibility (i.e. visibility from the cockpit in the direction of flight) of 800 meters, and a cloud base not lower than 150 meters above ground. In individual cases, pilots fly with

Piloten eine wichtige Hilfe. Diese Informationen können vom Rettungsdienst oder der Polizei vor Ort gegeben werden, die in Deutschland die gleichen Funkgeräte benutzen. Ist die Sonne am Notfallort sichtbar, der Himmel also nicht von Nebel oder Wolken bedeckt, kann diese Information ebenfalls für die Flugwegplanung von Bedeutung sein.

Der RTH fliegt mit einer Geschwindigkeit von 200 bis 250 Kilometer pro Stunde, d.h. mehr als 3 bis 4 Kilometer in der Minute zur Einsatzstelle. Wer selten mit RTH zusammenarbeitet, ist daher immer wieder überrascht, wie schnell der RTH den Notfallort erreicht. Sofern die Versorgung des Notfallpatienten dies zulässt, sollte im bodengebunden Fahrzeug deshalb immer jemand über Funk ansprechbar sein.

Auffinden des Notfallortes

Sind Polizei, Rettungsdienst oder Feuerwehr vor dem RTH am Notfallort, schaltet der RTH grundsätzlich auf den Funkkanal des Funkfahrzeuges vor Ort. So wird eine Einweisung über Funk möglich.

Eine Einweisung des RTH über Funk sieht etwa so aus:

RTW: „Christoph 3, fliegen Sie mehr nach links, jetzt geradeaus. Sie fliegen jetzt genau auf mich zu. Noch etwa 500 Meter."

Richtungsangaben sollten bezogen auf die Flugrichtung gegeben werden, oder ergänzt werden durch den Zusatz: „Aus meiner Sicht rechts..."

Diese Einweisung des RTH über Funk hat sich in der Praxis gut bewährt. Wenn die Sicht am Boden durch hohe Hindernisse wie etwa Hochhäuser eingeschränkt ist, wird auch der Pilot die Einsatzstelle am Boden erst sehr spät erkennen können. Deshalb sollte man den Piloten bereits dann informieren, wenn man den RTH hört, und wenn man der zunehmenden Lautstärke entnehmen kann, dass sich der RTH nähert, oder der abnehmenden Lautstärke entnehmen kann, dass sich der RTH entfernt und möglicherweise an der Einsatzstelle vorbeifliegt.

Rotierende Blaulichter sind aus der Luft erst sehr spät zu erkennen, da die Reflektoren parallel zur Erdoberfläche ausgerichtet sind. Das Einschalten von Fahrlicht und Warnblinkanlage verbessert die Erkennbarkeit. Wenn ein Einsatzfahrzeug unter einer Brücke, in einer Werkshalle oder mitten im Wald steht, wird der RTH dieses Fahr-

a lesser visibility or a lower cloud cover in the interest of saving human life.

Under borderline weather conditions, information on the weather conditions at the emergency site is an important input for the pilot. This information can be provided by the rescue service or police at the scene; in Germany police and rescue services use the same radio equipment. If the sun is visible at the emergency site, i.e. the sky is not covered by fog or clouds, this information can also be useful for planning the flight path.

The rescue helicopter flies at a speed of 200 to 250 kilometers per hour, i.e. more than 3 to 4 kilometers per minute, to the emergency site. People with little experience of rescue helicopters are often amazed at how fast the RH reaches the site. For this reason, as far as is possible in light of the necessity to provide emergency medical care, there should always be someone who can be reached by radio in the land-based rescue vehicle.

Locating the scene of the emergency

If police, rescue services or fire services arrive at the scene of the emergency ahead of the rescue helicopter, the helicopter pilot automatically switches to the radio channel used by the rescue vehicles on the ground. The helicopter can then be guided to the site by radio.

This could sound something like this:

Rescue ambulance: "Christoph 3, fly a little more to the left, now fly straight ahead. You are heading straight toward me. Just another 500 meters."

Directional information should be based on the direction of flight or supplemented by the remark "From my point of view..." The technique of guiding the helicopter down by radio has proved its worth in actual practice. When visibility on the ground is restricted by obstacles such as high-rise buildings, the pilot cannot recognize the emergency site until the helicopter is almost there. For this reason, rescue workers on the ground should give instructions to the helicopter pilot as soon as they notice that the helicopter is approaching the site (increasing noise level) or has possibly flown past the site (decreasing noise level).

zeug ohne die wichtige Information „Wir stehen unter der Brücke!" nicht finden können.

Bei Notfällen an Badeseen ist die Funkeinweisung besonders wichtig, weil oft nicht alle Rettungsmittel eine Sonderkarte mit Planquadraten haben.

Landeanflug

Sobald der Pilot den Notfallort gesichtet hat, wird er den gewählten Landeplatz überfliegen, um alle Hindernisse erkennen zu können, die dem RTH gefährlich werden können. Gefährlich sind für RTH Freileitungen und Masten aller Art. Diese Leitungen und Drähte sind vom Boden aus vor dem hellen Hintergrund des Himmels leicht zu erkennen. Aus der Luft, vor dem dunklen Hintergrund des Erdbodens, sind sie häufig schwierig zu erkennen. Auch hier sollte diese wichtige Warninformation zur Erhöhung der Flugsicherheit vom bodengebundenen Fahrzeug an den RTH weitergegeben werden.

Den geeigneten Landeplatz sucht sich der Pilot grundsätzlich selbst aus. Die Eignung des Landeplatzes ist dabei abhängig von Windrichtung- und stärke, Temperatur, Höhe über NN, Hindernissen, Untergrund und Neigung der Landefläche und der Erfahrung des Piloten. Die Mindestgröße sollte 30 x 30 Meter sein, im Einzelfall kann auch ein wesentlich kleinerer Platz ausreichend sein. Landungen auf Aschenplätzen, Sandflächen oder Pulverschnee werden, so weit möglich, gemieden. Durch den Rotorabstrahl wird der lose Untergrund aufgewirbelt und der Pilot kann den Sichtkontakt zum Boden verlieren. Lose herumliegende Teile werden vom RTH aufgewirbelt und können Personen am Boden, aber auch dem RTH gefährlich werden. Fahrzeugtüren sollten geschlossen werden, Dienstmützen abgenommen und festgehalten werden.

Auf Straßen wird nur gelandet, wenn keine andere Möglichkeit gegeben ist. Hier muss dann der Verkehr angehalten werden! Oft sind hinter den Häusern Landemöglichkeiten vorhanden, die von der Straßenseite aus nicht zu erkennen sind.

Solange die Rotoren drehen, sollte man nicht an den RTH herantreten! Hier sollte man auf eindeutige Zeichen des Piloten warten! In keinem Fall darf man in die Kreisfläche des Rotors hineinfahren! Man sollte sich nie bei drehendem Rotor vom Heckrotor aus dem Piloten nähern, da dieser schnelldrehende Rotor kaum optisch

The revolving blue lights atop German police cars cannot be seen from the air until the last minute since the reflectors are arranged parallel to the earth's surface. Turning on automobile lights and hazard blinkers makes it easier for the pilot to recognize the vehicle. If a rescue vehicle is standing under a bridge, inside a factory or in the woods, the rescue helicopter will not be able to find it without an important piece of additional information such as "We are standing under the bridge!"

This radio guidance is especially important at emergency sites located on recreational lakes since not all rescue vehicles possess special cartographic material with map squares.

Approach to landing

As soon as the pilot sees the emergency site, he or she will fly over the selected landing site in order to identify any obstacles which could be hazardous for the rescue helicopter. Overhead lines and masts of all kinds are dangerous for the rescue helicopter. From the ground, these lines are easy to recognize as dark lines against the light sky. From the air, they appear as dark lines against a dark background and are thus hard to see. Here again, land-based rescue workers are called upon to convey this important warning information to the rescue helicopter to increase flight safety.

The job of choosing a suitable landing spot is left strictly up to the pilot. The suitability of a landing spot depends on a number of factors: wind direction and strength, temperature, height above sea level, obstacles, ground consistency, inclination of the landing site, and pilot experience. The spot should have minimum dimensions of 30 x 30 meters although a much smaller site can suffice in individual cases. If at all possible, the pilot avoids setting down on cinders, sand or powder snow. The downwash from the rotors stirs up loose soil and can cause the pilot to lose sight of the ground. Any loose items lying around are sent flying by the downwash, which can also be dangerous for people or vehicles on the ground. Rescue workers should close all vehicle doors and hold onto their caps or hats.

The rescue helicopter lands on roads or highways only as a last resort. In this case, traffic must be halted before the landing. Frequently, there are landing possibilities behind a row of houses which are not visible from the road.

wahrzunehmen ist und der Pilot diese Person nicht sehen kann!

Flüge in der Nachtzeit

Alle RTH sind für den Nachtflug zugelassen, die Piloten im Nachtflug ausgebildet. Jedoch kann mit Bordscheinwerfern alleine eine sichere Hinderniserkennung nicht gewährleistet werden. Damit wird der Landeanflug zum unbekannten, nicht erkundeten Notfallort zum unkalkulierbaren Risiko. Erst mit der Einführung von Nachtsehhilfen (Bildverstärkerbrillen, engl.: Night Vision Goggles) und elektronischen Hinderniswarnsystemen wird die Luftrettung in naher Zukunft auch bei Nacht nahezu uneingeschränkt operieren können.

Der Rückflug vom Notfallort nach Einbruch der Dunkelheit zum Standortkrankenhaus ist jedoch problemfrei durchzuführen.

Sekundärtransporte, Verlegungen von einem Krankenhaus in eine Spezialklinik, sind jedoch dann möglich, wenn für den Nachtflug geeignete Landeplätze vorhanden sind und die Wetterminima die Flugdurchführung erlauben. Die Wetterminima bezogen auf die Flugsicherheit und die Wolkenuntergrenze müssen deutlich über den Mindestwerten am Tage liegen, da eine sichere Hinderniserkennung in Bodennähe nicht gewährleistet ist.

Landestellen für den RTH

Krankenhäuser, die regelmäßig von RTH angefolgen werden, sollten von einem Sachverständigen begutachtet werden, ob die bisher genutzte Landestelle ohne Gefahren zu benutzen ist. Gefährliche Hindernisse müssen optisch gekennzeichnet oder wo dies möglich ist, entfernt werden. Industriewerke mit vielen Beschäftigten sollten in ihrem Werksgelände ständig einen Platz für Landungen von RTH freihalten. Anderenfalls ergeben sich bei Notfällen im Werksgelände unnötige Verzögerungen, weil der Pilot des RTH sich erst einen geeigneten Landeplatz suchen muß.

Eine Katalogisierung von Landeflächen in Städten erscheint dagegen nicht sinnvoll, weil erfahrungsgemäß die Flexibilität des Einsatzes des RTH dadurch erheblich leidet. Das schnelle Rettungsmittel RTH würde gelähmt werden.

An important rule to remember is: don't approach a rescue helicopter as long as its rotors are turning! Wait for a clear-cut signal from the pilot! Do not under any circumstances drive into the area circumscribed by the turning rotors of a helicopter! Furthermore, never walk toward the pilot from the tail rotor if this rotor is turning: this fast-moving rotor is hardly visible and the pilot cannot see a person at this location!

Night flights

All rescue helicopters are approved for night flights and the pilots have undergone training for nighttime aviation. However, obstacles cannot be reliably recognized with the helicopter's spotlights alone. At night, the approach flight is transformed from a flight to a unknown emergency site to an incalculable risk. Only after the introduction of visual aids for night flight (e.g. image-intensifying glasses or night vision goggles) and electronic obstacle-warning systems in the near future will air rescue teams be able to operate with practically no restrictions at night.

Nevertheless, the return flight from the emergency site to its hospital base can be carried out without any problems, even after sunset.

However, secondary transports, i.e. transfer of patients from a normal hospital to a specialized medical center, can be carried out at night if suitable landing sites are available and the minimal weather requirements for flight are met. These minimal weather requirements must be considerably higher than the corresponding values during the day since reliable identification of obstacles near the ground cannot be guaranteed at night.

Landing sites for the rescue helicopter

Hospitals which are flown to regularly by the rescue helicopter should be inspected by an expert to ascertain whether the landing site used to date is still safe. Dangerous obstacles have to be optically identified or – if that is not possible – removed. Industrial plants with a large labor force should reserve a spot for helicopter landings on the factory or plant grounds. This prevents unnecessary delays in the event of an accident while the rescue helicopter pilot searches for a suitable landing spot.

Ausblick

Die heute verfügbaren Technologien hinsichtlich Navigation, Nachtsichtgeräten und Hinderniserkennung erlauben in sehr naher Zukunft eine tageszeitunabhängige Verwendung von RTH.

Wie schnell diese Einsatzmöglichkeiten in die Praxis umgesetzt werden, sind aufgrund der damit verbundenen deutlichen Mehrkosten für Personalaufstockung, Training dieses Personals und Beschaffung der neuen Technologie Fragen, die Gesellschaft und Staat beantworten müssen.

Schlussbetrachtung

Der RTH ist dem bodengebundenen Rettungsmittel weit überlegen in bezug auf Schnelligkeit und auch in Bezug auf die Vibrationsarmut beim Transport von Verletzten. Der RTW oder NAW sind deutlich überlegen in bezug auf die Unabhängigkeit von Wetter und sind bei Nacht ohne wesentliche Einschränkungen einsetzbar. Der integrierte Einsatz von RTH zusätzlich zu den bodengebundenen Rettungsmitteln, die durch zentrale Rettungsleitstellen eingesetzt werden, hat sich uneingeschränkt bewährt.

In contrast, drawing up a directory of landing sites in cities is contraindicated; experience has shown that this approach hampers the flexibility of the rescue helicopter substantially. Forcing this fast rescue resource to abide by such a directory would clip its wings severely.

Outlook

In the very near future, new technologies for navigation, night vision and obstacle recognition will permit round-the-clock operation of the rescue helicopter. The speed with which these new possibilities become reality will depend on the willingness of society and the government to meet the significantly increased costs for additional personnel, personnel training and new equipment purchases.

Concluding remarks

The rescue helicopter is far superior to land-based rescue vehicles as a fast and low-vibration mode of patient transport. On the other hand, the rescue ambulance or the emergency physician car are distinctly superior with respect to their virtual imperviousness to weather conditions; these two vehicles can also be used at night without any major limitations. Today rescue helicopters are employed in addition to the land-based rescue vehicles dispatched from the central coordination centers. The soundness of this concept can be attested to without any reservations.

Der Rettungshubschrauber ist einsatzbereit.
The Rescue Helicopter is ready for duty.

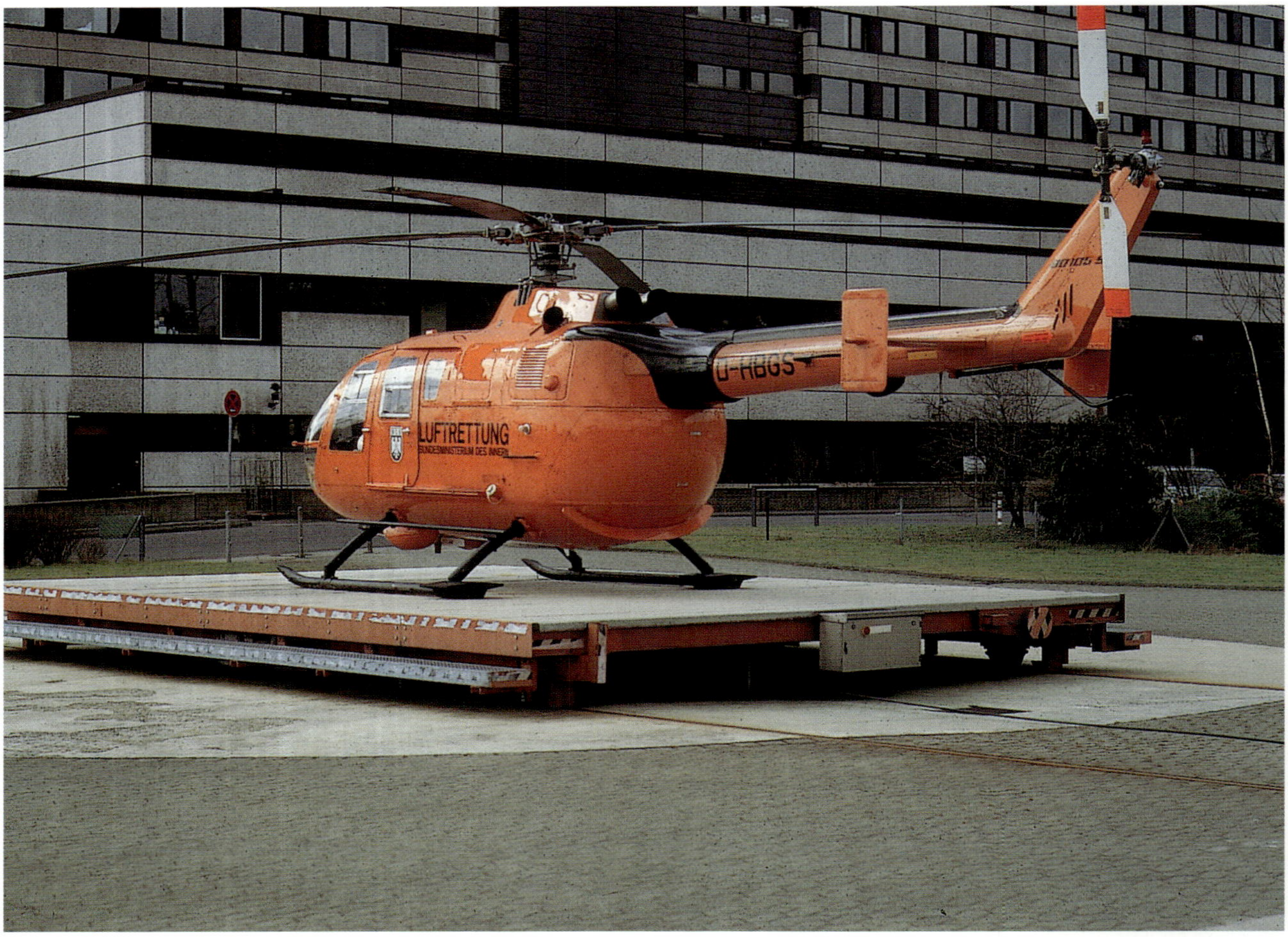

Der Rettungshubschrauber wird mit einer elektrisch angetriebenen Plattform auf seine Startposition aus dem Hangar gefahren.

The rescue helicopter is pushed out of the hangar to its starting position with an electric platform.

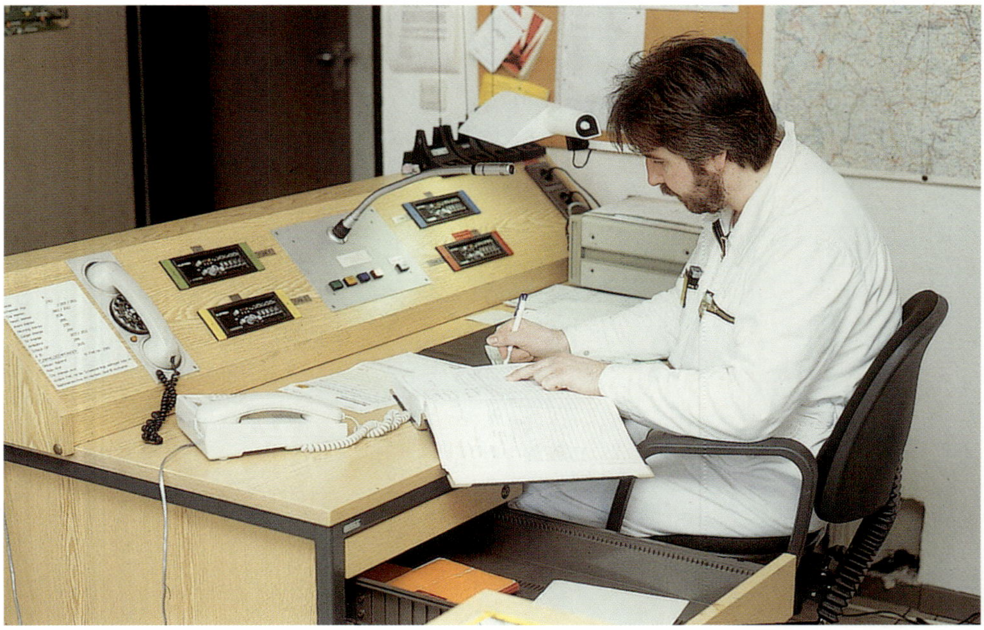

Der Rettungsassistent trägt in das Wachbuch die Namen der Besatzung ein und bereitet den Einsatztag vor.

The paramedic enters the names of the crew members in the duty book and makes preparations for the operational day.

Luftrettung – Gemeinsam sind wir stark.
Air Rescue – Together we are strong.

von/by Bertil Bouillon

Die Luftrettung ist ein wichtiges Glied in der Kette zur Rettung von Notfallpatienten. Durch einen Unfall und dadurch hervorgerufene Verletzungen oder eine akute Erkrankung können lebenswichtige Funktionen des Körpers bedroht oder akut beeinträchtigt werden. Ohne rasche ärztliche Hilfe können gravierende bleibende Schäden oder der Tod die Folge sein. Der durch das akute Ereignis ausgelöste gesundheitliche Schaden (Primärschaden) kann zwar nicht rückgängig gemacht werden, eine rasch einsetzende und optimale Therapie vom Notfallort bis zur Rehabilitation kann aber die Folgeschäden (Sekundärschäden) so niedrig wie möglich halten. Dabei ist der Gesamterfolg nur so gut wie das schwächste Glied dieser Rettungskette. Eine gute erste Laienhilfe, der korrekte Notruf, ein enges Rettungsnetz und die qualifizierte Versorgung durch das Rettungsteam vor Ort sind dabei ebenso wichtig wie eine rasche Diagnostik und bestmögliche Therapie in der Klinik bzw. Praxis einschließlich Rehabilitation.

Ziel eines Notarzteinsatzes ist es, in möglichst kurzer Zeit Arzt, Rettungsassistent und Material zum Notfallpatienten zu bringen, damit rasche ärztliche Hilfe möglich wird. Nach Stabilisierung der lebenswichtigen Funktionen, ist ein schneller und schonender Transport in eine geeignete Klinik, zur definitiven Diagnostik und Therapie wichtig.

Die Einsatzmöglichkeiten des Rettungshubschraubers ergeben sich aus den technischen bzw. logistischen Vorteilen: Schnelligkeit, erschütterungsarmer Transport und gerade Wege ohne Hindernisse. Von der Auslösung des Alarmes bis zum Eintreffen am Notfallort vergehen im Durchschnitt 9 Minuten, 80% der Einsatzorte werden innerhalb von 12 Minuten erreicht.

Die drei wichtigsten Einsatzmöglichkeiten sind der Einsatz als primäres Rettungsmittel, die Nachalarmierung zum Transport vom Notfallort in ein Zentrum und der Einsatz zum Transport von einer erstversorgenden Klinik zur Weiterbehandlung in ein Schwerpunktkrankenhaus (Sekundärtransport). Dabei soll er den bodengebundenen Notarztwagen ergänzen, nicht mit ihm konkurrieren. Damit jeder Notfallpatient das

Air rescue is an important link in the chain of events leading to the rescue of an emergency patient. As a consequence of an accident and the resulting injuries or of an acute illness, vital body functions may be endangered or acutely impaired. Without rapid emergency medical care, the patient may suffer serious permanent damage or even death. Although the damage to health triggered by the acute event – the so-called primary damage – cannot be undone, the rapid administration of optimal treatment in a chain of events stretching from the accident site to rehabilitation can minimize the consequential damage or "secondary damage". In this context, the overall outcome can only be as good as the weakest link in the rescue chain. High-quality first aid, a correctly placed emergency call, a tightly meshed rescue network and the provision of qualified care by the first rescue team on the scene are just as important as rapid diagnosis and optimal therapy (including rehabilitation) at a doctor's office or hospital.

The objective of every mission involving a physician with emergency & rescue certification is to bring the physician, a paramedic and medical supplies to the emergency patient as quickly as possible so that the patient receives prompt medical attention. After the patient's vital functions have been stabilized, the next important step is to transport the patient quickly but gently to a suitable hospital for definitive diagnosis and treatment.

The possibilities for using the rescue helicopter are a direct consequence of its technical and logistic advantages: high speed, low-vibration transport, and straight transport paths unimpeded by obstacles. In Germany the response time between the placing of the emergency call and the arrival of a rescue team at the emergency site is 9 minutes on the average; rescue teams reach 80 % of the emergency sites within 12 minutes.

The three most important functions performed by the rescue helicopter are: employment as a primary rescue resource, the transport of emergency patients from the emergency site to a medical center (notification by other rescue teams), and the transport of a patient from a hospital providing the first medical care to another

optimale Rettungsmittel erhält, ist eine Koordinierung bzw. Zuweisung aller Rettungsmittel durch eine zentrale Rettungsleitstelle notwendig.

Grundsätzlich kann der Rettungshubschrauber zu jedem Notarzteinsatz herangezogen werden. Ist der Notfallort entfernt gelegen oder sind bodengebundene Notarzteinsatzfahrzeuge bereits anderswo im Einsatz, dann ist ein primärer Einsatz des Rettungshubschraubers sinnvoll. Dies gilt sowohl für Einsätze in ländlichen Gebieten als auch in Städten und Großstädten. Dies gilt weiterhin für Verletzungen wie für akute Erkrankungen. Viele kennen den Rettungshubschrauber als Rettungsmittel nach schweren Unfällen, aber auch oder gerade bei einem akuten Lungenödem kommt es auf die rasche ärztliche Hilfe an. Heute entfallen etwa 50% aller Rettungshubschraubereinsätze auf Unfälle, 40% auf akute Erkrankungen und 10% sind Fehleinsätze.

Vor Ort steht die Stabilisierung der Vitalfunktionen und die Herstellung der Transportfähigkeit des Patienten im Vordergrund, nicht die Erstellung einer kompletten Diagnose und auch nicht die endgültige Therapie. Das Rettungsteam untersucht jeden Notfallpatienten vor Ort nach einer Checkliste und wird dann die notwendigen ersten Behandlungsschritte einleiten. Dabei kann das Team neben der körperlichen Untersuchung bei der Diagnostik und Therapie auch auf eine Reihe technischer Untersuchungsmethoden zurückgreifen. Neben dem Stethoskop steht den Luftrettern das gleiche Equipment wie im bodengebundenen Notarztwagen zur Verfügung: automatische Blutdruckmessung, EKG, Puloxymetrie, Defibrillator, Herzschrittmacher, Beatmungsmaschine, Sauerstoff, Infusionen, Medikamente, Lagerungshilfen und jedes Jahr kommen neue Materialien hinzu.

Der Transport in die Klinik kann je nach Erkrankung des Patienten und der Entfernung des Krankenhauses mit dem Rettungshubschrauber oder dem Notarzt- bzw. Rettungswagen, bei Bedarf in Begleitung des Hubschrauberarztes, durchgeführt werden. Ziel dabei ist der schnellste und schonendste Transport in die nächstgelegene Klinik, die eine optimale Diagnostik und Therapie des Patientens ermöglicht.

Dabei werden Patienten mit akuten Erkrankungen (Herzinfarkt, Lungenödem, Asthmaanfall usw.) meist bodengebunden transportiert. Das enge Netz internistischer Kliniken mit einer Intensivstation, die eine gute Behandlung dieser

medical center providing further care (secondary transport). In all of these scenarios, the rescue helicopter should complement – and not compete with – the rescue ambulance carrying a physician with emergency & rescue certification on the ground. To ensure that every emergency patient has access to the optimal rescue resources, coordination and assignment of rescue resources by a rescue coordination center is vital.

The rescue helicopter can in principle be called in on any mission requiring a physician with emergency & rescue certification. In situations where the physician with emergency & rescue certification is some distance away or the land rescue vehicles are already on missions, it is good practice to use the rescue helicopter for a primary mission. This applies to both missions in rural areas and missions in towns and cities regardless of whether the patient has an injury or an acute disease. Many people associate the rescue helicopter with severe accidents; however, a patient with acute pulmonary edema is equally in need of rapid medical assistance. Today accidents account for 50 % of all rescue helicopter missions; acute diseases (40 %) and false alarms (10 %) make up the other 50 %.

The most urgent task facing the rescue team at the scene of an emergency is to stabilize the patient's vital functions and to prepare him or her for transport – not to make a complete diagnosis or administer the definitive treatment. The rescue team examines every emergency patient at the emergency site according to a checklist; on the basis of the examination results, it then institutes the first treatment steps. In addition to performing a physical examination with traditional instruments such as the stethoscope, the team uses a wide range of medical equipment for diagnosis and treatment. Like their colleagues on the ground, the rescue helicopter team has access to automatic blood-pressure measurement devices, pulse oximetry, an EKG machine, defibrillator, pacemakers, respirators, oxygen, infusions, medications and positioning aids; new items are continually added to this list.

Depending on the particular disease or injury – and the distance to the hospital – the patient can be taken to the hospital by rescue helicopter or rescue ambulance (with or without a physician with emergency & rescue certification aboard). To achieve optimal diagnosis and treatment for the patient, the goal of the rescue team must be to transport him or her to the nearest hospital in the fastest and most gentle way possible.

Patienten gewährleistet, ermöglicht kurze bodengebundene Transportzeiten. Weiterhin besteht für diese Patienten die Gefahr in einer akuten Dekompensation ihrer Kreislauf- oder Atmungsfunktion. Eine dann notwendige Reanimation im Hubschrauber wäre aufgrund der räumlichen Enge erschwert.

Bei schweren Verletzungen (Polytrauma, Schädel-Hirn-Trauma, Wirbelsäulenverletzungen, Amputationsverletzungen, Verbrennungen und Starkstromverletzungen) steht in der Regel der schnelle und schonende Transport in ein vom Notfallort entfernter gelegenes Zentrum oder eine Spezialklinik im Vordergrund. Bei einer Amputationsverletzung eines Unterarmes kann der rasche Transport in ein Zentrum mit der Möglichkeit einer sofortigen Replantation unter Nutzung mikrochirurgischer Operationsmöglichkeiten den Erfolg der Replantation und das Ausmaß der Folgeschäden (Sekundärschaden) maßgeblich beeinflußen. Aber auch bei akuten Erkrankungen wie speziellen Intoxikationen und kindlichen Notfällen kann ein rascher Transport in ein Zentrum sinnvoll sein.

Das optimale Zielkrankenhaus wählt der Notarzt in Abstimmung mit der Rettungsleitstelle. Neben medizinischen Kriterien können auch logistische Überlegungen die Wahl des Zielkrankenhauses beeinflussen. Bei 20% aller Einsätze erfolgt der Transport des Notfallpatienten mit dem Rettungshubschrauber.

Falls sich bei einem Patienten, der bereits in einer Klinik erstversorgt wurde, die Notwendigkeit einer raschen und schonenden Verlegung in ein Zentrum zur weiteren Diagnostik oder Therapie ergibt, kann ein Hubschraubertransport sinnvoll sein. Dies kann bei einem Unfallpatienten notwendig werden, der in einer chirurgischen Klinik zunehmend eintrübt und eine neurologische Syptomatik entwickelt. Der Patient sollte dann rasch in ein Zentrum mit der Möglichkeit zur Computertomographie und anschließender neurochirurgischen Therapie transportiert werden.

Und ... hinter jedem Glied stehen Menschen ... Ersthelfer, Leitstellenmitarbeiter, Polizisten, Piloten, Rettungsassistenten, Notärzte: Nur gemeinsam sind wir stark!

Transport times on land are usually short, thanks to the tightly meshed network of hospitals with intensive care units offering optimal possibilities for treating emergency patients. Another reason for transporting these patients on land is the danger of an acute decompensation of their cardiovascular or pulmonary functions. In the cramped quarters aboard a rescue helicopter, it would be more difficult to carry out the necessary resuscitation measures.

For patients with severe injuries (e.g. polytrauma, craniocerebral trauma, vertebral column injuries, amputation injuries, burns and high-voltage injuries), rescue efforts are focused on transporting the patient quickly but gently to a specialized hospital or medical center some distance from the accident site. In a patient with an amputation injury of the lower arm, for example, rapid transport to a medical center with possibilities for immediate reattachment of the severed arm via microsurgical techniques can be crucial for the success of the surgical treatment and the severity of the sequelae (secondary damage). However, rapid transport to a medical center may also be the best choice for many patients with acute disease (e.g. certain kinds of intoxication and pediatric emergencies).

The physician with emergency & rescue certification chooses the optimal hospital for the patient in cooperation with the Coordination Center. In addition to medical criteria, logistic considerations may also play a role here. In 20 % of all rescue missions, the emergency patient is transported by rescue helicopter.

If a patient who has received initial medical treatment at one hospital needs to be transported quickly but gently to another hospital or medical center for further diagnostic or therapeutic measures, the rescue helicopter may be the transport vehicle of choice. A good example of this situation is an accident victim who has been admitted to a Division of Surgery but is now exhibiting neurological symptoms. If his condition starts to deteriorate, he needs to be transported quickly but gently to a medical center with possibilities for computer tomography and subsequent neurosurgical treatment.

Behind every link in the rescue chain are dedicated individuals: first aiders, Coordination Center staffers, police, pilots, paramedics, rescue workers, and physicians with emergency & rescue certification. Together we are strong.

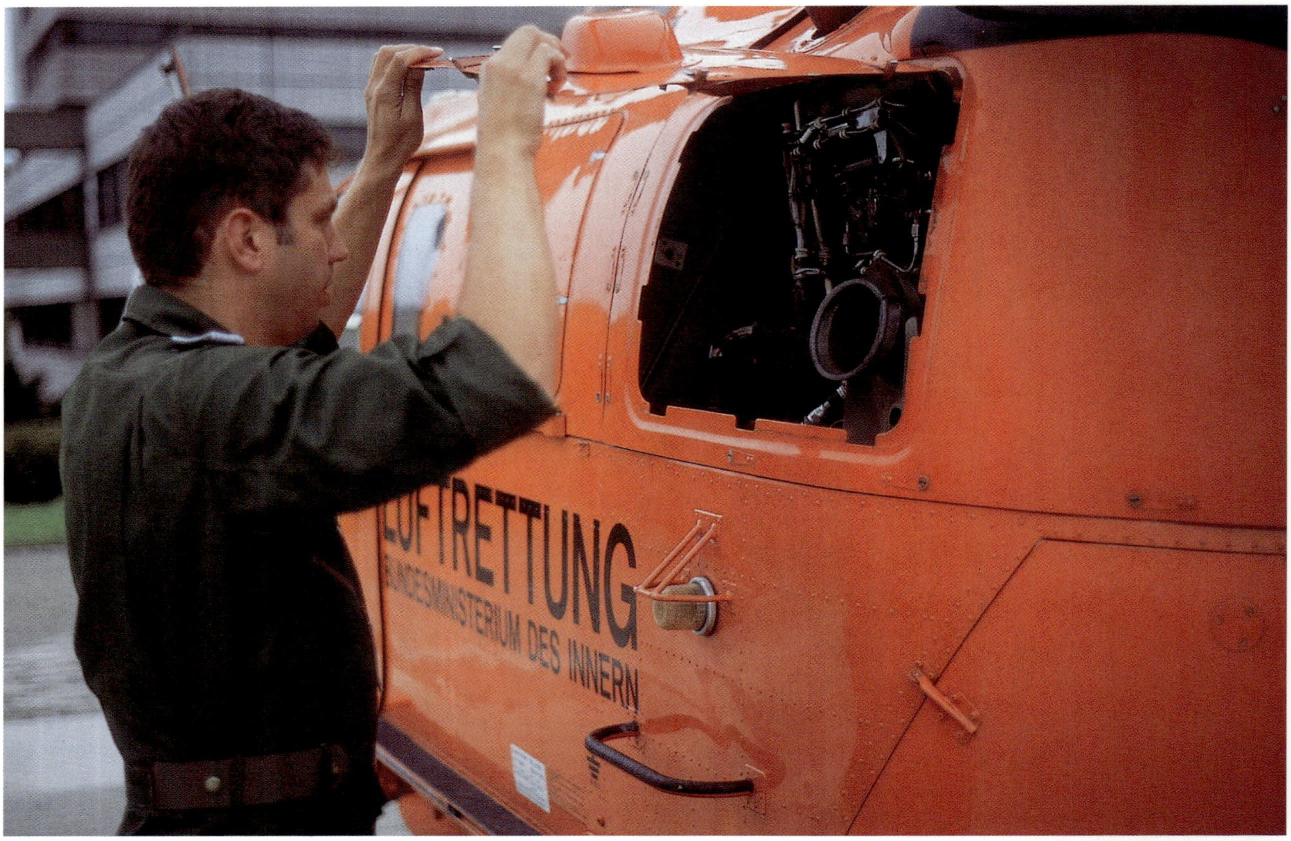

Good Airmanship – Sichtkontrolle nach der Landung am Einsatzort und nach Rückkehr zur Station.

Good Airmanship – A visual inspection is performed after the landing at the emergency site – and again after the return to base – to make sure that the rescue helicopter is airworthy.

Einsatz für den Rettungshubschrauber
Mission for the Rescue Helicopter

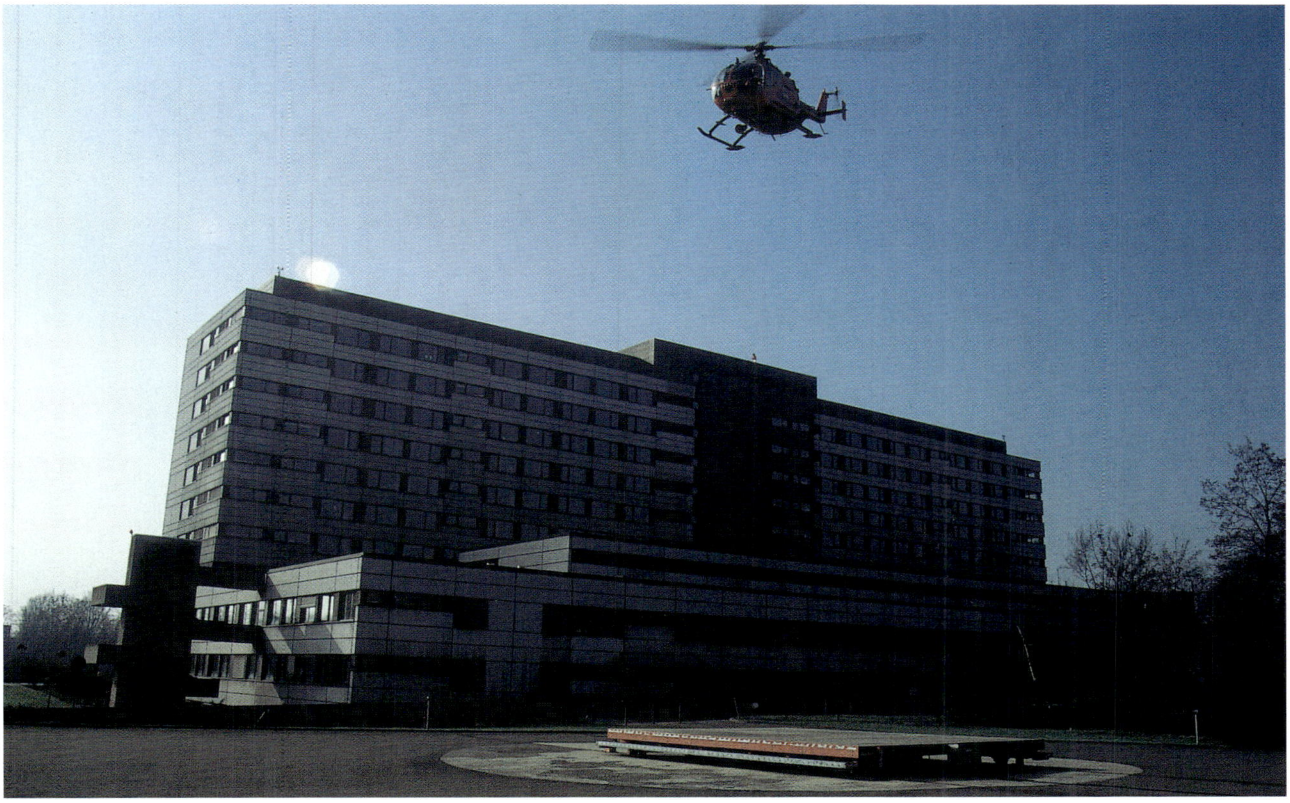

Verkehrsunfall auf der Autobahn.

Traffic accident on the autobahn.

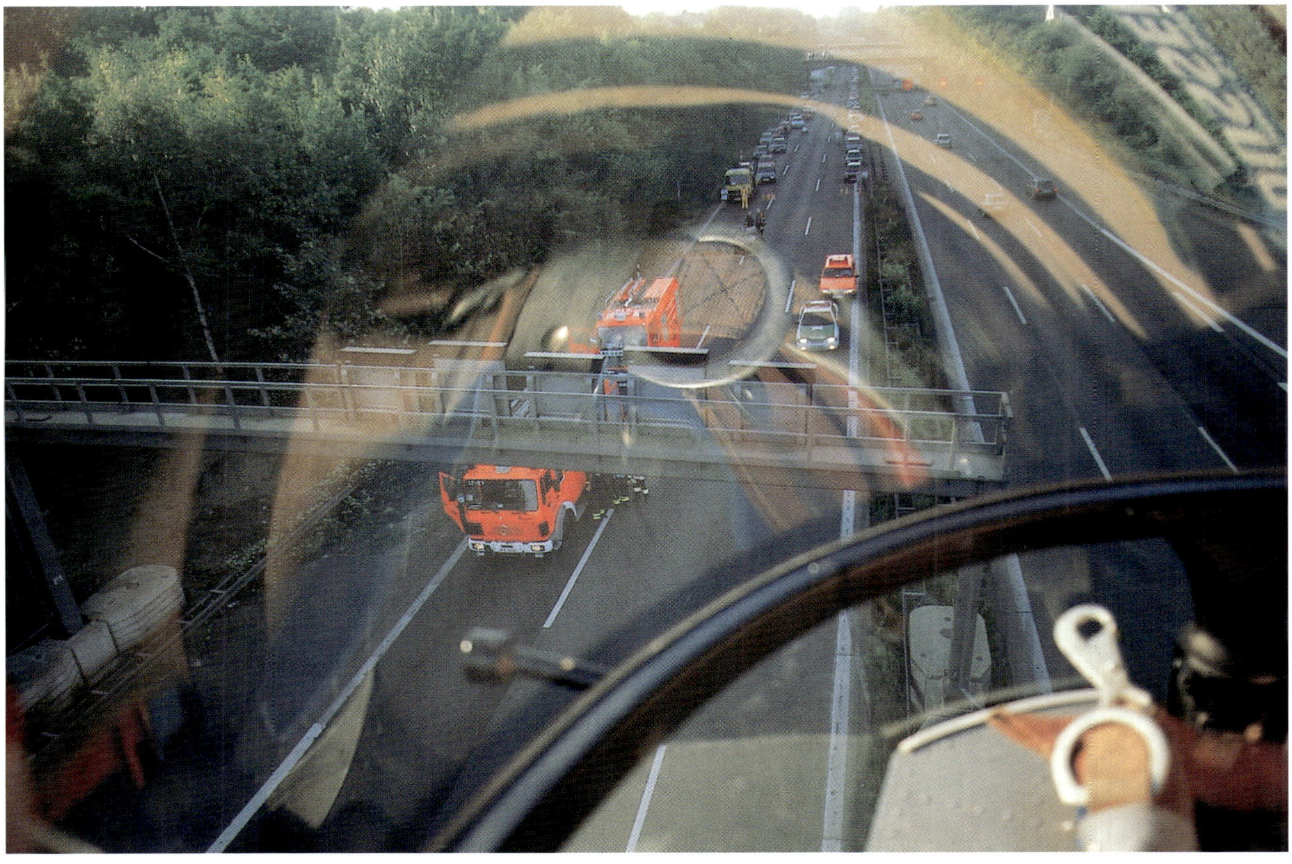

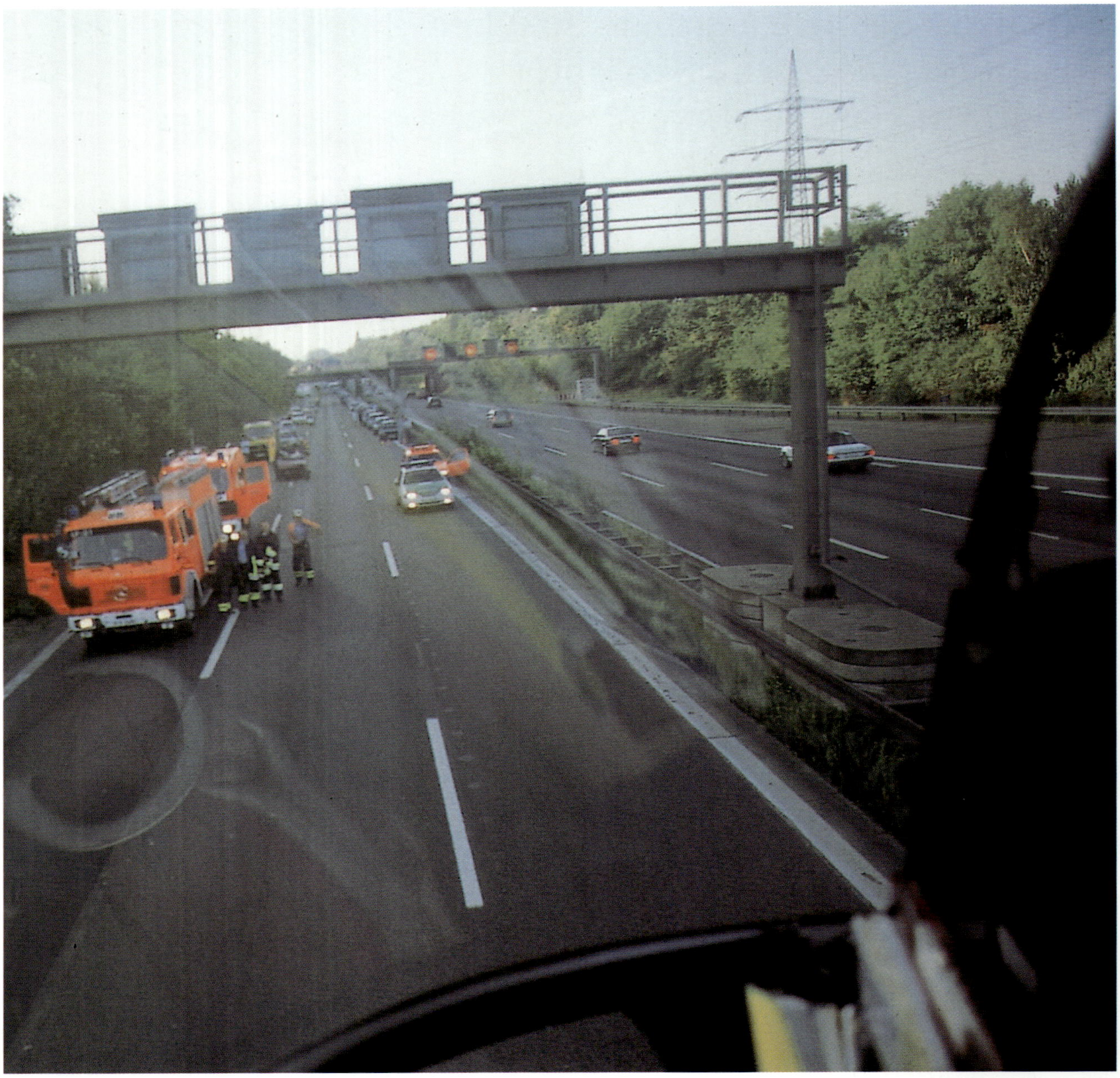

Im Anflug ist erkennbar, dass die Autobahn gesperrt ist. Der Rettungshubschrauber kann vor den Einsatzfahrzeugen der Feuerwehr und Polizei landen. Es wird mitgeteilt, dass der Fahrer, der nur leicht verletzt ist, angibt, eine weitere Person sei in seinem PKW mitgefahren und aus dem PKW geschleudert worden. Sofort suchen der Rettungshubschrauber sowie die Einsatzkräfte der Feuerwehr und Polizei am Boden die Einsatzstelle weiträumig ab, finden jedoch keinen weiteren Verletzten. Die Aussage eines Augenzeugen, der zwischenzeitlich der Polizei mitgeteilt hat, dass er gesehen hat, dass kein weiterer Insasse in dem PKW gefahren ist, veranlasst die Leitstelle zu entscheiden, dass der Rettungshubschrauber den Einsatz abbricht, nachdem der Patient versorgt und dem Rettungswagen übergeben worden ist.

During the approach, it is already evident that the autobahn is blocked. The rescue helicopter is able to land in front of the police and fire service vehicles. During the approach the helicopter crew is informed that the driver of the automobile involved in the accident has only mild injuries; however, he reports that a passenger was thrown out of the car. The rescue helicopter and the rescue workers (police and fire service personnel) on the ground immediately mount a wide-area search of the accident site without finding another injured person. In the meantime, an eyewitness to the accident has informed the police that there was no passenger in the automobile; the helicopter crew is told to terminate its mission after the patient has been treated and loaded into the rescue ambulance.

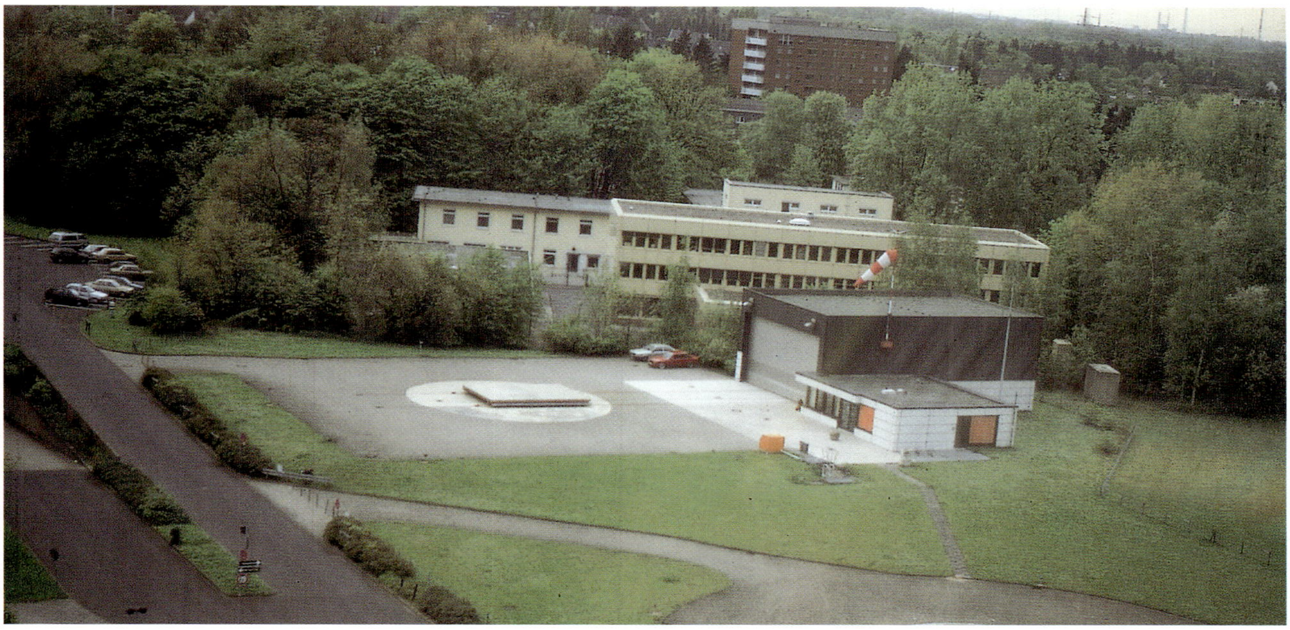

Im Anflug auf die Landeplattform vor dem Hangar.

During the approach to the landing platform in front of the hangar.

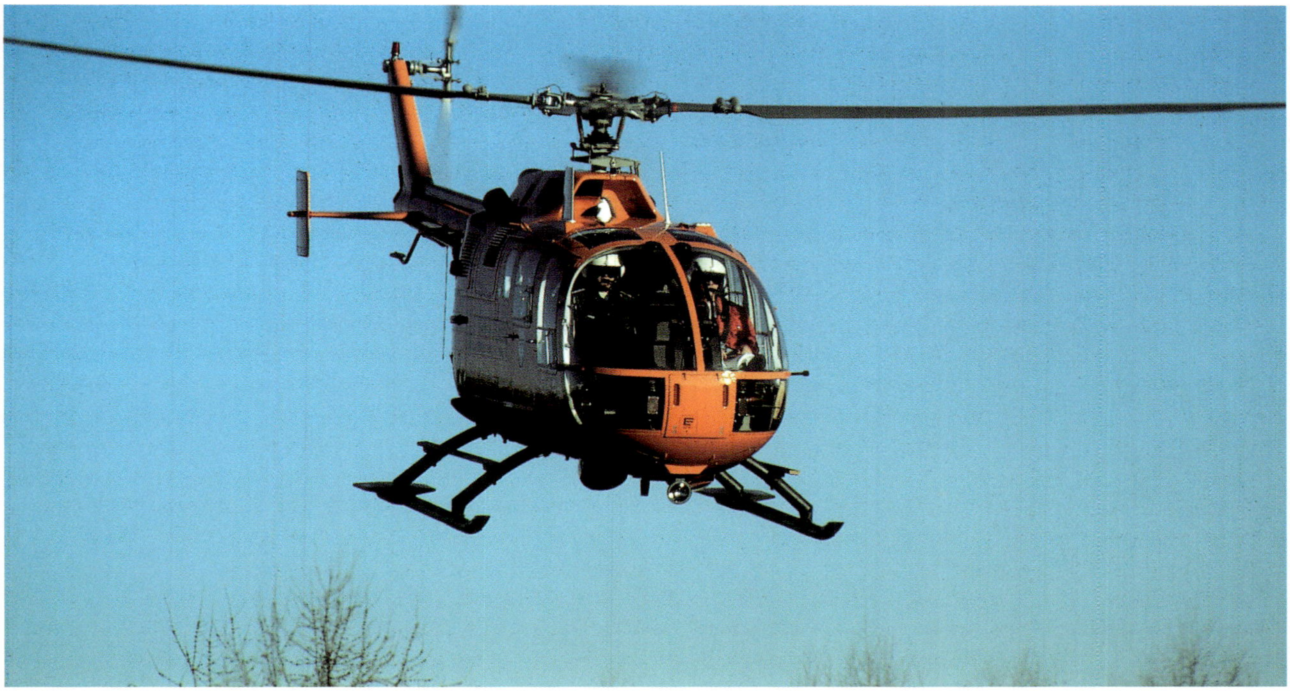

Der Rettungshubschrauber kehrt zur Station zurück.

The rescue helicopter returns to base.

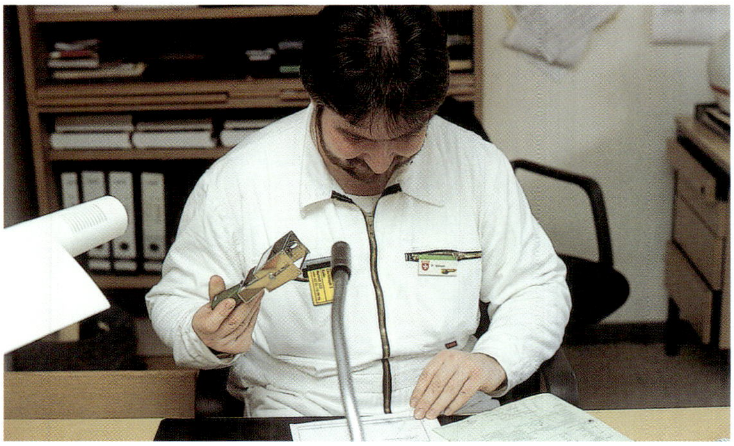

Der Einsatz wird dokumentiert.

The mission is documented: a report is drawn up.

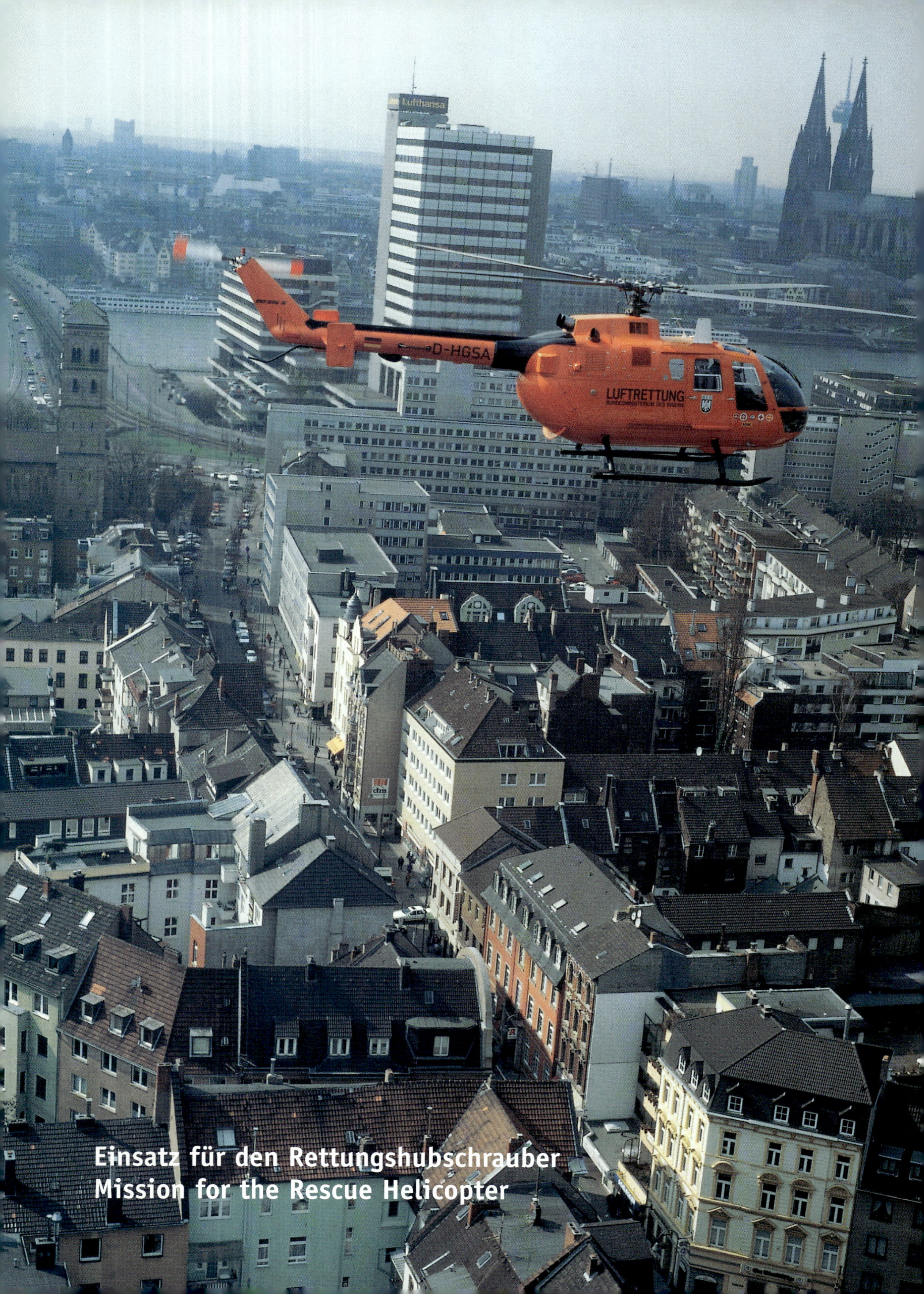

Einsatz für den Rettungshubschrauber
Mission for the Rescue Helicopter

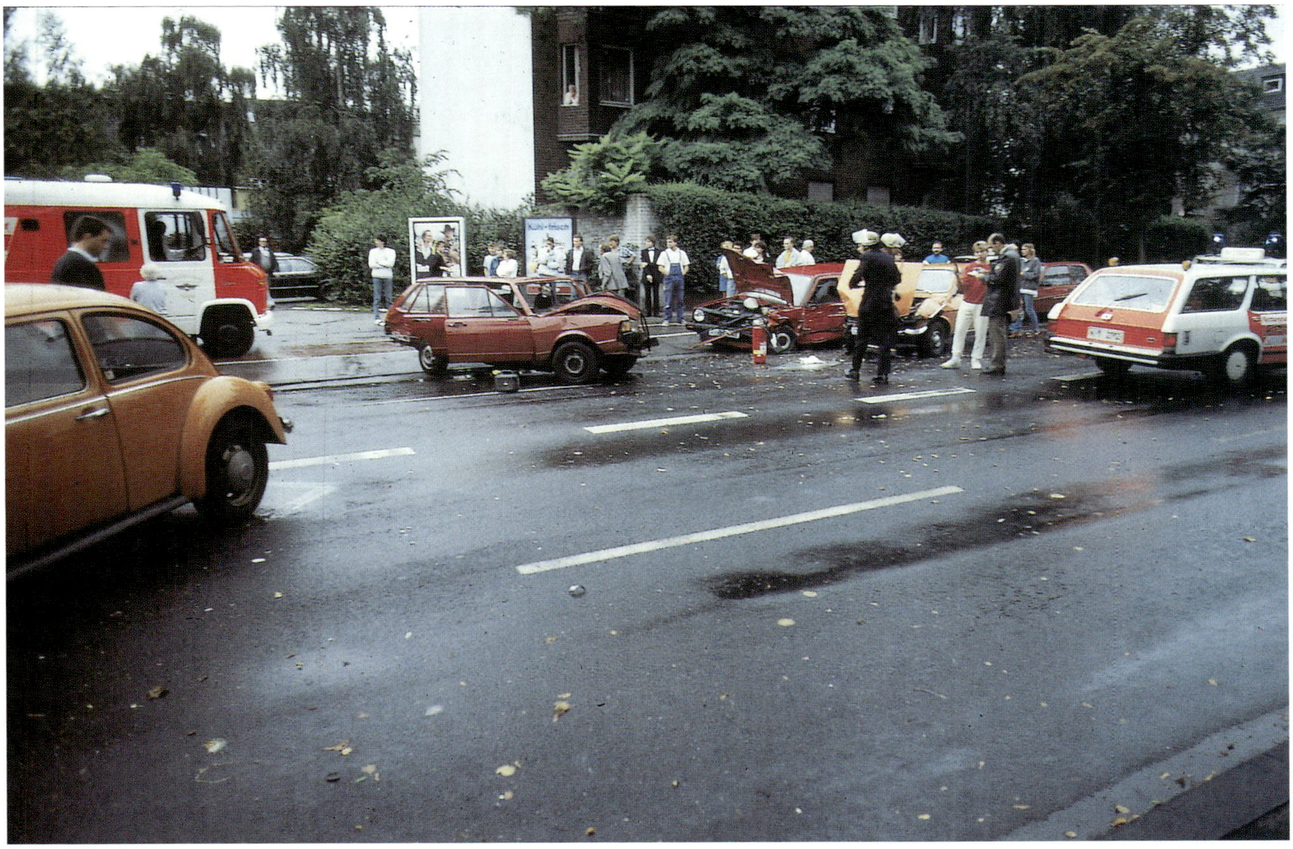

Mehrere PKW sind zusammengeprallt. Für den Rettungshubschrauber gibt es jedoch keine Arbeit, da alle Insassen nur leicht verletzt sind und mit dem Rettungswagen ins Krankenhaus gefahren werden können.

Several automobiles have collided. There is no work for the rescue helicopter, however: all of the drivers and passengers suffered only minor injuries and were taken to the hospital in a rescue ambulance.

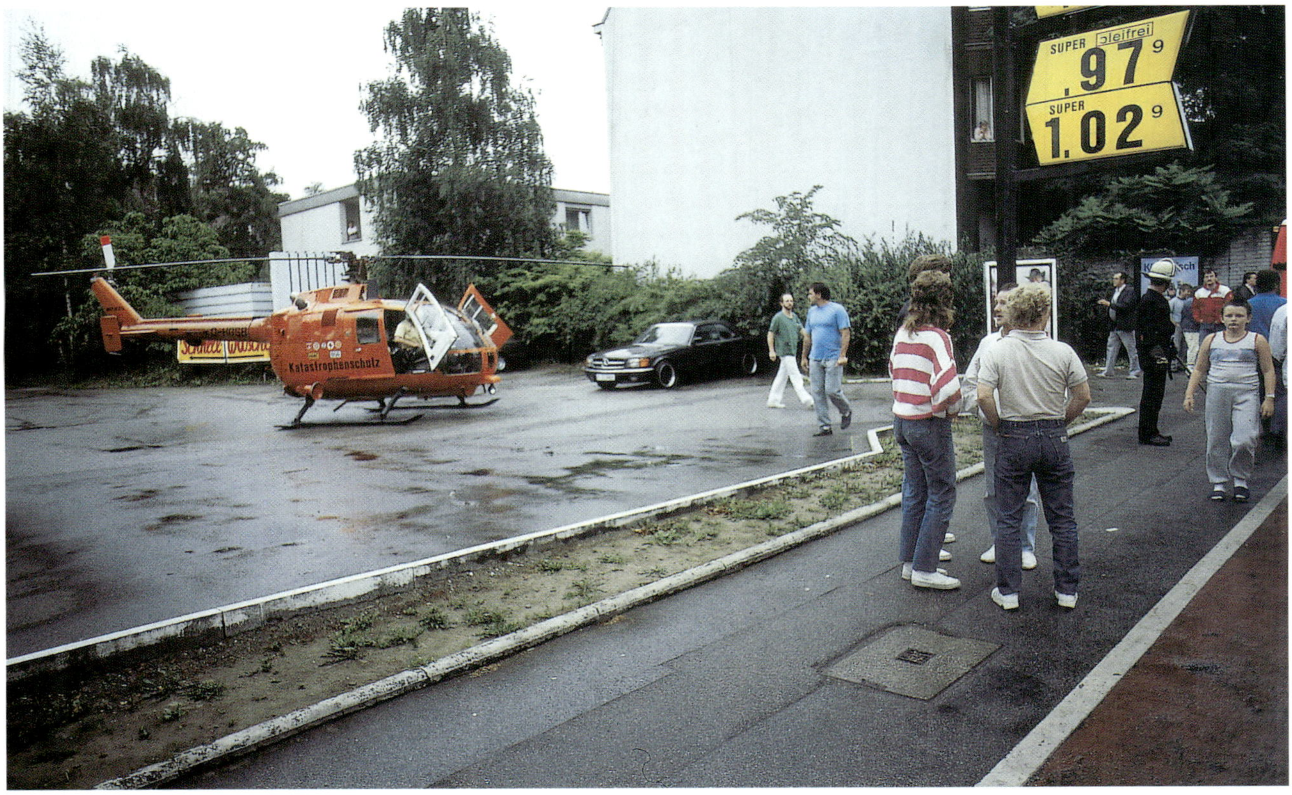

Der Rettungshubschrauber landet unmittelbar neben der Einsatzstelle auf einem Tankstellengelände.

The rescue helicopter lands on the grounds of a filling station directly next to the accident site.

Einsatz für den Rettungshubschrauber
Mission for the Rescue Helicopter

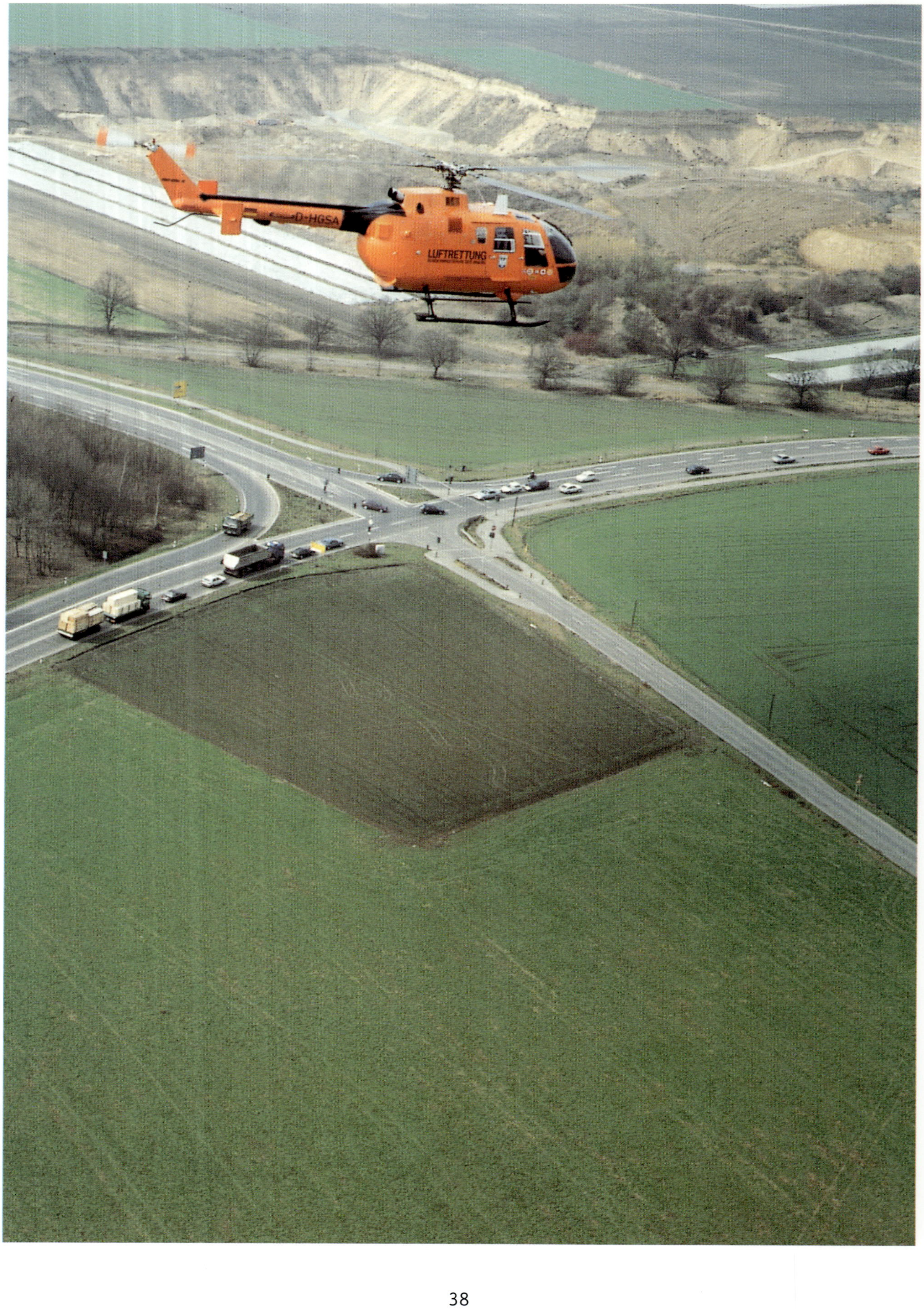

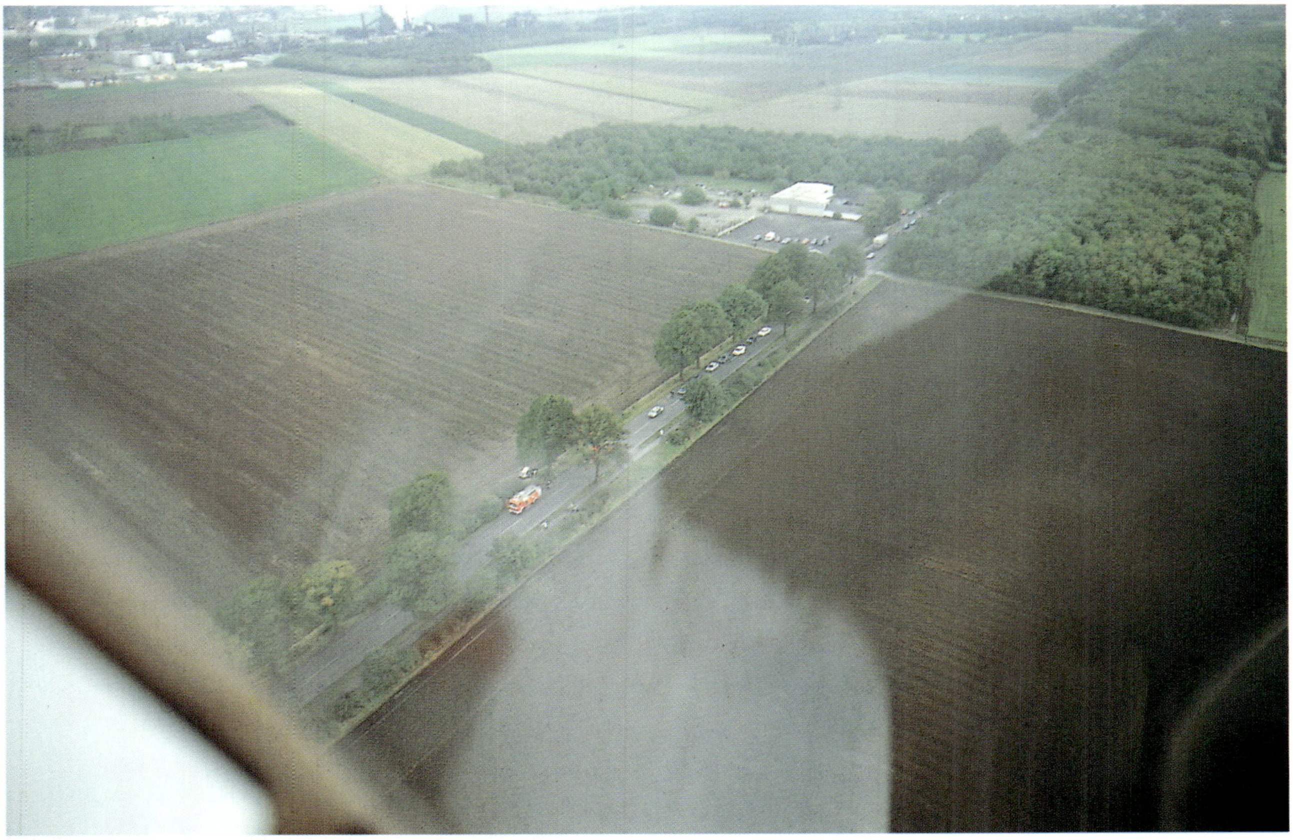

Im Anflug auf die Einsatzstelle auf der Landstraße.

During the approach to the accident site on a country road.

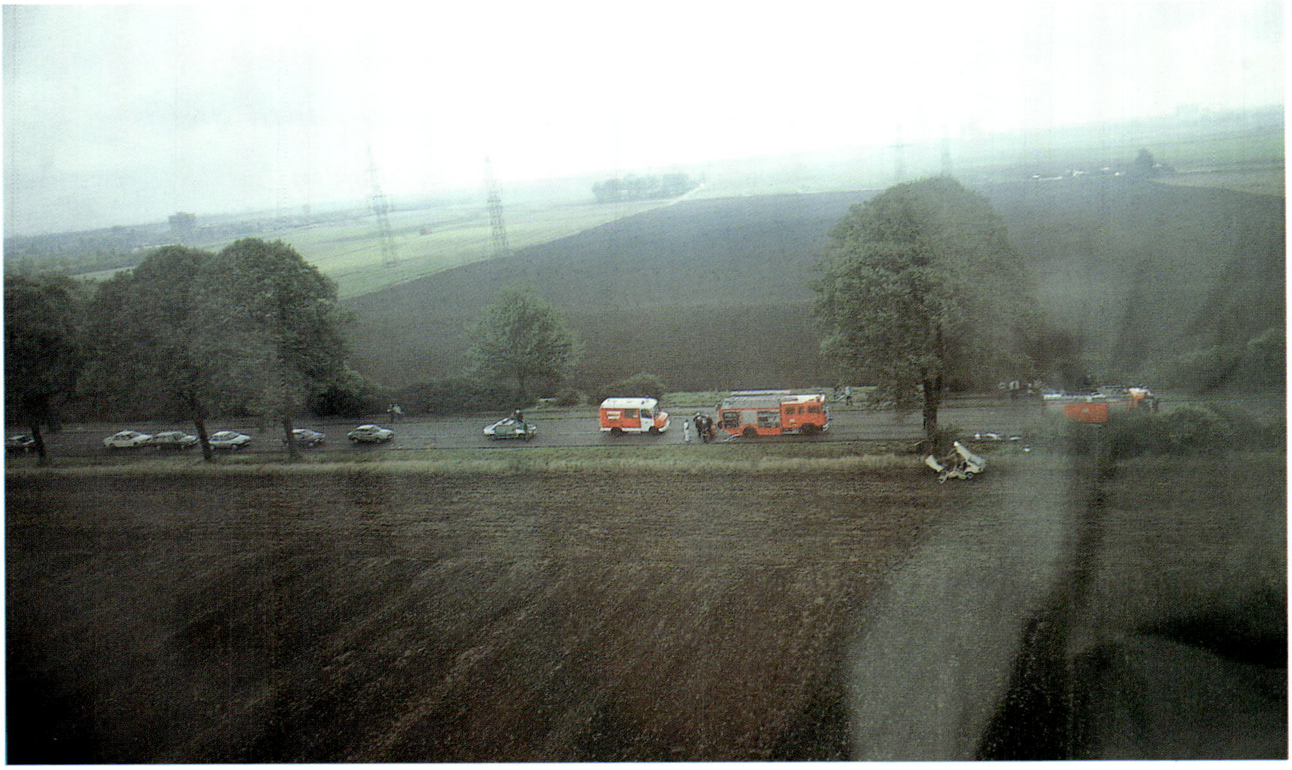

Das Unfallgeschehen ist erkennbar. Ein PKW ist offensichtlich gegen einen Baum geprallt. Über Funk wird mitgeteilt, dass Personen eingeklemmt sind, die von der Feuerwehr mit Hydraulikscheren, mit denen Sie das Dach des PKWs abtrennt, geborgen werden.

It is obvious what has happened here: an automobile has run into a tree. The fire service radios us that people are trapped in the car. They are attempting to rescue them by cutting the car roof open with hydraulic shears.

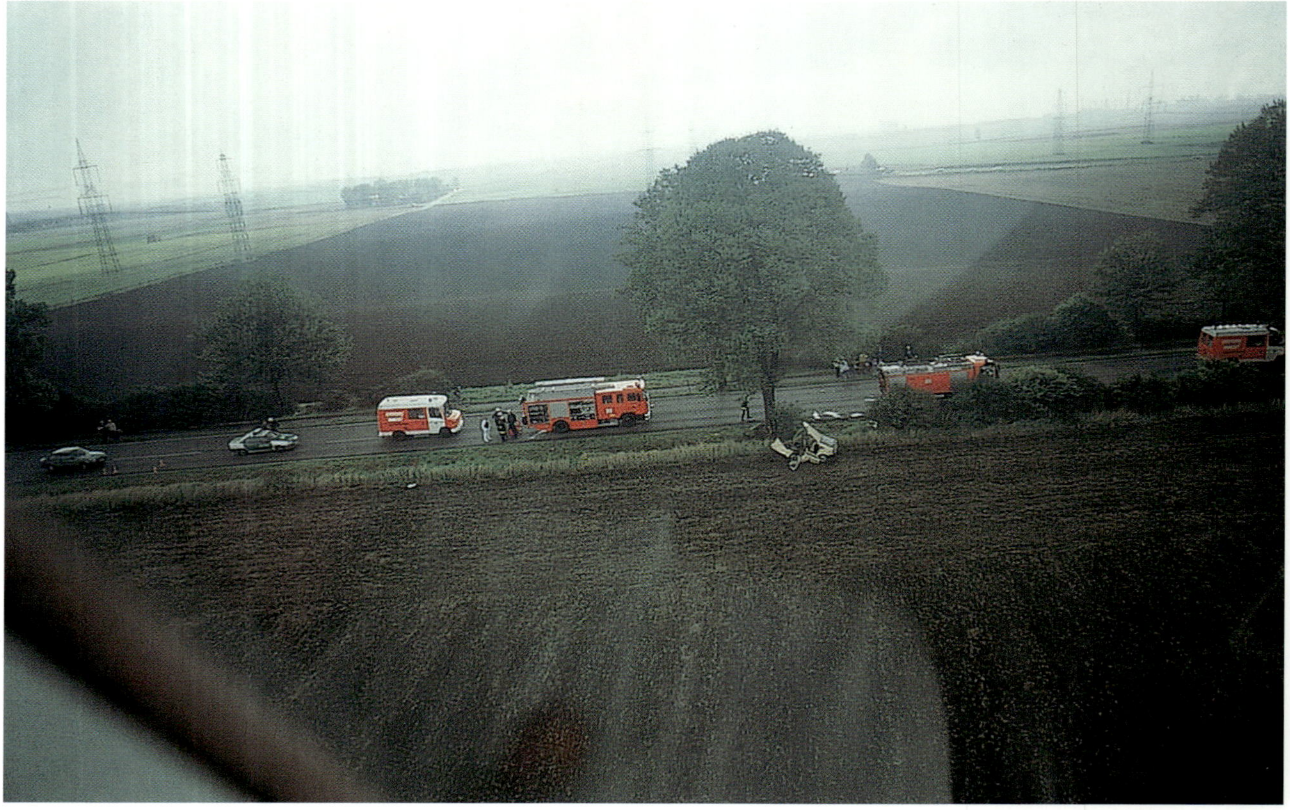

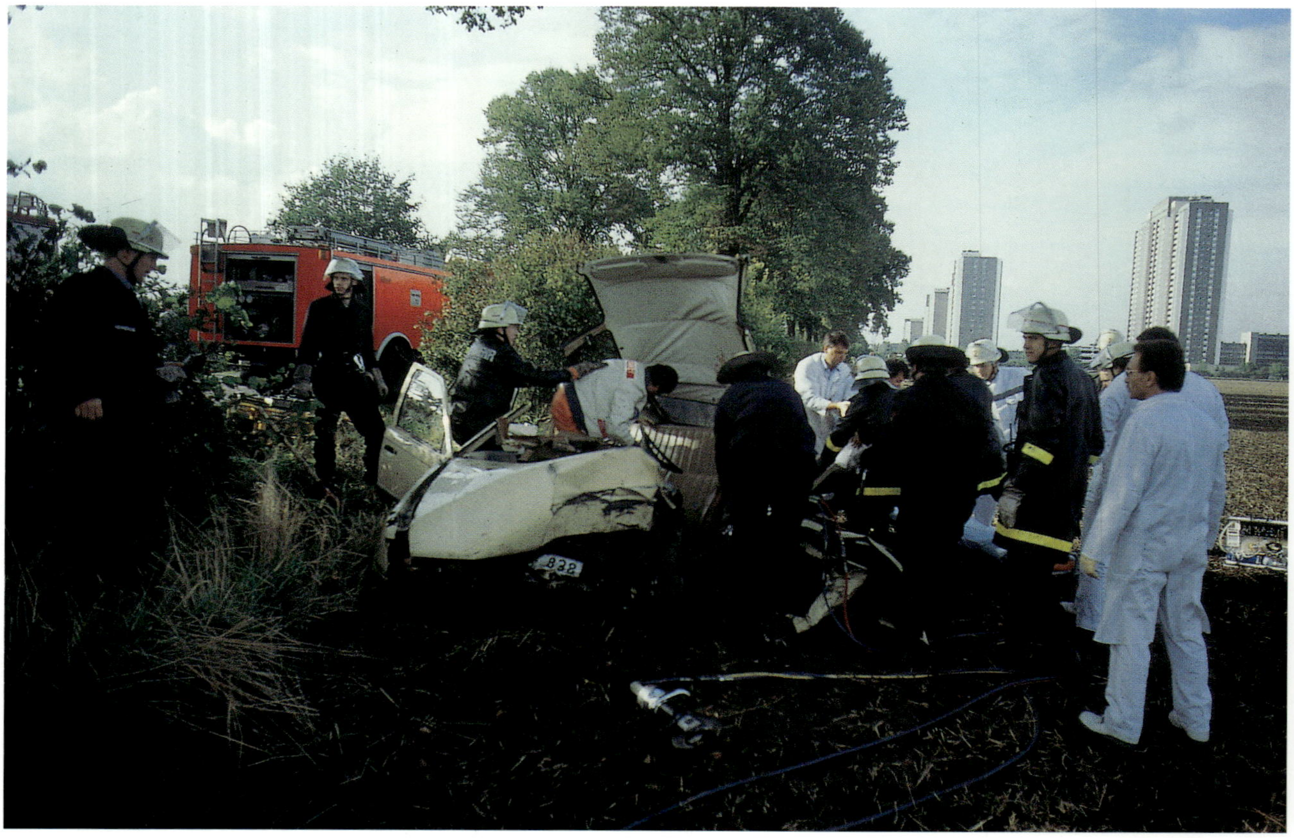

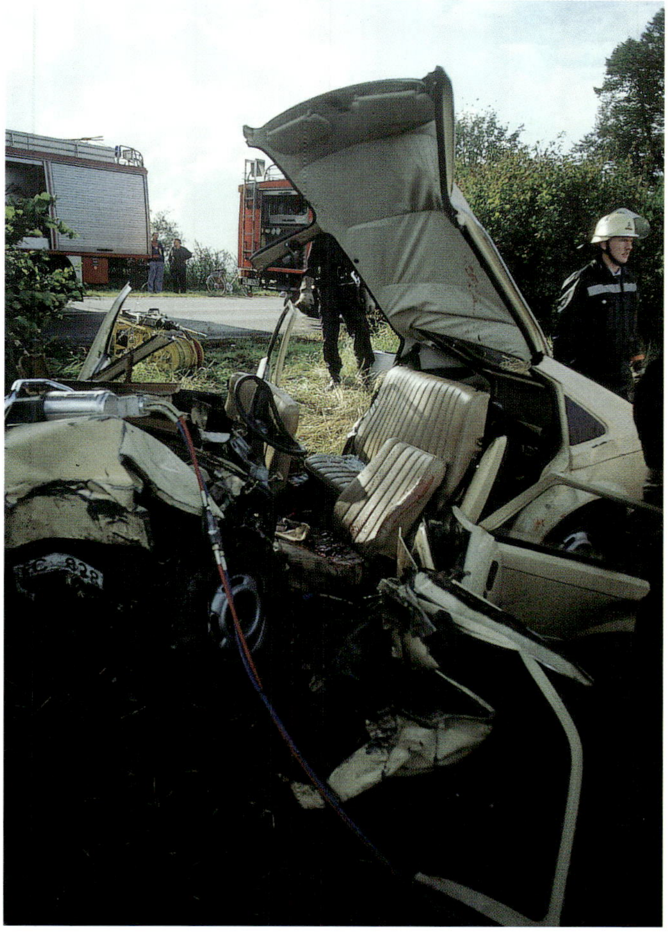

Die Patienten sind aus dem PKW befreit.

The trapped accident victims have been rescued from their automobile.

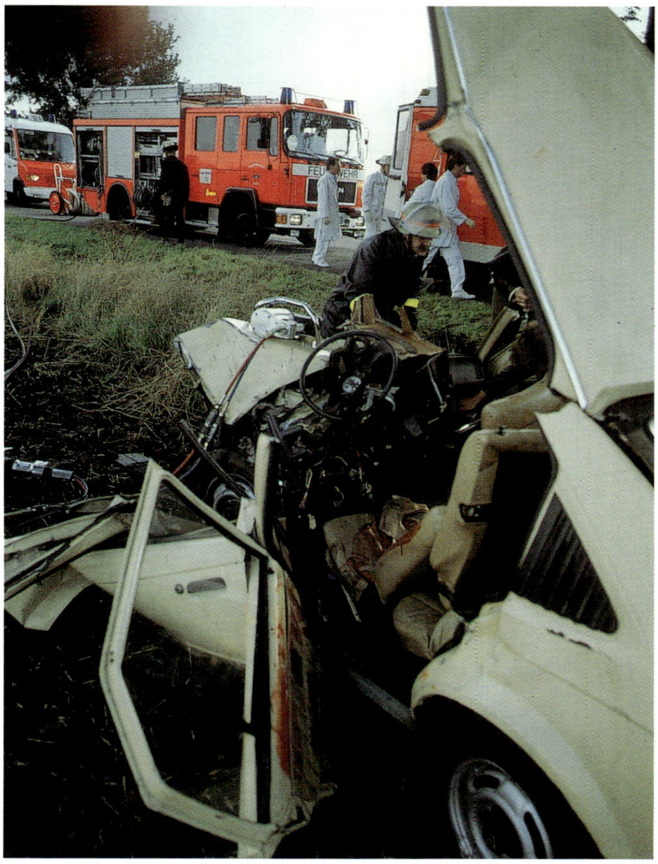

Mit Rettungswagen und Rettungshubschrauber werden die Verletzten in Krankenhäuser zur Weiterversorgung gebracht.

The patients are transported to the hospital by rescue ambulance and rescue helicopter for further medical care.

Einsatz für den Rettungshubschrauber
Mission for the Rescue Helicopter

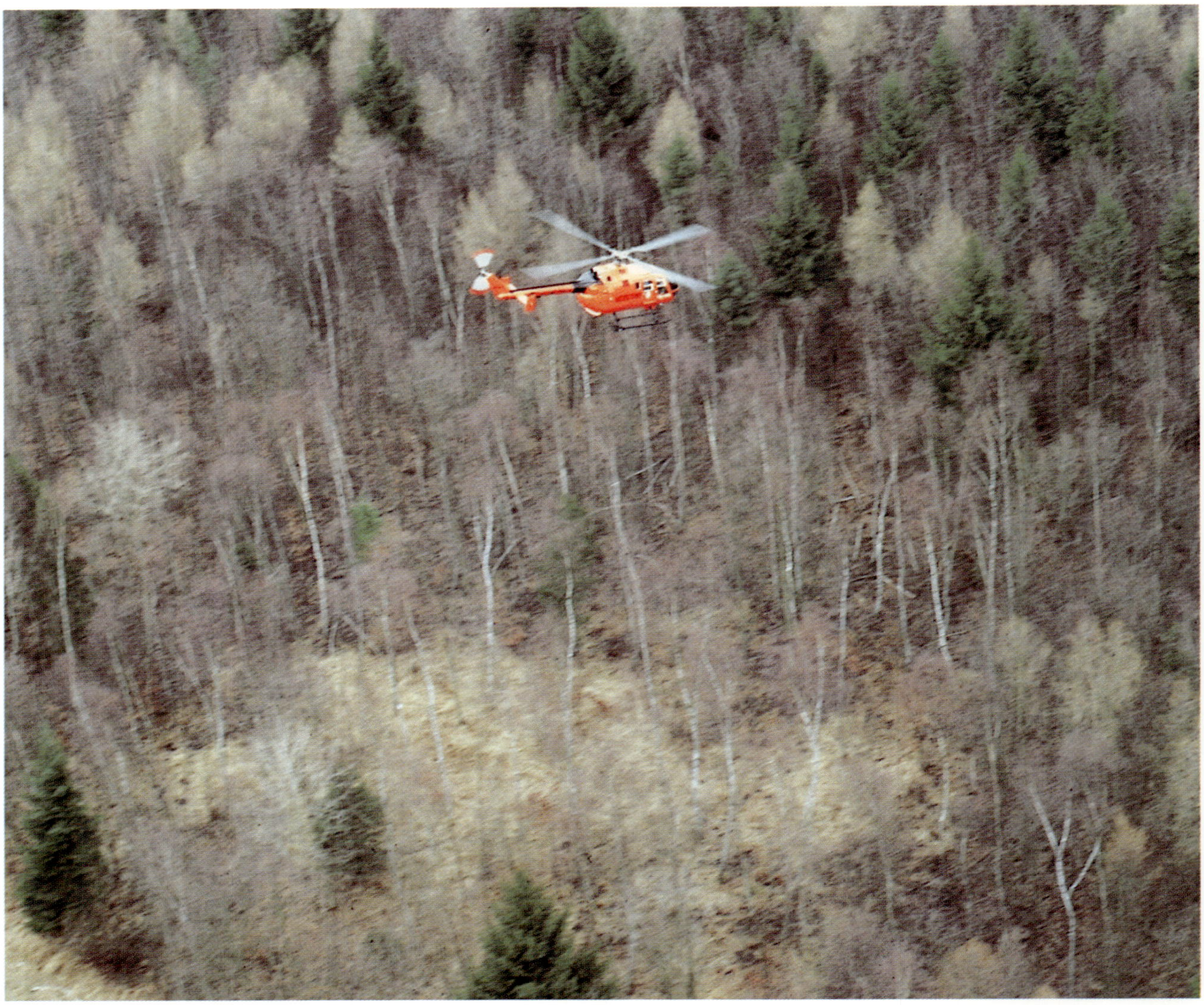

Immer, wenn Rettungshubschrauber zu Suchflügen eingesetzt werden, heißt das natürlich, dass, wenn die Person, die gesucht wird, gefunden worden ist, sie der ärztlichen Hilfe zugeführt wird. Die Versorgung kann die RTH-Besatzung durchführen. Sie kann aber auch die Koordinierung der Hilfskräfte und deren Führung zum Verletzten übernehmen (siehe dazu „Segelflugzeug-Notlandung").

Whenever rescue helicopters are assigned to search flights, this means that the persons the helicopters are looking for will be given medical attention once they have been found. Search flights are by definition rescue flights. The rescue helicopter crew can provide this emergency medical care. In some situations, however, they coordinate the rescue workers and lead them to the injured patient (Refer to "Glider Emergency Landing").

Augenblicke

Wiederbelebung. In der Wohnung. Patient liegt in der Küche auf dem Boden. Am Körper EKG-Verkabelung, Beatmungsschlauch, Herzdruckmassage. Die Angehörigen suchen Blickkontakt. Wird es gut ausgehen? Schaffen Sie das? Das Bild ist eindeutig. Die Reanimation wird abgebrochen. Der Patient ist tot. Der fragende Blick wird zu einem traurigen.

Snapshots

Resuscitation scene inside an apartment. A patient is lying on the kitchen floor surrounded by EKG leads, infusion lines and respiratory equipment. Cardiac massage. Relatives seeking eye contact. An imploring look asking: "Will everything be alright? Can you pull him through?" The clinical picture leaves no room for interpretation; the patient is dead. Resuscitation efforts are terminated. The questioning look is transformed into tragic certainty.

Im Cockpit wird die Einsatzstelle auf der Karte ermittelt. Pilot, Rettungsassistent und Notarzt fliegen in das Suchgebiet. Die Leitstelle teilt mit, dass ein älterer Herr aus einem Altenheim nicht nach Hause gekommen ist und man nun annimmt, ihm sei etwas zugestoßen.

Inside the cockpit, the crew locates the accident site on the map. The pilot and the paramedic with a physician with emergency and rescue certification fly into the specified area. The Coordination Center reports that an elderly man has failed to return to the Old People's Home where he lives. The staff and the other residents are worried that something has happened to him.

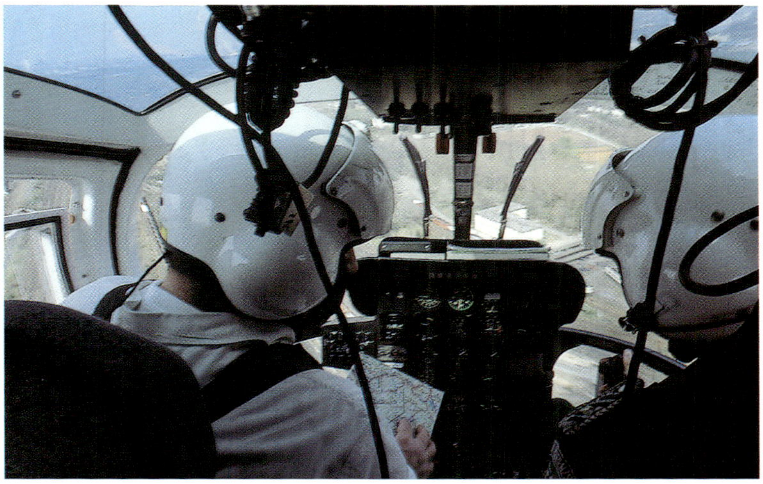

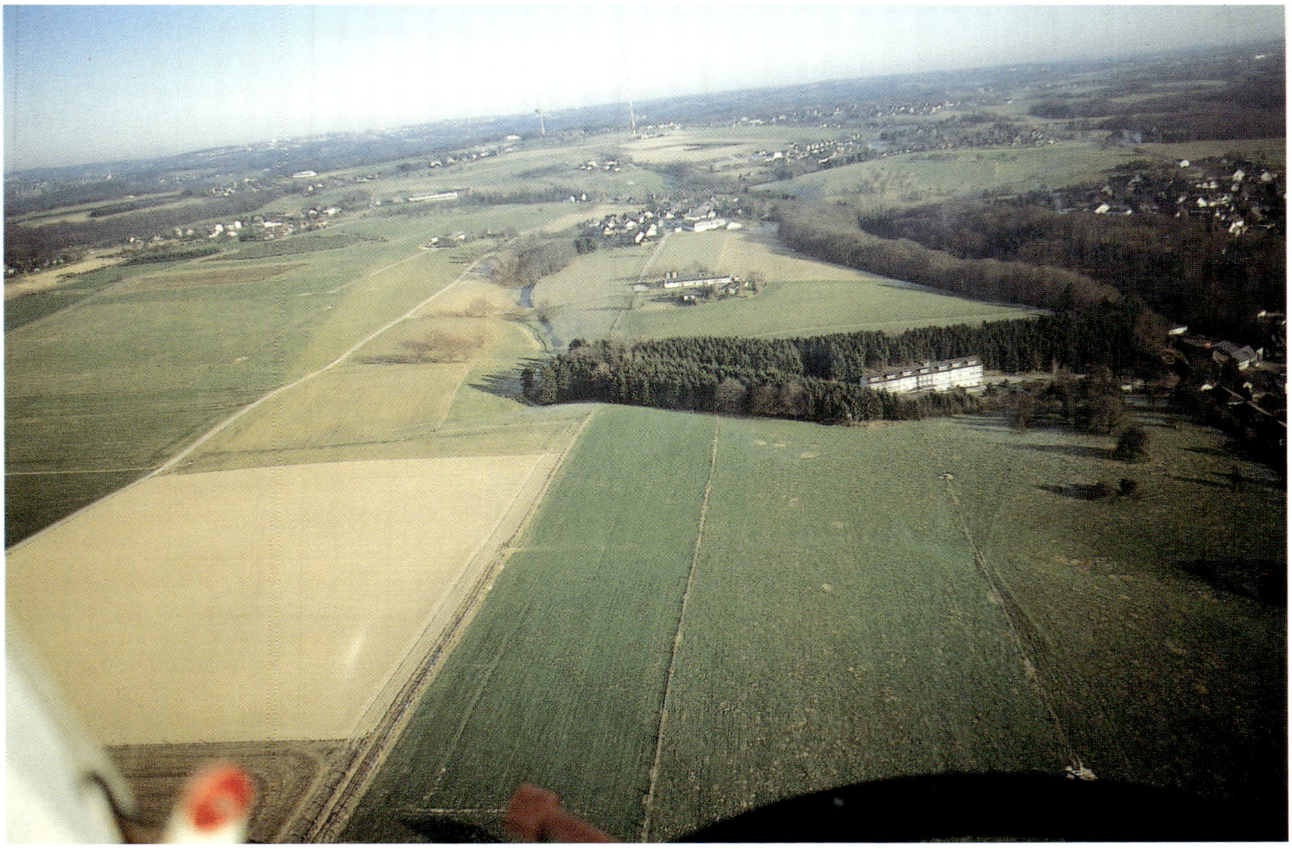

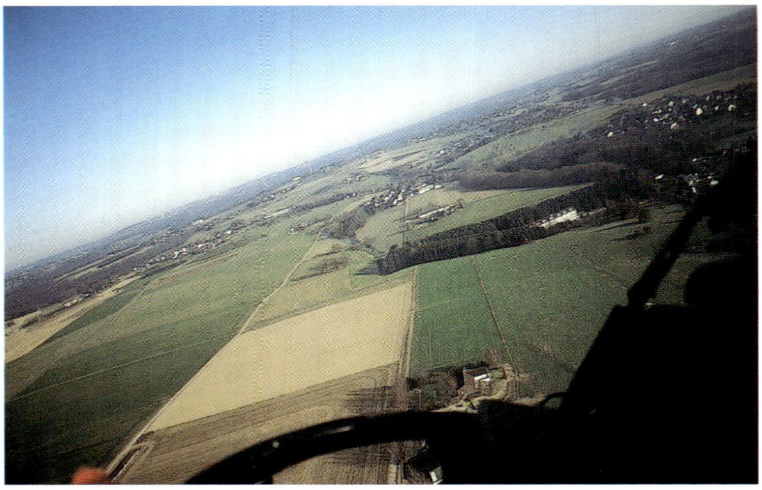

Im Anflug wird dann weiter mitgeteilt, dass sich in der Nähe eines Waldrandes zwei Personen bemerkbar machen, um den Rettungshubschrauber einzuweisen.

During the approach the crew is notified that two people are waiting at the edge of the woods. When the helicopter arrives at the scene, these helpers draw attention to themselves and direct the helicopter to a landing site.

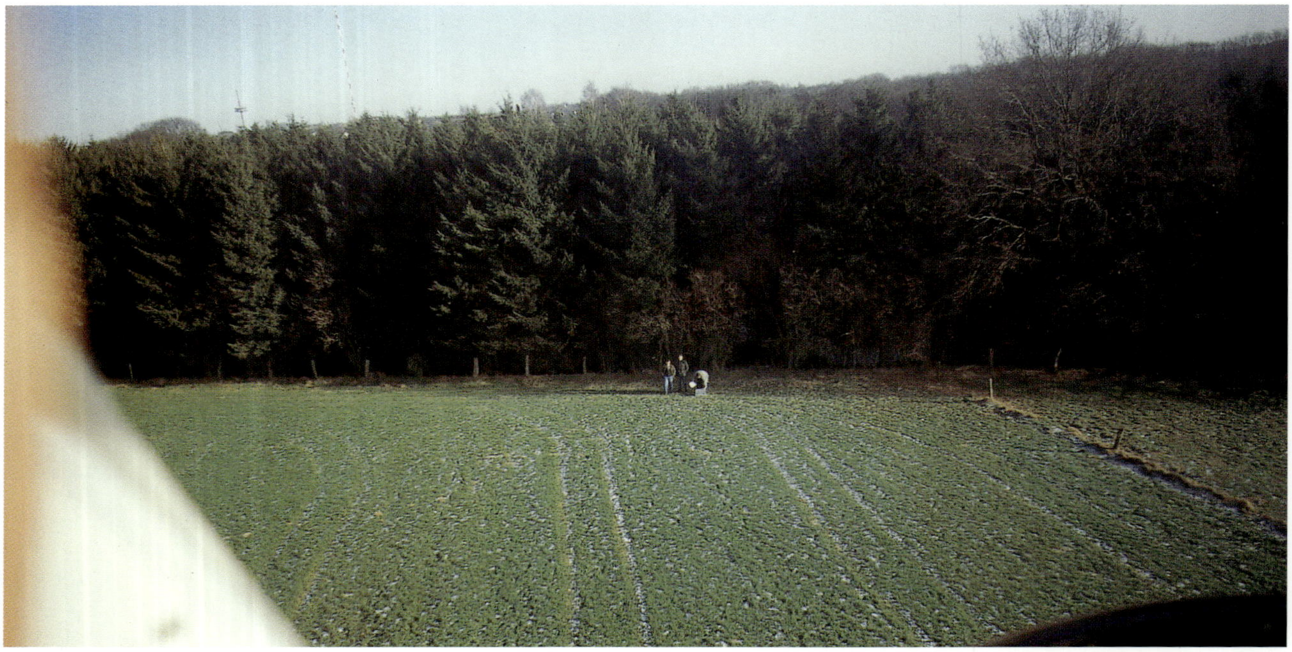

Die Personen, die den leblosen Patienten gefunden haben, führen die Besatzung des Rettungshubschrauber zur Fundstelle.

The persons who have found the lifeless patient lead the helicopter crew to the site.

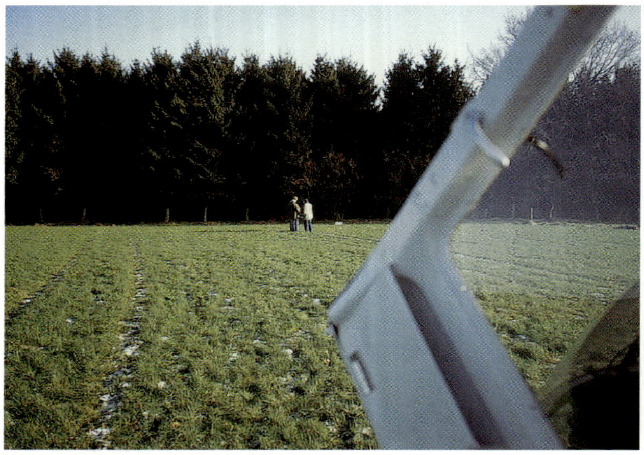

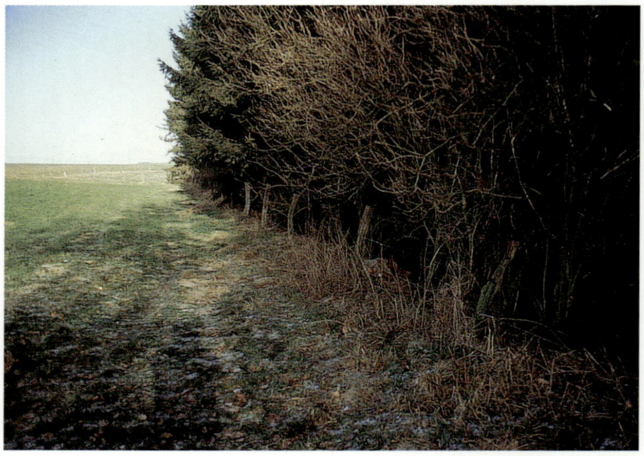

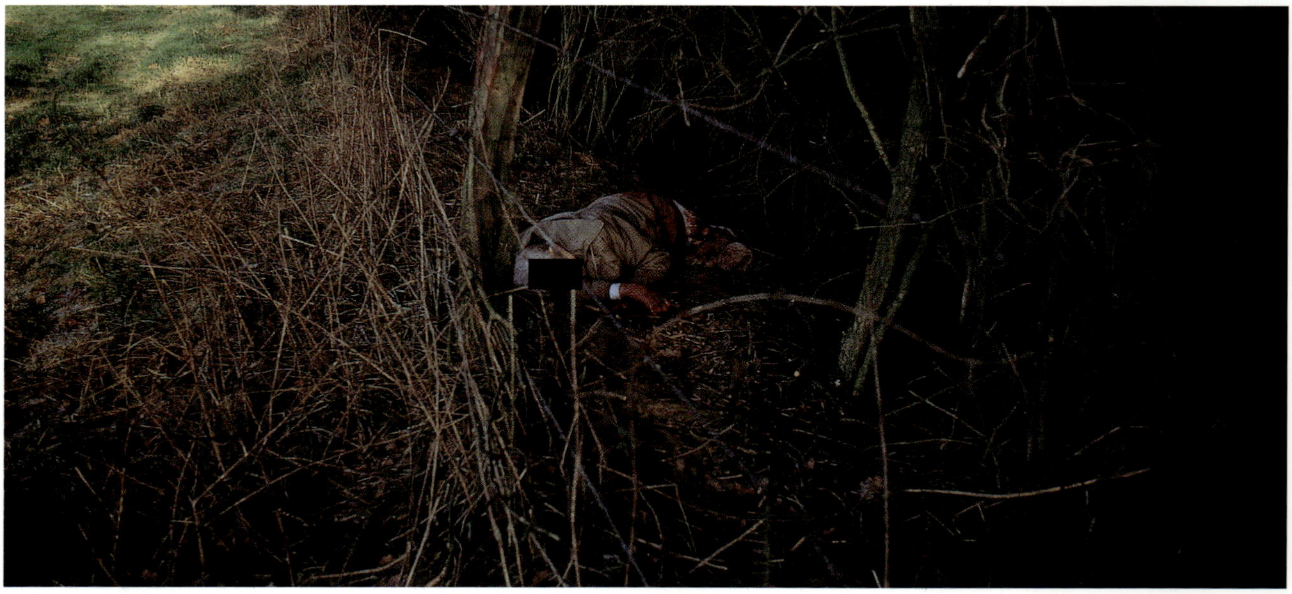

Dem Patienten kann nicht mehr geholfen werden. Die Einsatzstelle wird der Polizei übergeben.

There is nothing the crew can do for the lifeless patient. The site is turned over to the police.

Einsatz für den Rettungshubschrauber
Mission for the Rescue Helicopter

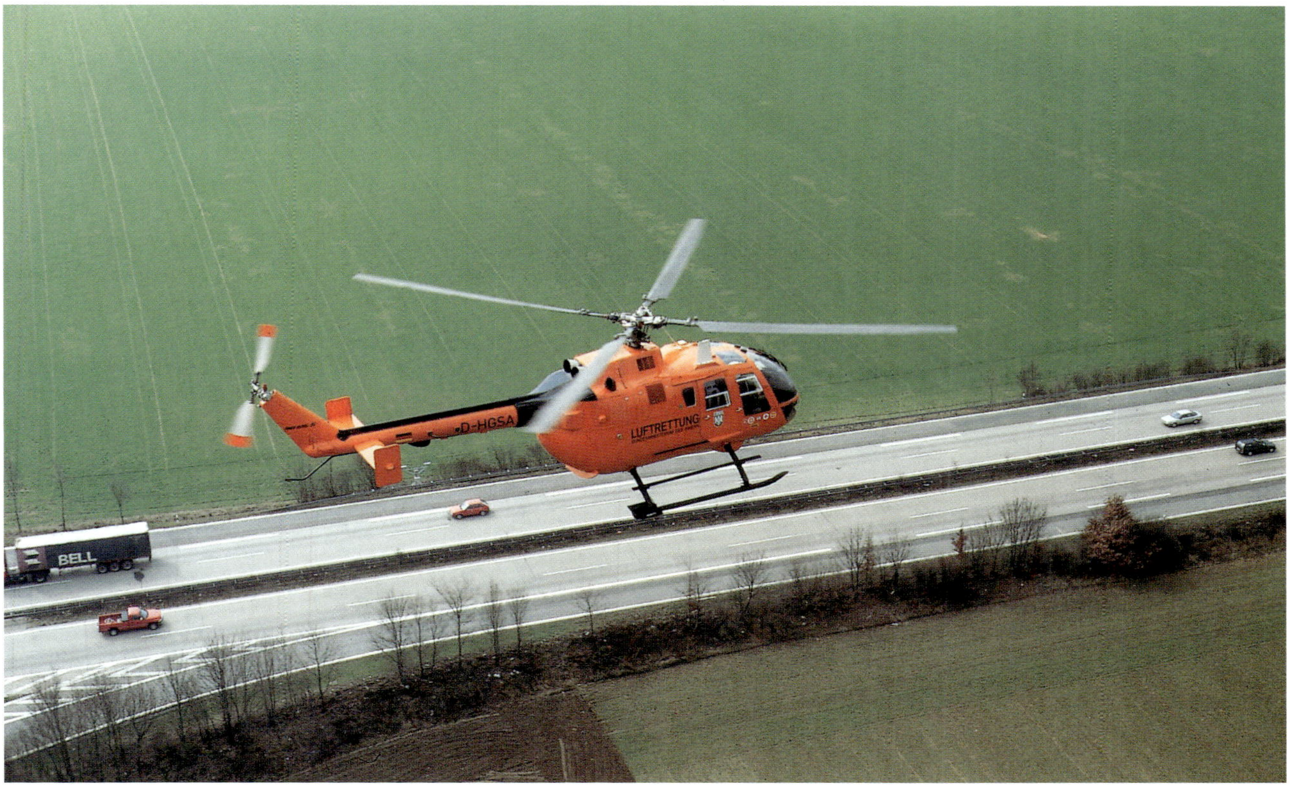

Ein PKW-Fahrer hat einen Herzinfarkt auf der Autobahn erlitten und sitzt in seinem Fahrzeug auf dem Standstreifen.

A motorist has suffered a heart attack on the autobahn; his car is stopped in the emergency lane.

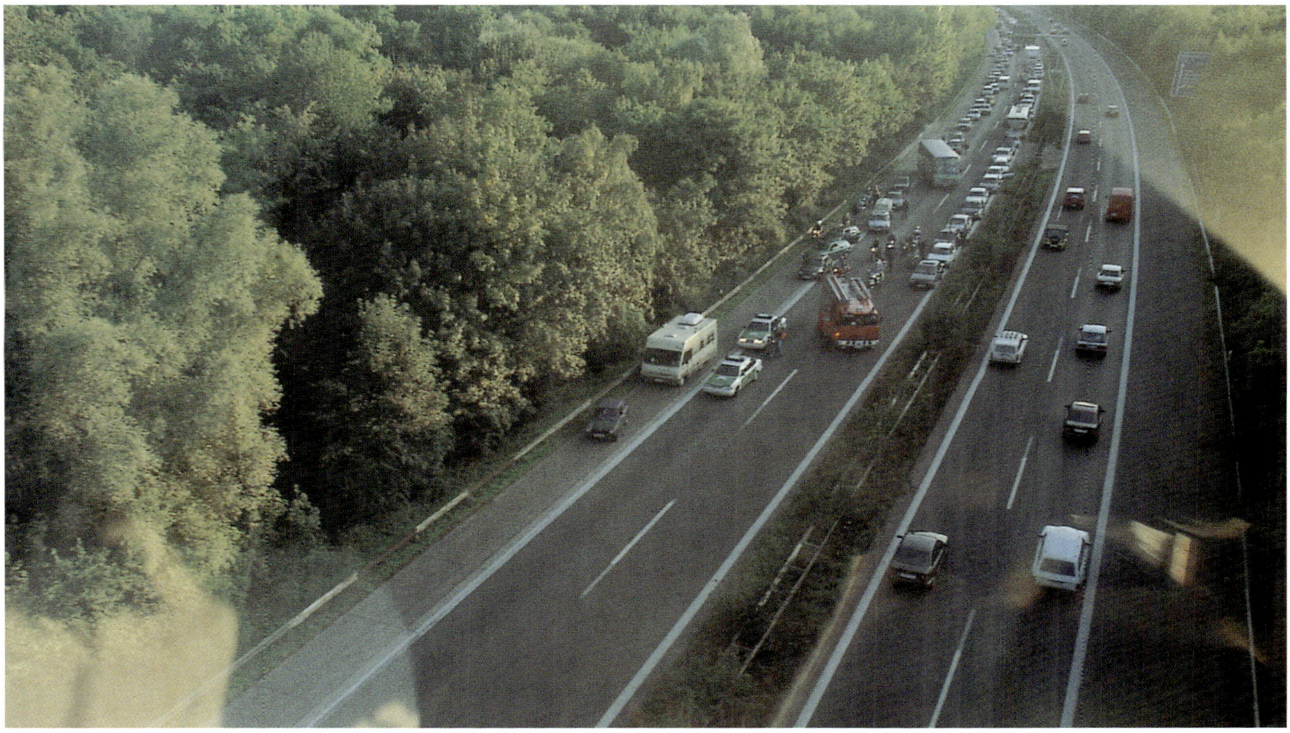

Nach der Versorgung wird der Patient mit einem Rettungswagen ins Krankenhaus gebracht. Der Hubschrauber startet zu einem neuen Einsatz.

The patient is given emergency medical care and then transported to the hospital in a rescue ambulance. The helicopter takes off – ready for a new mission.

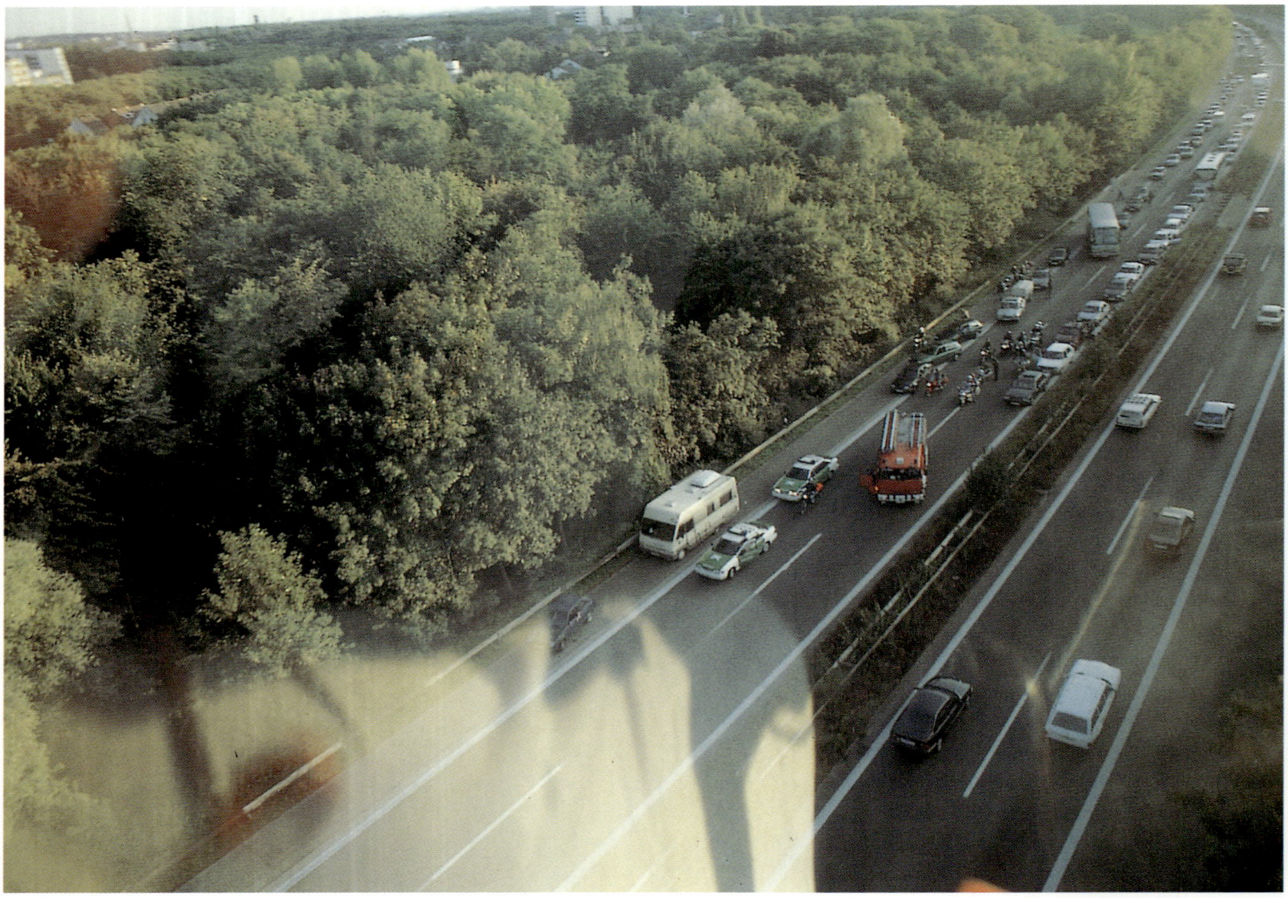

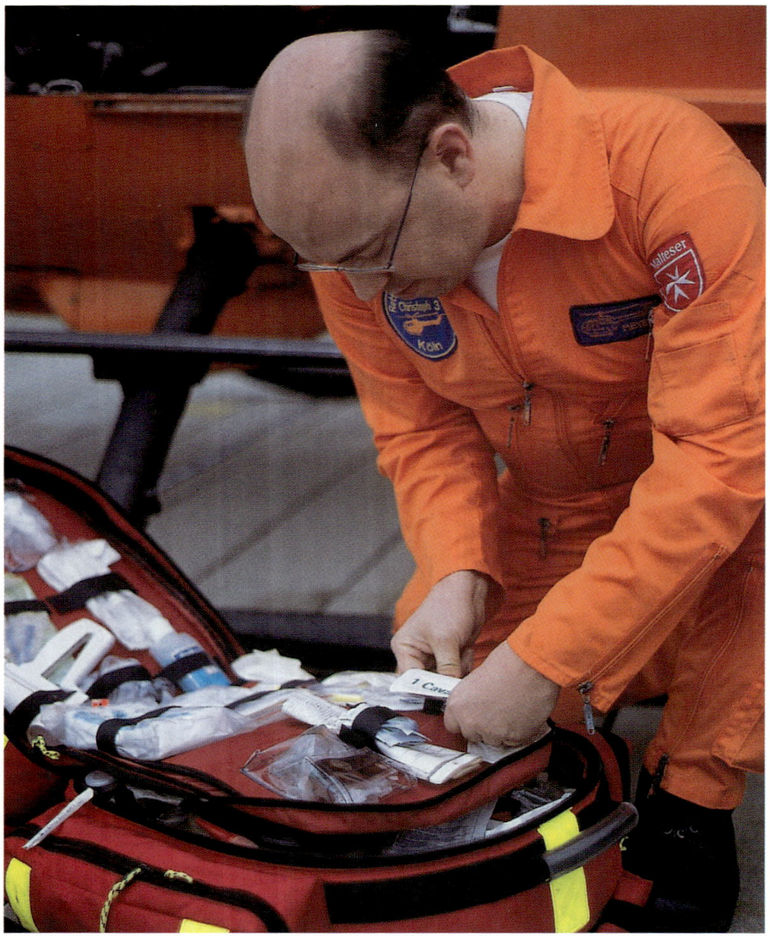

Verbrauchtes Material wird aufgefüllt.

The supply of consumables is replenished.

Augenblicke

Einsatzbefehl: in der Wohnung 1112 im sozialen Brennpunkt. Dort in der Wohnung zwei Männer, die über Computer miteinander sprechen, wobei der eine den anderen töten will. Eintreffen an der Einsatzstelle. Mehrere Gebäudekomplexe jeweils mit Hausmeister. Hausmeister in Loge abgetrennt mit PC. Zwei Streifenwagen, ein Rettungswagen, in dem die Hubschrauberbesatzung nun ist, suchen. Ist bei Ihnen Wohnung 1112? Nein. Der zweite Streifenwagen meldet: Wohnung 1112 auf der Rückseite. Einmal um das Gebäude herumfahren. Mit Aufzug erreichen wir Wohnung 1112. Vor der Türe ein junges Mädchen. Sagt. „In der Wohnung ist mein Freund und dessen Freund, die über PC miteinander reden. Mein Freund will den anderen erschießen." Vor der Tür erscheint der Hausmeister. Wir fragen noch einmal: „Was ist in der Wohnung genau los?" Das Mädchen wiederholt den gleichen Text. Plötzlich: Die Aufzugstür öffnet sich. Ein schwarz gekleideter Herr, Borsalinohut, schwarzer Anzug steigt aus. Er öffnet den Schlauchschacht und rollt in Sekundenbruchteilen den Feuerwehrschlauch aus. Auffällig: Der Schwarzgekleidete hat weder Hemd noch Schuhe an. Der Hausmeister kennt ihn: „Hau ab." Der Aufzug geht auf. Der Schwarzgekleidete verschwindet. Die Polizei fragt erneut: „Was genau ist in der Wohnung los." Das Mädchen wiederholt den gleichen Text. Der Einsatzleiter der Polizei erscheint. „Müssen wir ein Sondereinsatzkommando bestellen?" Der Sanitäter des Rettungswagens lauscht an der Tür. Plötzlich: Die Tür geht auf. Das Mädchen: „Das ist er." Der Sanitäter hinter der Tür haut ihm ins Kreuz. Ein dünnes Männlein fällt in den Flur. Handschellen. Polizisten betreten die Wohnung. Tatsächlich ein zweites unscheinbares Männlein. In der Wohnung zwei PC. Wirre Texte. Kaum Einrichtung. Holzkisten. Über der Tür zwei rostige gekreuzte Schwerter. Patient befragt. Keine Antwort, die die Situation weitergehend erklären würde. Patient in den RTW. Gefesselt mit Handschellen zur Psychiatrie. Auch am Einsatzende keine Aufklärung.

Snapshots

An emergency mission to apartment no. 1112 in a deprived area. Inside no. 1112 two men are talking to each other by computer; one of them wants to kill the other. The rescue crew arrives at the scene. There are several building complexes, each with a building manager. The building manager has a separate office equipped with a PC. Two police cars and a rescue ambulance (containing the helicopter crew) search for no. 1112. "Is this number in your building?" No. The second police car radios: "no. 1112 is in the rear of the building." We drive around to the back, enter the building, and take the lift to no. 1112. A young girl waiting in front of the door tells us: "My boyfriend and his friend are inside, talking to each other by PC. My boyfriend wants to shoot the other guy." The building manager appears on the scene. We ask again: "What exactly is going on in there?" The girl repeats her statement. Suddenly, the lift door opens. A man wearing a Borsalino hat and black suit emerges from the lift – sans shirt and sans shoes. Without saying a word to us, he opens the hose box and unrolls the fire hose in a matter of seconds. The building manager recognizes him and barks: "Get lost!" The lift door opens and the man in black disappears as quickly as he appeared. The police ask once again: "What exactly is going on in there?" The girl repeats her story. The police officer in charge of the police action arrives and asks us: "Do we have to call in a SWAT team?". The emergency medical technician from the rescue ambulance puts his ear to the door. Suddenly, the door opens. The girl says: "That's him!" The EMT delivers a well-aimed punch in the back. An unassuming man of small stature collapses in the hallway. Handcuffs. The police enter the apartment, where they find a second unassuming man of small stature. There are two PCs in the apartment, with incomprehensible texts on the monitors. Beside a few orange crates, there is hardly any furniture. Above the door are two rusty crossed swords. The patient is questioned. He does not give any answers which shed light on the bizarre situation. The patient is brought to the rescue ambulance and transported in handcuffs to a psychiatric ward. At the end of the mission, we leave without ever finding out what was going on in no. 1112.

Einsatz für den Rettungshubschrauber
Mission for the Rescue Helicopter

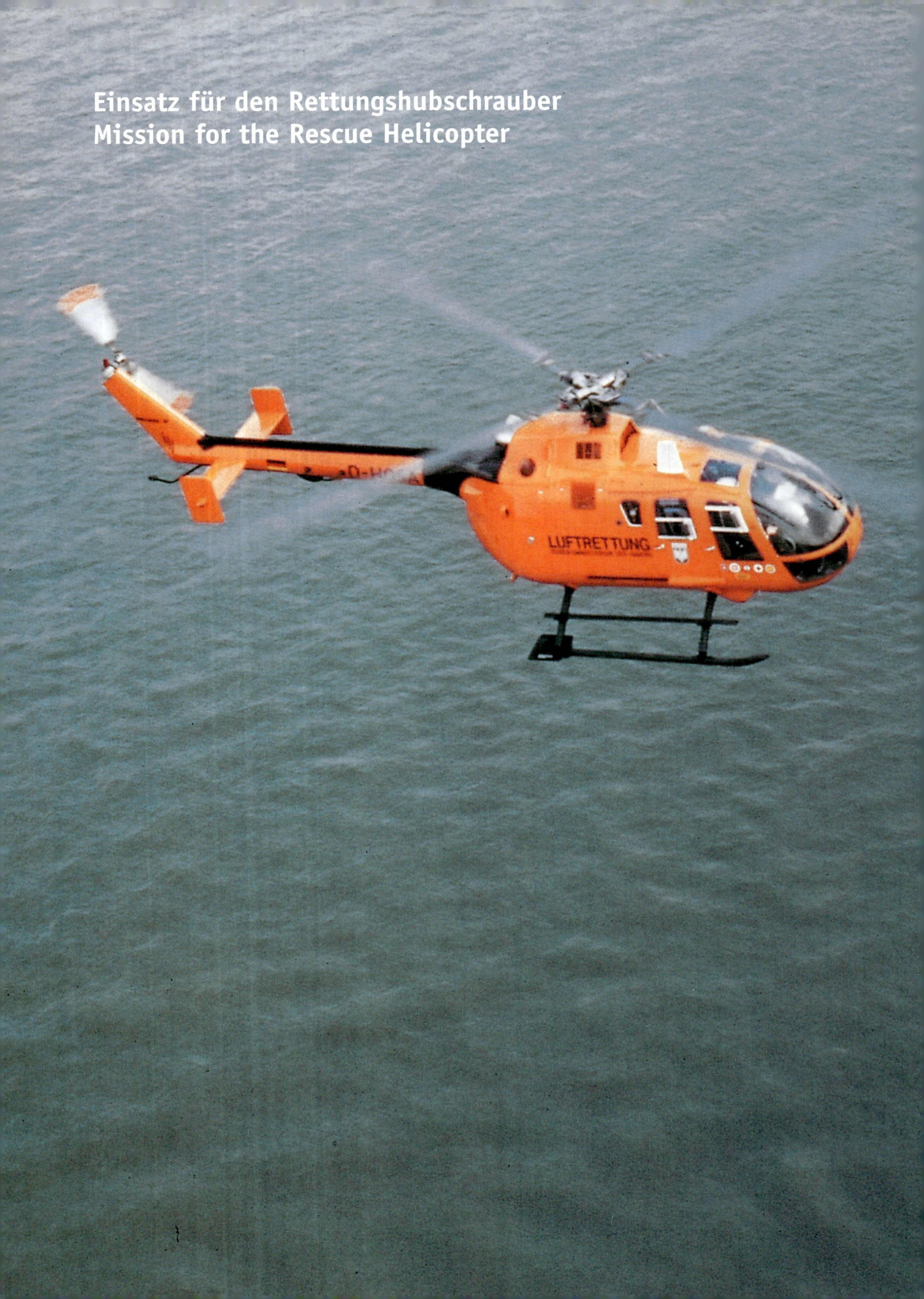

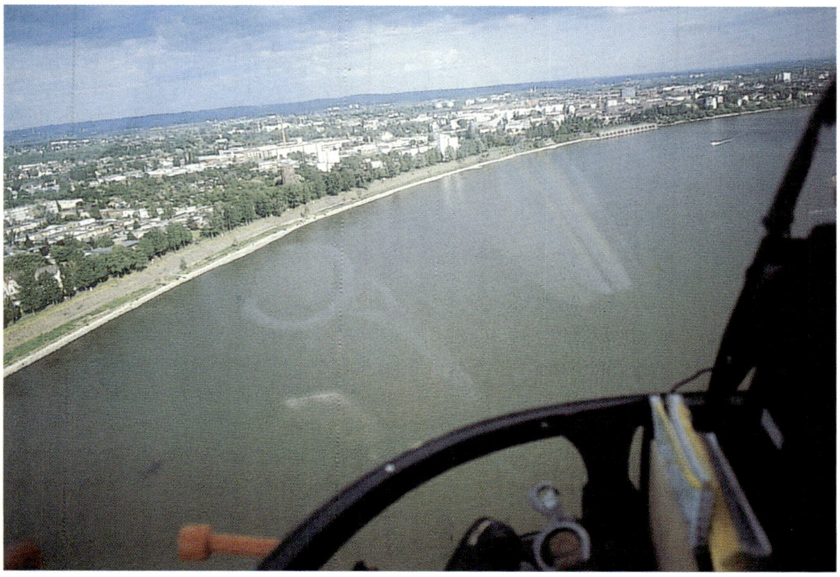

Feuerwehrboot und Rettungshubschrauber sowie Einsatzkräfte an beiden Uferseiten suchen nach einer Person, die sich im Wasser befinden soll.

The rescue helicopter and a fire service boat, together with rescue workers on both sides of the river, search for a person reported to be in the water.

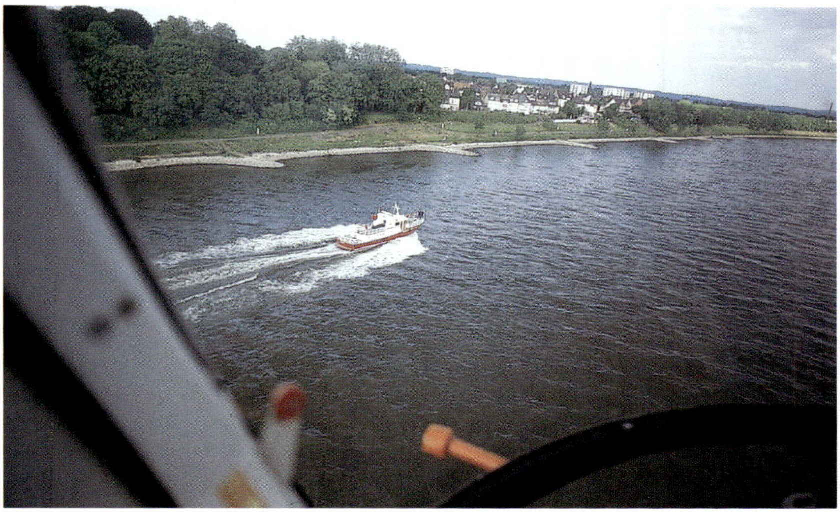

Rettungsboot und Rettungshubschrauber sind auf gleicher Höhe, finden aber keinen Anhalt für eine Person im Wasse-.

The rescue helicopter is now directly over the rescue boat; neither of them see any signs of a person in the water.

Aus unterschiedlichen Gründen gehen Leute ins Wasser: Sie springen aus Übermut von Brücken; sie springen in suizidaler Absicht ins Wasser; sie versuchen, den Strom zu überqueren; sie gehen einer Wette nach und betreten das unsichere Element Wasser ohne zu wissen, welch hohe Strömung Flüsse haben können.

People who go into the water do so for a wide variety of reasons: they brashly jump from bridges, they dive into a river with suicidal intent, or they overestimate their swimming ability and try to swim across a river. Still others dive into water, a very dangerous element, in response to a dare or bet without realizing that rivers contain very strong invisible currents.

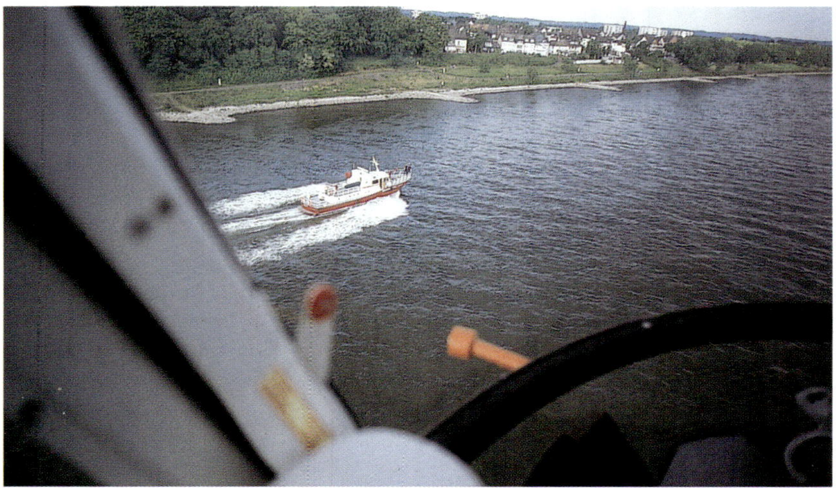

Die Suche wird nach zwanzig Minuten ergebnislos abgebrochen.

The search is broken off without results after 20 minutes.

Einsatz für den Rettungshubschrauber
Mission for the Rescue Helicopter

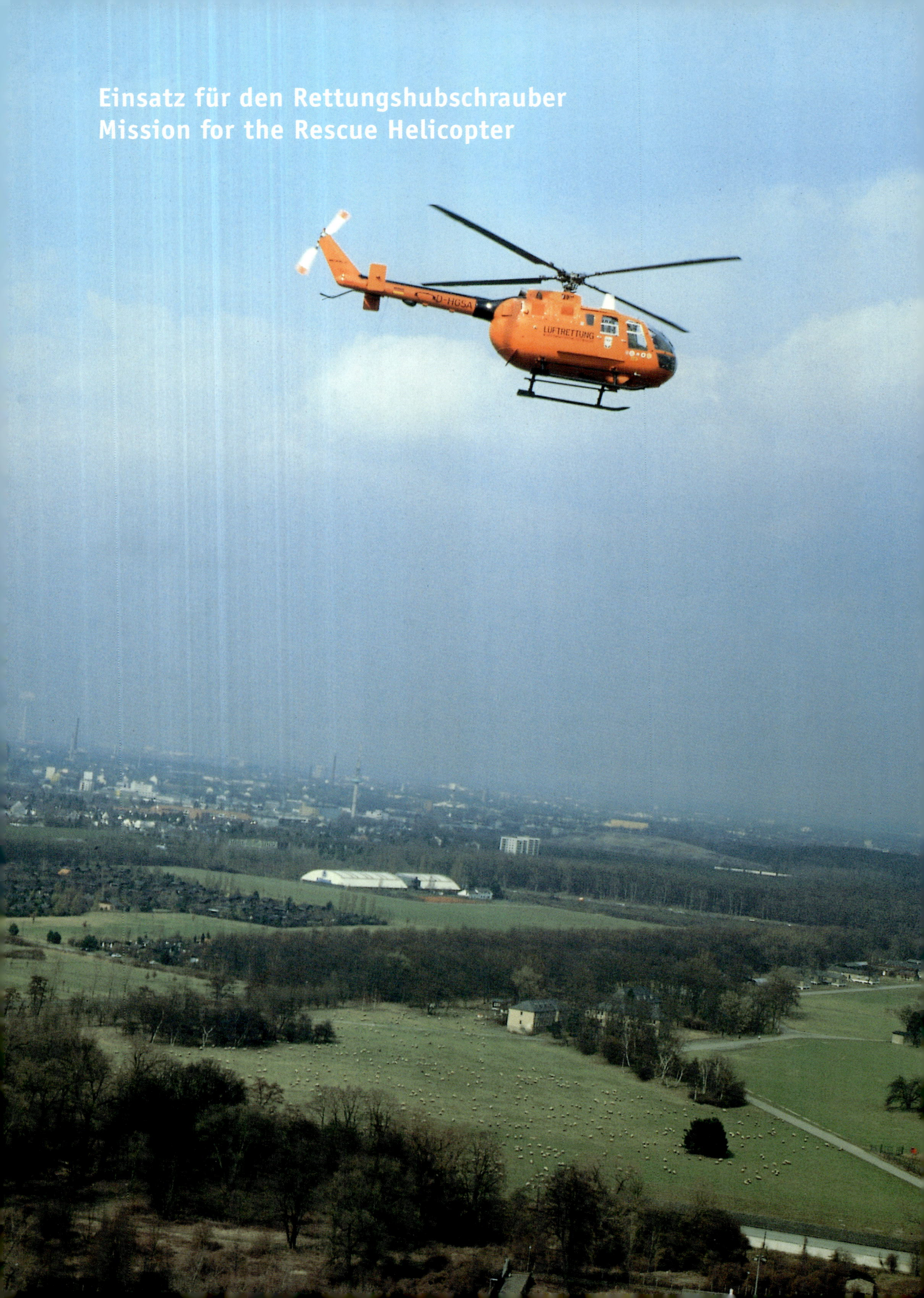

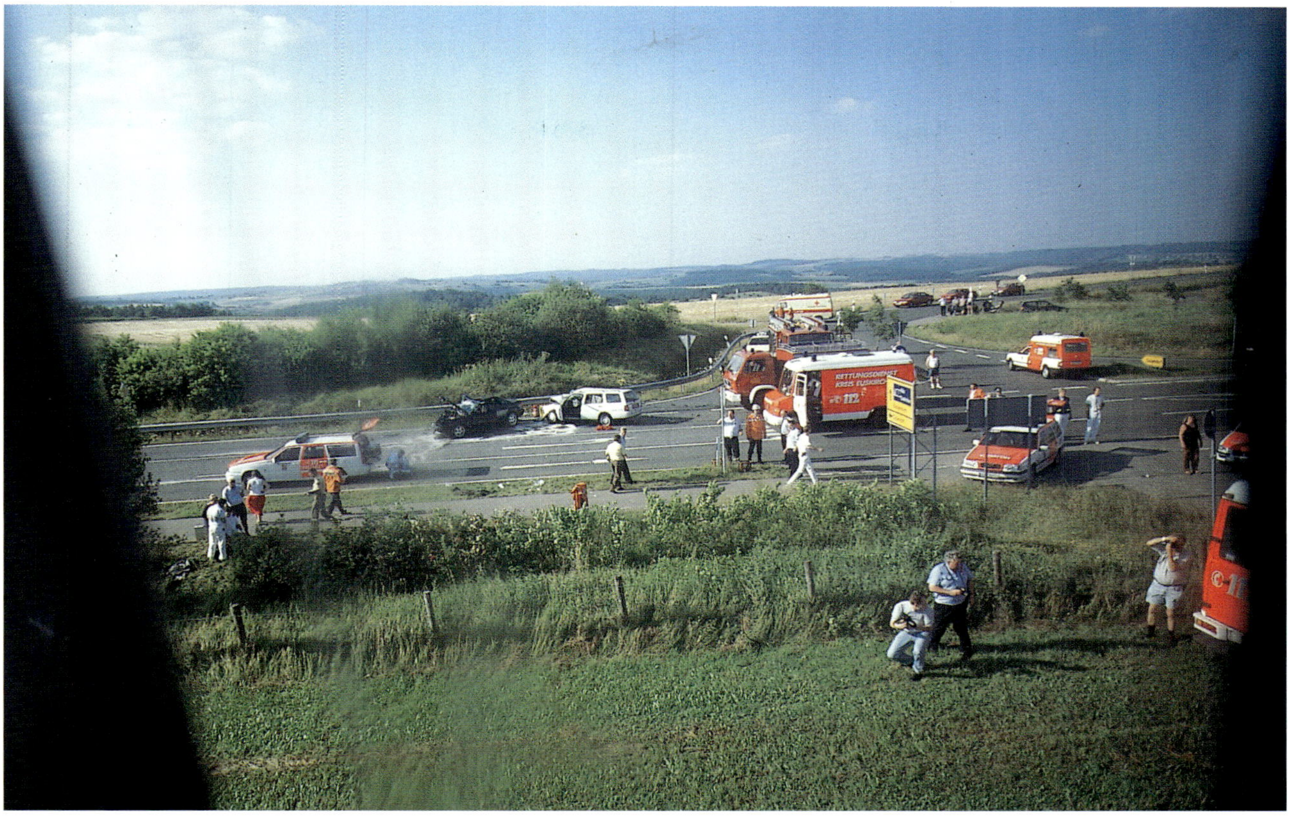

Auf einer Kreuzung sind PKW zusammengestoßen. Mehrere bodengebundene Notärzte sowie zwei Rettungshubschrauber bringen die z.T. schwerverletzten Patienten in verschiedene Krankenhäuser.

A number of automobiles have crashed into each other at an intersection. Several land-based physicians with emergency & rescue certification, as well as two rescue helicopters, transport the accident victims, some of whom have serious injuries, to various hospitals.

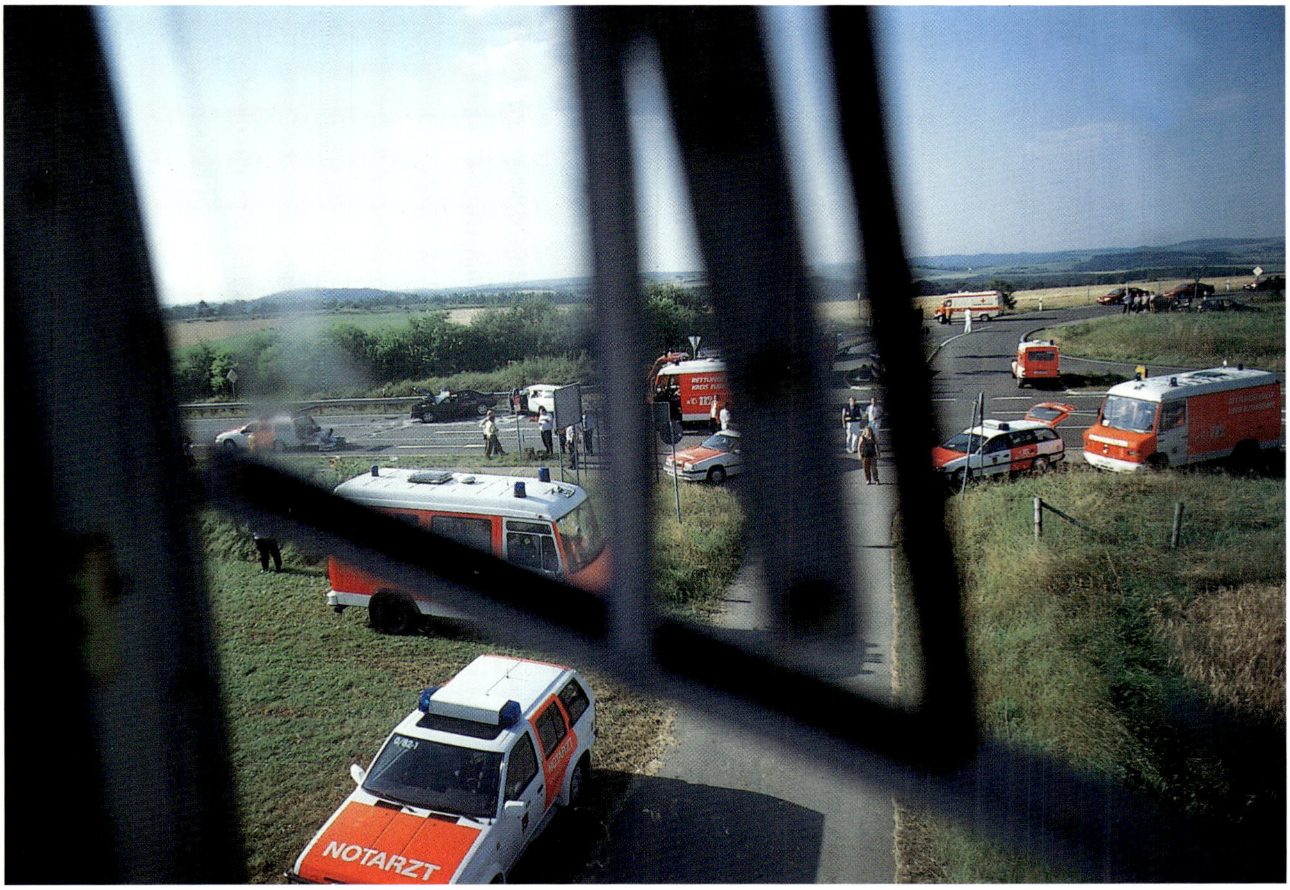

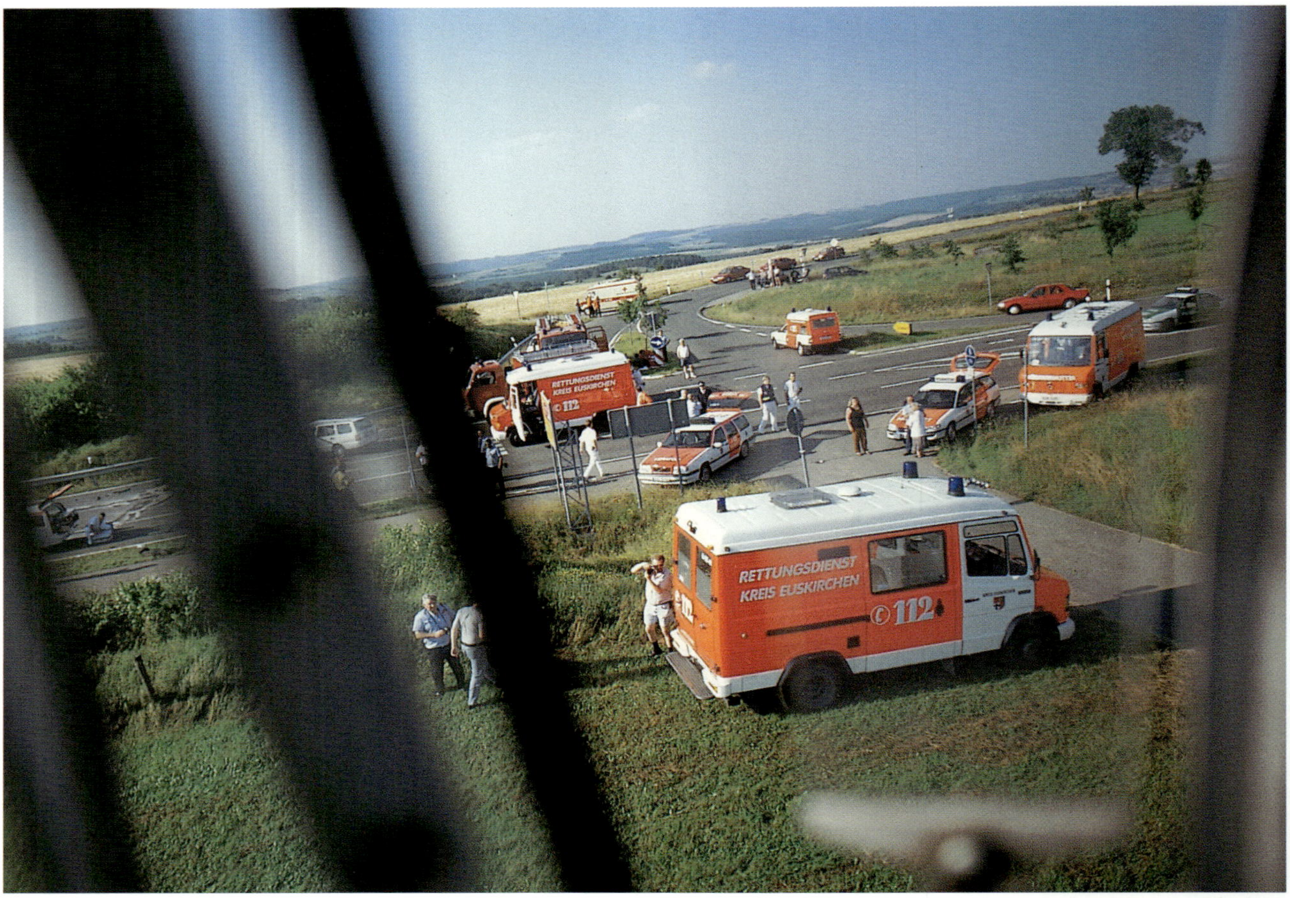

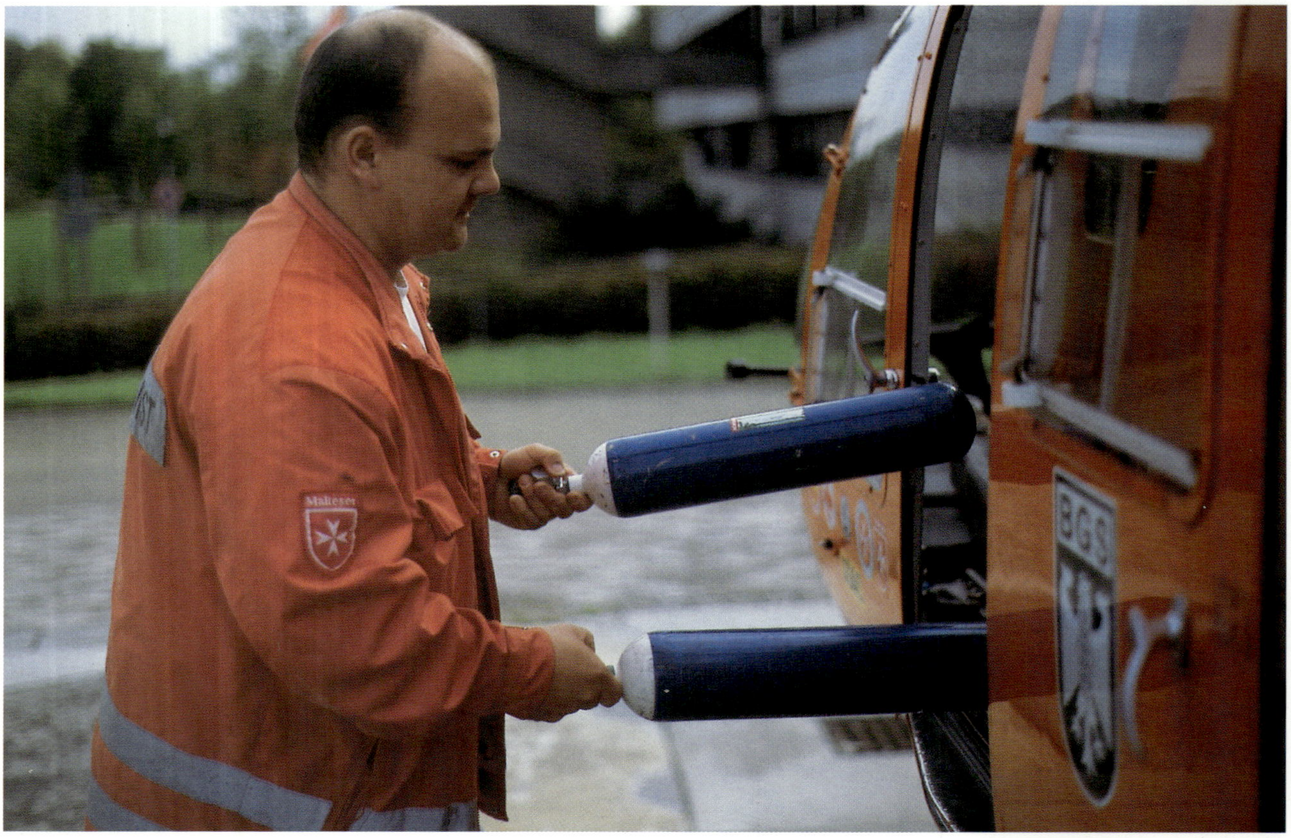

Lebenswichtiger Sauerstoff wird aufgefüllt.

The supply of vital oxygen is replenished.

Einsatz für den Rettungshubschrauber
Mission for the Rescue Helicopter

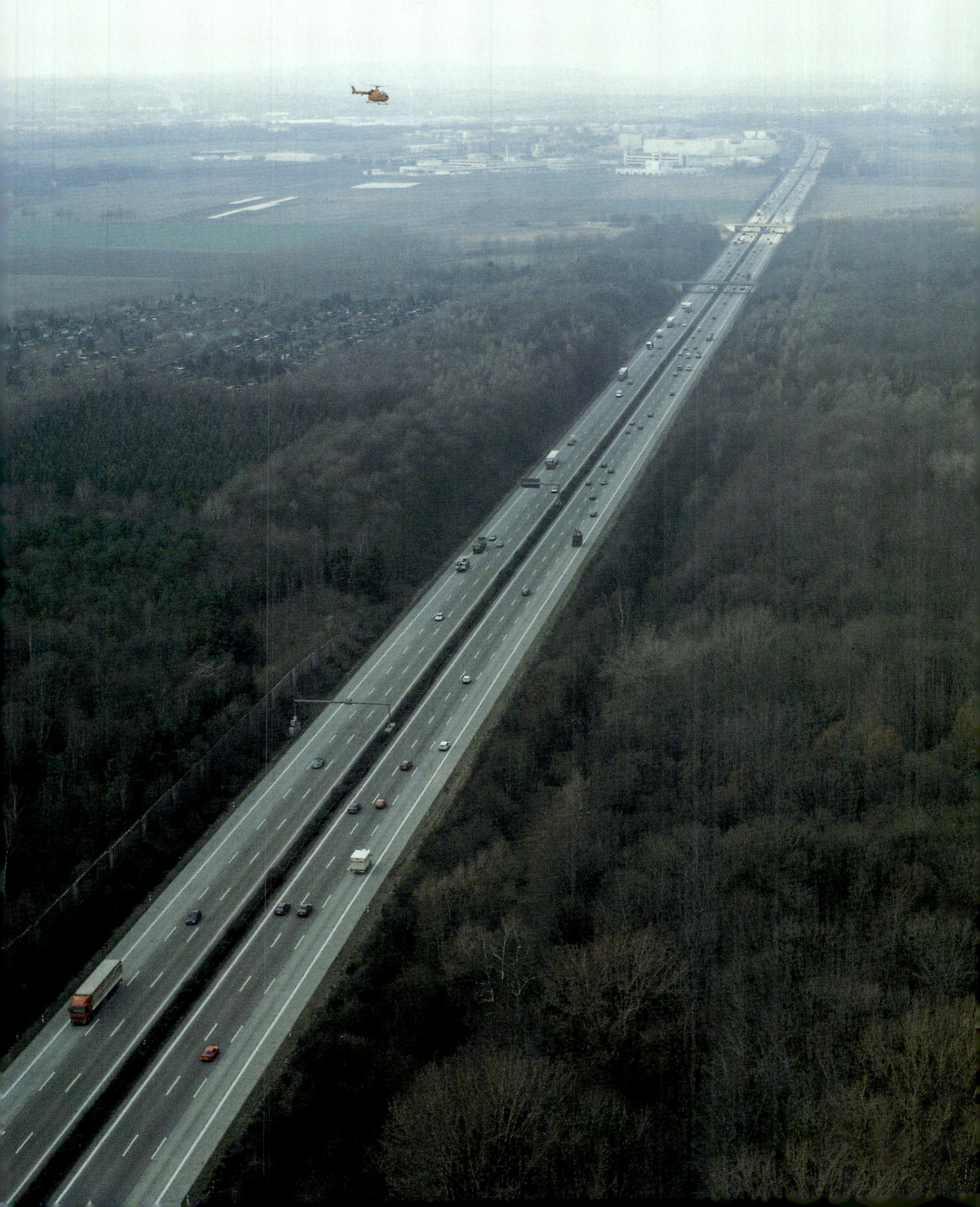

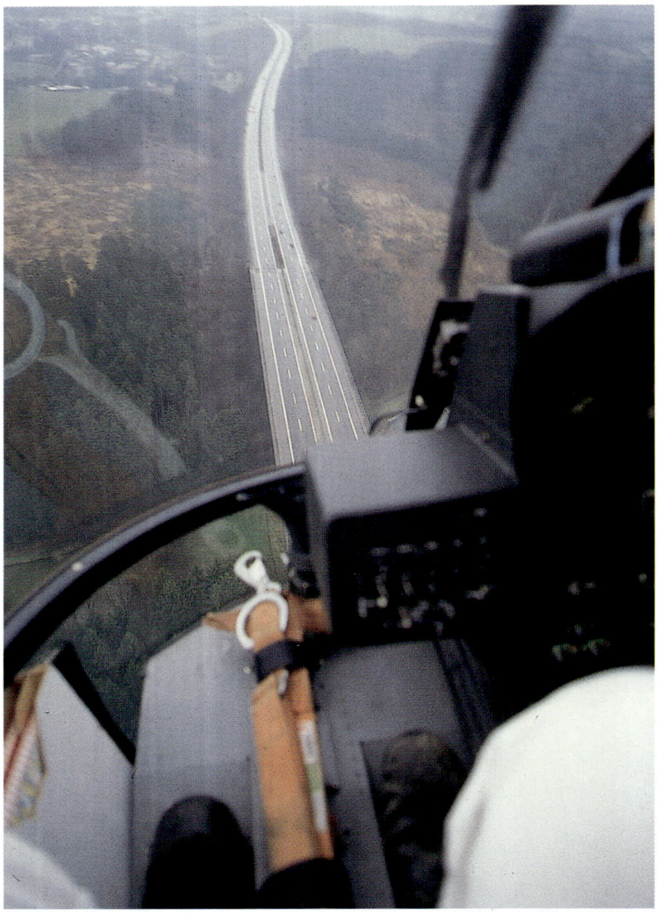

Autobahnen sind zur Orientierung einfache Linien. Piloten nennen sie Bauernlineale!

Seen from the air, autobahns are simple orientation lines. Pilots call them "the farmer's ruler".

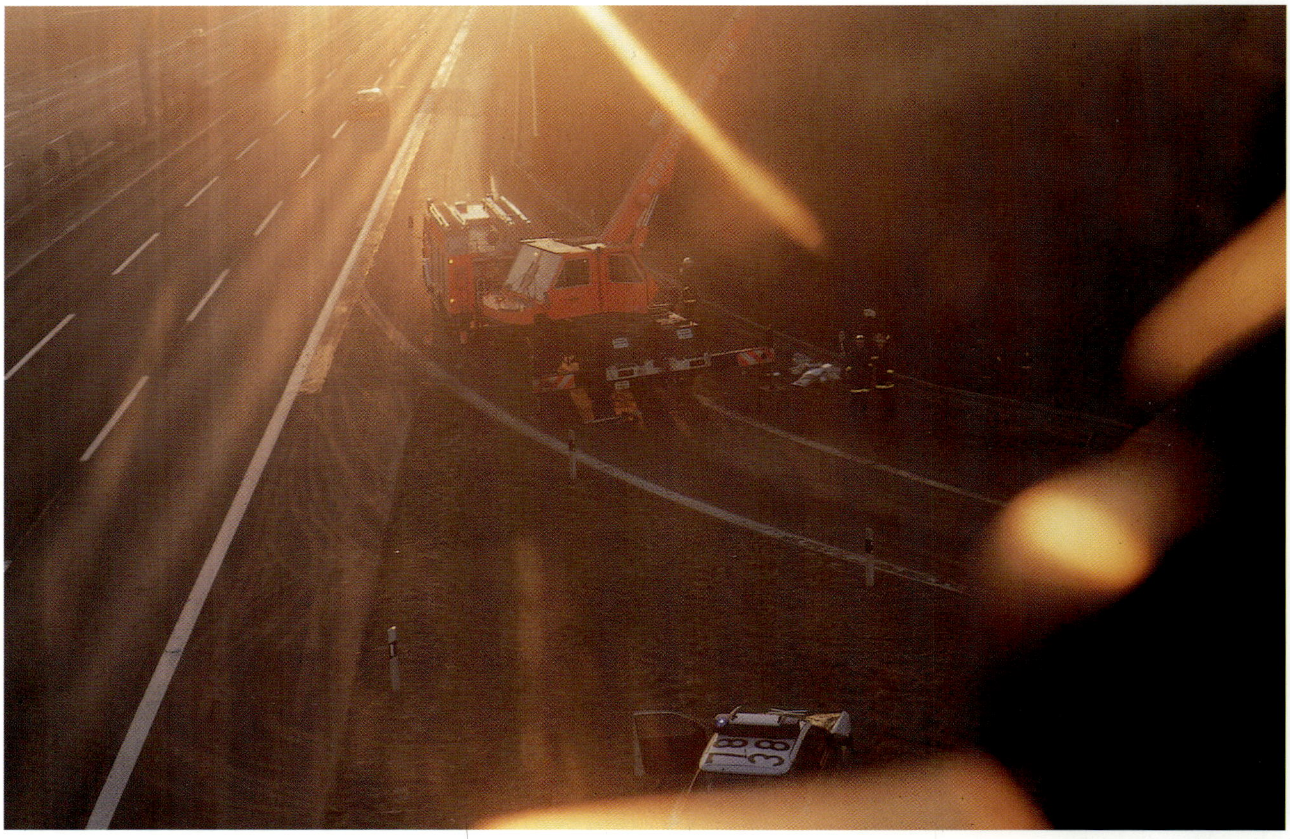

Ein PKW ist ins Schleudern geraten und eine Böschung hinuntergestürzt.

The driver of this automobile lost control, and the vehicle plunged down an embankment.

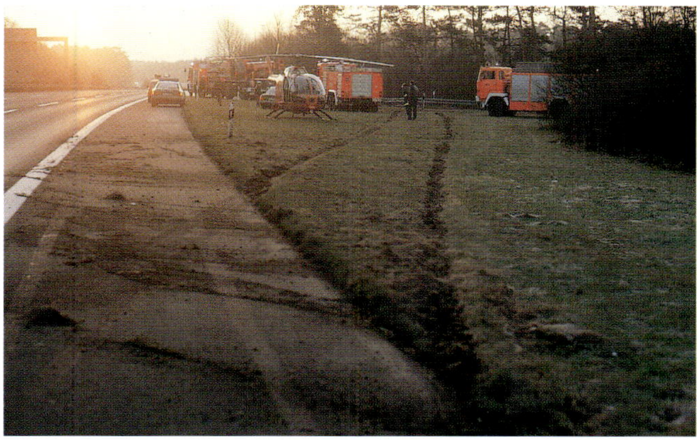

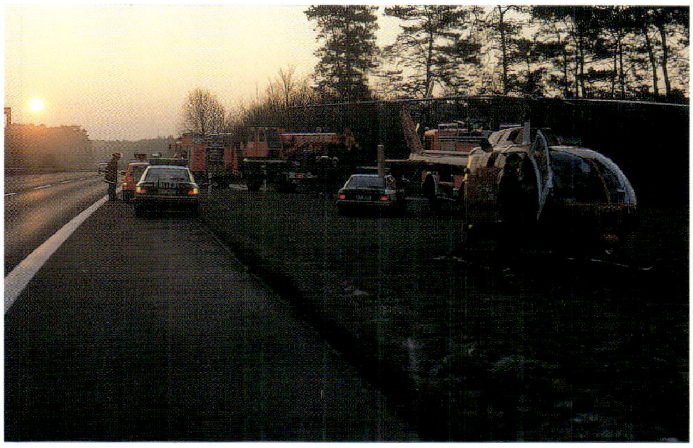

Die Spuren zeigen uns den Weg.

The skid marks show the way.

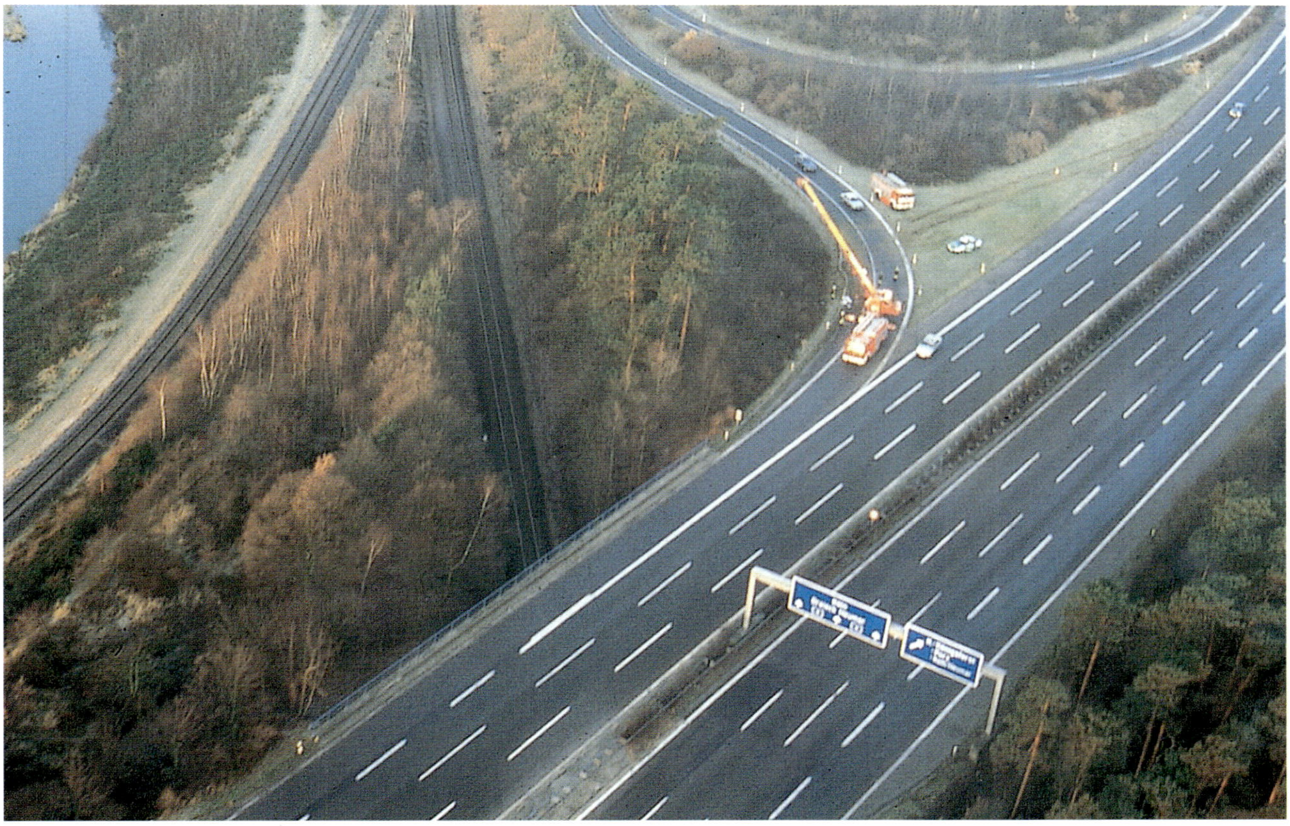

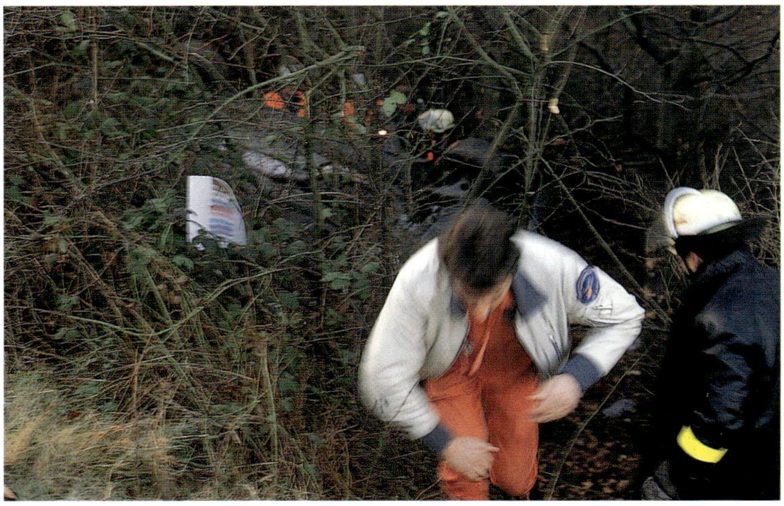

Der Patient ist nur leicht verletzt. Das Auto wird mit dem Kran geborgen.

The patient is only slightly injured. The car is hoisted by a crane.

Einsatz für den Rettungshubschrauber
Mission for the Rescue Helicopter

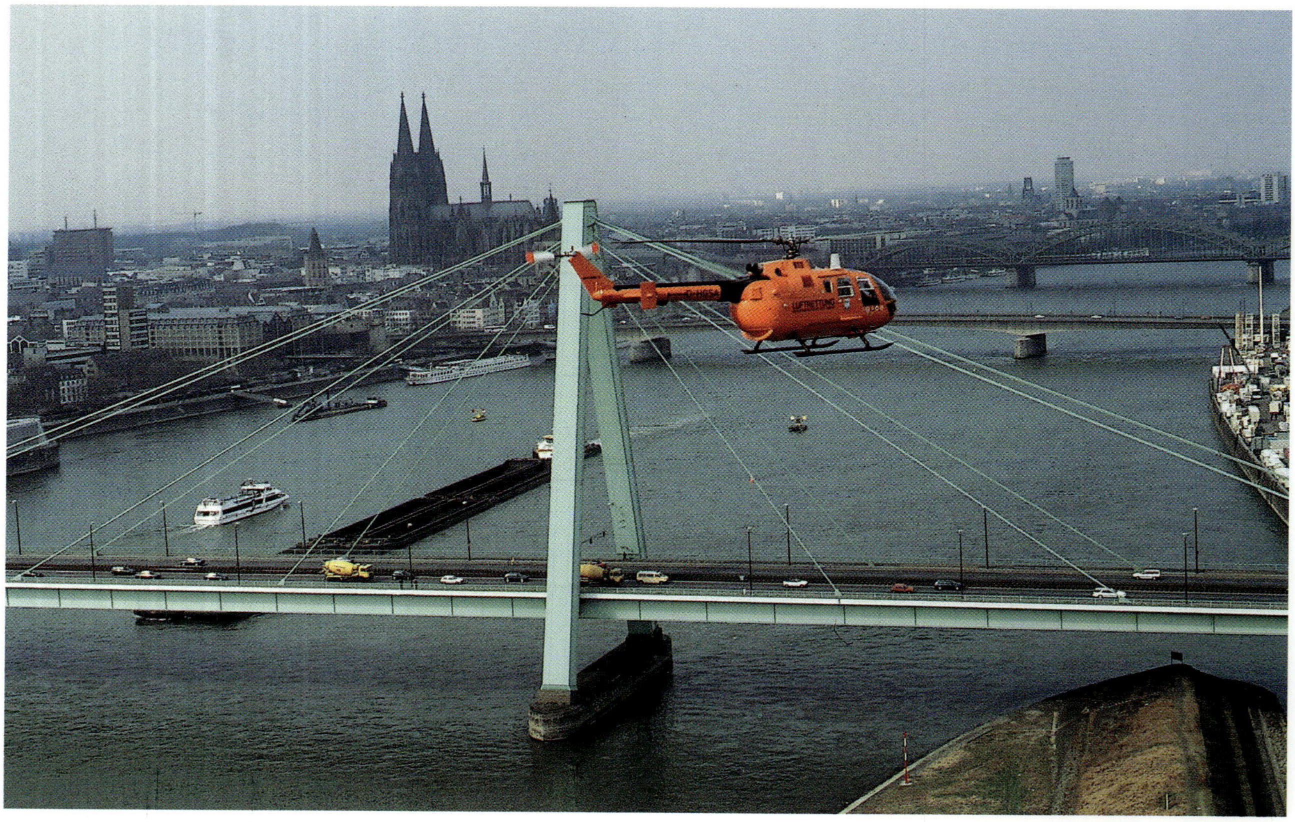

Gebrochenes Bein, allerdings auf einer Brücke.

Im Überflug erkennen wir, dass ein Gerüstarbeiter auf der Hohenzollernbrücke, die in Köln Eisenbahnbrücke ist, ein Bein gebrochen hat und geborgen werden muß. Wir können nicht an der Einsatzstelle landen, sondern gehen am nahegelegenen Ufer zur Landung. Wir klettern am Außengerüst hoch, in den Jackentaschen Schmerzmedikamente, Infusionen und Beinschienen.

Patient with a broken leg: a routine case if he weren't waiting for help on a bridge.

During the fly-over we can see that a scaffold worker on the Hohenzollern Railway Bridge in Cologne has broken his leg and is awaiting rescue. Since we cannot land at the accident site, we touch down on the nearby riverbank. With painkillers, infusions and leg splints in our pockets, we climb up the outer scaffolding.

Augenblicke

Karneval. Karnevalsmorgen. In einer Garage Pkw mit leblosem Patienten. Patient als Clown verkleidet. Hat Autoabgase in den Innenraum geleitet. Frage an die Hausbewohner und die Ehefrau: „Haben Sie den die ganze Nacht laufenden Wagen nicht gehört?" „Nein." Es erscheint ein Mann, der sich auffällig um die Ehefrau kümmert. Todesfeststellung. Totenschein. Rückflug.

Snapshots

German Carnival (Mardi Gras). An automobile with a lifeless patient in a garage. The dead man is dressed as a clown. He had directed auto exhaust fumes into the car interior. Question posed to the neighbors and the man's wife: "Didn't you hear a running motor all night?" "No." A man appears on the scene and makes a big show of consoling the widow. The man in the clown costume is declared dead. The Death Certificate is filled out. We climb into the helicopter and fly off.

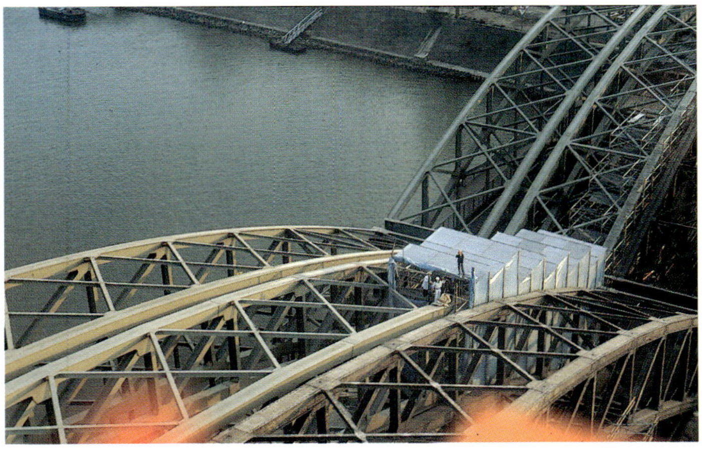

Der Patient wird versorgt. Die Bergung: Wir können ihn nicht auf eine der Rheinseiten abseilen, weil es zu gefährlich ist. Wir können ihn auch nicht nach unten abseilen, weil dort die Stromkabel der Bundesbahn verlaufen. Die Leitungen sind mittlerweile ohne Strom.

Wir bestellen von oben einen Bundeswehrhubschrauber mit einer Winde. Der Patient wird aufgenommen, hochgehievt und zum nahen Ufer geflogen. Von dort ist alles einfach. Transport mit dem Rettungswagen in das Krankenhaus.

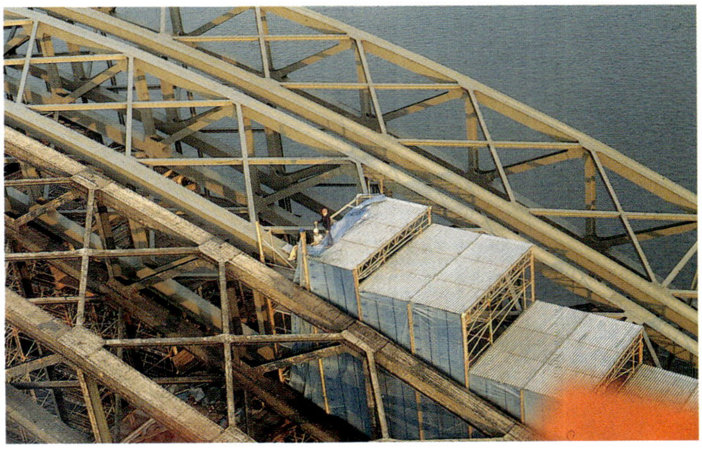

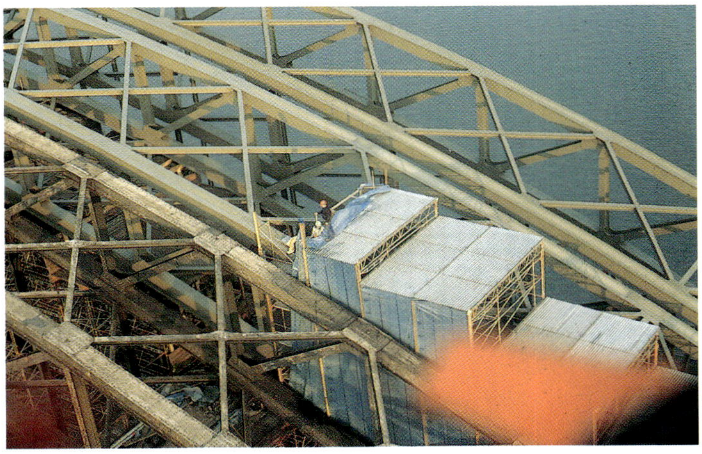

The patient receives emergency medical care. But how to rescue him? Lowering him by rope on either side of the Rhine would be too risky. Lowering him straight down would be dangerous since he would have to cross the power lines of German Rail.

However, the power lines are now dead. From the air we request a German Army helicopter with a winch. The army helicopter drops down a rescue rope, winches up the patient, and flies him to the nearest shore. From there it's all very simple. The helicopter unloads the patient and a rescue ambulance transports him to a hospital.

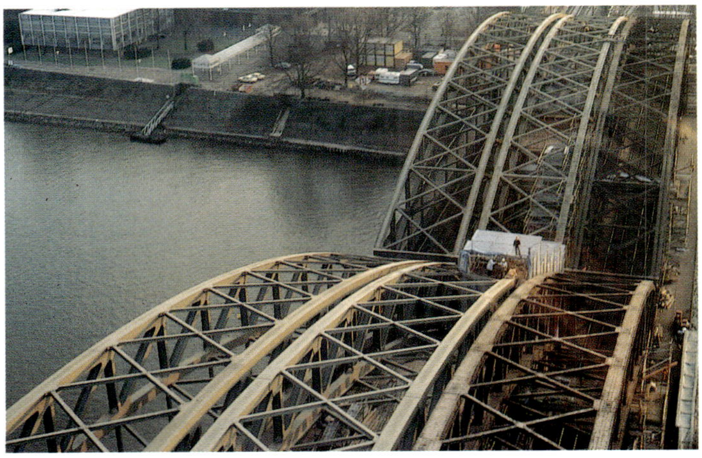

Einsatz für den Rettungshubschrauber
Mission for the Rescue Helicopter

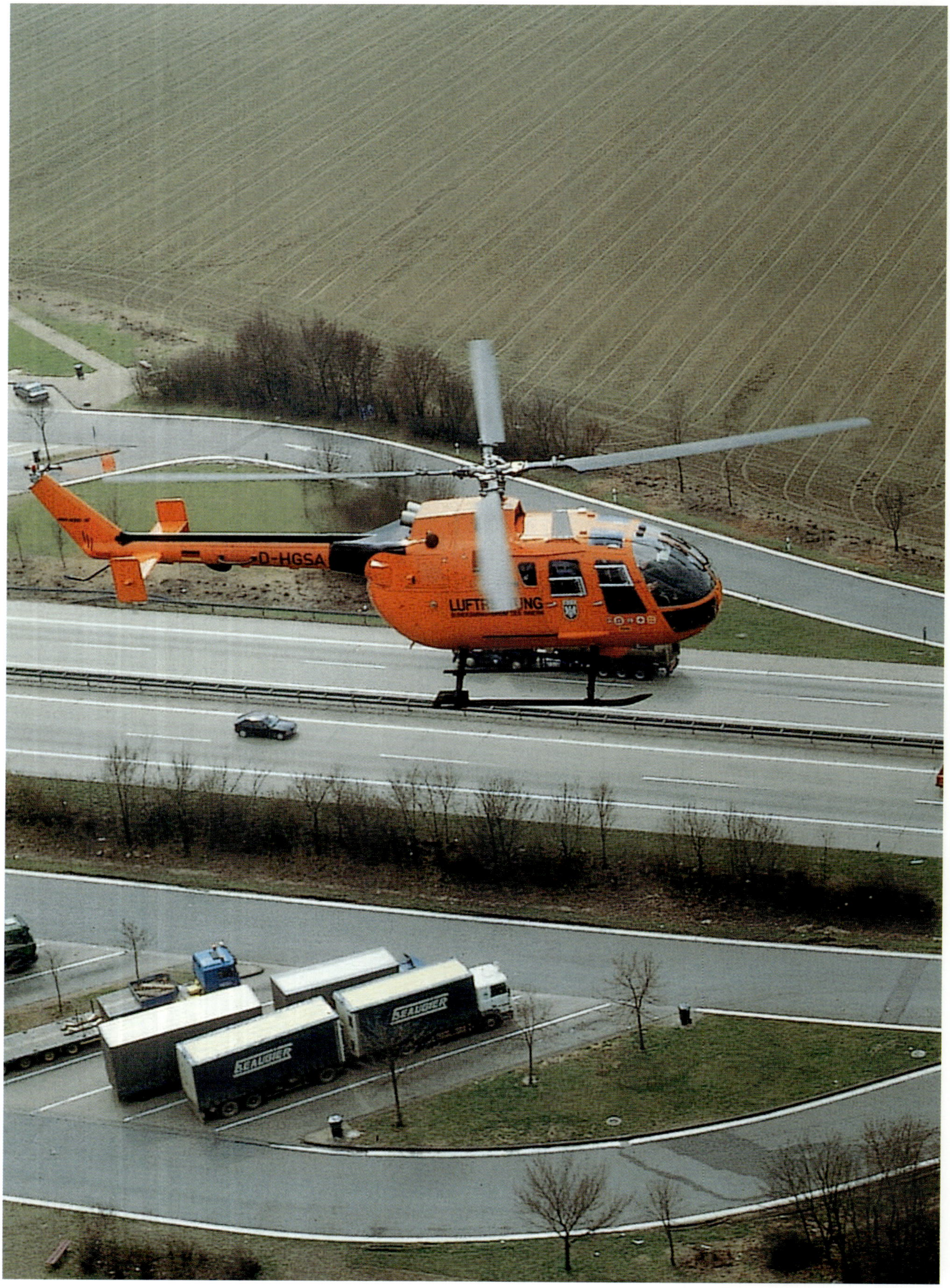

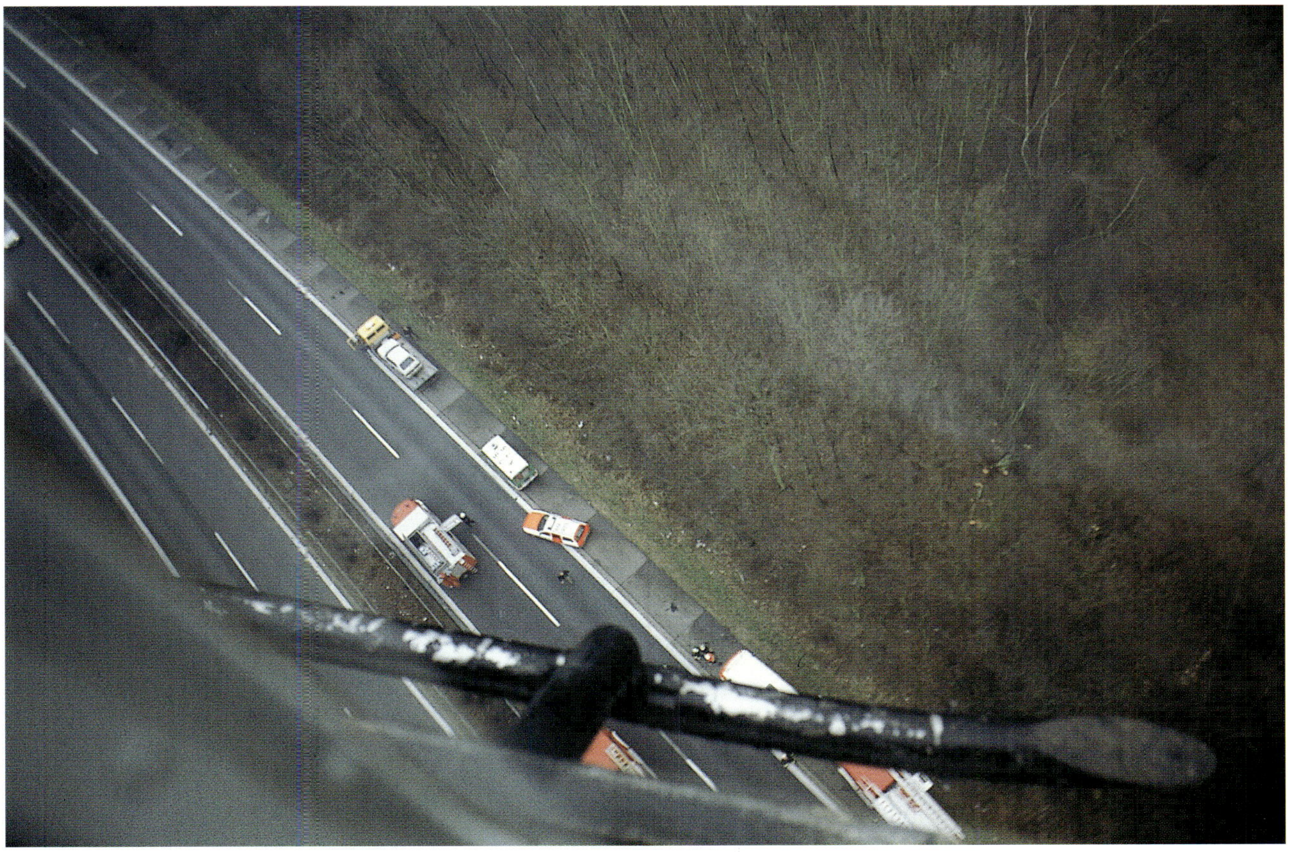

Ein Motorradfahrer hat die Kontrolle über sein Motorrad verloren und ist eine Böschung entlanggerast. Dabei hat sich sein Motorrad überschlagen. Er hat mehrere Ober- und Unterschenkelfrakturen erlitten.

A motorcyclist has lost control of his bike and plunged down an embankment. The motorcycle turned over several times and the rider suffered multiple fracture of the femur and lower leg bones.

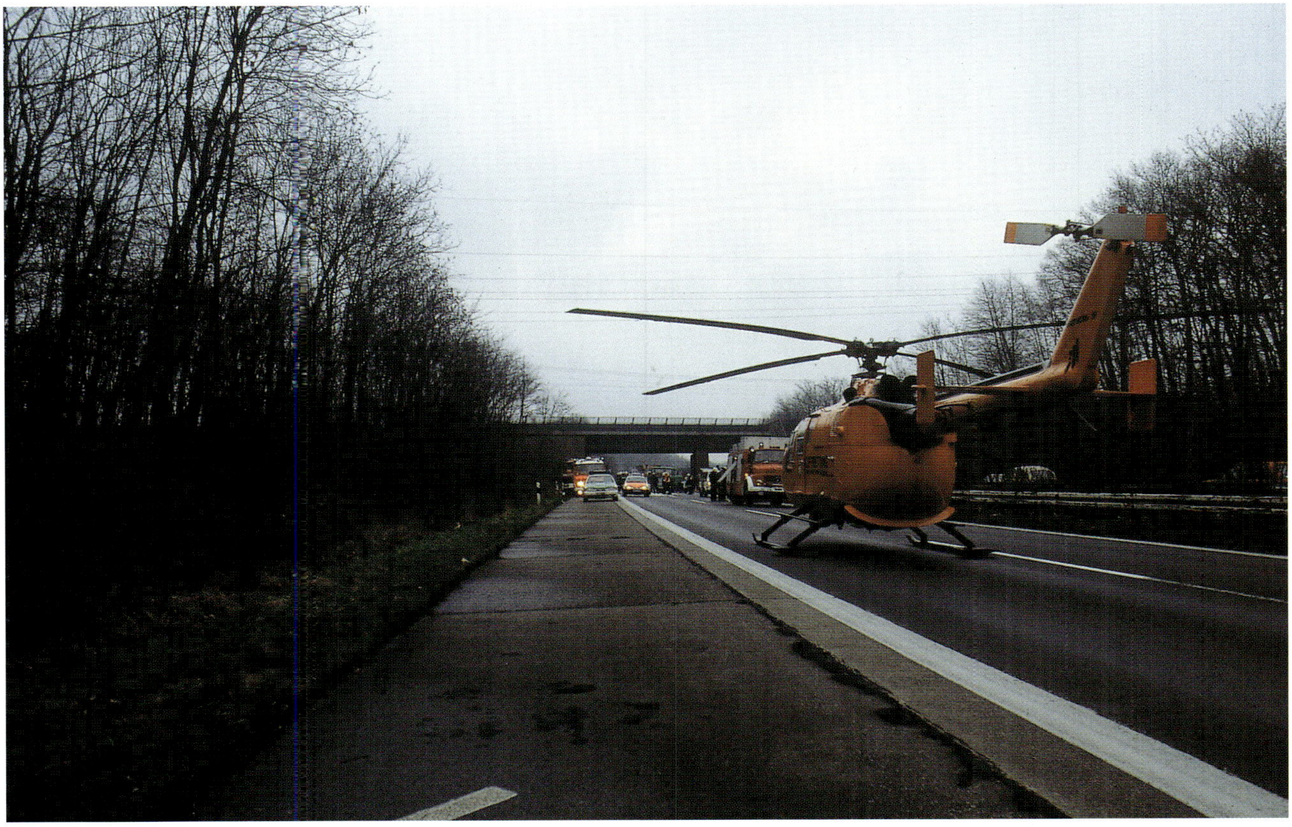

Der Hubschrauber landet unmittelbar vor der Einsatzstelle.

The helicopter lands directly in front of the accident site.

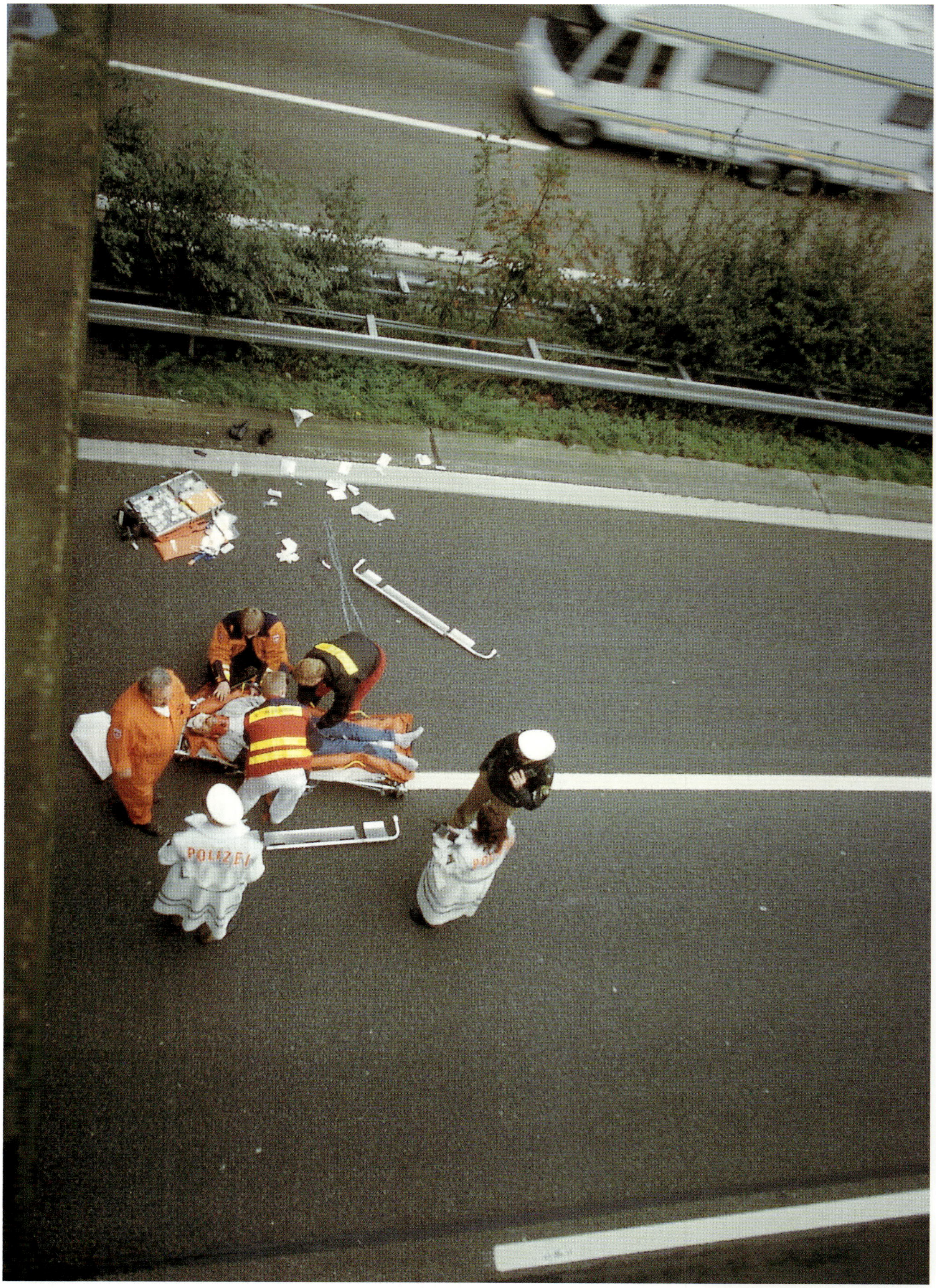

Der Motorradfahrer wird in eine Vakuummatratze gebettet, die einen schonenden Transport ins Krankenhaus ermöglicht. Der Patient wi-d zum Transport im Hubschrauber vorbereitet.

The motorcyclist is placed on a vacuum mattress to ensure gentle transport to the hospital. He is prepared for transport in the rescue helicopter.

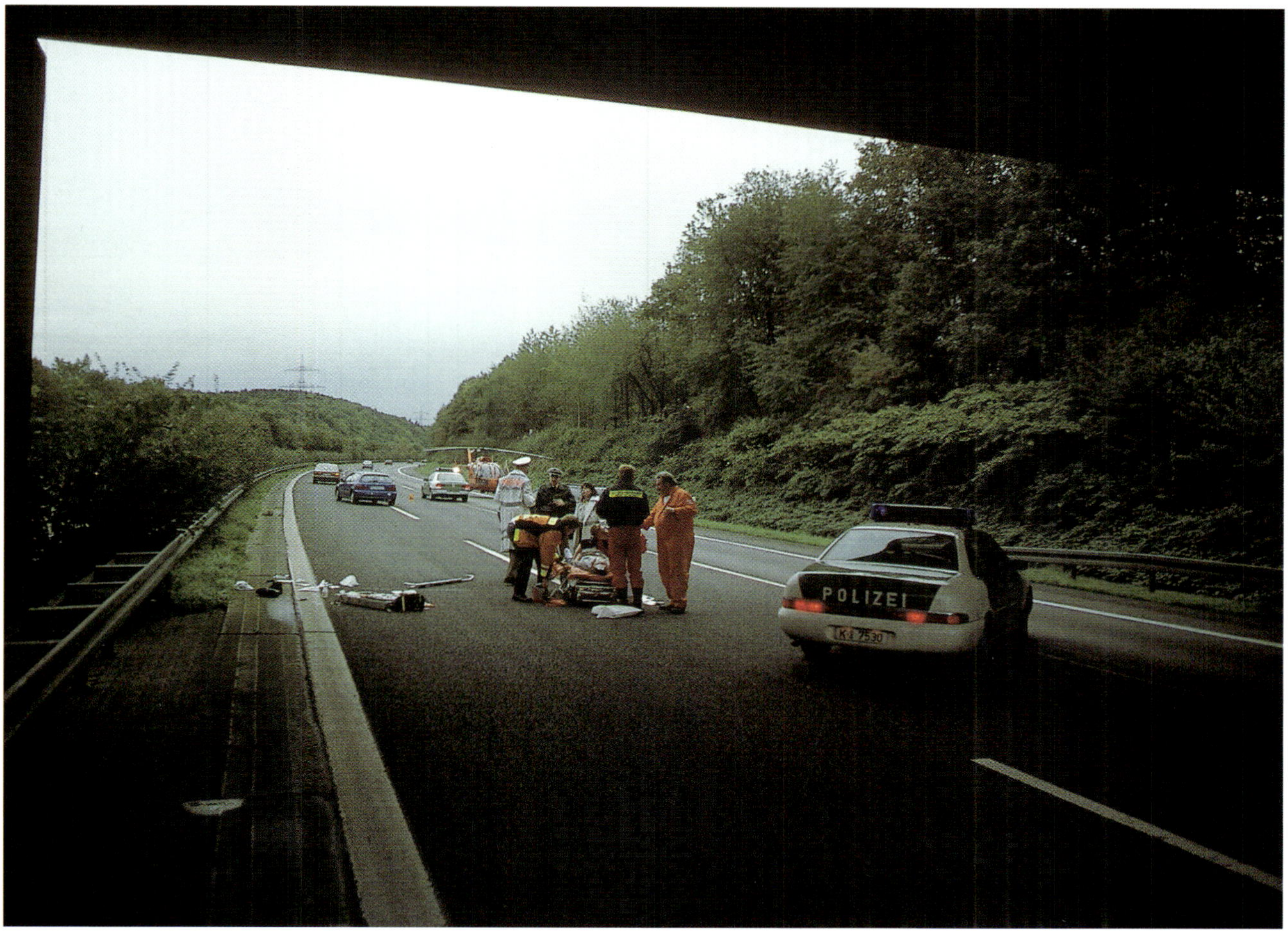
POLIZEI

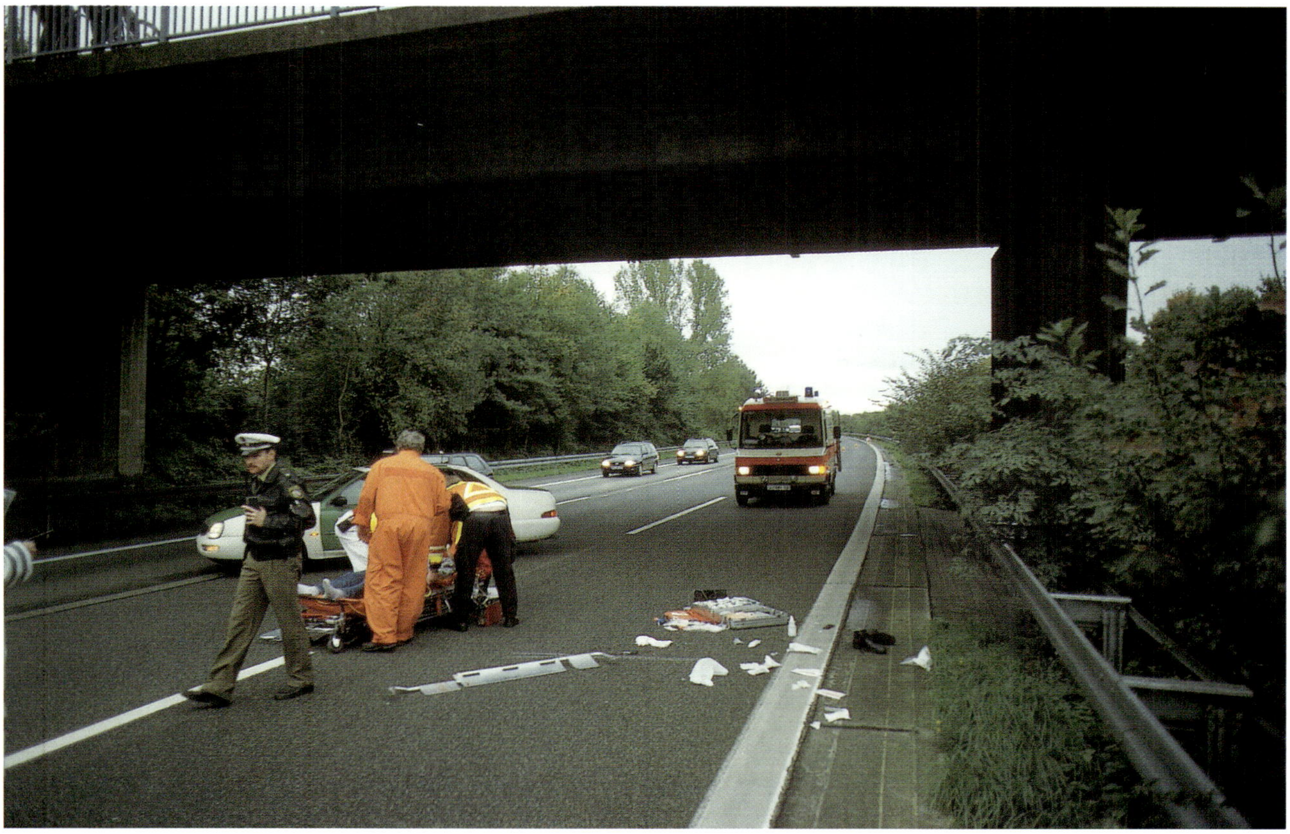

Einsatz für den Rettungshubschrauber
Mission for the Rescue Helicopter

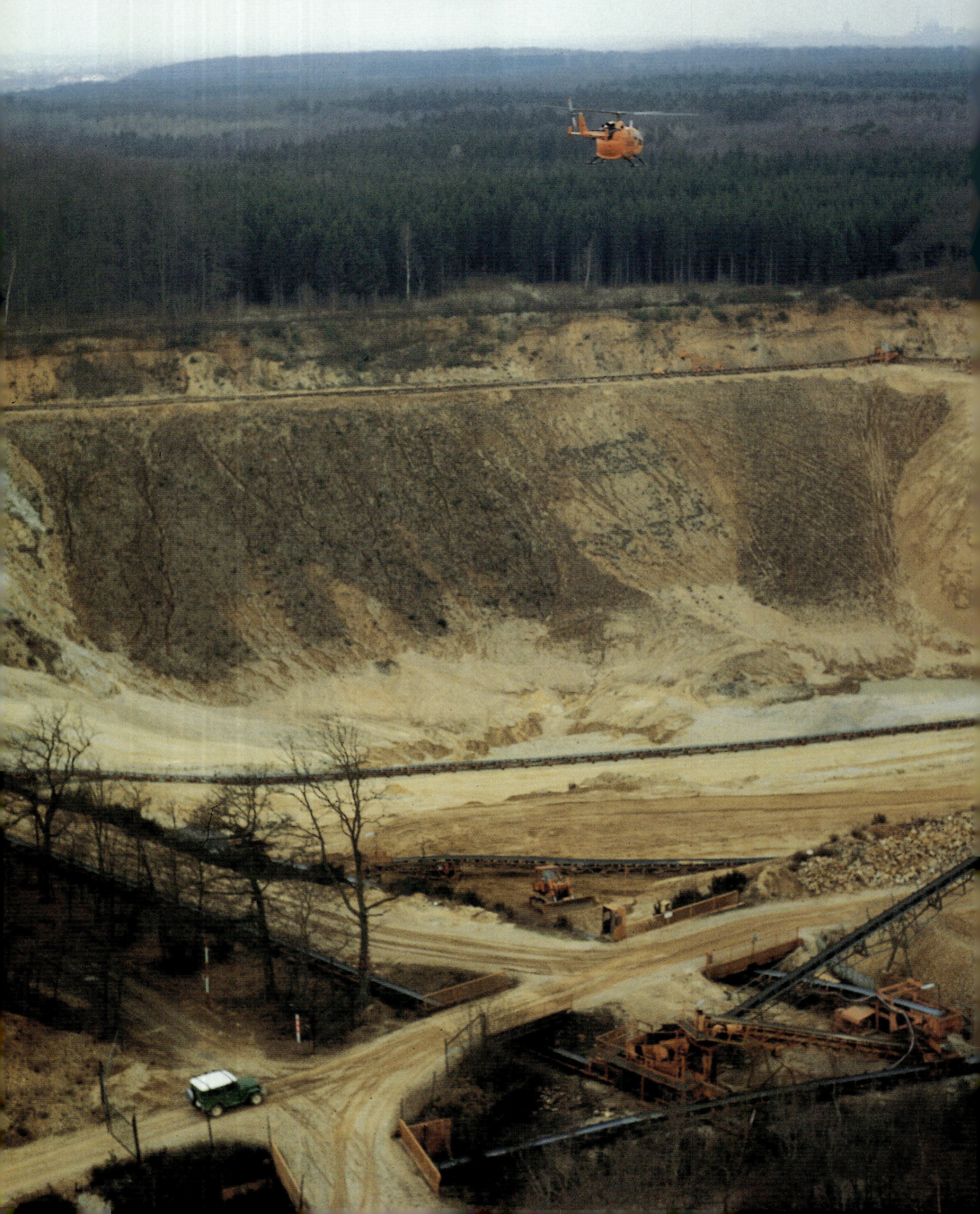

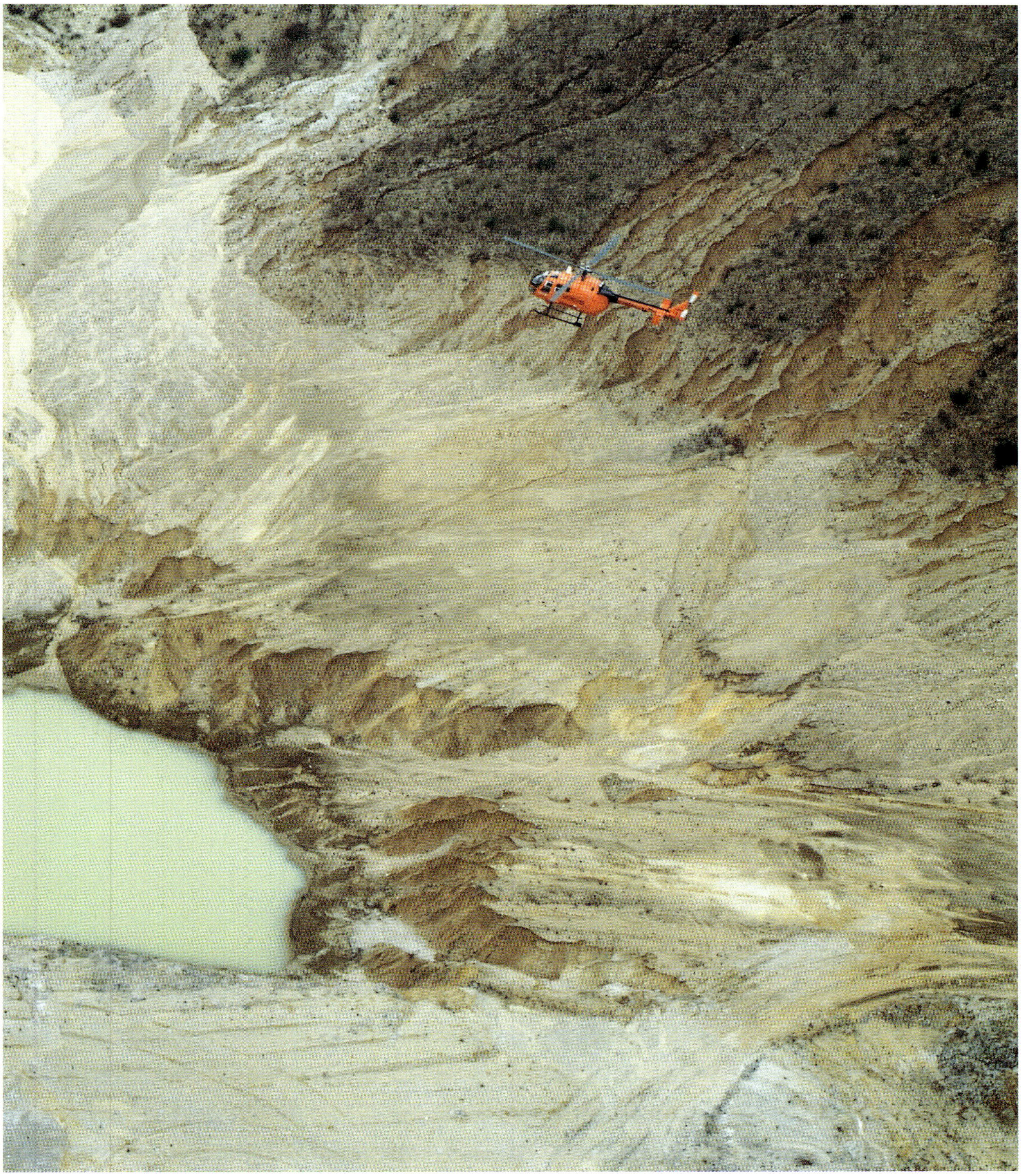

Spielende Kinder haben in einem Tagebaugebiet, das sie nicht betreten durften, eine Höhle gebaut. Einer der Jungen wird von zusammenstürzenden Sandmassen begraben und von nachrutschenden weiteren Erdmassen bedeckt. Sein mitspielender Gefährte versucht schnell, ihn zu befreien, sieht aber, dass ihm das nicht gelingt. Er klettert mühsam den Weg zurück, um in einer nahegelegenen Bäckerei die Rettungskette in Gang zu setzen. Er erklärt der Bäckersfrau, was im Tagebau passiert ist. Der Rettungshubschrauber findet die Einsatzstelle recht schnell und kann in unmittelbarer Nähe des Geschehens landen. Die Rettungskräfte können nur langsam und mühsam in dem unwegsamen Gebiet ihre Suche und Bergung des schwer verletzten Jungen fortführen.

Several children have dug a cave while playing in an open-cast mining area their parents had declared "off limits". One of the boys is suddenly buried under masses of sand as a sand pile collapses, triggering a further landslide. His buddy immediately tries to rescue him but realizes at once that the task is too big for him. He arduously retraces their steps out of the mine. At a nearby bakery he tells the baker's wife what has happened. The rescue helicopter finds the accident site fairly quickly and touches down in the direct vicinity of the accident. Nevertheless, the rescue workers are hampered in their search and rescue activities by the difficult terrain.

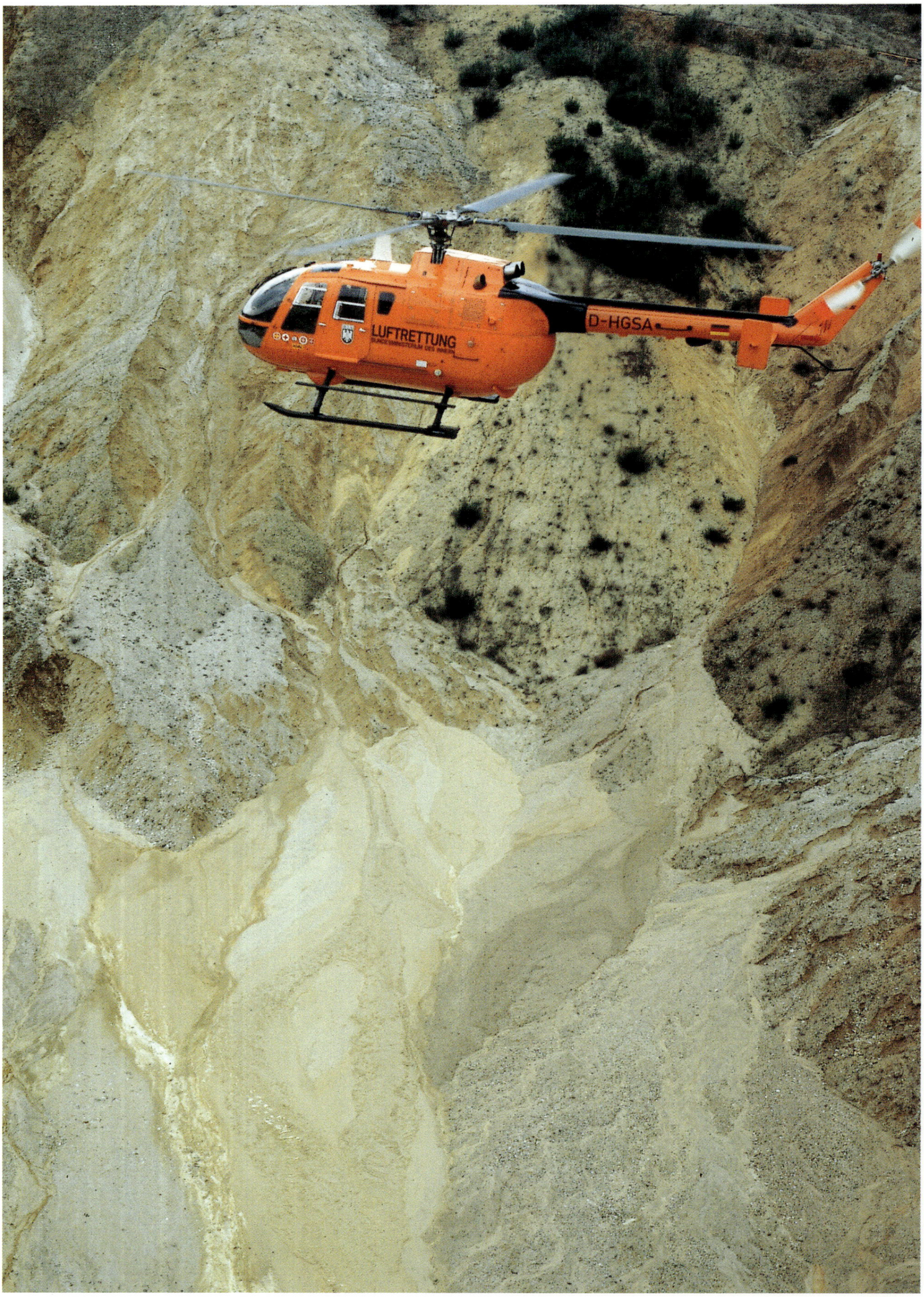

Der Junge wird mit dem Rettungshubschrauber in die Klinik geflogen.

The injured boy is flown to the hospital in the rescue helicopter.

Augenblicke

Unfall auf der Autobahn. PKW in Böschung. Im PKW lebloser Patient. Patient im PKW tot. „Kümmere dich um die Ehefrau, die sitzt im grünen Auto!" Ich gehe zur Ehefrau. Ehefrau erzählt: „Wir wollten ein befreundetes Ehepaar abholen. Mein Mann sagte, steig in das andere Auto, falls wir uns auf der Autobahn verlieren, dann kannst du die Leute weiterführen. Wir fahren im Abstand von ca. 200 m voreinander her. Ich sehe, wie ein anderer Pkw den Pkw meines Mannes touchiert. Der Pkw meines Mannes überschlägt sich sofort und fliegt in die Böschung. Was ist mit meinem Ehemann los?" Ich bleibe ein paar Minuten bei der Frau sitzen und erzähle mit ihr und höre ihr still zu.

Snapshots

Accident on the autobahn. An automobile has rolled down the embankment. Inside the car we find a lifeless patient. "Take care of the wife; she's in the green car." I go to the wife, who relates the events leading up to the accident: "We wanted to pick up another couple we are friends with. My husband told me to get in the other car. 'If we lose sight of each other on the autobahn, you can guide them the rest of the way,' he said. We were driving approx. 200 m behind my husband. I watched as another automobile hit my husband's car. His car turned over right away and plunged down the embankment. What's wrong with my husband?" I stay with the woman for a few minutes and explain that her husband is dead.

Einsatz für den Rettungshubschrauber
Mission for the Rescue Helicopter

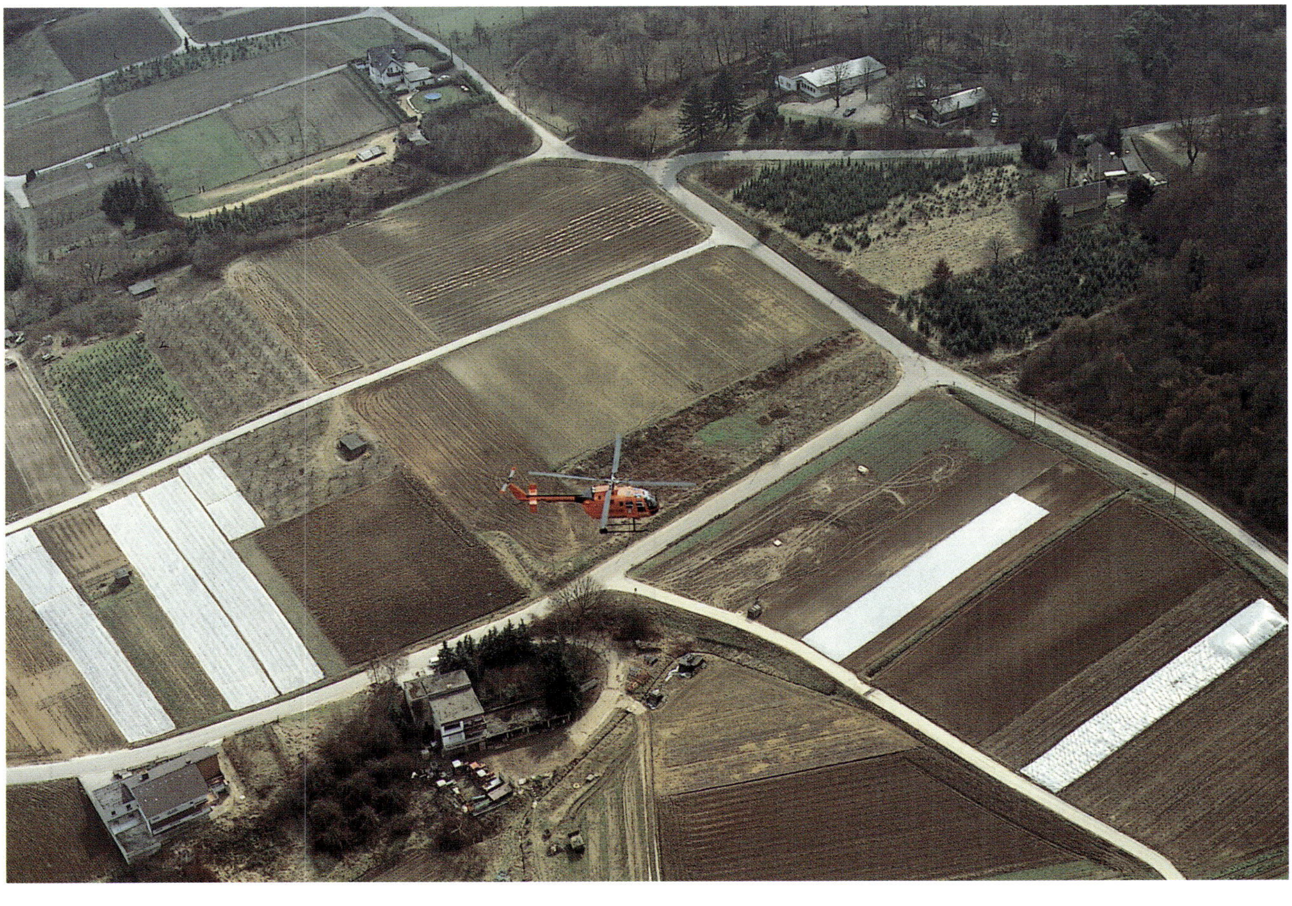

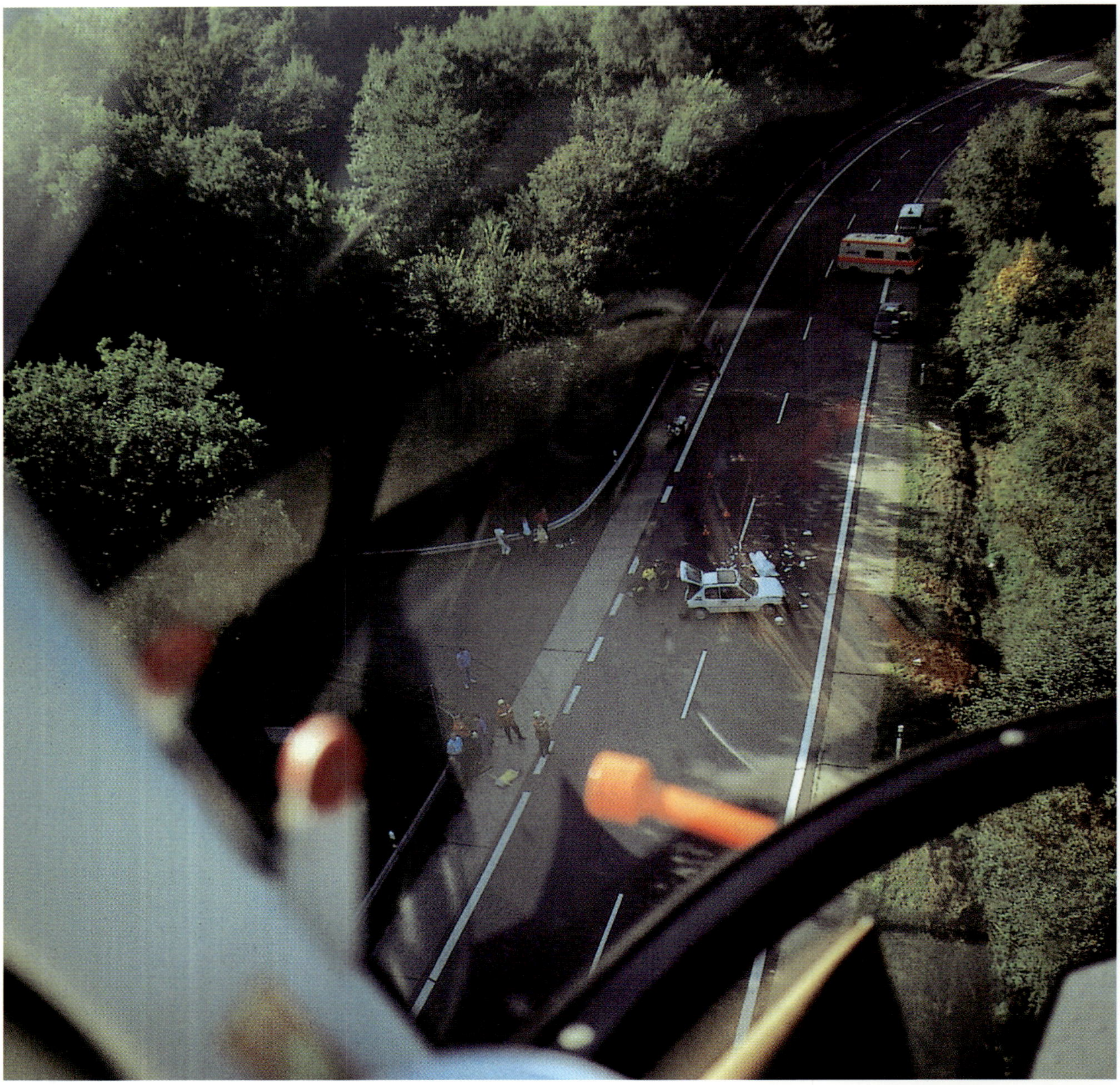

Landeanflug auf die Einsatzstelle auf der Landstraße.

The helicopter descends to land at an accident site on a country road.

Auf einer Einmündung:
Eine junge Frau fährt mit ihrem schreienden Kind auf dem Rücksitz auf diese Einmündung zu. Sie versucht, ihr Kind zu beruhigen und ihm einen Schnuller in den Mund zu stecken. Sie dreht sich dabei nur für den Bruchteil einer Sekunde zurück zu ihrem Kind, rollt mit dem PKW aber weiter auf die Kreuzung zu. Ein aus der anderen Richtung fahrender Motorradclub älterer Herren fährt auf das Auto auf. Der erste Motorradfahrer hat keine Chance.

Tragic accident at a T-junction. A young woman approaches the T-junction with a screaming child in the back seat. She tries to calm the child by giving him a pacifier. While she turns toward the back seat for a split second, the car continues to move toward the intersection. A group of motorcyclists, members of a senior citizens' motorcycle club, approaches the intersection from the other direction. The first motorcyclist doesn't have a chance.

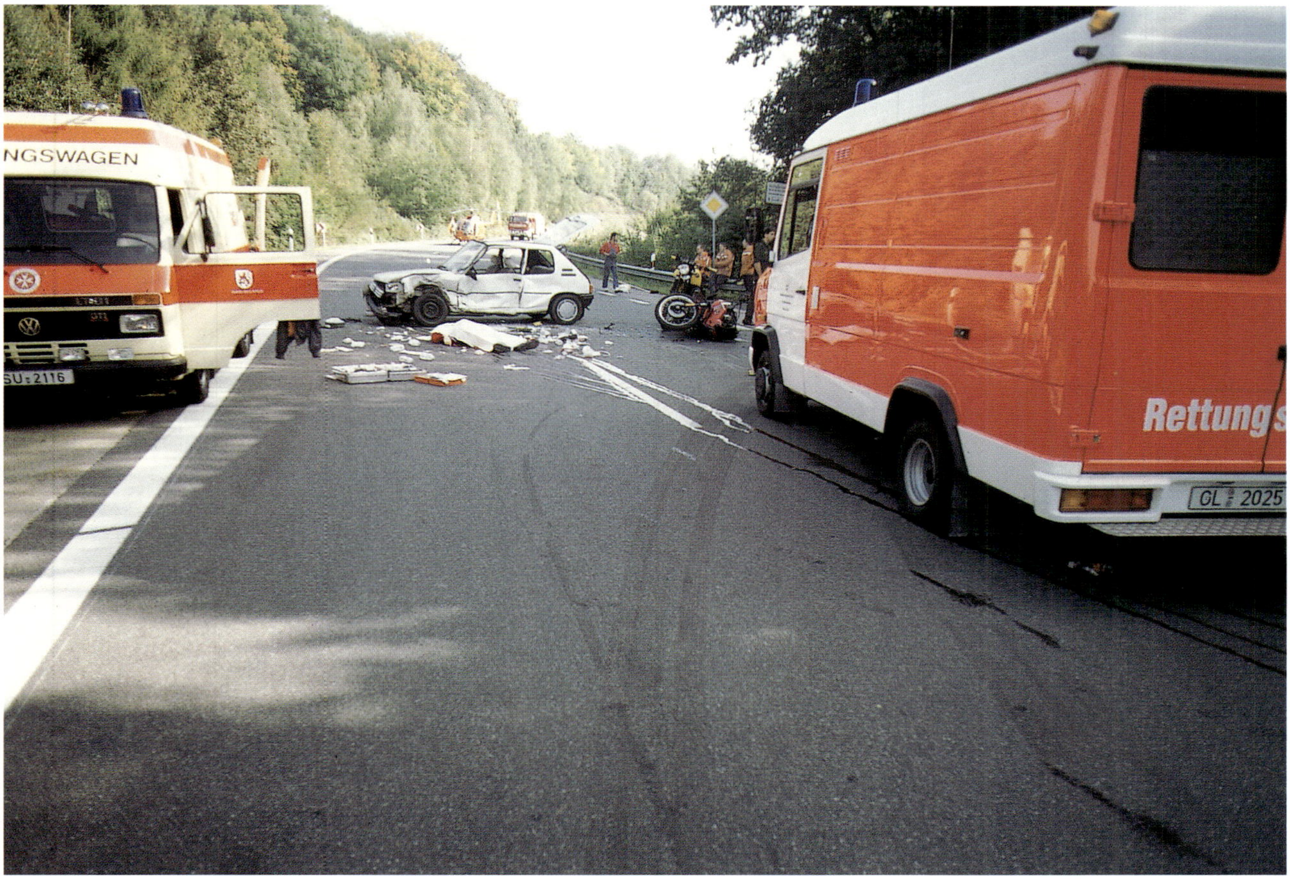
NGSWAGEN
Rettungs
GL 2025

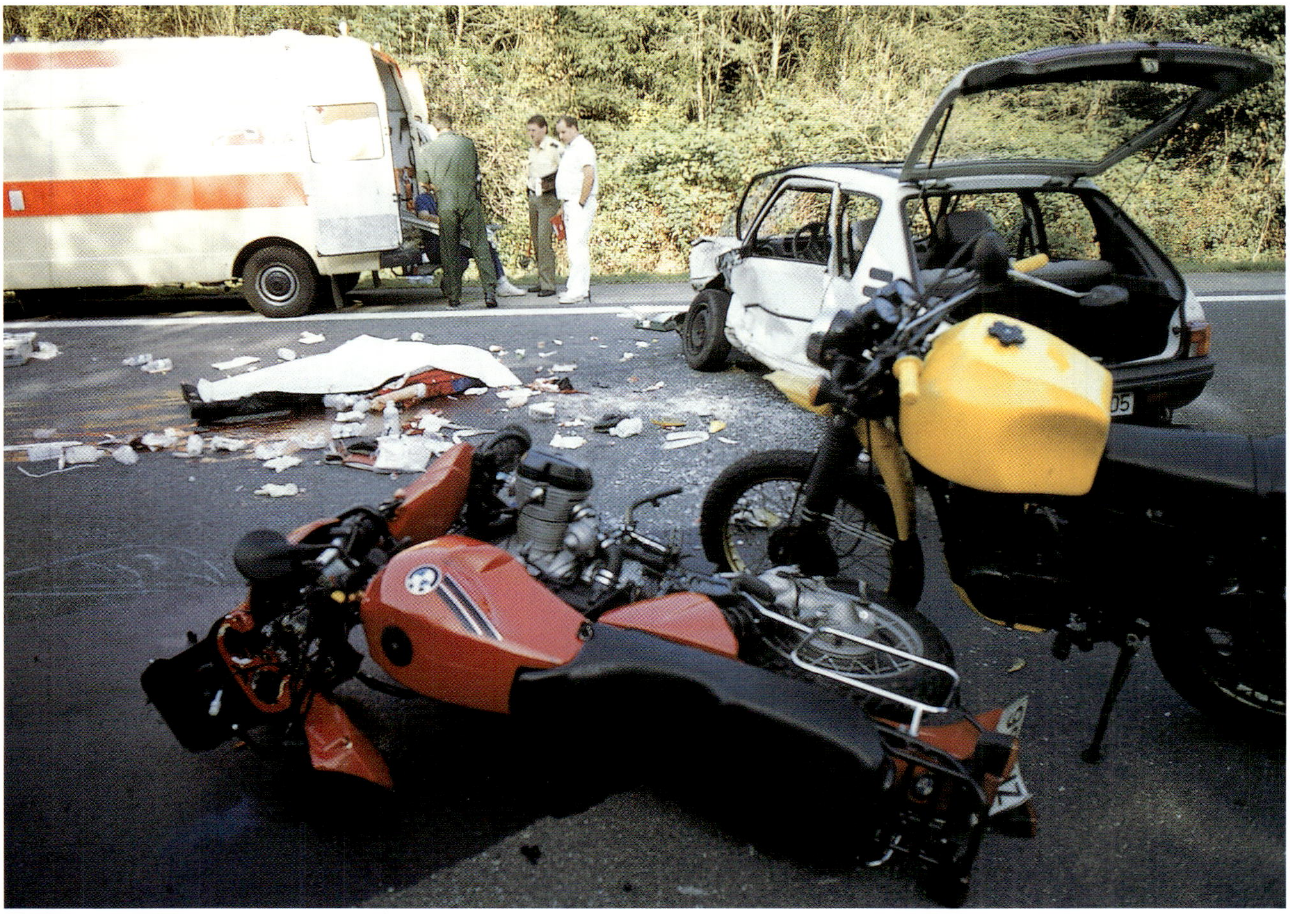

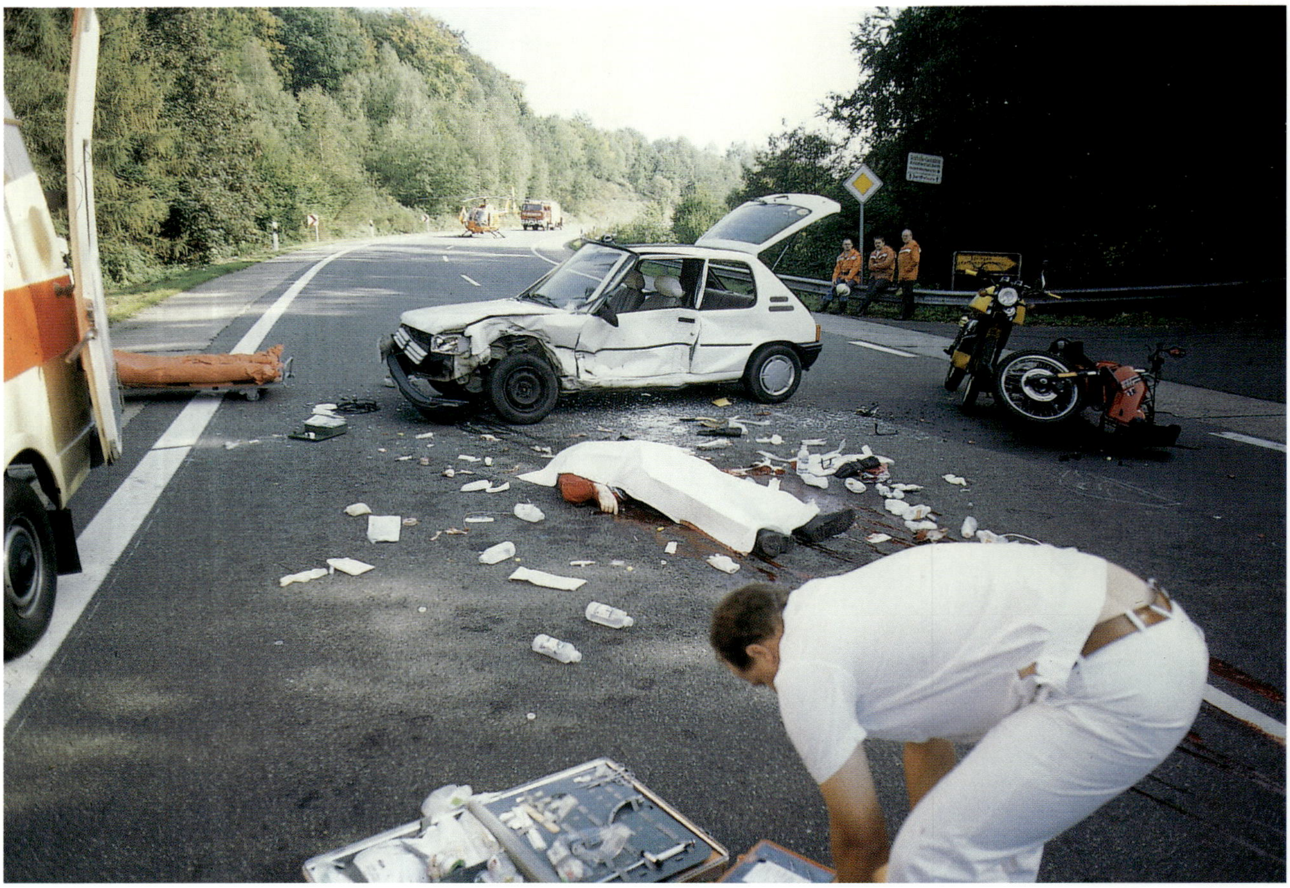

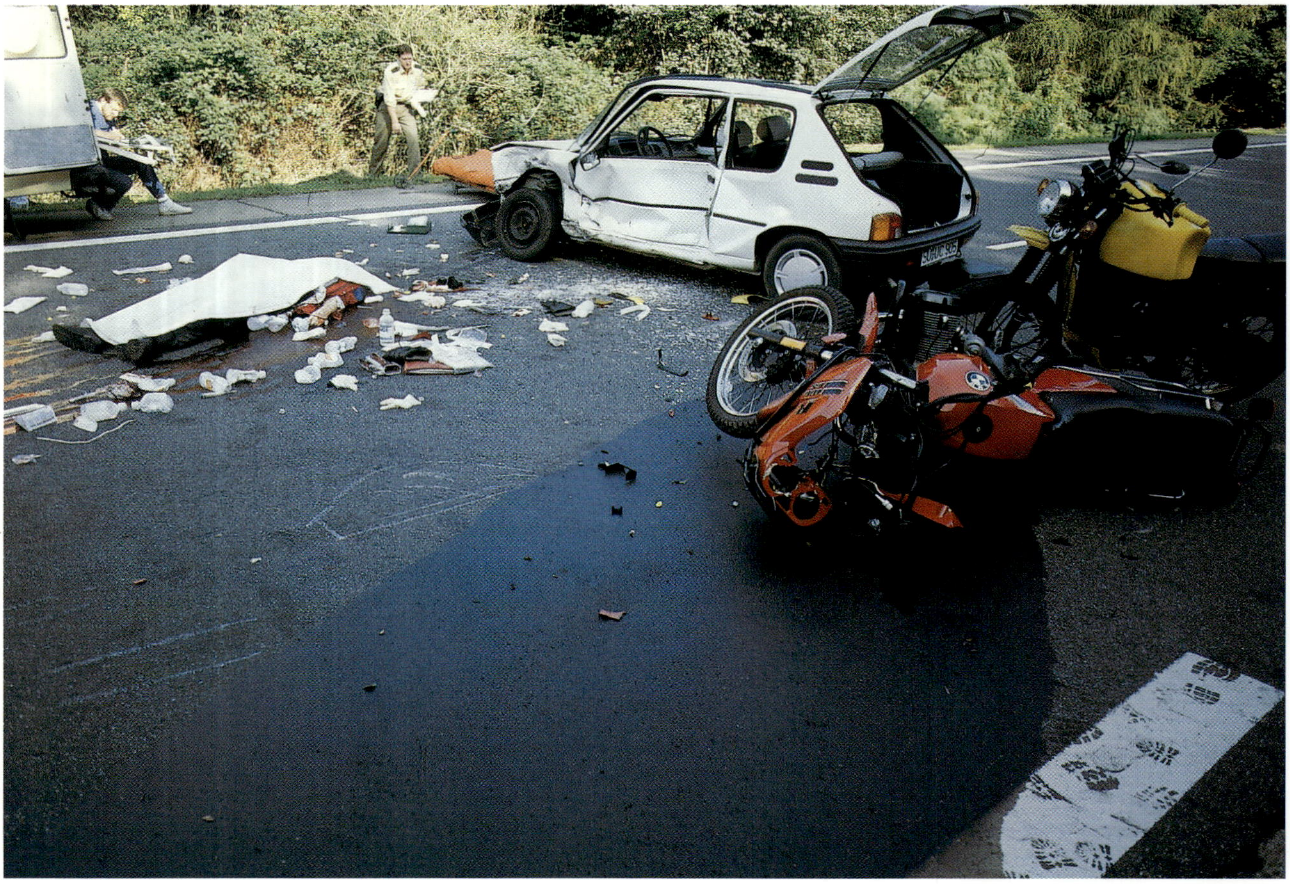

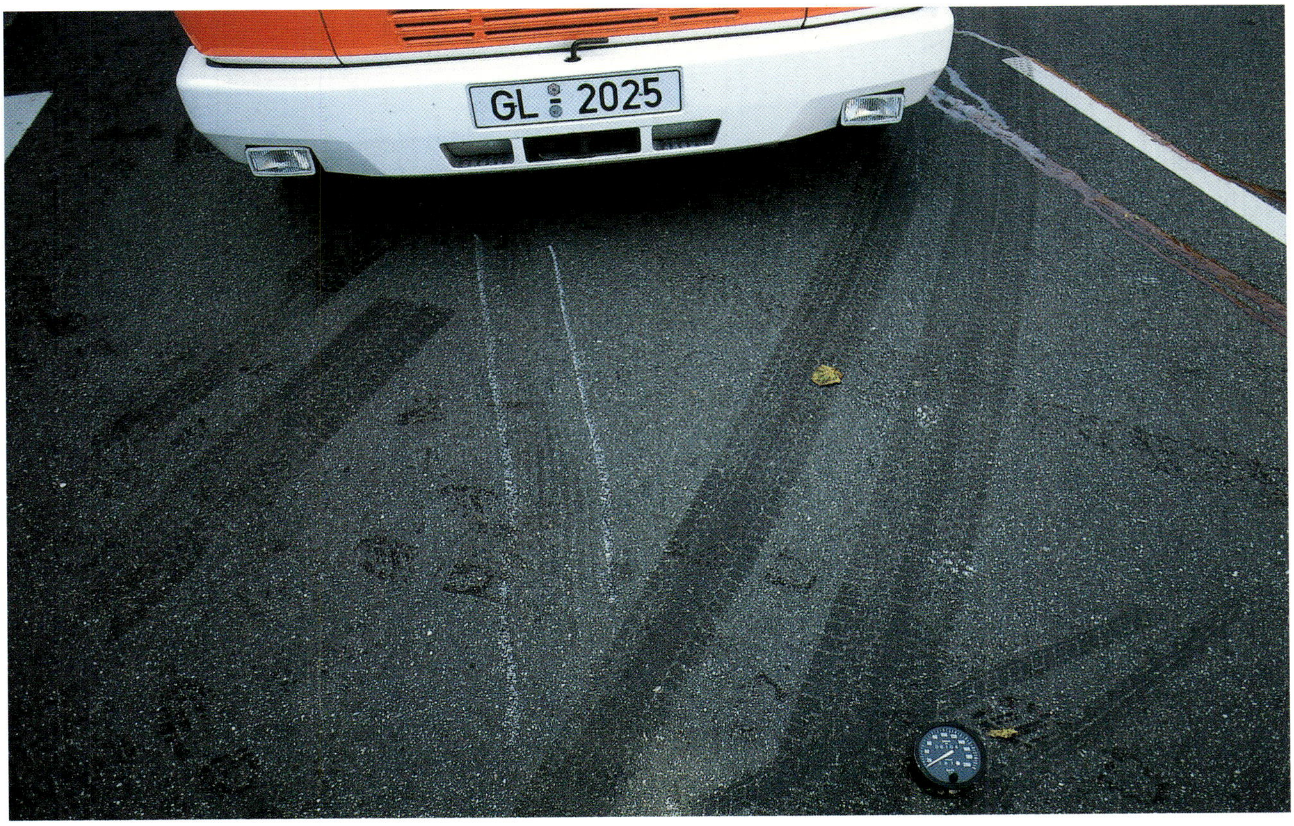

Der Tacho des Motorrads und die Bremsspuren.

The motorcycle's tachometer and the skid marks.

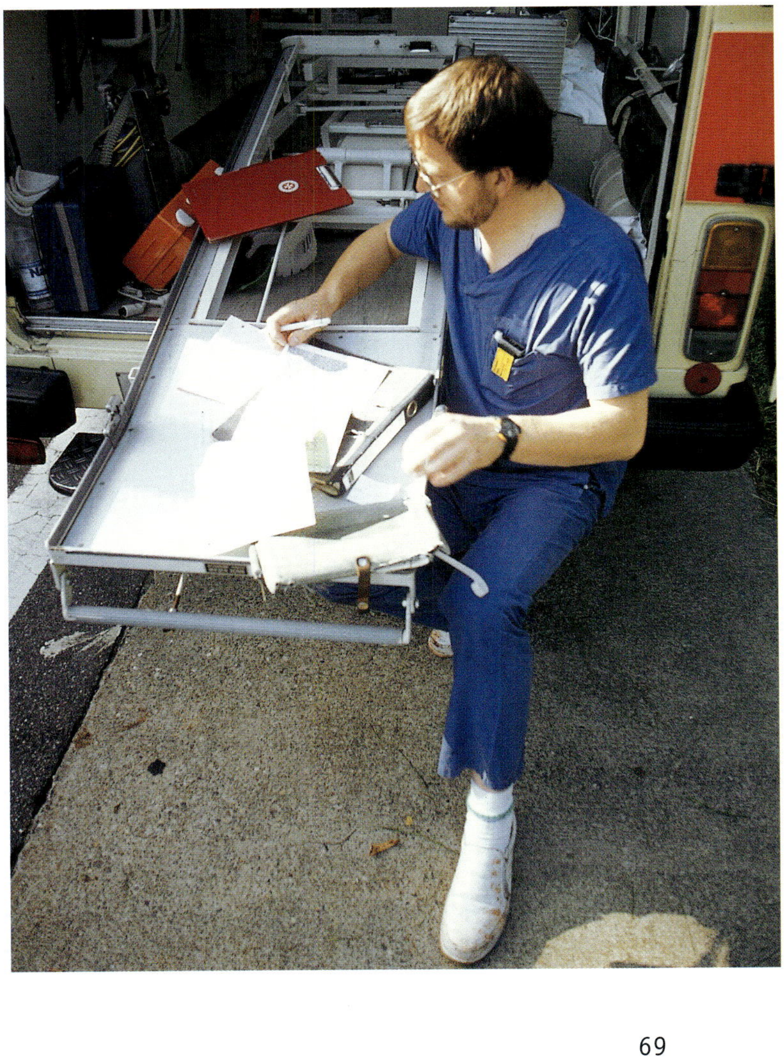

Dokumentation nach dem Einsatz

Documentation after the mission.

Einsatz für den Rettungshubschrauber
Mission for the Rescue Helicopter

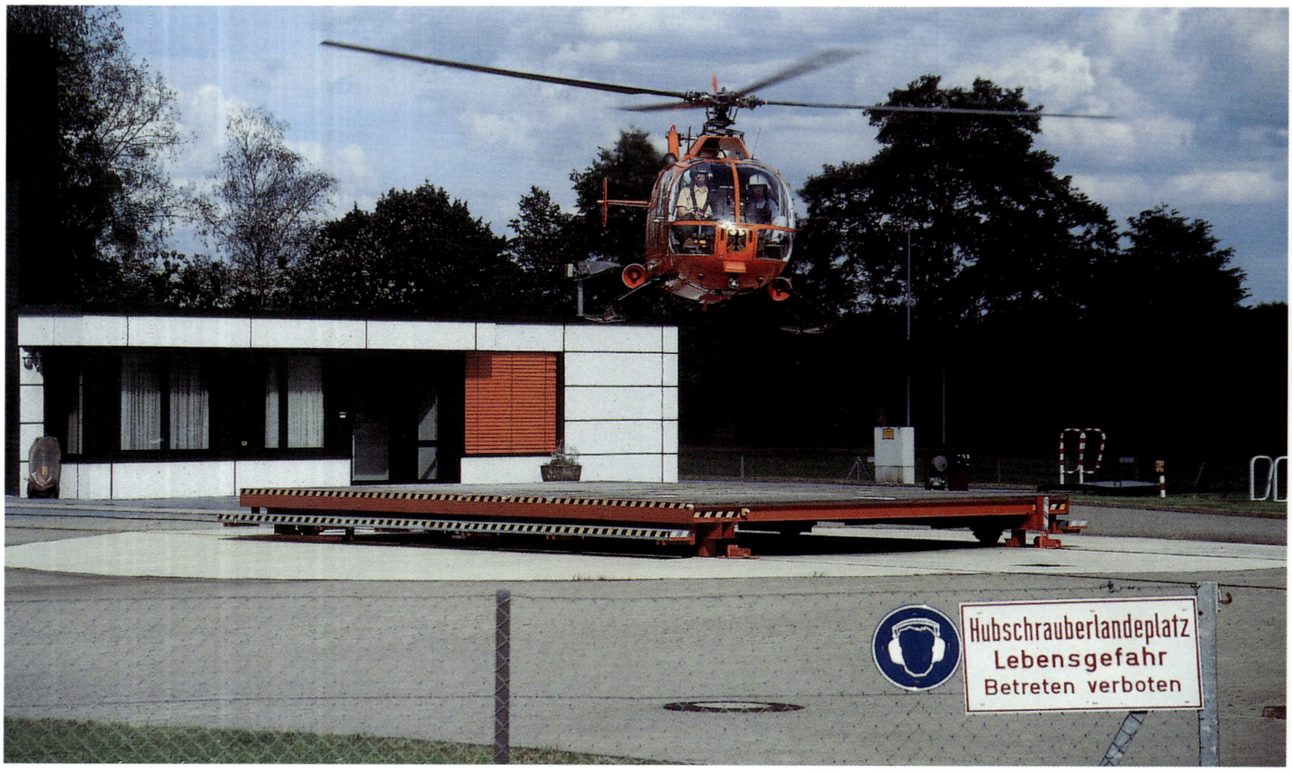

Augenblicke

Sommertag: viele Einsätze. Wir sind mit einem Patienten zur Begleitung im Rettungswagen zur Klinik unterwegs. Die Maschine wird vom Piloten alleine zum Krankenhaus gesteuert. Plötzlich Anfrage: „Kann der Hubschrauber bei der Suche nach einem ertrunkenen Kind helfen?" Der Pilot dreht sofort ab Richtung Bootshafen. Die Taucher der Feuerwehr sind unterwegs. Wir treffen am Krankenhaus ein, übergeben unseren Patienten, sprechen ab, wo der Hubschrauber uns aufnehmen kann. Die Taucher haben das Kind drei Meter unter dem Boot gefunden, bringen es zur Wasseroberfläche. Der Hubschrauber holt uns vom Krankenhaus ab. Ein zweiter Notarzt ist mittlerweile eingetroffen, beginnt mit der Wiederbelebung. Wir steigen in die Maschine um, kurzer Flug zur Einsatzstelle, wir landen. Beide Ärzte entscheiden: das Kind ist tot. Die Mutter – 100 m entfernt – schaut mich an. Ohne sie anzusprechen, erzählt sie mir. „Ich habe das geträumt. Gestern Nacht. Ich habe es so geträumt. Gestern Nacht." Rekonstruktion. Zwei- und fünfjährige Kinder auf dem Schiff. Zweijähriges Kind ohne Schwimmweste. Fällt über Bord. Fünfjähriges Kind Schock. Es dauert bis die Familie die Situation erkennt.

Snapshots

A summer day with emergency calls non-stop. We are accompanying a patient to the hospital in a rescue ambulance. The pilot is alone in the helicopter on his way to the hospital when he gets a call: "Can the helicopter assist in the search for a drowned child?" The pilot immediately changes course and heads toward the marina. The fire department divers are already on their way to the scene. We reach the hospital, deliver our patient, and arrange a location where the helicopter can pick us up. The divers have found the child three meters under the boat; they bring it to the surface. The helicopter picks us up at the hospital. In the meantime, a second physician with emergency & rescue certification has arrived on the scene and initiated resuscitation procedures. We climb into the helicopter and land at the scene after a short flight. Both physicians with emergency & rescue certification decide: the child is dead. The mother – standing 100 m away – looks at me. Before I can say anything, she says: "I dreamt it last night. Just the way it happened." Reconstruction of events: two children on the boat, aged two and five. The two-year-old falls overboard without a life vest. The five-year-old child is in a state of shock. It takes a while before the family comprehends the tragic reality.

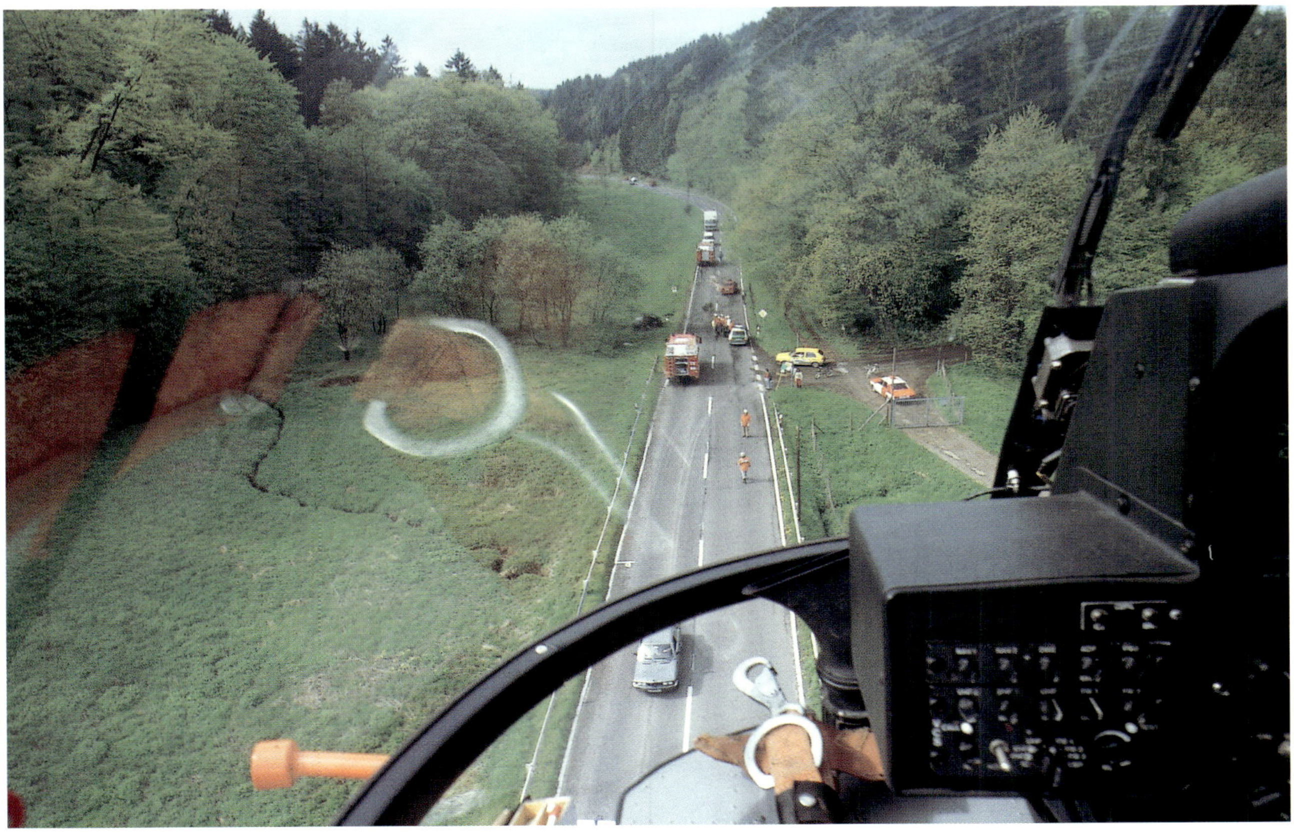

Anflug auf die Einsatzstelle.

Approach to the accident site.

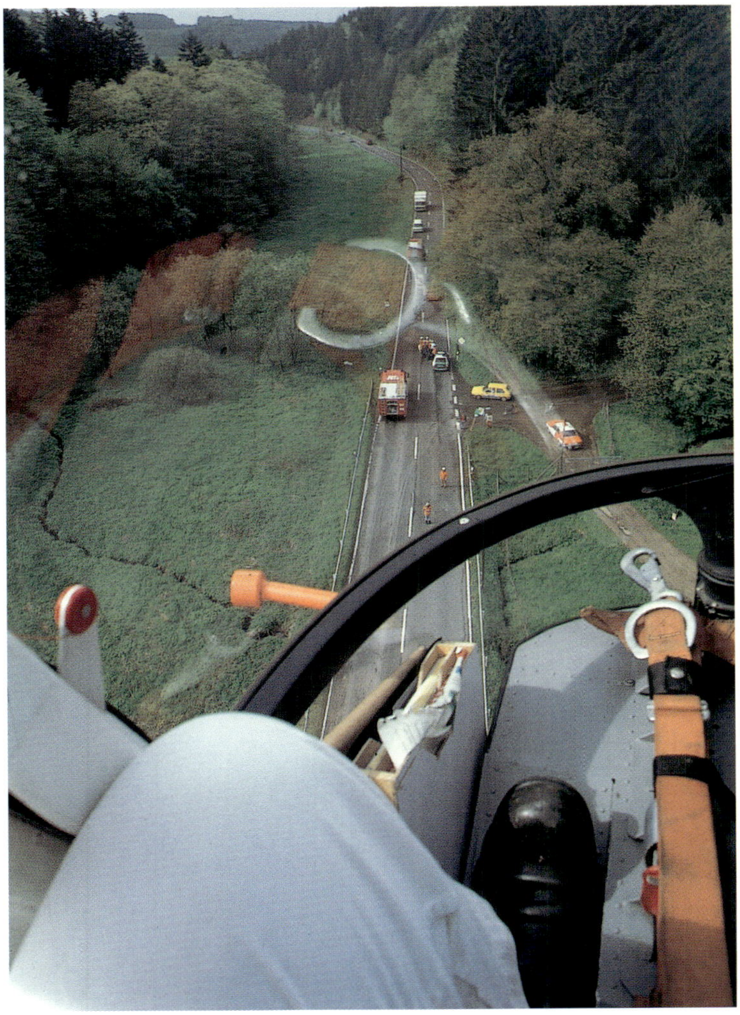

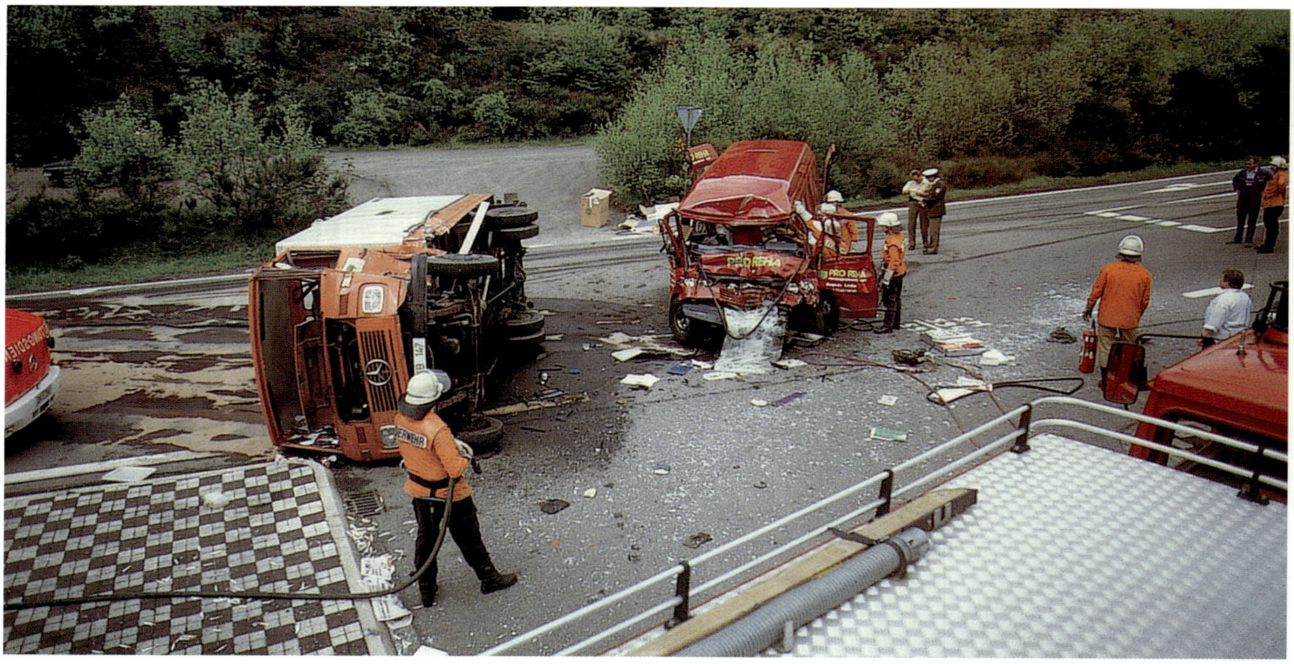

Augenblicke

In der Kneipe. Älterer Mann ca. 60. Schmerzen, Schwindel. Hat Bier getrunken. Sagt: „Ich habe Leberzirrhose im Endstadium. Welchen Rat kann man geben“?

Snapshots

We answer an emergency call from a pub, where an older man around 60 years of age complains of pain and dizziness. He has apparently been drinking beer. He tells us: “I have terminal liver cirrhosis“. What advice can we give him?

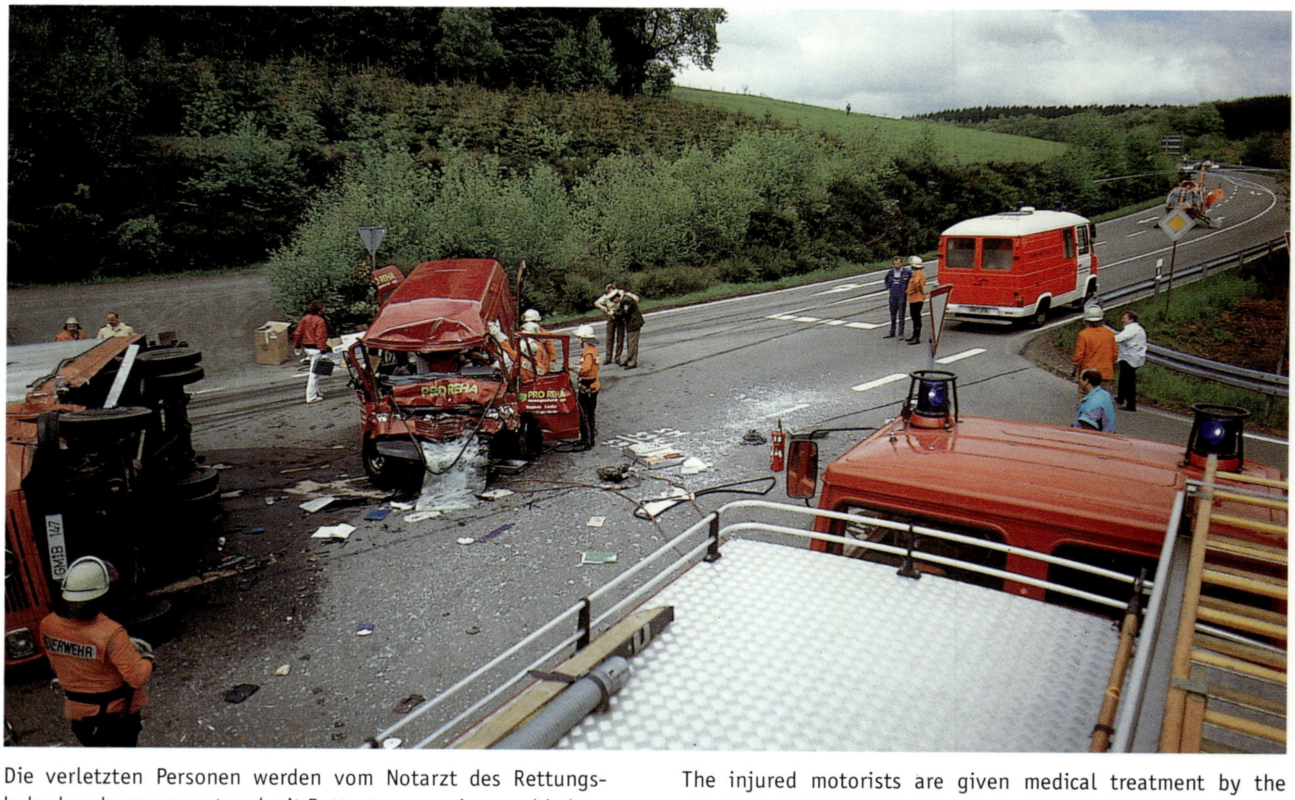

Die verletzten Personen werden vom Notarzt des Rettungshubschraubers versorgt und mit Rettungswagen in verschiedene Krankenhäuser gebracht.

The injured motorists are given medical treatment by the physician with emergency & rescue certification flying with the rescue helicopter and are transported by rescue ambulance to various hospitals.

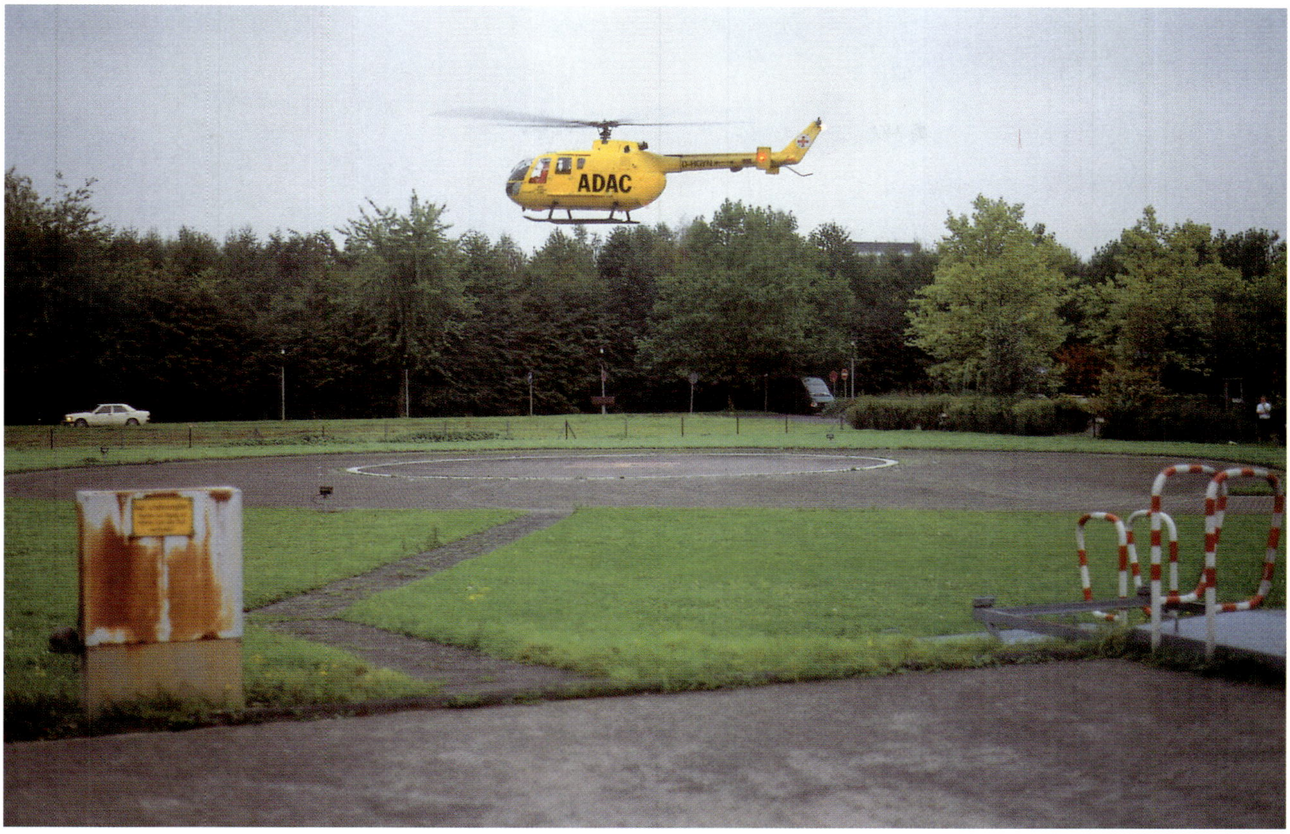

RTH anderer Stationen bringen Patienten.

A patient is brought to the hospital by a rescue helicopter from another base.

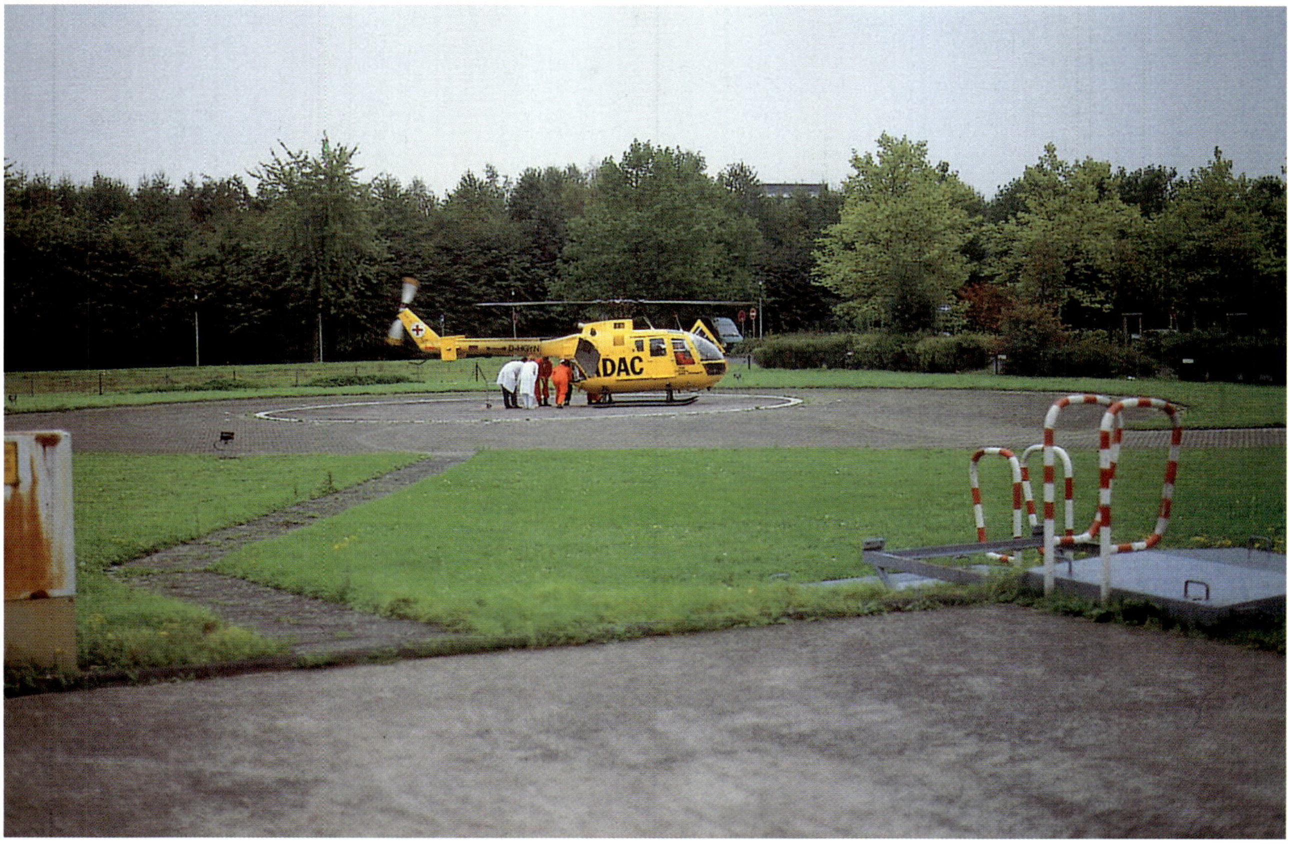

Der Luftrettungsassistent

The Air Rescue Paramedic

von/by Bernd Falk

Philosophie

Luftrettung besteht aus den Kernkomponenten „Flugbetrieb und Notfallmedizin". Demnach gehören zur personellen Ausstattung eines Rettungshubschraubers (RTH) wie auch der meisten Intensivtransporthubschrauber (ITH) neben Pilot, ggf. Bordwart und Notarzt ein Luftrettungsassistent (LRA). Dieser bildet zusammen mit dem Notarzt die medizinische Besatzung. Hinter dieser Konstellation verbirgt sich die Philosophie des „fliegenden Notarztwagens": Bei Erstankunft am Notfallort soll eine suffiziente Versorgung der Notfallpatienten stattfinden können. Im Bedarfsfall soll der Transport in eine geeignete Klinik möglich sein. Für diese beiden wesentlichen Funktionen ist ein medizinisches Team und damit auch nichtärztliches Assistenzpersonal erforderlich. Zugleich sollte der Assistent (oder auch die Assistentin) Aufgaben übernehmen, die den Piloten bei seiner Arbeit während des Fluges und am Boden unterstützen. Der LRA ist also als eine Funktion ausgelegt, die zunächst medizinische wie flugbetriebliche Aufgaben umfasst. Über die Jahre hat sich aber auch eine Funktion herauskristallisiert, die so etwas wie das Bindeglied innerhalb der Besatzung des Hubschraubers und den Besatzungen der bodengebundenen Rettungsmittel ist. Eine oftmals unterschätzte Funktion. Das eingesetzte Personal wird in der Regel von den Rettungsorganisationen Arbeiter-Samariter-Bund (ASB), Deutsches Rotes Kreuz (DRK), Johanniter-Unfallhilfe (JUH), Malteser-Hilfsdienst (MHD) wie auch von Feuerwehren oder Kliniken gestellt. Bundesweit dürften etwa 500-700 LRA im Einsatz sein. Zumeist werden sie alternierend auch im bodengebundenen Rettungsdienst oder als Disponenten eingesetzt, was dem „Blick über den Zaun" sehr zuträglich ist. Die Idealzahl der LRA pro Station liegt bei 5-6 Personen, so daß ein kontinuierlicher Praxiseinsatz gegeben ist.

Der LRA hat sich im Team der fliegerischen wie medizinischen Hubschrauberbesatzung in den zurückliegenden 30 Jahren Luftrettung in Deutschland außerordentlich bewährt. Er hat einen hohen Anteil daran, daß sich die deutsche Luftrettung einen Ruf als eines der besten Systeme der Welt und als Premiumprodukt des Rettungsdienstes erworben hat.

Philosophy

Air rescue consists of the components of "flight operation and emergency medicine". In conformance with this definition, the crew of a rescue helicopter (RH) – like the crew of most intensive care transport helicopters (ITH) – includes a pilot, in some cases a flight technician, a physician with emergency & rescue certification, and an air rescue paramedic. The ARP and the physician with emergency & rescue certification constitute the medical crew of the aircraft. Underlying this constellation is the philosophy of the "airborne rescue ambulance". In keeping with the philosophy behind the rescue helicopter, its crew should be able to provide emergency care to patients if they are the first to arrive at the scene. A second important idea is that they should be able to transport the patient to a suitable hospital if necessary. To carry out both of these important functions, a medical team – and thus auxiliary medical personnel – is necessary. At the same time, the paramedic (male or female) should be able to perform tasks which assist the pilot in the air and on the ground. It is evident, therefore, that the responsibilities of the air rescue paramedic should include both medical and flight-related tasks. Over the years a position has evolved which serves as a link between the helicopter crew and the crews on ground. The importance of this linking function is often underestimated. The personnel trained for this position are usually supplied by the rescue organizations Arbeiter-Samariter-Bund (ASB), German Red Cross (DRK), Johanniter-Unfallhilfe (JUH) and Malteser-Hilfsdienst (MHD) as well as the fire services and hospitals. There are around 500-700 air rescue paramedics working throughout Germany. They are usually assigned alternately to work as land rescue personnel or as dispatchers. This helps them to gain experience beyond the confines of their own scope of responsibility. Ideally, each base station should have 5-6 air rescue paramedics to guarantee the constant availability of ARPs for aeromedical missions.

During the past 30 years of air rescue in Germany, the air rescue paramedic has proved to be a valuable addition to the aeromedical crew of the rescue helicopters. In fact, the air rescue paramedics deserve a large share of the credit for the reputation the German aeromedical service enjoys today of being one of the best in the world – the

Historie

Als 1970 die ADAC-Luftrettung mit Christoph 1 in München den ersten Rettungshubschrauber vom Typ BO 105 zum Einsatz brachte, war dieser mit einem Rettungssanitäter des Bayrischen Roten Kreuzes besetzt. Es folgte Ende 1971 mit Christoph 3 (heute Standort Köln) der erste RTH des Bundesinnenministeriums, seit Anfang an besetzt von Rettungsfachpersonal des Malteser-Hilfsdienstes. Die ersten Sanitäter im Luftrettungsdienst waren wie die meisten Luftretter ausgeprägte Idealisten (auch dies ist ein über die Jahre gebliebenes Merkmal). Sie nahmen Wind und Wetter, undichte Hubschrauber und bescheidene Unterkünfte in Kauf. Professionelle Improvisation könnte man den damaligen Zustand in den Kinderschuhen der Luftrettung nennen. Infusionslösungen und Endotrachealtuben wurden in Ermangelung eines Hangars während der Wintermonate in der Fliegerjacke am Mann getragen, um körperwarm bzw. biegsam zum Patienten zu gelangen. Und wenn der Wasserhahn an der vorläufigen Unterkunft wieder einmal zugefroren war, dann kochte der „Sani“ die Frühstückseier eben mit einer Kochsalzlösung. Eines ist aus dieser Pionierzeit unbeirrbar geblieben: Die Einstellung zum Notfallpatienten, ausschließlich zu dessen Wohlergehen in oftmals misslicher oder gar lebensbedrohlicher Situation da sein zu wollen. Dieses Berufsethos des Sanis (es gab damals schließlich noch kein Berufsbild für den Sanitäter) ist bis heute unverändert geblieben, auch wenn man in der Luftrettung ein wenig aufpassen muß, daß durch die Faszination der Technik „Hubschrauber“ der Notfallpatient nicht in den Hintergrund gerät.

Ausbildung

1978 erschien in erster Auflage in der ADAC-Schriftenreihe Straßenverkehr mit der Nr. 22 „Der Sanitäter im Luftrettungsdienst“. Dieser erste Leitfaden war Resultat verschiedener Hubschrauberfachtagungen des ADAC in Schliersee. Eine Arbeitsgruppe unter Mitwirkung verschiedener Organisationen hatte dieses historische Ausbildungswerk erarbeitet. Im wesentlichen umfasste die damalige Qualifikation auf der Grundlage einer Rettungssanitäterausbildung (damals keineswegs 520 Stunden) nachfolgende Inhalte:

top-of-the-line product of the overall German rescue system.

History

When the ADAC Air Rescue Service put the first rescue helicopter of the type BO 105, Christoph 1, into service in Munich in 1970, the crew included an emergency medical technician from the Bavarian Red Cross. Christoph 1 was followed by Christoph 3 (now stationed in Cologne) in late 1971. Christoph 3 was the first rescue helicopter operated by the Federal Minister of the Interior and was staffed by professional rescue personnel from the Malteser-Hilfsdienst. The first EMTs working in the air rescue service were – like most air rescue personnel – dyed-in-the-wood idealists; fortunately, this attitude has not changed over the years. They put up with wind and weather, drafty helicopters and modest accommodations. "Professional improvisation" is a good description of the early days of air rescue. In the absence of hangars, the aeromedical personnel carried infusion bottles and endotracheal tubes in their pockets in the winter so that the solutions would be at body temperature and the tubes still pliable when they reached the patient. When the water faucets in the temporary quarters were frozen as usual during the winter, the EMTs boiled eggs for the crew's breakfast in physiological saline. One feature of those early days that has not changed over the years is the attitude toward the emergency patient: even in dangerous or life-threatening situations, the well being of the patient is the foremost concern of air rescue personnel. The professional ethics of the EMTs (members of a profession which did not exist back then) have remained constant over the years, even if today's air rescue personnel have to be careful not to relegate the patient to a minor role out of sheer fascination with helicopter technology.

Professional training

In 1978 a publication with the title "The Emergency Medical Assistant in the Air Rescue Service" was published as No. 22 of the ADAC series on motor vehicle traffic. This first printing was the result of several helicopter conferences held by the des ADAC in Schliersee, Germany. A task force composed of representatives of various organizations prepared this historic educational work. At that time the professional training of an EMT assigned to air rescue was based on the education of an EMT on the ground (which definitely did not

- Flugtechnik und Flugsicherheit in Theorie und Praxis 36 Stunden
- Organisation 12 Stunden
- Medizin 6,5 Stunden

Gesamt: 54,5 Stunden

Die damalige Idee war ein wirkliches Qualitätsmerkmal und machte den zukünftigen Rettungssanitäter mit den besonderen Gegebenheiten des Hubschraubers und des Luftrettungseinsatzes vertraut. Dieses Prinzip und der hohe Anspruch an den Flugsanitäter hat sich bis heute erhalten.

So wundert es nicht, daß eine Arbeitsgruppe am 1.10.1998 wiederum einen Meilenstein in Sachen Qualifikation des jetzt genannten LRA mit der Herausgabe eines „Einweisungsplans für Besatzungsmitglieder bei medizinischen Hubschraubernoteinsätzen" gelegt hat. Die Gruppe, bestehend aus Vertretern der gemeinnützigen ADAC-Luftrettung GmbH, der Bundesgrenzschutz (BGS)-Fliegergruppe, der Deutsche Rettungsflugwacht (DRF e.V.), des DRK Landesverbandes Rheinland-Pfalz und der Malteser-Werke gGmbH, hat quasi als Fortschreibung der Ausarbeitung von 1978 einen neuen Gegenstandskatalog vorgelegt. Hierfür gibt es einen rechtlichen Hintergrund durch die Harmonisierung europäischer Vorschriften in der Zivilluftfahrt. Bereits 1991 wurde empfohlen, „im Rahmen der gemeinsamen Verkehrspolitik technische Vorschriften und Verwaltungsverfahren in bezug auf die Sicherheit und den sicheren Betrieb von Luftfahrtzeugen auf der Grundlage der JAR-Vorschriften (Joint Aviation Requirements) der JAA (Joint Aviation Authorities) zu harmonisieren." Es wurden Regelwerke in Form der so genannten JAR-OPS 3 (OPS steht für Operations) gefertigt, die auch für den LRA erhebliche Auswirkungen mit sich bringen und seit dem 1.10.1998 Anwendung finden sollen. Denn für die Luftrettung mit Hubschraubern ist seitdem grundsätzlich ein Besatzungsmitglied vorgeschrieben, das den Piloten während des Einsatzes zu unterstützen hat. Hierzu ist eine entsprechende Einweisung erforderlich, die hinsichtlich der flugbetrieblichen Erfordernisse im Anhang 1 zu JAR-OPS 3.005 (d) für medizinische Hubschraubernoteinsätze (HEMS – Helicopter Emergency Medical Service) festgelegt ist. In den meisten Fällen wird in der Luftrettung der Rettungsassistent eine Doppelfunktion sowohl als Assistent des Piloten wie auch des Notarztes

include 520 hours of instruction back then) and consisted of the following components:

- Flight technology and safety: theory and practice 36 hours
- Organization 12 hours
- Medicine 6.5 hours

Total: 54.5 hours

The basic idea developed back then was a genuine quality milestone. The training based on this idea familiarized the future EMTs with the special features of helicopters and helicopter rescue operations. This principle and the high standards set for EMTs in the aeromedical service are still valid today.

It is not surprising therefore that a later task force laid another milestone in the qualifications of what is now called an air rescue paramedic with the publication of an "Instruction Plan for Crew Members Taking Part in Helicopter Medical Emergency Missions" on 1 Oct. 1998. This task force – which consisted of representatives of ADAC-Luftrettung GmbH, the Aviation Group of the German Border Police, DRF e.V., the German Red Cross chapters in the state of Rhineland-Palatinate, and Malteser-Werke gGmbH – had drawn up a new list of requirements by reworking the requirements set down in 1978. The legal background to this accomplishment was the harmonization of European regulations concerning civil aviation. As early as 1991 a recommendation was made "to harmonize technical regulations and administrative procedures related to safety and the safe operation of aircrafts on the basis of the Joint Aviation Requirements (JAR) issued by the Joint Aviation Authorities (JAA) within the scope of joint traffic and transport policy." Books of regulations were prepared in the form of so-called JAR-OPS 3 (OPS stands for operations); these books of regulations have been in force since 1 Oct. 1998 and have had substantial consequences for the ARP. Since this date it is specifically prescribed by law that a rescue helicopter must carry a crew member who assists the pilot during the mission. This crew member has to receive corresponding instruction; information on aviation requirements is contained in Annex 1 to JAR-OPS 3.005 (d) for emergency medical missions performed by rescue helicopters (HEMS – Helicopter Emergency Medical Service). In most cases the air rescue paramedic performs a double role during air rescue operations as an assistant to both the pilot and the physician with

wahrzunehmen haben. Hierfür sind klare und auch konsequente Qualifikationswege notwendig.
So beginnt der Weg in den Luftrettungsdienst an einer staatlich anerkannten Rettungsschule mit der in der Regel zweijährigen Ausbildung zum Rettungsassistenten. Hiernach schließt sich zumeist bodengebundene Praxis auf einem Einsatzfahrzeug an. Zweifelsohne entwickelt sich dann sehr schnell beim Absolventen einer Rettungsassistentenschule der Wunsch, in der Luftrettung tätig sein zu wollen. Eine verständliche Absicht, die sicherlich auch mit der Faszination des Fliegens zu tun hat. Leider besteht ein krasses Mißverhältnis zwischen den zur Verfügung stehenden Arbeitsplätzen in der Luftrettung und der tatsächlichen Nachfrage. Jeder Rettungshubschrauber wäre leicht mehrfach mit Rettungsfachpersonal auszustatten, wenn es nach der Anzahl der Bewerber ginge. Der Weg zum Luftrettungsdienst erfolgt fast immer über eine Rettungsorganisation. Dort ist der Rettungsassistent in der Regel angestellt und versieht seinen Einsatzdienst. Ist die betreffende Organisation an der Gestellung von Personal für einen RTH beteiligt, kann ein Tag kommen, den der Rettungsassistent vielleicht lange ersehnt hat: Er wird für den Luftrettungsdienst vorgesehen. Jetzt beginnt die Ausbildung zum zum HEMS Crew Member (HCM) bei einer Luftrettungsorganisation. Der ADAC führt solche Kurse über das von ihm mitinitiierte und geführte Europäische Schulungszentrum für Luftrettung und bodengebundenen Rettungsdienst EUCREW durch. In einem neuntägigen Crash-Kurs wird der künftige LRA intensiv auf seine künftige Tätigkeit vorbereitet. Im einzelnen umfasst der Kurs folgende Schwerpunkte:

- Luftrecht
- Crew Coordination Concept (CCC)
- Navigation
- Meterologie
- Hubschraubertechnik
- Flugphysiologie
- Medizinische Besonderheiten der Luftrettung
- Cockpit-/Kabineneinweisung
- Vorbereitung für den Soforteinsatz
- Betankung des Hubschraubers
- Hubschraubertransport am Boden
- Einweisung in Rettungs- und Sicherheitsgeräte, Verhalten in besonderen Situationen

emergency & rescue certification. To prepare the air rescue paramedic for this role, clear and consistent educational programs are required.

The first step toward a career as an air rescue paramedic is to complete a period of training, which usually takes about two years, at a state-licensed school for paramedics. After completing this training, the paramedic is usually assigned to land rescue vehicles to gain his or her first experience. It cannot be denied that most paramedic school graduates very soon develop the wish to work in air rescue. This is an understandable wish which is undoubtedly connected with the fascination of flying. Unfortunately, there is a glaring disproportion between the number of jobs open in air rescue and actual demand. Every rescue helicopter could be manned several times with trained rescue personnel if hiring was geared to the number of applicants. The path to a job in the aeromedical service almost invariably starts out at a rescue organization. As a rule the paramedic is employed by this organization and is sent on rescue missions by the organization. If the organization in question participates in sending personnel to the aeromedical service, the long-awaited day may come for the paramedic on which he or she is recommended for the aeromedical service. The candidate can now enter a training program making him or her eligible to work as an HEMS crew member (HCM) at an air rescue organization. The ADAC holds such courses at the European Training Center for Air and Land Rescue Services (EUCREW); the ADAC is one of the initiators and sponsors of EUCREW. During the 9-day intensive course, the future air rescue paramedic is prepared for his or her future responsibilities. The main topics covered by the course are:

- aviation law
- crew coordination concept (CCC)
- navigation
- meteorology
- helicopter technology
- flight physiology
- special medical features of air rescue
- cockpit & cabin instructions
- preparation for the emergency mission
- refuelling the helicopter
- helicopter transport on the ground
- instruction on the use of rescue and safety equipment, rules of conduct for special situations.

Lehrkräfte sind zumeist erfahrene Einsatzpiloten. Bei der ADAC-Luftrettung beinhaltet der Lehrgang auch noch das Flugfunkzeugnis BZF II. Nach einer Erfolgskontrolle über den gesamten Stoff erfolgt die praktische Einweisung in den Flugbetrieb mit mindestens 10 Einsätzen an mindestens 3 Tagen. Jetzt endlich ist es so weit: Der LRA ist „clear for take off", bereit zum Einsatzdienst auf einem RTH / ITH. Ein Traumjob? Für eine Weile ganz bestimmt. Aber das war der Einsatz auf dem Notarztwagen zunächst auch. Das Fliegen, die sehr intensive Teamarbeit, die Besonderheiten einer Hubschrauberstation, die vielfältigen Aufgaben, der weite Einsatzbereich, vielleicht auch die Qualität der Notfälle haben sicher ihre dauerhafte Wirkung. Aber auch das Besondere wird schnell zur Normalität. Das Wichtigste aber und Verhaltensregel Nr. 1 für alle LRA ist: Der Hubschrauber ist ein „fliegender Notarztwagen", nicht mehr und nicht weniger. Daran muß sich das Verhalten des Rettungsassistenten (wie auch der gesamten Besatzung) orientieren. Dezente Zurückhaltung ist angesagt, Überblick bewahren, keinesfalls den RTW „besetzen". Wer sich korrekt verhält, wird gerne wieder angefordert.

Damit der HCM up to date bleibt, ist für ihn jährlich ein zumeist eintägiger Refresher-Kurs obligatorisch. Dies ungeachtet der medizinischen Fortbildungen, die länder- oder organsiationsspezifisch vorgeschrieben oder aus Eigeninitiative heraus besucht werden.

Für LRA auf ITH kommt noch das Erfordernis hinzu, über intensivmedizinische Erfahrungen verfügen zu müssen. Insofern hat Fachpersonal der Intensivpflege einen unbestreitbaren Vorteil, wenn es sich darüberhinaus zum Rettungsassistenten und anschließend zum HCM ausbilden lässt.

Aufgaben

Die Aufgaben des LRA sind vielschichtig. Er ist eigentlich Allrounder. Auf der einen Seite Assistent des Notarztes, auf der anderen Assistent des Piloten und zu guter letzt Büroorganisator, Materialbeschaffer, Desinfektionsdurchführender und einiges mehr. Die beste Übersicht gibt der Rettungseinsatz wohl selbst.

Beim Eingang des Alarms

- nimmt der LRA den Einsatz über Funk auf,
- sucht den Einsatzort auf der Karte, legt einen

The teachers are generally experienced pilots who have flown many missions. The ADAC Air Rescue Training Program also includes a course leading to the attainment of the BZF II aviation radio license. After passing examinations on the entire body of material covered in the courses, the students receive practical instruction on aviation; they must fly at least 10 missions taking place on at least three days. Finally, the big day arrives: the ARP is "cleared for take off", i.e. is ready to serve on a rescue helicopter or intensive care transport helicopter. A dream job? For a while at any rate. However, the work on the rescue ambulance with a physician with emergency & rescue certification aboard was a dream job at first, too. The flying, the very intensive teamwork, the special qualities of a helicopter base, the diversified tasks, the wide range of responsibilities, and perhaps even the special quality of emergency work: all of these undoubtedly make a lasting impression. However, even very unusual work soon becomes routine. Be that as it may, the no. 1 rule of conduct for all air rescue paramedics is: the helicopter is nothing more (and nothing less) than an airborne rescue ambulance with a physician with emergency & rescue certification aboard." The conduct of the paramedics (and of the entire crew) must reflect this realization. An attitude of respectful reticence is appropriate; the crew members should always have the entire situation under control but should avoid "occupying" the rescue helicopter. A crew member who displays correct conduct will be asked to come aboard again.

To ensure that the skills of the HCMs are constantly up to date, a refresher course (usually lasting for one day) is compulsory. This is in addition to any continued education events prescribed by the individual German states or the various rescue organizations or to any courses the crew members attend on their own initiative.

In addition, air rescue paramedics working on intensive care transport helicopters have to possess experience in intensive care medicine. In this respect, medical personnel with specialized training in intensive care have an undisputed advantage when applying for further training to become a paramedic and eventually an HCM.

Scope of Responsibility

The responsibilities of the air rescue paramedic are highly diversified. He or she is actually a versatile all-rounder. On one hand, the ARP is the assistant of the physician with emergency & rescue certi-

Kursstrich an und berechnet Kurs sowie Entfernung und Flugzeit, und

- läuft zur Maschine, beobachtet den Anlaßvorgang, prüft den Verschluss der Passagiertüren und -gurte, steigt ein und informiert den Piloten.

Während des Fluges

- führt er als HCM den Funkverkehr im BOS-Bereich und ggf. im Bereich des Flugfunks,
- liest Checklisten,
- beobachtet den Luftraum,
- leistet Navigationshilfe,
- hilft beim Einsprechen der Einsatzstelle, d. h. Landeinformationen für den Piloten geben, und
- beobachtet den Raum hinter und ggf. unter der Maschine.

Am Notfallort wird er zum Assistent des Notarztes und

- leistet lebensrettende Maßnahmen alleine oder auf Anordnung des Notarztes,
- steht dem Notarzt bei der Versorgung des Notfallpatienten zur Seite,
- hält sich je nach Engagement und Können der bodengebundenen Kollegen eher diskret zurück,
- kümmert sich um Angehörige oder körperlich offensichtlich Unverletzte,
- unterstützt die Verbringung des Patienten in den Hubschrauber und
- beschafft Personalien.

All dies kann je nach Einsatzstelle stark variieren.

An der Hubschrauberstation

- dokumentiert der LRA Teile des Einsatzes,
- bereitet die Ausrüstung auf, überprüft und verzurrt diese und
- reinigt den Hubschrauber.

Umfeld / Team

Der LRA ist Teamarbeiter. Vielleicht sogar noch etwas intensiver als auf einem Notarztwagen. Auch wenn der Pilot letztendlich für den Hubschrauber im Rettungseinsatz allein verantwortlich ist, so wird er sich doch meistens darauf verlassen, wenn der LRA den Abstand der laufenden Rotorblätter zu den benachbarten Bäumen bei der Landung angibt. Das Wirken in

fication. On the other hand, he or she is the assistant of the pilot and, last but certainly not least, a good office manager, material procurement expert, disinfection specialist, etc. The best description of his or her tasks is provided by a chronological description of the rescue mission itself. When an emergency call comes in:

- The ARP accepts the incoming call by radio.
- He or she looks for the emergency site on the map, plots a course, and calculates the distance and flying time to the scene of the emergency.
- He or she sprints to the aircraft, observes the starting-up procedure, checks the closing of the passenger doors and belts, boards the helicopter, and informs the pilot that he or she is now aboard the craft.

During the flight:

- In his or her capacity as an HCM, the ARP is responsible for radio communication in the police and rescue and sometimes in the aviation radioband.
- The ARP reads the checklists.
- He or she observes the air space.
- He or she assists with navigation.
- He or she provides the pilot with information required for landing.
- He or she keeps an eye on the space in front of the aircraft and possibly underneath it as well.

At the scene of the emergency the ARP becomes the assistant of the physician with emergency & rescue certification. In this capacity he or she performs the following tasks:

- carries out life-saving procedures on his or her own initiative or under the supervision of the physician with emergency & rescue certification
- assists the physician with emergency & rescue certification in providing emergency care to the patient
- depending on the commitment and capability of the land-bound colleagues, assumes an attitude of discrete reticence
- looks after relatives and people who obviously have no physical injuries
- assists in loading the patient into the helicopter
- takes down the patient's personal data.

All of the above activities can vary greatly, depending on the particular emergency site.

At the helicopter base station the ARP:

- documents the role played by the ARP during the mission

verschiedenen Rettungsdienstbereichen, mit freiwilligen und Berufsfeuerwehren, mit verschiedenen Polizeiinspektionen, Notfallseelsorgern, technischen Rettungseinheiten usw. erfordert ein hohes Maß an sozialer Kompetenz und Integrationsfähigkeit. Aber auch Einfühlungsvermögen ist in hohem Maße gefordert, insbesondere natürlich im Umgang mit den Patienten, Angehörigen oder sonstigen Betroffenen eines Notfalles. In der Luftrettung wird die Besatzung häufiger als im bodengebundenen Rettungsdienst mit Leid und Tod konfrontiert. Umso wichtiger sind funktionierende kollegiale und familiäre Verhältnisse, um das Erlebte besprechen und verarbeiten zu können.

Ausblick

Immer einmal wieder wird darüber diskutiert, ob das Primat des Notarztes in Frage zu stellen sei. Ganz bestimmt nicht, denn zum einen hat sich der bundesdeutsche Rettungsdienst für den Notarzt entschieden, zum anderen wäre es unsinnig, auf viele engagierte Notärzte zu verzichten. Ein Rettungshubschrauber ohne Notarzt ist somit nicht vorstellbar. Auf der anderen Seite benötigt die Ausbildung zum Rettungsassistenten eine Reformierung. Diese muß eine dreijährige Ausbildung ebenso wie eine duale Ausbildungstätigkeit mit Prüfungen am Ende der Ausbildung beinhalten. In dieser Kombination macht die kleine „Luftrettungsreform" des HCM noch mehr Sinn. Die Frage nach der Sinnhaftigkeit des Rettungsassistenten im Rettungsdienst stellt sich somit ebenfalls nicht. Das gilt auch und insbesondere für den Luftrettungsdienst. Getreu dem Motto „never change a winning team" ist ein Rettungshubschrauber ohne LRA nicht vorstellbar.

- prepares, checks and lashes the equipment
- cleans the helicopter.

The Rescue Environment and the Rescue Team

The ARP is a team player. This aspect of the job is perhaps even more pronounced in a rescue helicopter than in a rescue ambulance. Ultimately, the pilot bears the sole responsibility for the rescue mission; nevertheless, he or she will usually take the ARP's word for it when the latter states the distance between the moving rotor blades and nearby trees during a helicopter landing. The necessity to work together with various sectors of the rescue service – i.e. with volunteer and professional fire-fighters, police, pastors working on telephone counseling hot lines, members of technical rescue units, etc. – demands highly developed social and integrative skills. In addition, a high degree of empathy is called for, especially when dealing with patients, relatives or other persons affected by an emergency. Crews involved in air rescue operations are confronted more frequently with suffering and death than are rescue crews on the ground. In this situation, a well-functioning network of colleagues, family and friends is all the more important so that the crew member can work through his or her experiences by talking about them.

Outlook

Repeatedly, the question is raised as to whether the physician with emergency & rescue certification should continue to play the leading role during rescue operations. This role should not be tampered with: firstly, the Federal Rescue Service has decided in favor of retaining this primacy and secondly, it would make absolutely no sense at all to dispense with the work of so many dedicated physicians with emergency & rescue certification. For this reason, a rescue helicopter without a physician with emergency & rescue certification is inconceivable. On the other hand, the education of paramedics is in need of reform. The new curriculum must consist of a three-year training period and two-track educational activities followed by examinations. In this combination the small "aeromedical reform" embodied by the HCM makes even more sense. As a result, the role played by the rescue paramedics in the rescue service is not questioned, either. This also applies, in particular, to the aeromedical service. In keeping with the motto "never change a winning team", a rescue helicopter without an ARP is equally inconceivable.

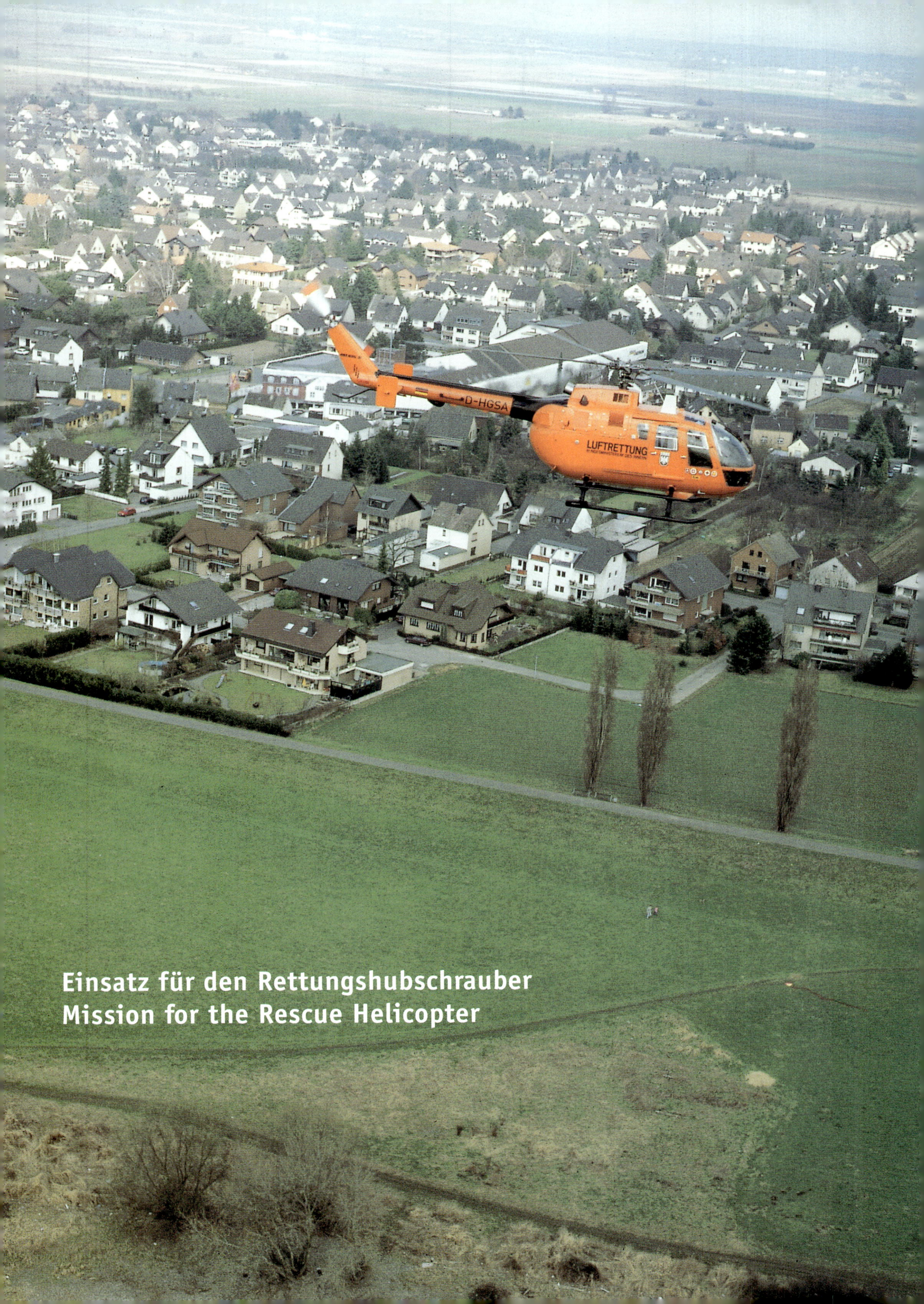

Einsatz für den Rettungshubschrauber
Mission for the Rescue Helicopter

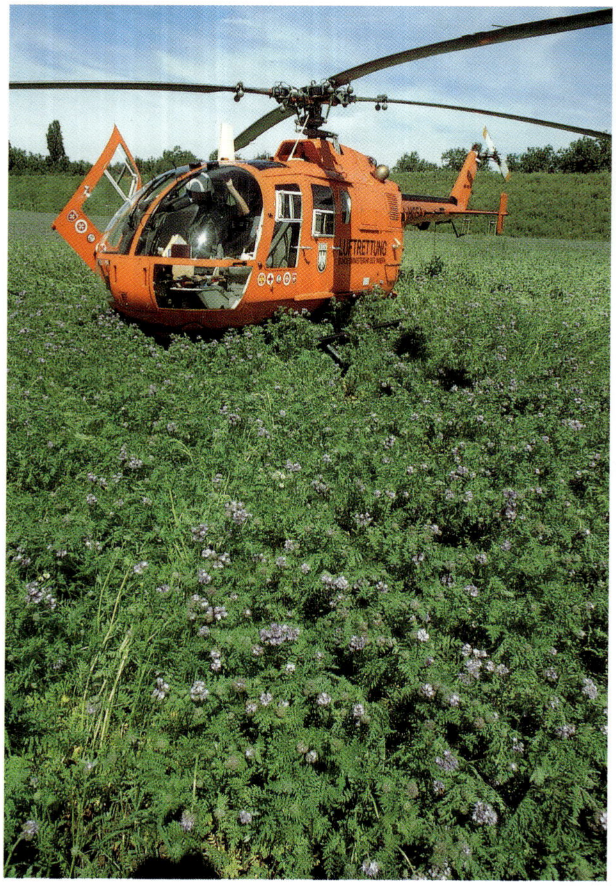

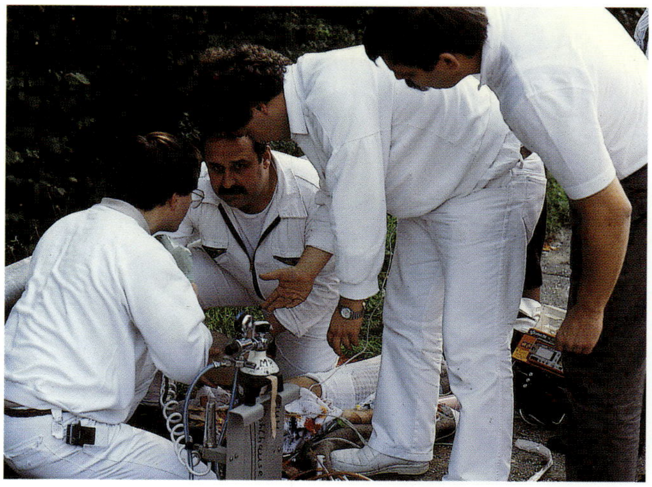

Ein Kind ist aus einem PKW geschleudert worden. Die Besatzung des Rettungshubschraubers bemüht sich mit sofort eingeleiteten Maßnahmen das Kind mit Sauerstoff zu beatmen und mit Infusionen zu versorgen.

A child has been thrown out of an automobile. The crew of the rescue helicopter initiate life-saving measures immediately; they administer oxygen and infusions to stabilize the child's circulation.

Der Hubschrauber landet auf einer nahegelegenen Wiese.

The helicopter lands on a nearby meadow.

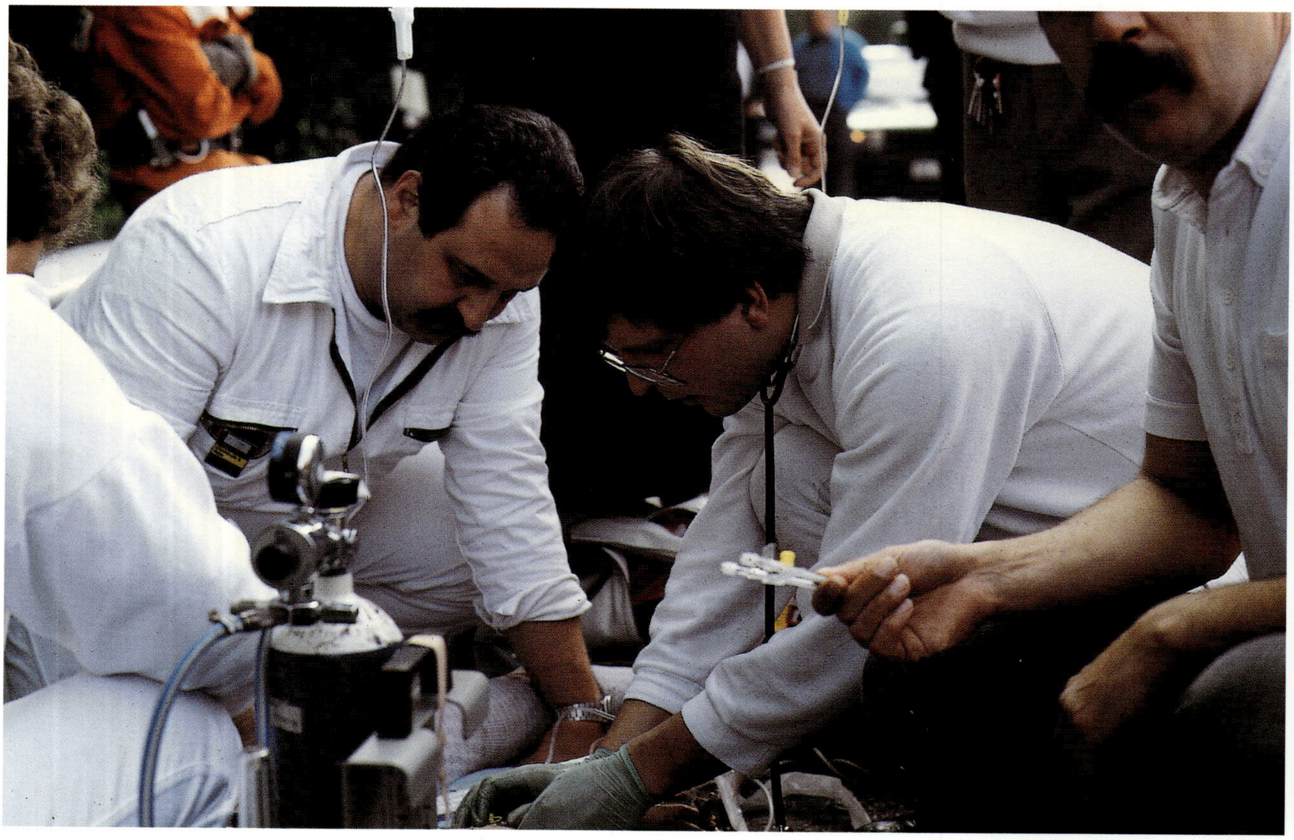

Die reibungslose Zusammenarbeit mit bodengebundenen Einsatzkräften optimiert die Rettungskette zum Wohle des Patienten.

The smooth collaboration with the rescue workers on the ground optimizes the rescue chain; this kind of teamwork is in the patient's best interests.

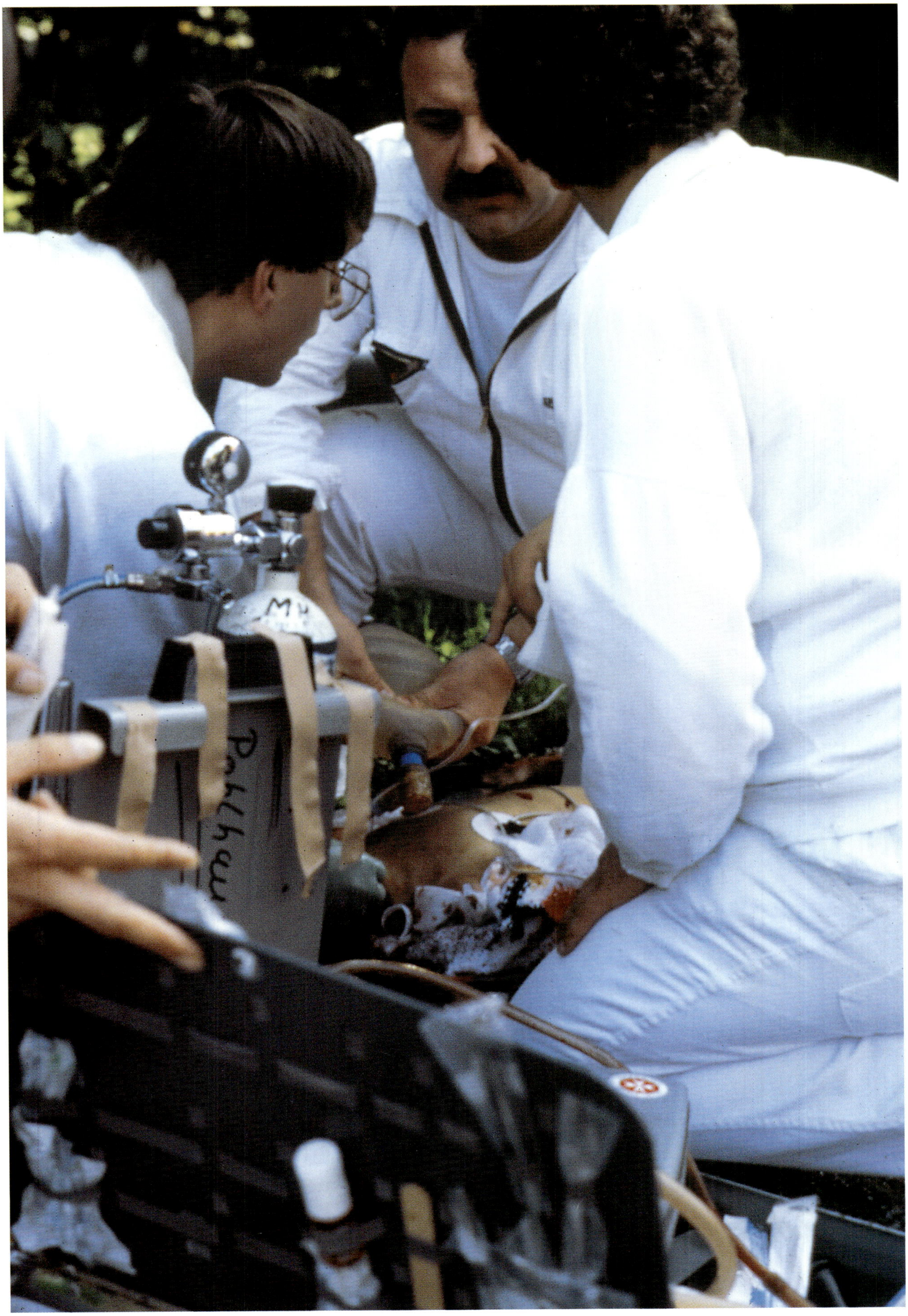

Einsatz für den Rettungshubschrauber
Mission for the Rescue Helicopter

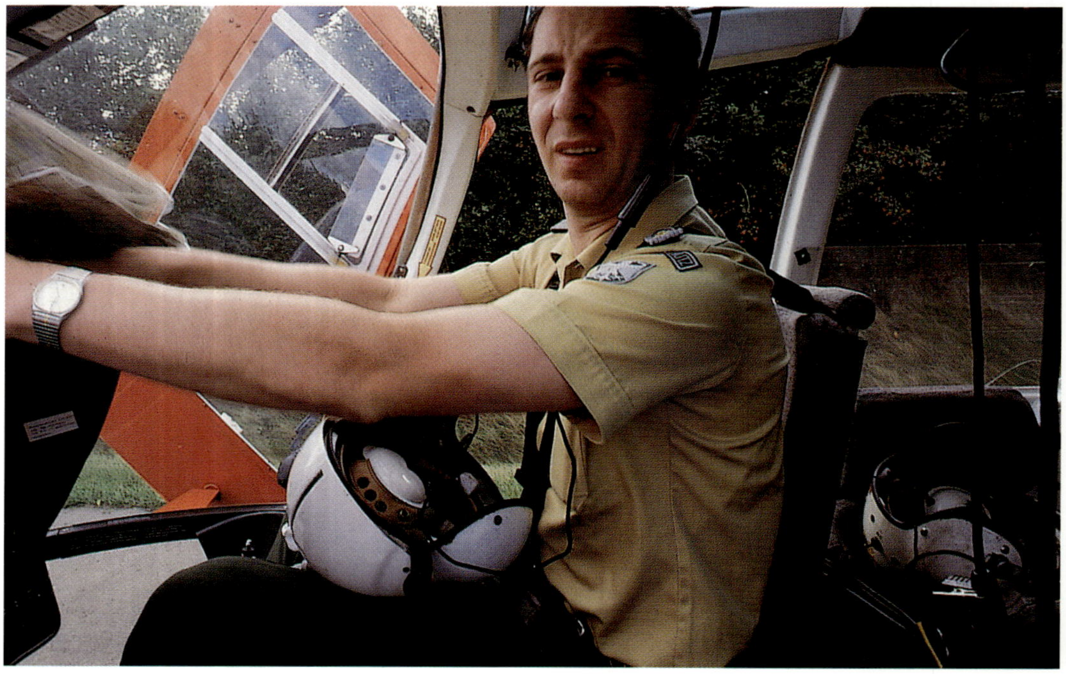

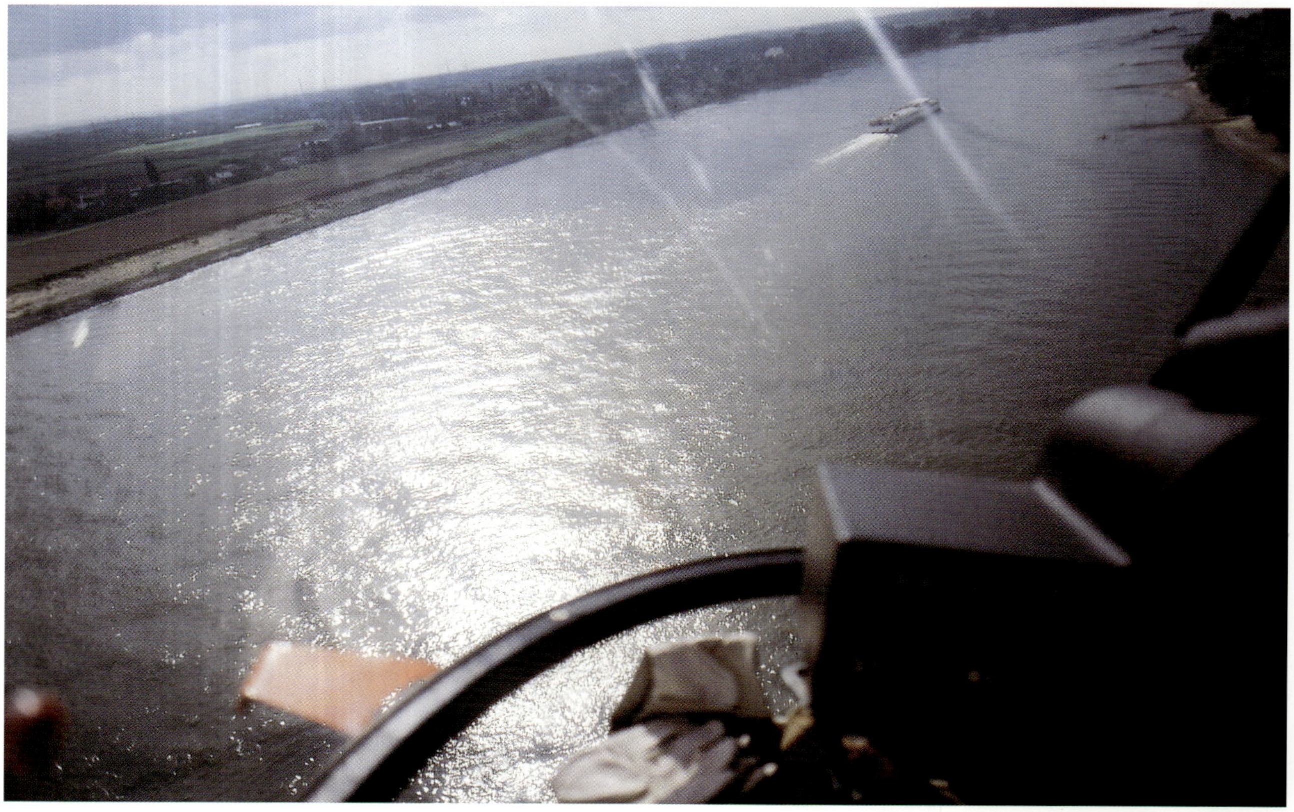

Auf einem Passagierschiff, das im Strom kurzfristig keine Anlegestelle erreichen kann, hat ein Patient, der bereits mehrere Herzinfarkte erlitten hat, plötzlich die gleichen Schmerzen, die ihm schon von seinen anderen Herzinfarkten bekannt sind.

Die Besatzung des Rettungshubschraubers macht das Schiff im Strom aus.

On a passenger ship underway between two ports of call, with no immediate possibility to dock, a patient who has had several heart attacks in the past suddenly experiences chest pain which he identifies as the first sign of a myocardial infarction.

The crew of the rescue helicopter locates the ship from the air.

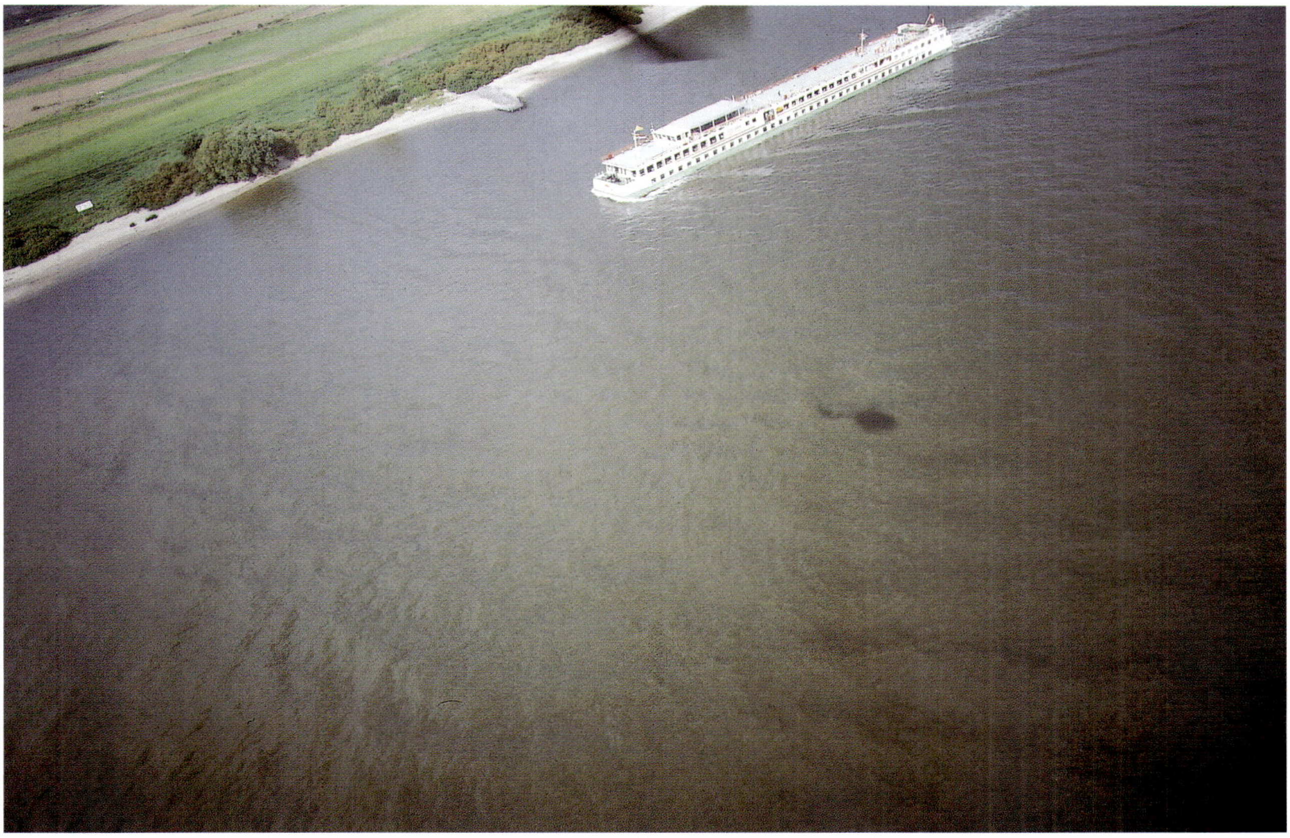

Es wird geprüft, ob das Deck für eine Landung freigeräumt ist und eine Landung dort möglich ist.

They inquire whether the deck has been cleared for a possible helicopter landing and whether the helicopter can land there.

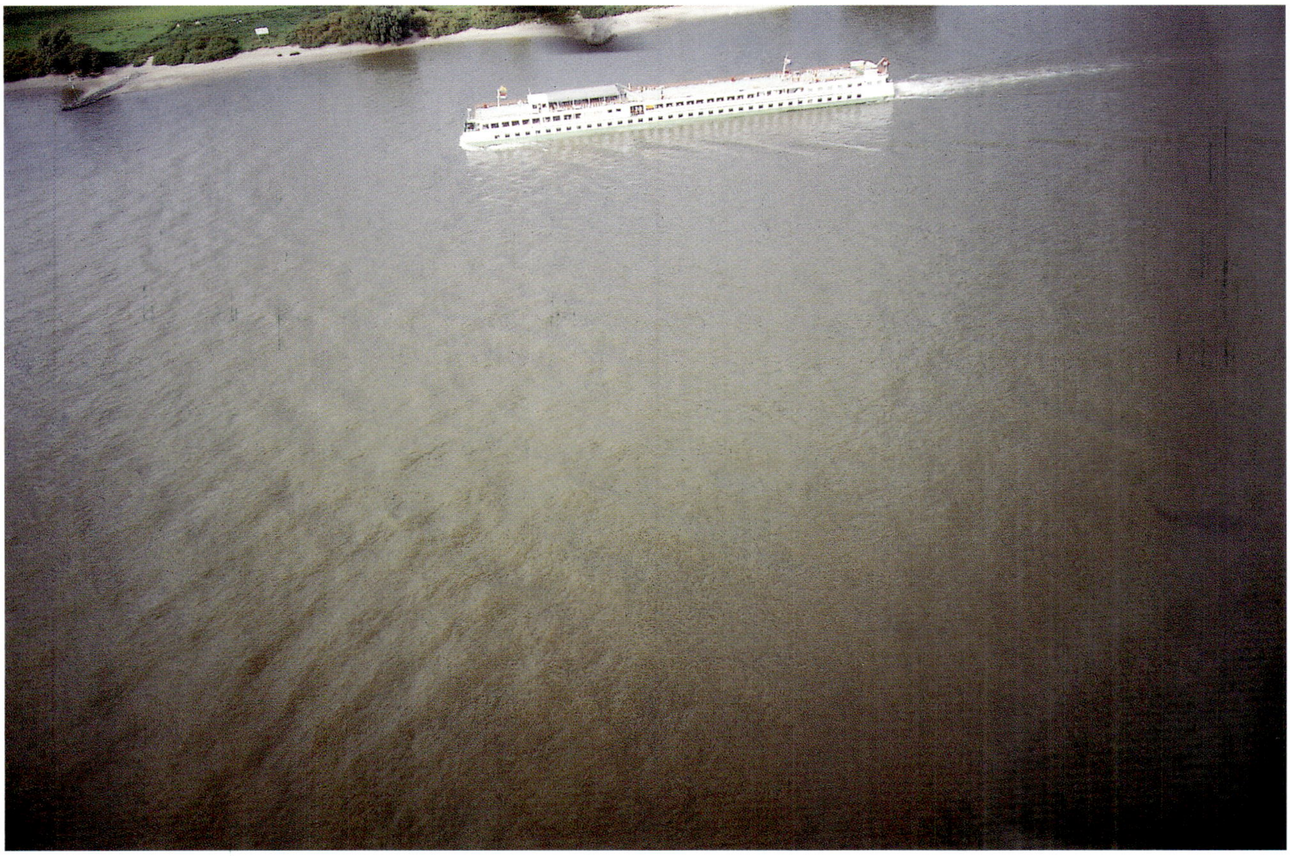

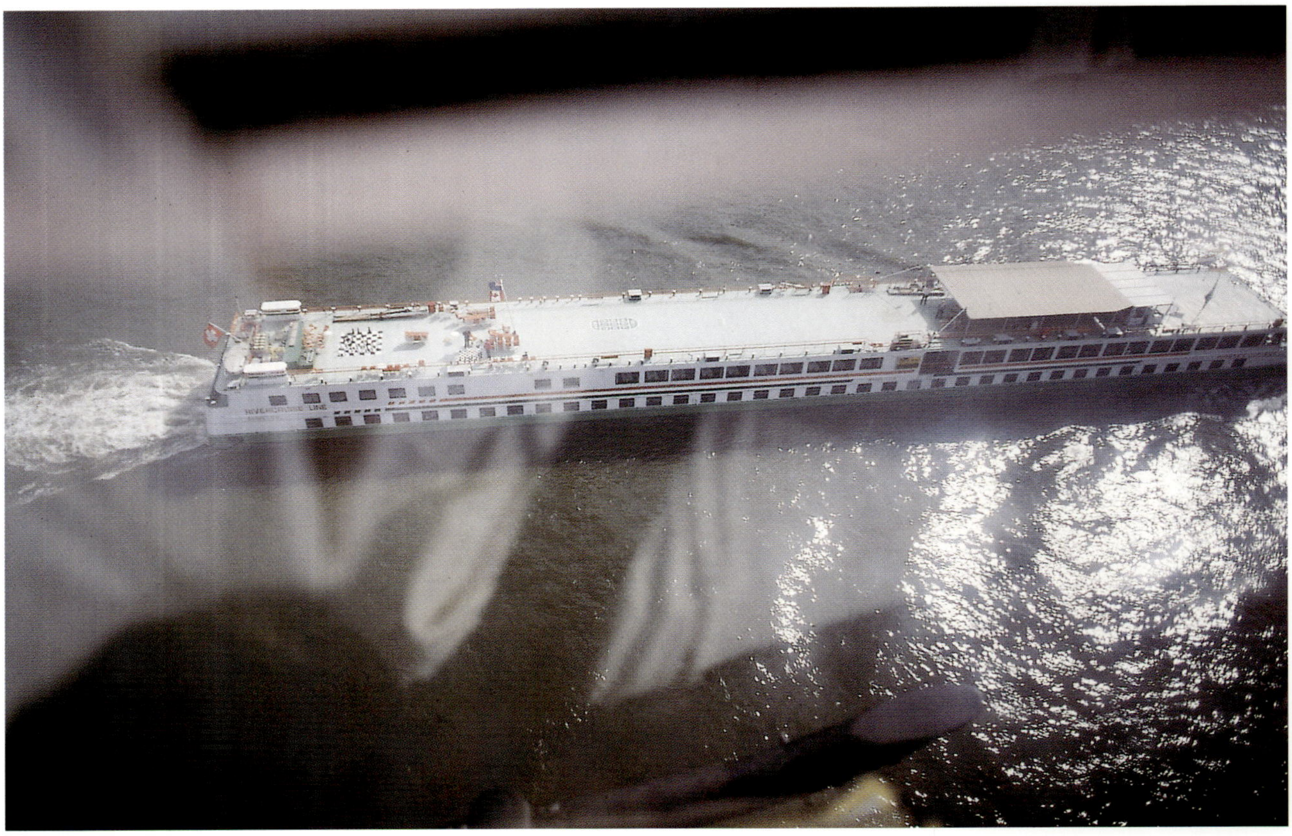

Beim Überflug wird über die Leitstelle dem Kapitän des Passagierschiffes mitgeteilt, dass er das Deck noch weiter freiräumen möge.

During the fly-over the captain of the passenger ship is requested, by the Coordination Center, to clear a larger area on the deck.

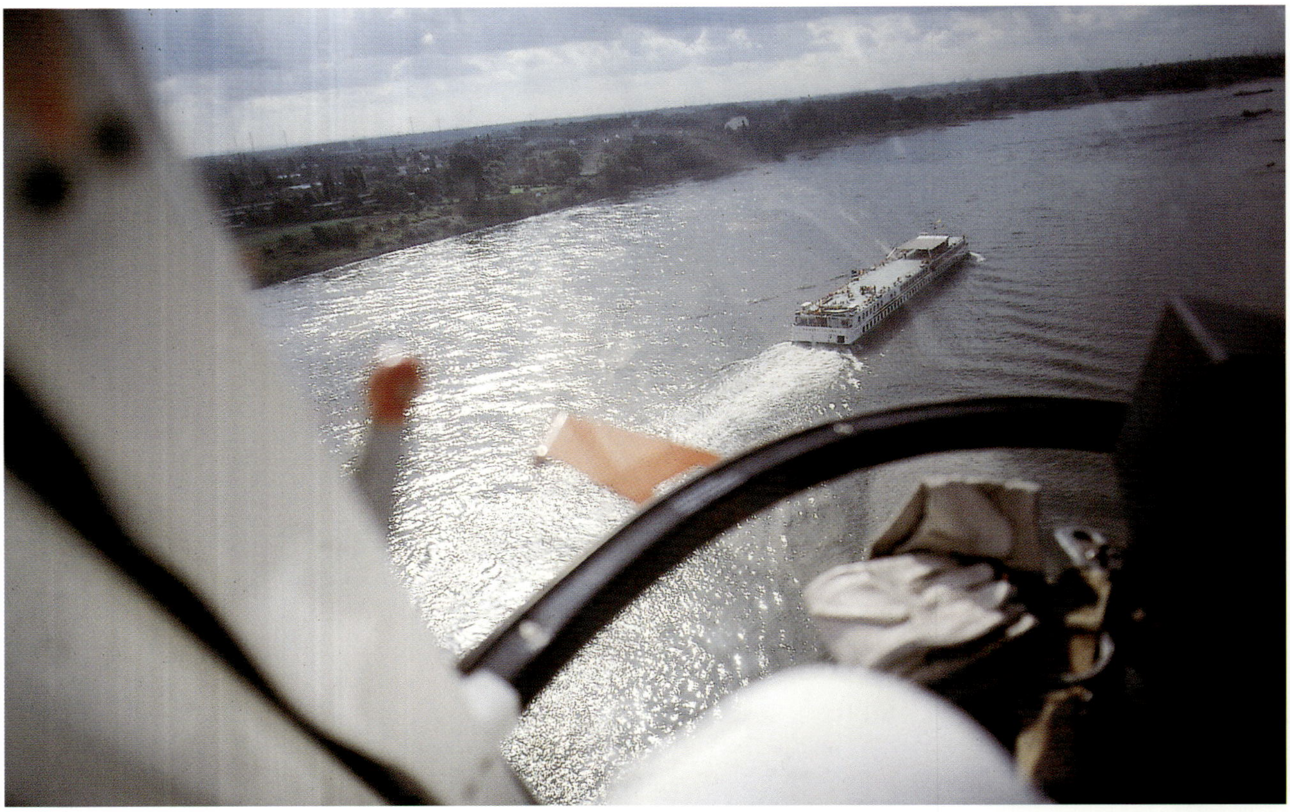

Das Deck ist freigeräumt und ein Anflug zur Landung wird probiert. Die Frage ist, ob das Schiffsdeck den Hubschrauber trägt.

The deck has now been cleared and the helicopter makes a trial approach flight. The question is: will the deck hold the helicopter?

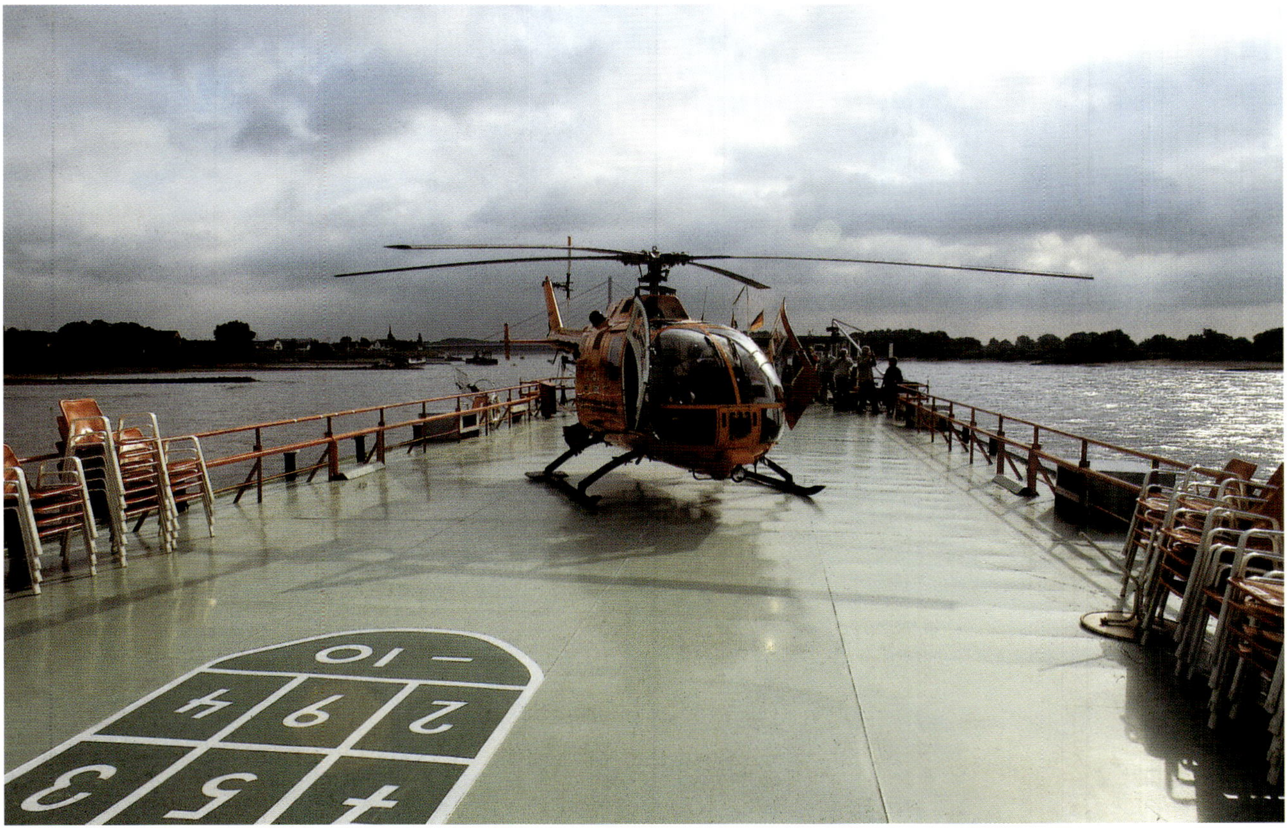

Der Rettungshubschrauber ist auf dem Passagierdeck gelandet. Der Rest ist Routine.

The rescue helicopter has landed on the passenger deck. The rest is routine.

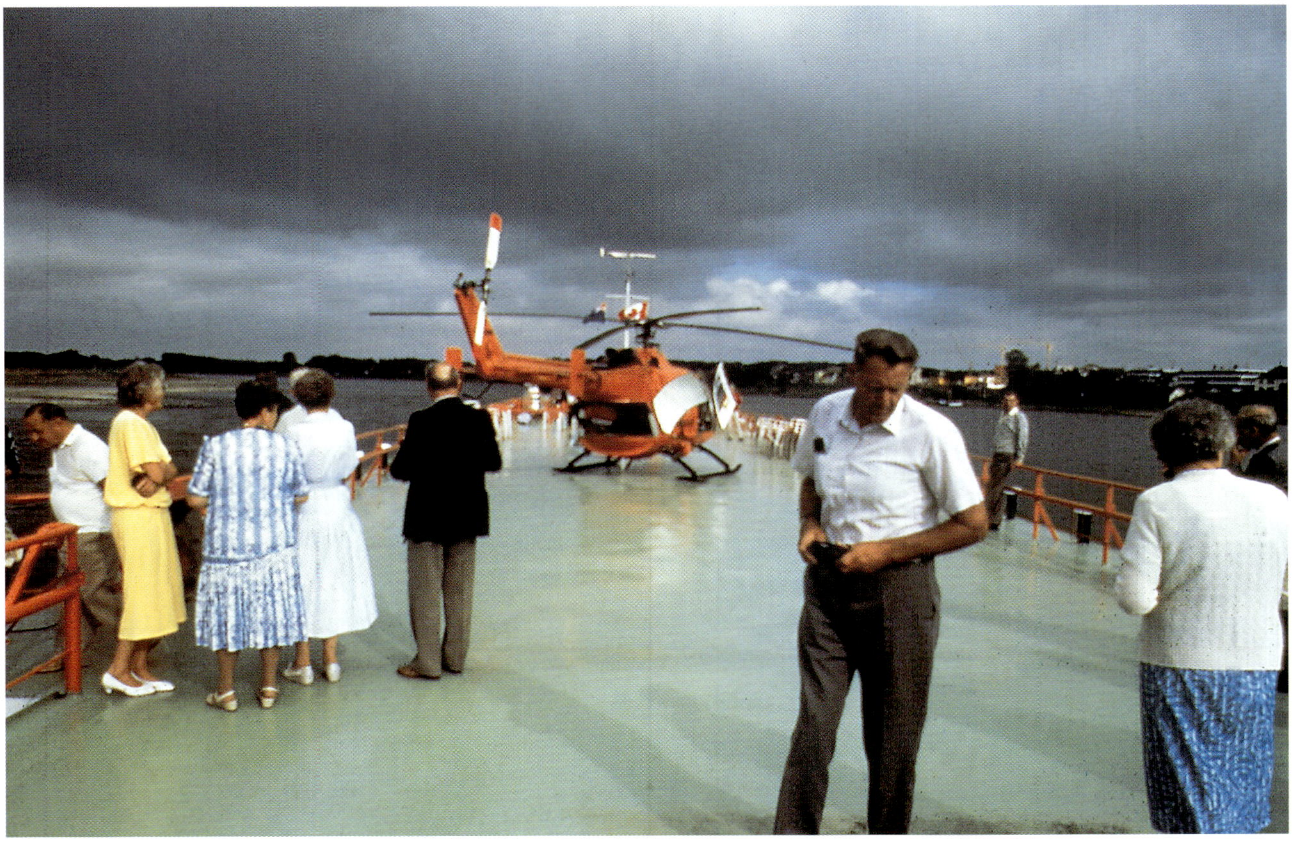

Der Hubschrauber wird vorbereitet zum Patiententransport.

The helicopter is prepared for the patient transport.

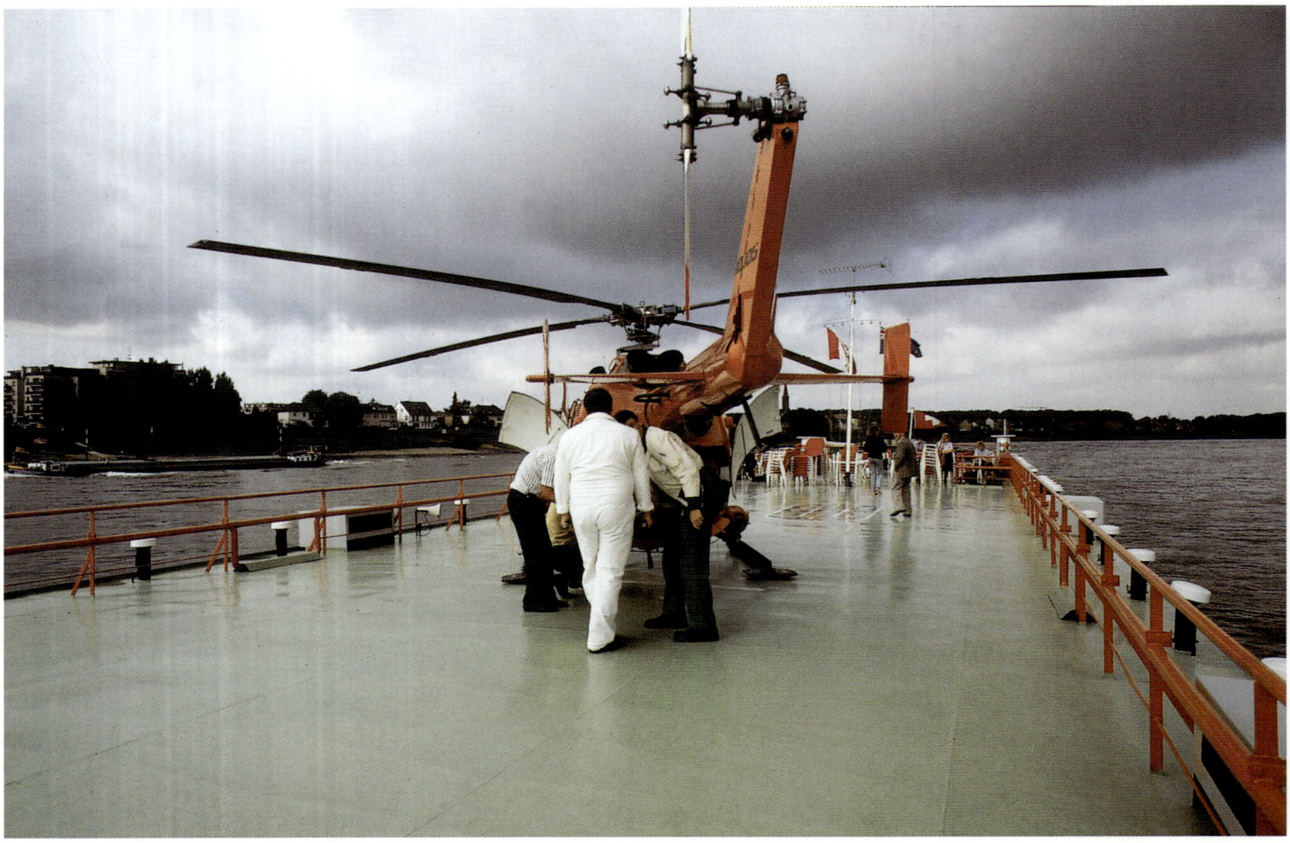

Der Patient wird durch die Heckklappe eingeladen.

The patient is taken aboard through the rear door of the helicopter.

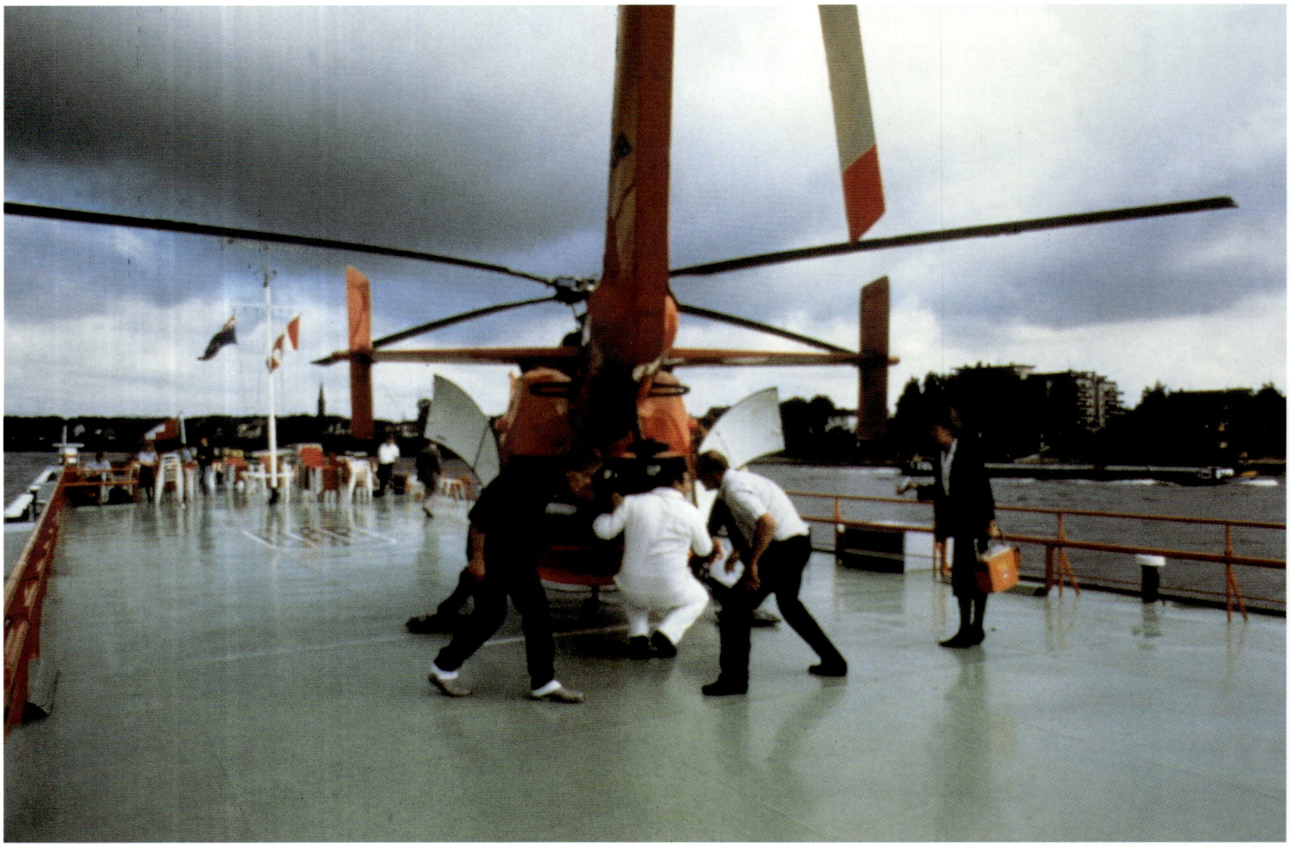

Der Hubschrauber startet wenige Minuten später und bringt den Patienten in eine Spezialklinik.

The helicopter takes off several minutes later and transports the patient to a specialized hospital.

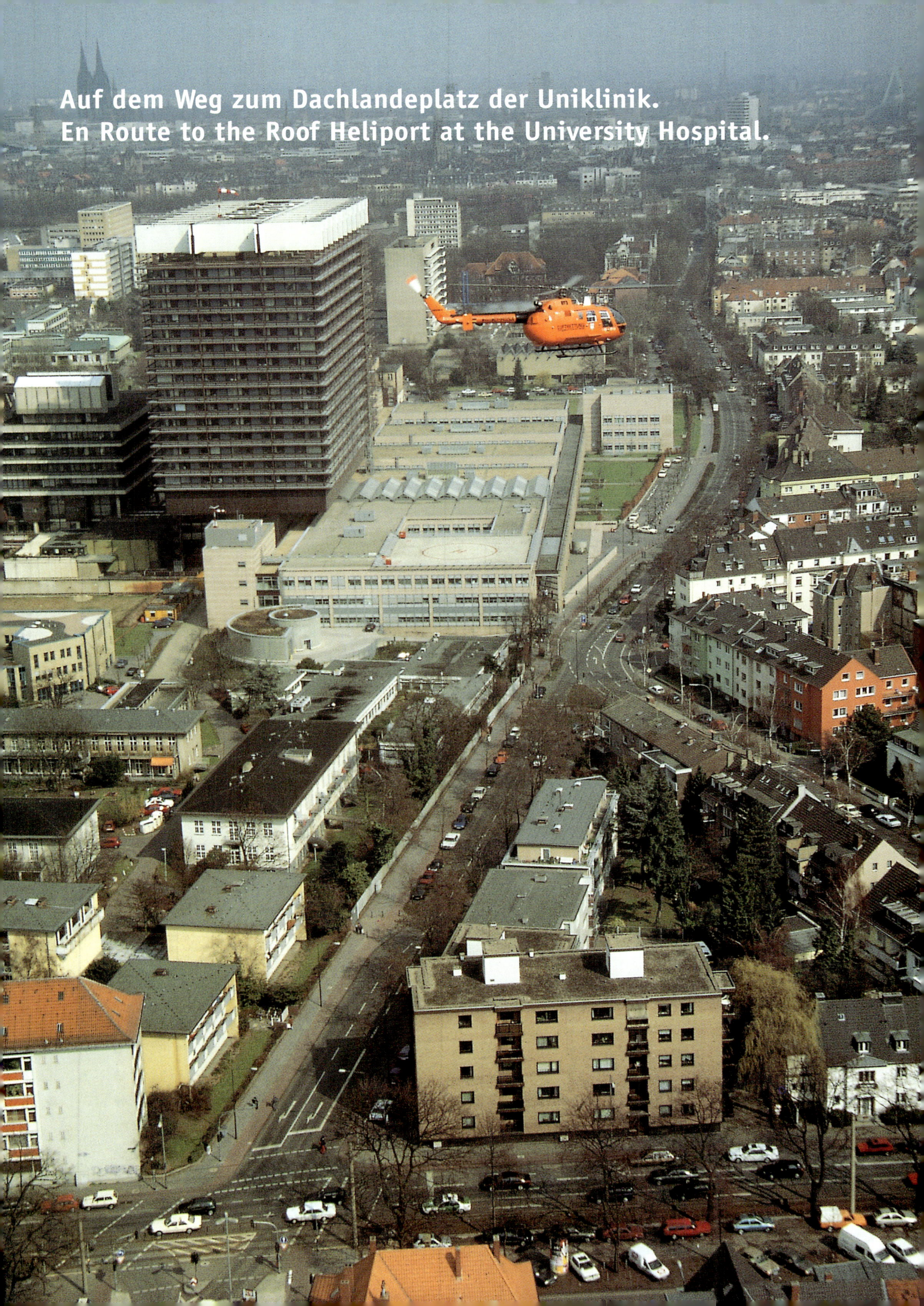

Auf dem Weg zum Dachlandeplatz der Uniklinik.
En Route to the Roof Heliport at the University Hospital.

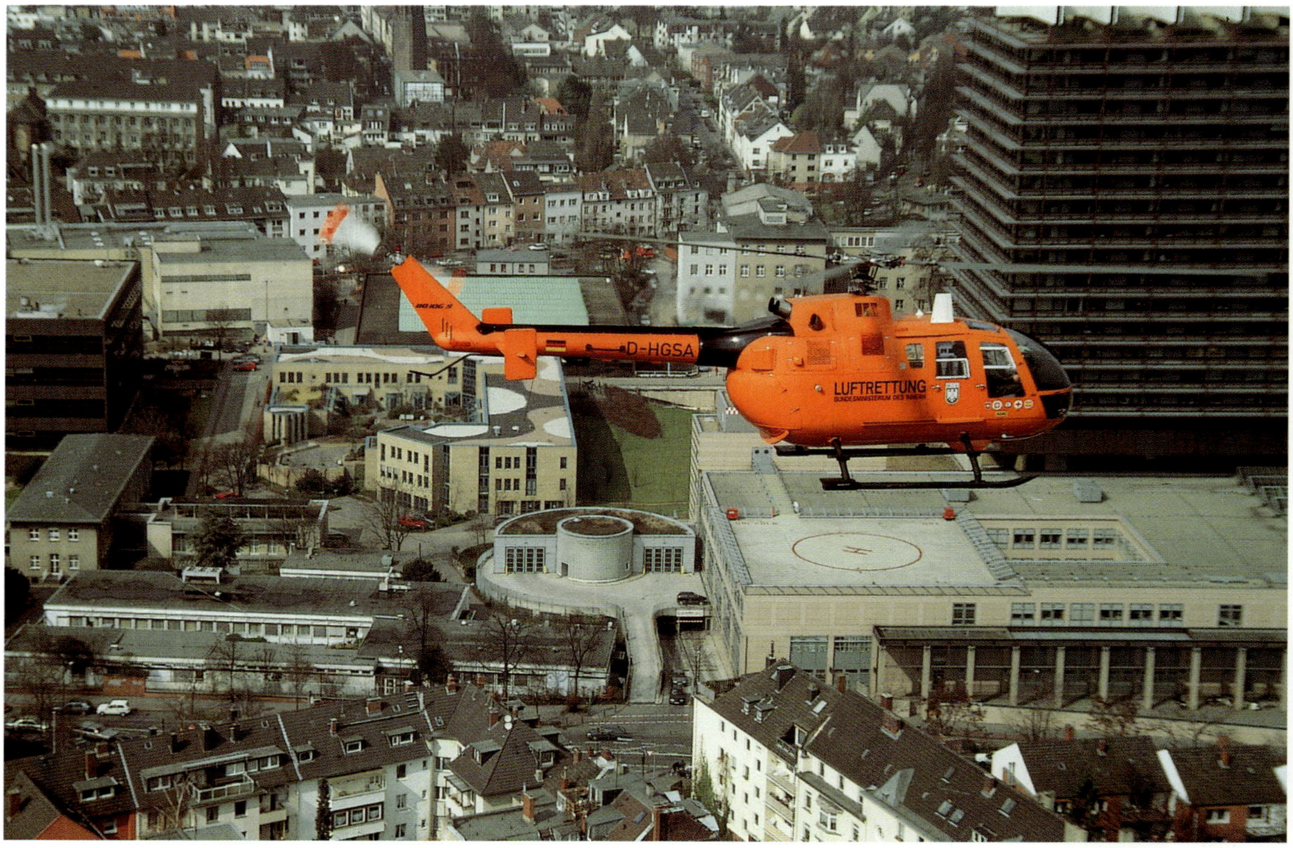

Heliports an Krankenhäusern: Voraussetzungen für eine effiziente Luftrettung

Hospital Heliports: A Prerequisite for Efficient Air Rescue

von/by Gunter Carloff

Einleitung

Die Luftrettung mit Hubschraubern beginnt und endet häufig an einem Krankenhaus, sofern dort Landemöglichkeiten vorhanden sind. Zum Wohle des Patienten soll das Umladen von einem Transportmittel (hier RTH) auf ein weiteres (hier RTW) auf das unumgängliche Mindestmaß reduziert werden. Daher werden vorhandene - Freiflächen an Krankenhäusern – so weit rechtlich zulässig und flugbetrieblich möglich – für Landungen mit RTH genutzt, um Zwischentransporte mit Rettungsfahrzeugen zu vermeiden. Somit sind Landplätze an Krankenhäusern unmittelbare limitierende Faktoren.

Entwicklung des neuen Luftrechts

Es lohnt der Blick auf die Entwicklung des neuen Luftrechts für den Betrieb von Hubschraubern.

Introduction

Air rescue flights involving helicopters frequently originate and terminate at a hospital, provided that there are possibilities for landing. In the interests of the patient, transfers from one rescue vehicle (in this case a rescue helicopter) to another (such as a rescue ambulance) are kept to a minimum. For this reason, available open areas at hospitals are used for rescue helicopter landings – insofar as law and the aviation requirements permit – to prevent secondary transports in other rescue vehicles. From this discussion, it becomes clear that the availability of landing areas at hospitals constitutes an immediate limiting factor on rescue helicopter operation.

Start und Landung kennzeichnen Beginn und Abschluss des Fliegens. Gerade Starts und Landungen, die sich im Gegensatz zu der übrigen Nutzung des Luftraumes im Spannungsfeld zwischen Rechten und Interessen von vorwiegend nicht am Luftverkehr beteiligten Dritten abspielen, sollten auf besondere Verkehrswege konzentriert bleiben.

Start- und Landephase sind mit erhöhten Risiken verbunden. Daher sind diese grundsätzlich an Flugplätze gebunden, die bauliche Mindestvoraussetzungen erfüllen, damit auch bei Betriebsstörungen des Hubschraubers oder ungünstigen Wetterbedingungen ohne Gefahren für Dritte sicher am Boden gelandet werden kann. Dieser Grundsatz des Flugplatzzwangs gilt prinzipiell in Deutschland.

Die Rechtsprechung in Deutschland hat schon mehrfach entschieden, dass dieser Flugplatzzwang nicht unter Hinweis auf Sonderrechte,

Development of the New Aviation Law

It is informative to take a look at the impact of the new Aviation Law on the operation of helicopters. Take-off and landing mark the beginning and end of a flight. In contrast to the other uses of air space, aircraft take-off and landing, in particular, take place in a highly charged area between the requirements of air traffic and the rights and interests of third parties who are, for the most part, not involved in aviation. This is the reason why take-off and landing are restricted to special locations.

The take-off and landing phases are associated with heightened risks. Consequently, they are always restricted to airfields which satisfy certain minimum structural requirements to ensure that – even in the event of helicopter malfunction or unfavorable weather conditions – helicopters can be safely set down without endangering third parties. This basic principle of

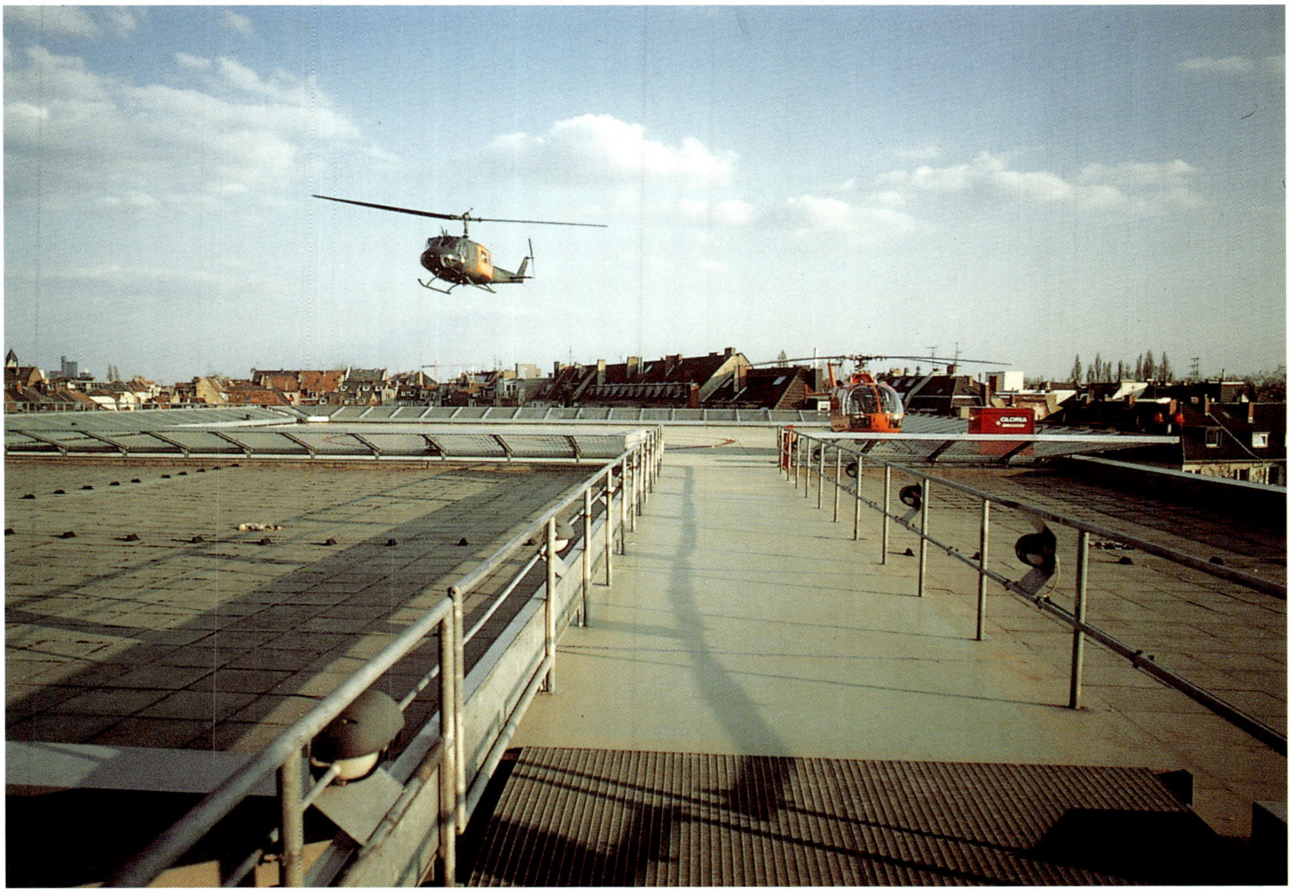

Kurze Zeit später landet die Bundeswehr mit einer SAR-Hubschrauber vom Typ Bell UH-1D, auf dem Dachlandeplatz der Uni. Kurz nach dem die Bundeswehr gelandet ist, meldet sich ein Rettungshubschrauber des ADAC mit einem weiteren Verletzten an und landet ebenfalls.

Shortly afterwards, a German Airforce helicopter – a German Air Force SAR-Helicopter, type Bell UH-1D – also lands at the rooftop heliport at the university hospital. A few minutes later a rescue helicopter of the ADAC – the German Automobile Club – carrying another injured person joins the other two rescue helicopters.

z.B.Hilfeleistung bei Gefahr für Leib und Leben einer Person umgangen werden darf. Daher ist überall dort, wo fortgesetzt und regelmäßig an einem Ort gelandet werden soll – z.B. an einem Krankenhaus – die Einrichtung eines Flugplatzes grundsätzlich erforderlich.

Die bisher in Deutschland gültigen baulichen Anforderungen an einen Flugplatz sind in den Richtlinien des Bundesministeriums für Verkehr aus dem Jahr 1969 für Hubschrauberlandeplätze veröffentlicht.

Flugbetriebsflächen und Hindernisfreiheit in zwei Abflugsektoren waren so bemessen, dass die damals vorhandenen Hubschrauber einen sicheren Flugbetrieb durchführen konnten. Die zumeist einmotorigen Hubschrauber waren in der Lage, die zulässigen Hindernishöhen in den Abflugsektoren (Steigung ca.16,7%) mit ausreichendem Abstand zu überfliegen. Eine mögliche Triebwerkstörung blieb außer Betracht. Diese Regelungen haben sich unter der Sicherheitsphilosophie der 1960er Jahre insgesamt bewährt.

In den 1980er Jahren wurden von der Internationalen Zivilluftfahrtorganisation (ICAO) Standards für grenzüberschreitenden Flugbetrieb mit Hubschraubern entwickelt. Sie wurden in der 2.Fassung als ICAO Annex 6 Part III „International Operations – Helicopters" im Juli 1990 veröffentlicht. Hierin sind erstmals Leistungsanforderungen für Hubschrauber festgelegt, die auch bei Triebwerksstörungen sichere Notlandungen oder Startabbruch bzw. Fortsetzung des Fluges bis zu einem geeigneten Landeplatz verlangen. Parallel wurden Bauvorschriften für mehrmotorige Hubschrauber und Hubschrauberflugplätze definiert. Selbst bei Ausfall eines Triebwerkes mussten die Hubschrauber in der Lage sein, eine sichere Notlandung durchführen zu können. Wo keine Notlandeflächen verfügbar sind, müssen mehrmotorige Hubschrauber verwendet werden, die nach Kategorie A (Tabelle 1) zugelassen sind und entsprechend Flugleistungsklasse 1 (Tabelle 2) betrieben werden können. Das heißt, die zulässigen Hindernishöhen in den Abflugsektoren von Heliports dürfen nur so flach steigen, dass auch bei Störung eines Triebwerks mit dem verbleibenden Triebwerk Hindernisse sicher überflogen werden können (Steigungswinkel 4,5%).

allowing take-off and landing only at airfields applies all over Germany.

German courts have repeatedly ruled that the principle of limiting take-offs and landings to airfields may not be circumvented by claiming special privileges, e.g. for the provision of emergency assistance in situations where human life and health are endangered. For this reason, an airfield has to be erected at all locations where aircraft continually and regularly take off and land, e.g. at hospitals.

The structural requirements applicable to heliports in Germany to date were set down in the Guidelines of the German Minister of Transport published in 1969. Aviation operations areas and the absence of obstacles in two departure sectors were defined to ensure that the helicopters in service at that time could carry on flight operation safety. These helicopters, which usually had only one engine, were able to clear the obstacle heights permitted by law in two take-off sectors (angle of climb: approx. 16.7%). Possible engine failure was not taken into account. These regulations were on the whole sufficient for the safety philosophy of the 1960s.

In the 1980s the International Civil Aviation Organization (ICAO) developed standards for cross-border flight operations with helicopters. These standards were published in July 1990 in the 2nd Edition of the ICAO, Annex 6, Part III "International Operations – Helicopters". This standard is the first to contain performance requirements which stipulate safe emergency landing, abortion of take-off, or continuation of the flight to a suitable landing area even in the event of engine failure. Parallel to this, structural regulations were defined for multi-engine helicopters and for heliports. Even with one engine inoperative, the helicopter must be able to make a safe landing. In areas where no emergency landing areas are available, multi-engine helicopters must be employed which are licensed for Category A (Table 1) and can be operated according to Performance Class 1 (Table 2). This means that the permitted obstacle heights in the departure sectors must allow the helicopter to rise so slowly that – even in the event of a failure of one engine, the helicopter can safely clear any obstacles with the remaining engine (angle of climb: 4.5 %).

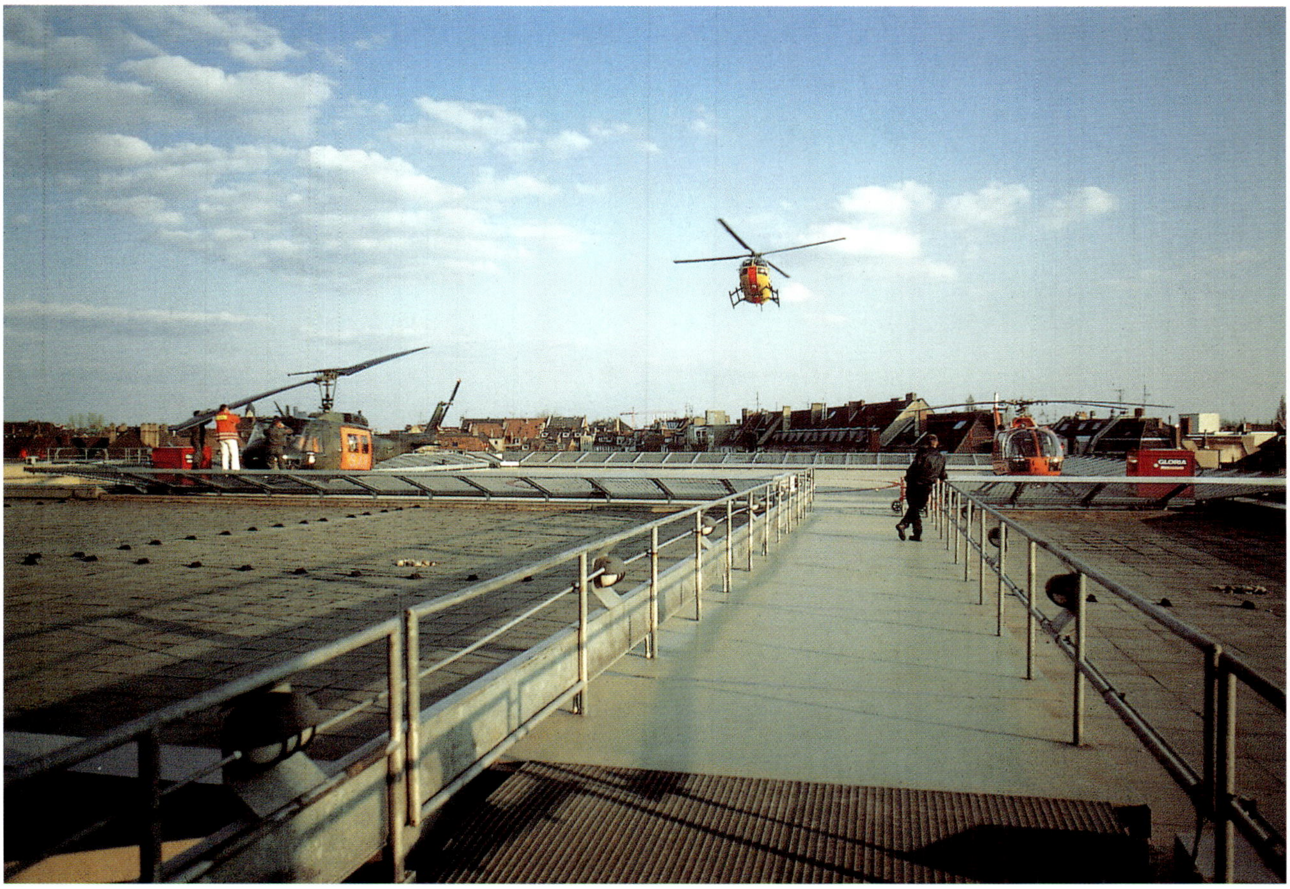
GLORIA

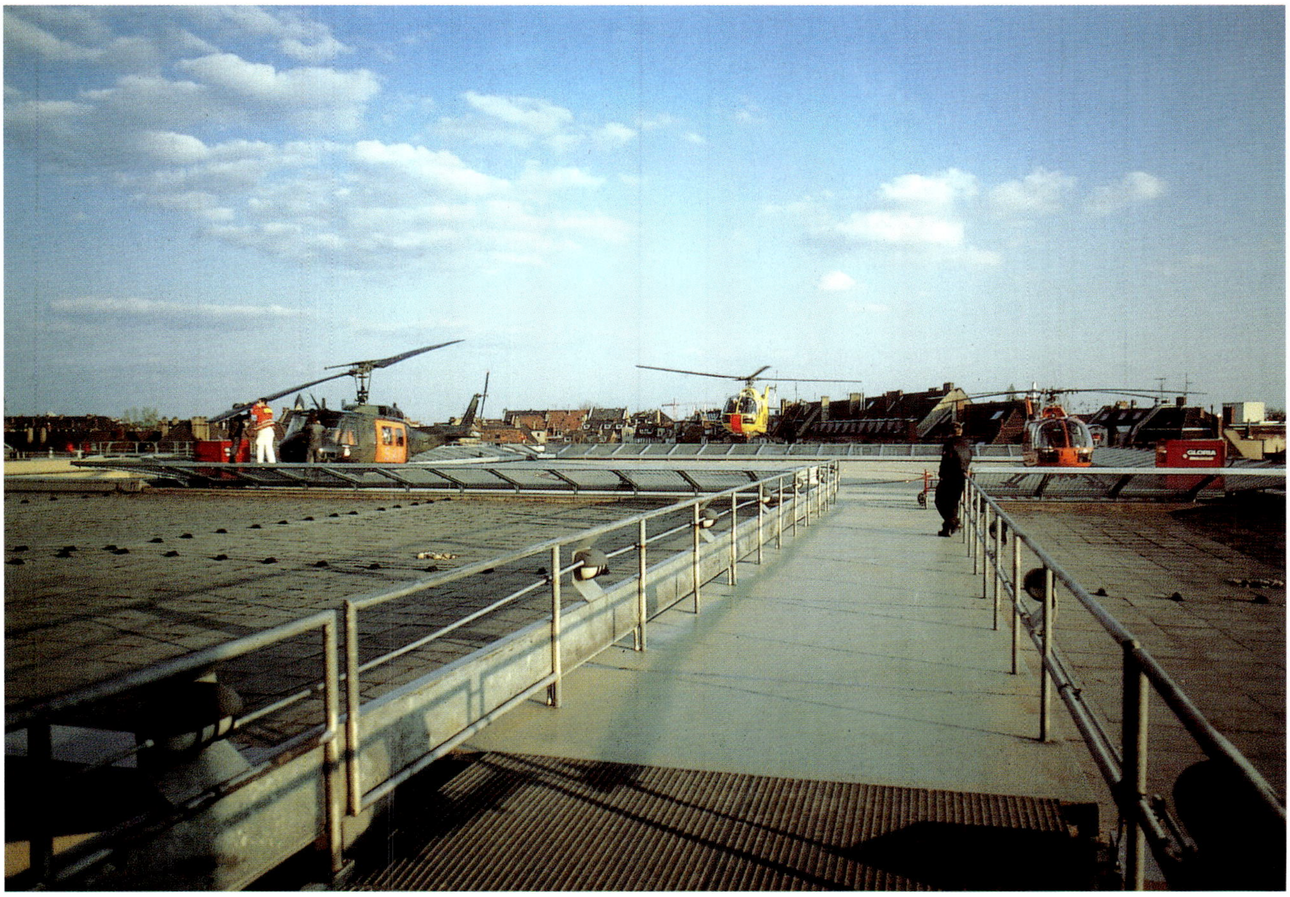
GLORIA

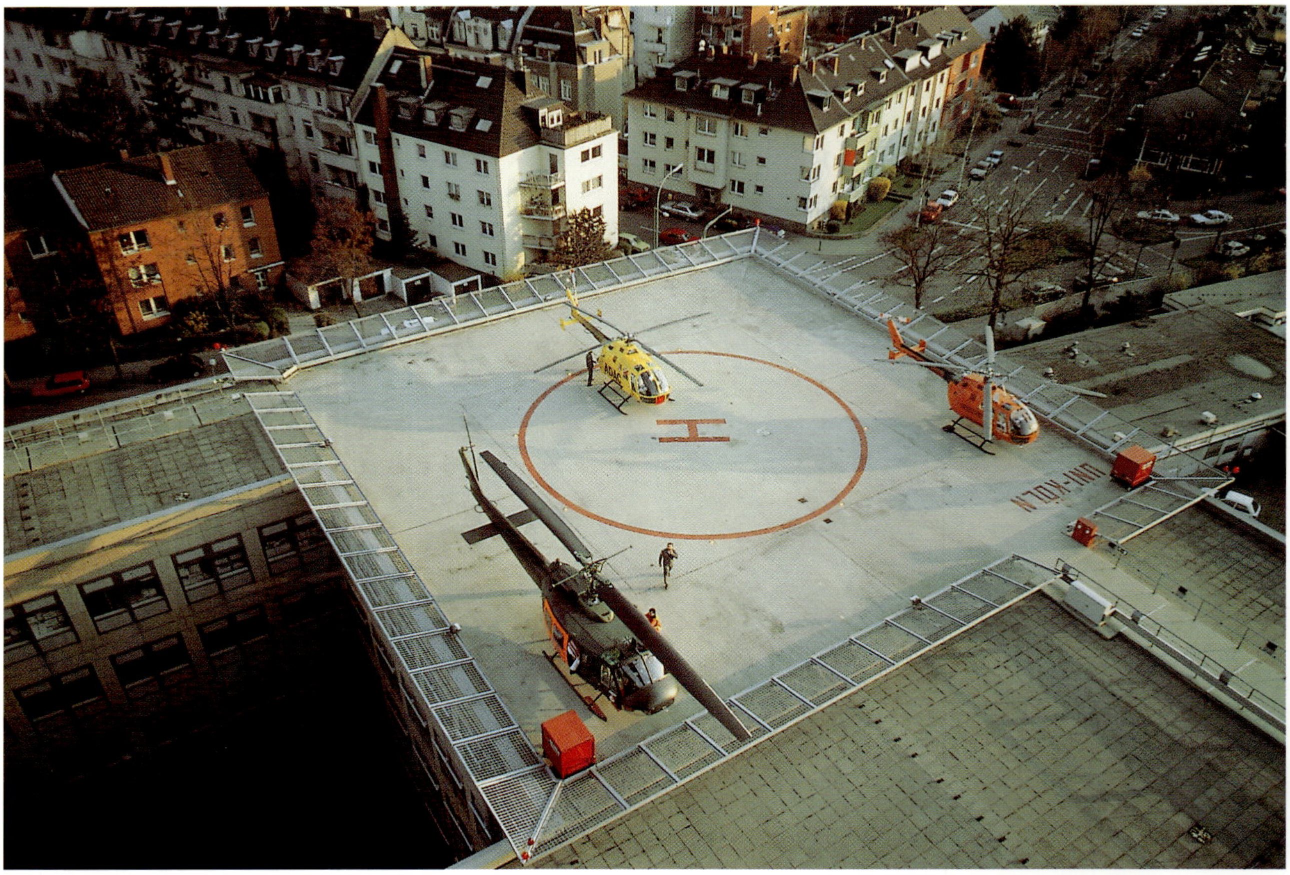

Drei Rettungshubschrauber unterschiedlicher Betreiber friedlich vereint auf dem Dachlandeplatz der Kölner Uni.

Three rescue helicopters, each operated by a different organization, form a harmonious trio on the rooftop heliport of the University Hospital Cologne.

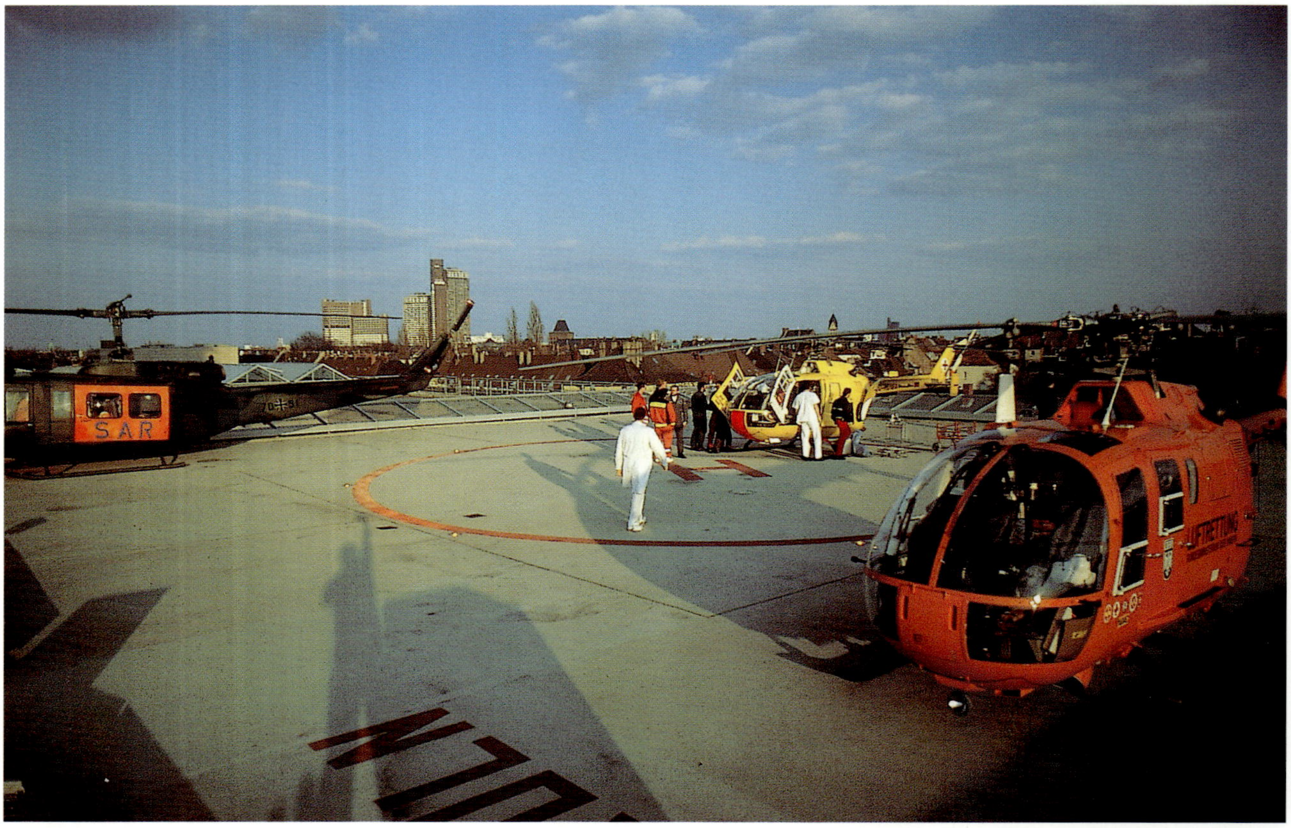

Es bleibt nur kurze Zeit für einen Informationsaustausch und Small Talk.

There's only a few minutes for an exchange of information and some small talk.

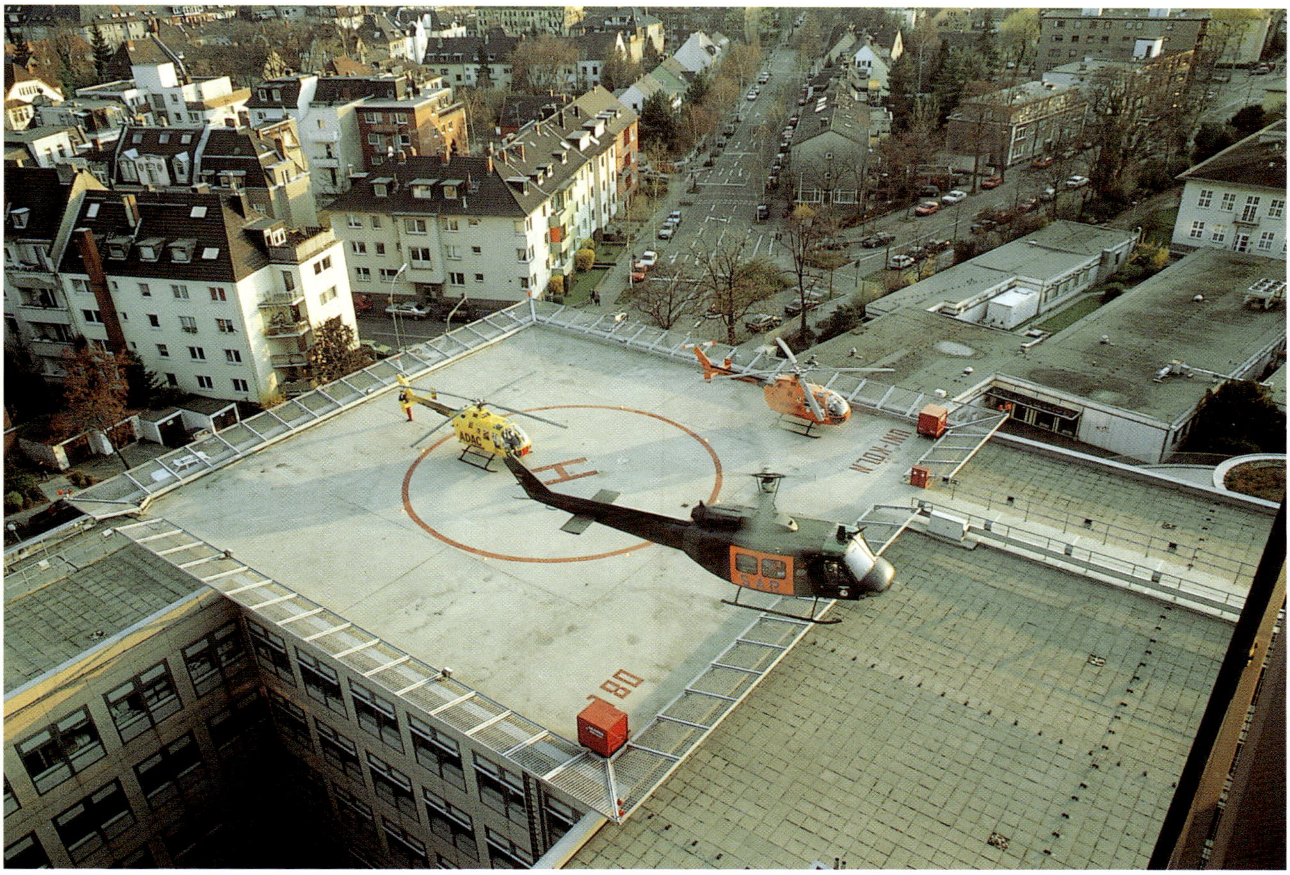

Der neue Einsatz beendet das Gespräch schnell.

An emergency call puts an abrupt end to the conversation.

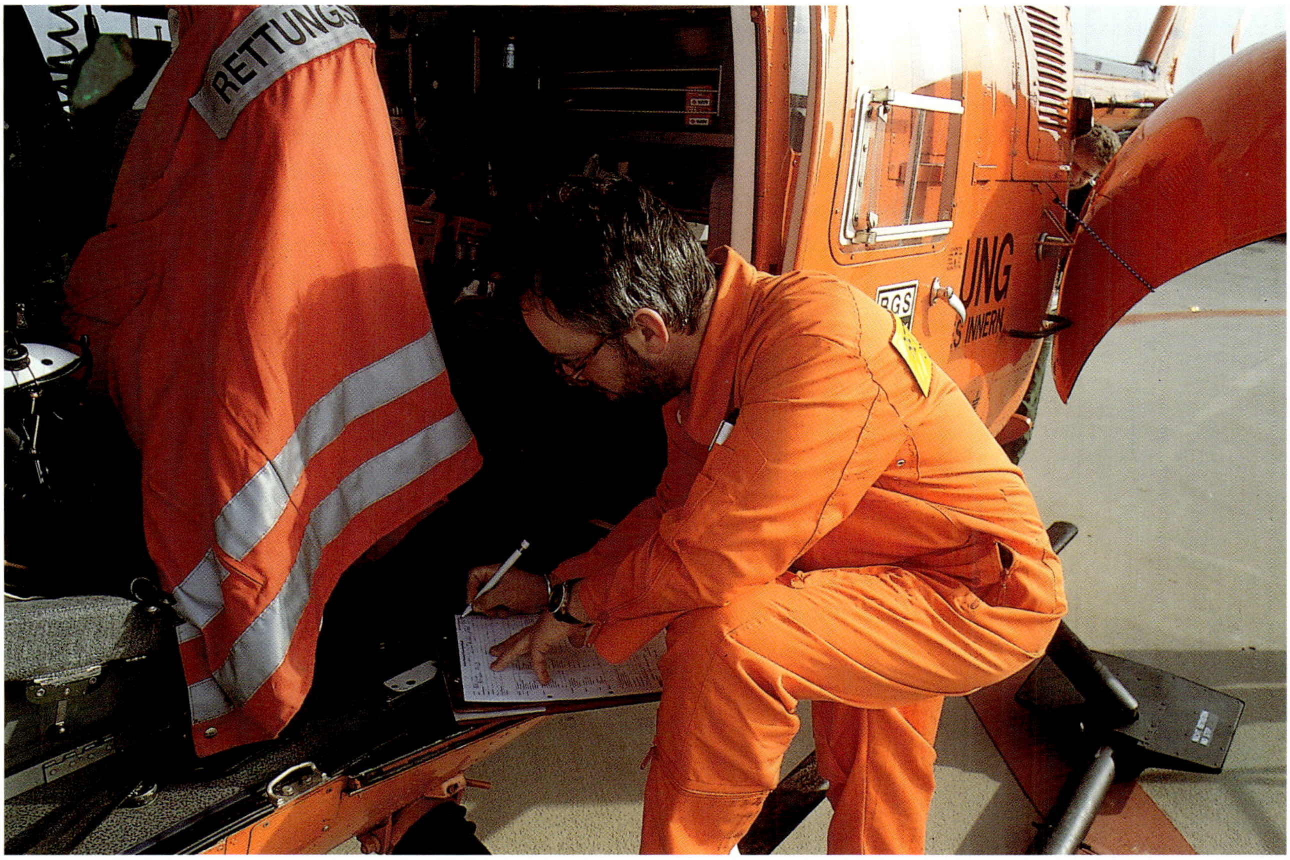

Die Dokumentation wird zu Ende geführt.

The documentation is completed.

Zulassung von Hubschraubern nach JAR 27/29
Certification of Helicopters in Conformance with JAR 27/29

Kategorie A (Cat.A)	Kategorie B (Cat.B)
Mehrmotorige Hubschrauber, ausgestattet mit voneinander unabhängigen Triebwerken und Systemen, die bei Ausfall des kritischen Triebwerkes sicheren Startabbruch oder sichere Fortsetzung des Fluges gewährleisten.	Ein- oder mehrmotorige Hubschrauber, die nicht alle Anforderungen der Kategorie A vollständig erfüllen. Nach einem Triebwerkausfall kann eine Notlandung erforderlich werden.
Category A (Cat.A)	Category B (Cat.B)
Multi-engine helicopters equipped with independent engines and systems to ensure safe abortion of take-off or continuation of the flight in the event of a failure of the critical engine.	Single-engine or multi-engine helicopters which do not completely satisfy all the requirements set for Categroy A. Helicopters in this category may have to make an emergency landing if there is a failure of one engine.

Seit Beginn der 90er Jahre wurden von der Arbeitsgemeinschaft der europäischen Luftfahrtbehörden (Joint Aviation Authorities, JAA) u.a. Betriebsvorschriften für den gewerblichen Transport von Personen und Sachen (Joint Aviation Requirements, JAR-OPS 3) entwickelt. Sie wurden durch die Verordnung des Bundesministeriums für Verkehr, Bau- und Wohnungswesen (BMVBW) mit Wirkung vom 01.10.1998 als „JAR-OPS 3 deutsch" rechtskräftig.

Diese europäische Vorschrift darf keine geringeren Standards definieren, als die international im Rahmen der ICAO vereinbarten. Daher ist die Einführung der ICAO-Standards nunmehr unvermeidlich geworden.

Since the early 1990s the European Joint Aviation Authorities (JAA), among others, have developed operating regulations for the commercial transportation of persons and goods (Joint Aviation Requirements, JAR-OPS 3). These regulations went into law in Germany on 1 Oct. 1998 in the form of an Ordinance issued by the Minister of Transport, Building and Housing (BMVBW) with the name "JAR-OPS 3 German".

This European regulation may not define any standards less stringent than the international standards established within the framework of the ICAO. For this reason, the introduction of the ICAO standards has now become unavoidable.

Die luftrechtliche Situation heute

Mit Einführung von „JAR-OPS 3 deutsch" hat seit Oktober 1998 der gewerbliche Betrieb mit Hubschraubern zur Beförderung von Personen oder Sachen eine neue Grundlage. Auf begründeten Antrag können Luftfahrtunternehmen die Übergangsphase bis zur Anwendung des neuen Luftrechts bis Ende 2001 strecken.

Das Ziel der Gesetzgebung für die Zivilluftfahrt – und damit auch von JAR-OPS 3 – ist, das weiteste Spektrum für den Flugbetrieb bei geringstmöglichem Risiko zu gestatten. Es lohnt der Blick darauf, wer oder was geschützt werden soll:

Present status of aviation law

The "JAR-OPS 3 German" introduced in October 1998 placed the commercial operation of helicopters to transport persons or goods on a new foundation. Operators may extend the transition period between the adoption and implementation of the new law to the end of 2001 by submitting an application containing valid reasons for this extension.

The objective of the new Civil Aviation Law – and thus of JAR-OPS 3 as well – is to permit the broadest possible spectrum of flying operations with the smallest possible risk. In particular, the JAR-OPS 3 protects:

Leistungsklassen für Hubschrauber gem. JAR-OPS 3

Leistungsklasse 1	Leistungsklasse 2	Leistungsklasse 3
Definition: Der Hubschrauber ist in der Lage, bei Ausfall eines Triebwerkes sicher innerhalb der Startabbruchstrecke zu landen oder den Flug zu einer geeigneten Landefläche fortzusetzen.	Definition: Die Leistung des Hubschraubers reicht aus, bei Ausfall eines Triebwerkes den Flug sicher fortzusetzen, jedoch kann in einer frühen Phase des Starts oder im letzten Teil des Anfluges eine Notlandung erforderlich werden.	Definition: Bei einmotorigen Hubschraubern folgt einem Triebwerkausfall eine Notlandung, bei mehrmotorigen Hubschraubern kann eine Notlandung erforderlich werden.
Zulassung nach Cat. A	Zulassung nach Cat. A oder Cat. B; Betrieb entsprechend Cat. A möglich	Zulassung nach Cat. A oder Cat. B
Notwendig für RTH-Station an einem Krankenhaus mit schwierigen Umgebungsbedingungen (keine Notlandelflächen vorhanden)	Notwendig Am Notfallort: Die Phase bis Erreichen der LK 1 soll nur kurz sein.	

Performance Classes for Helicopters in Accordance with JAR-OPS 3

Performance Class 1	Performance Class 2	Performance Class 3
Definition: In the event of the failure of one engine, the helicopter is able to land within the Startabbruchstrecke or to continue the flight to a suitable landing area.	Definition: The performance of the helicopter is sufficient to continue the flight safely in the event of the failure of one engine. However, an emergency landing may be necessary during the early phase of take-off or the late phase of the approach.	Definition: In single-engine helicopters, the failure of one engine necessitates an emergency landing. In multi-engine helicopters, emergency landing may be necessary.
Certification in Category A.	Certification in Category A or Category B Operation in accordance with Category A possible.	Certification in Category A or Category B
Necessary for rescue helicopter stations at a hospital with unfavorable environment conditions (i.e. no emergency landing areas available).	Necessary condition at the emergency site: The phase up to the attainment of Performance Class 1 shall be of only short duration.	

- Dritte (Sachen eingeschlossen),
- Passagiere (Patienten eingeschlossen) und
- Besatzungsmitglieder

Wo sehr viele Starts und Landungen erfolgen – am Betriebsstandort eines RTH (HEMS Operating Base) soll das technische Risiko Null betragen. Hier wird die Leistungsklasse 1 verlangt, wenn schwierige Umgebungsbedingungen herrschen, d.h. in dichtbesiedelten Gebieten ohne ausreichende Notlandeflächen. Am Einsatzort, dort wo der Notfallpatient aufgenommen wird, soll das Risiko so gering sein, wie es in die Praxis umsetzbar ist.

Landeflächen an Krankenhäusern, die nur selten oder gelegentlich angeflogen werden, können wie ein Einsatzort angesehen werden.

JAR-OPS 3 ist – wie bereits erwähnt – eine Betriebsvorschrift, die sich insbesondere an den Luftfahrtunternehmer und den verantwortlichen Luftfahrzeugführer (Piloten) richtet. Daher sucht man in dieser Vorschrift detaillierte Angaben hinsichtlich der baulichen Gestaltung für Hubschrauberflugplätze vergeblich. Die geforderten fliegerischen Verfahren sind jedoch ohne die baulichen Mindeststandards, die in ICAO Anhang 14, Band 2 definiert sind, grundsätzlich nicht zu erfüllen. JAR-OPS 3 und ICAO Anhang 14, Band 2 sind zwei Seiten einer Medaille!

Die Flugverfahren, die von JAR-OPS 3 dargestellt werden, ermöglichen die sichere Notlandung. Wie diese Start- und Landeverfahren im einzelnen exakt definiert sind, ist in der Betriebsanleitung des jeweiligen Hubschraubermusters (rechtlicher Fachbegriff aus der Luftverkehrszulassungsordnung;Hubschraubertyp), dem Flughandbuch (Flight Manual oder auch Rotorcraft Flight Manual) nachzulesen. Alle Hubschrauber, die nach Kategorie A zugelassen sind oder entsprechend betrieben werden können (z.B. EC BO 105 CBS-5), verfügen über ein zusätzliches Kapitel „CAT A-Verfahren“. Diese Verfahren unterscheiden sich hinsichtlich der einzuhaltenden Höhen bzw. Geschwindigkeiten zwischen den einzelnen Hubschraubermustern.

Aufgrund der beschränkten Triebwerks- bzw. Hauptgetriebeleistung und der gleichen aerodynamischen Bedingungen sind die grundsätzlichen Verfahren äußerlich jedoch sehr ähnlich.

Ist der Abflug frei von Hindernissen und sind Notlandeflächen verfügbar, wird bodennah

- third-parties (including goods)
- passengers (including patients)
- crew members.

At any location with a large number of take-offs and landings – e.g. the operating base of a rescue helicopter (HEMS Operating Base) – the technical risk should be equal to zero. Performance Class 1 is required at all locations with difficult or "hostile" conditions, e.g. in congested areas with insufficient emergency landing areas. At the emergency site itself, i.e. the site where the patient is loaded into the helicopter, the risk should be kept as low as is possible under emergency operating conditions.

Landing areas at hospitals with only infrequent rescue helicopter landings can be viewed as HEMS Operating Sites. As has already been mentioned, JAR-OPS 3 is a set of operating regulations aimed, in particular, at operators and pilots. As a result, these regulations do not contain any information on the structural design of heliports. However, the required aviation procedures cannot be carried out without the minimum structural standards defined in ICAO, Annex 14, Vol. 2. JAR-OPS 3 and ICAO, Annex 14, Vol. 2 are two sides of the coin!

Flight operations described in JAR-OPS 3 make safe emergency landings possible. Precise definitions of the individual take-off and landing procedures can be found in the operating instructions for the particular helicopter type, the Flight Manual or Rotorcraft Flight Manual. All manuals for helicopters which have been certificated for Category A – or which can be operated in accordance with Category A (e.g. EC BO 105 CBS-5) – have an additional chapter on „CAT A Procedures“. The procedures prescribed for the different types or classes of helicopters differ with respect to the speeds or altitudes to be maintained.

However, owing to the limited power of the engine or main gearbox and the uniform aerodynamic conditions, the basic procedures are externally very similar. If there are no obstacles impeding take-off and emergency landing areas are available, the helicopter accelerates close to the ground and then continues its departure at the safe take-off speed until it attains the best speed for climbing. It continues to climb at this speed (Vy ~ 60-70 kt) until it has reached the minimum safety height.

beschleunigt und mit der sicheren Startgeschwindigkeit weiter gestiegen, bis die Geschwindigkeit für bestes Steigen erreicht wird. Nun wird mit dieser Geschwindigkeit (Vy ~ 60-70 kt) der Abflug bis zur Sicherheitsmindesthöhe fortgesetzt.

Tritt vor Erreichen der sicheren Startgeschwindigkeit ein Leistungsverlust in einem Triebwerk ein, wird der Start auf den Notlandeflächen sicher abgebrochen. Erfolgt eine Triebwerkstörung nach Überschreiten dieser Geschwindigkeit, entscheidet der Pilot, ob er den Flug zu einem geeigneten Flugplatz fortsetzt oder den Flug sofort beendet.

Der Landeanflug erfolgt sinngemäß in umgekehrter Reihenfolge. Ist jedoch dann die Geschwindigkeit für den sicheren Start bereits unterschritten, wird eine Notlandung unvermeidlich.

Wird der Startplatz von Hindernissen umschlossen (Confined Area) oder sind Notlandeflächen nicht vorhanden, müssen die Startverfahren so ausgeführt werden, dass bei Triebwerkleistungsverlust die sichere Notlandung auf dem Startplatz möglich wird. Nach der Kontrolle der verfügbaren Leistung und der ordnungsgemäßen Funktion aller Systeme im Schwebeflug in einer Höhe von ca. 3 Metern über Grund steigt der Pilot gegen den Wind rückwärts auf bis zu einer Höhe von ca. 60 Metern über dem Startplatz bzw. oberhalb der Hindernisse. Die Länge der Rückwärtsbewegung ist u.a. abhängig von den Sichtverhältnissen des Piloten nach vorn unten. Er muss ständig Sichtverbindung zu seinem möglichen Notlandeplatz behalten. Ereignet sich vor Erreichen der Entscheidungshöhe eine Störung, wird der Startvorgang abgebrochen. Ist dieser Punkt bereits passiert worden, wird der Startvorgang fortgesetzt.

Die Startverfahren für Dachlandeplätze sind vom Ablauf her sehr ähnlich. Die Landeverfahren verlaufen wiederum sinngemäß in umgekehrter Reihenfolge.

Häufig wird die Frage gestellt, warum die Hubschrauber denn nicht senkrecht starten und landen würden. Dann könne man doch auch die Hindernisse außer Betracht lassen! Die Antwort: Technisch gesehen können Hubschrauber senkrecht starten. Nach Flughandbuch bewegt sich der Pilot dann jedoch in einem zu vermeidenden oder verbotenen Bereich. Weder ist dann eine sichere Einmotorenlandung noch eine Autorotation möglich. Beim Landeanflug besteht zusätz-

If a loss of power occurs in one engine before the helicopter has reached this safe take-off speed, take-off is safely aborted on the emergency landing area. If an engine failure occurs after this speed has been reached, the pilot makes the decision to continue the flight to a suitable heliport or to terminate the flight immediately. The approach flight is carried out, not surprisingly, in the reverse order. If the helicopter has already fallen below the speed for safe take-off, however, an emergency landing is unavoidable.

If the take-off site is in a confined area, i.e. enclosed by obstacles, or if emergency landing areas are not available, the take-off procedure must be carried out in a way ensuring that a safe emergency landing can be made on the take-off area in the event of a loss of engine power. After determining the engine power available and checking the correct functioning of all systems while hovering approx. 3 meters above the ground, the pilot ascends backwards against the wind to a height of approx. 60 meters above the take-off site or the obstacles. The length of the backwards movement depends on several factors, including the pilot's visibility in front of the aircraft. The pilot must maintain constant visual contact with a possible emergency landing site. If a malfunction occurs before the craft reaches the decision height, the take-off procedure is terminated. If the pilot has already flown past the decision height, the take-off procedure is continued.

The take-off procedures to be followed in rooftop heliports are very similar. The landing procedure is carried out, as one might expect, in the reverse order.

Helicopter pilots are frequently asked why helicopters cannot take off and land vertically since this would eliminate the problem of obstacles! The answer is: technically, helicopters are able to take off vertically. According to the Flight Manual, however, a pilot who takes off vertically moves into a prohibited sector or a sector that should be avoided. In this sector neither safe single-engine landing nor autorotation is possible. During a vertical approach to landing, there is the additional danger that the helicopter will suck up its own rotor wash and end up in a vortex ring. In this situation, a flight accident is inevitable. Since a safe emergency landing is the main prerequisite for flight operations in con-

lich die Gefahr, die eigene verwirbelte Luft erneut anzusaugen und in das Wirbelringstadium (Vortex Ring) zu geraten. Ein Flugunfall ist dann unvermeidlich. Weil die Voraussetzung für den Flugbetrieb nach JAR-OPS 3 die sichere Notlandung ist, bleiben senkrechte Start- und Landeverfahren daher ausgeschlossen!

Da mehr als 90 % der an Krankenhäusern vorhandenen Landemöglichkeiten in Deutschland den ICAO-Standard heute nicht erfüllen, sind weitergehende Erleichterungen notwendig, um die Zwecke der Luftrettung nicht zu gefährden.

Die meisten häufig angeflogenen Krankenhäuser liegen in dicht besiedelten Gebieten, wo geeignete Notlandeflächen nicht verfügbar sind. Vorhandene Bauwerke können nicht entfernt werden. Deshalb wurden für die Luftrettung durch das Helicopter Subcommittee JAR-OPS 3, das mit Spezialisten aus zahlreichen Ländern das Regelwerk fortentwickelt, folgende Erleichterungen vorgesehen:

- Einführung eines „kritischen Zeitraumes" (Exposure Time Concept),bei dem die Ausfallwahrscheinlichkeit eines Triebwerks aufgrund der nachgewiesenen Zuverlässigkeit unberücksichtigt bleiben kann und
- Einführung von Landeplätzen, die ausschließlich öffentlicher Widmung unterliegen (Public sites; z.B: Krankenhauslandeplätze).

Derartige Landeflächen werden – wo Hindernisse nicht entfernt werden können – zumindest den Standard der alten deutschen Richtlinie zu erfüllen haben. Eine Arbeitsgruppe des Bundesministeriums für Verkehr, Bau- und Wohnungswesen, der Luftfahrtbehörden der Länder, des Ausschusses Rettungswesen und von weiteren Experten wird Kriterien hierfür definieren. Hubschrauber, die entsprechend Kategorie A betrieben werden können, werden für einen angemessenen Übergangszeitraum auch weiterhin in der Luftrettung eingesetzt werden können.

Anforderungen an Landeplätze

Die wesentlichen Kriterien für Landeplätze sind wie folgt:

Start- und Landefläche:
Größe 35x35 Meter, mindestens ca. 25x25 Meter inklusive Sicherheitsstreifen; Tragfähigkeit: Grundsätzlich 10 t, mindestens 6 t, Höchstabflugmasse (MTOM)

formance with JAR-OPS 3, vertical take-off and landing procedures continue to be prohibited!

Since more than 90 % of present landing sites at hospitals in Germany do not satisfy the ICAO Standard, more extensive measures are necessary to avoid jeopardizing the aims of air rescue.

Most of the hospitals with frequent helicopter landings are located in congested areas where suitable emergency landing areas are not available. Moreover, existing structures cannot be torn down. For this reason, the experts from many different countries on the Helicopter Subcommittee JAR-OPS 3, which is revising this standard, has foreseen the following alleviations:

- introduction of an "exposure time concept" – during the exposure time the probability of engine failure can be disregarded on the basis of the demonstrated reliability
- introduction of landing areas reserved exclusively for public helicopter services (e.g. hospital heliports).

Landing areas of this kind – where obstacles cannot be removed – will have to satisfy at least the standards contained in the older German guidelines. A working party containing representatives from the Ministry of Transport, Building and Housing, the civil aviation authorities of the German states, the Ministry of the Interior and the Ministry of Social Affairs and other experts, will define the criteria to be used for this purpose. Helicopters which can be operated according to Category A will be allowed to carry out air rescue flights during a suitable transition period.

Requirements for heliports

The main criteria for heliports are given below:

Final approach and Take-Off Area (FATO):
35x35 m (at least 25x25 m), inclusive safety area;
Load baring capacity: 10 t (at least 6 t)
Maximum take-off mass (MTOM)

Departure sectors:
Normally at least two, must take account of main wind directions, angle of climb to clear obstacles in the departure sectors: 4.5 %.

Abflugsektoren:
Grundsätzlich mindestens zwei, Hauptwindrichtung berücksichtigt; zulässiger Steigwinkel von Hindernissen in den Abflugsektoren maximal 4,5%.

Anforderungen an Landemöglichleiten am Einsatzort

JAR-OPS 3 fordert hinsichtlich der Landestelle am Notfallort nur das, was auch heute möglich ist. Der Hindernisabstand soll ausreichend sein. Grundsätzlich soll die Landestelle nicht kleiner als zweimal die größte Länge des Referenzhubschraubers im Quadrat sein.

Sollten Landungen in der Dunkelheit erfolgen, erhöht sich die Länge der Landestelle auf viermal die größte Länge. Daraus ergibt sich für einen großen RTH eine Länge mal Breite von ca. 70 x 35 Metern.

Praktische Umsetzung

Mehr als 90 % der heute in Deutschland vorhandenen Landemöglichkeiten an Krankenhäusern erfüllen nicht die Anforderungen von ICAO 14 Anhang bzw. von JAR-OPS 3. Daher müssen in Abstimmung mit der örtlich zuständigen Luftfahrtbehörde die Landestellen durch Sachverständige geprüft und die Abweichungen dokumentiert werden. Hindernisse sind zu entfernen wo dies möglich ist. Bei ungeeigneten Plätzen ist zu prüfen, ob alternative Landemöglichkeiten (z.B: Rasensportplätze) in der Nähe verfügbar sind. Die Übergangsregelungen, die JAR-OPS 3 für Krankenhauslandeplätze bietet, sind zu nutzen.

Zur Hilfeleistung bei Gefahr für Leib und Leben eines Notfallpatienten dürfen heute vorhandene Landemöglichkeiten auch in Zukunft angeflogen werden.

Fazit für die Praxis

Die Einführung eines harmonisierten europäischen Luftrechts für gewerblichen Personentransport mit Hubschraubern führt auch in der Luftrettung zu deutlichen Veränderungen und insbesondere zu einem erhöhten Sicherheitsstandard. Neue Flugverfahren bei Start und Landung entsprechend den Flugleistungsklassen 1 und 2 machen die Bestandsaufnahme der

Requirements for possible landing sites at the HEMS operating site

With respect to the landing site at the scene of the emergency, the requirements set down in JAR-OPS 3 do not go beyond what is possible today. Obstacle clearance should be sufficient. The dimensions of the landing site should basically be at least twice the largest dimension of the reference helicopter squared.

For night landings, the length of the landing site is increased to four times the longest dimension. For a large rescue helicopter, this is equal to a landing site with dimensions of approx. 70 x 35 m.

Practical implementation

More than 90 % of the hospital heliports now in use in Germany do not satisfy the requirements contained in ICAO, Annex 14 or JAR-OPS 3. For this reason, these landing sites must be inspected by appointed experts in cooperation with the local aviation authorities; non-conformities must be documented. Obstacles are to be removed where possible. Moreover, a search should be made for alternative landing sites (e.g. grassy athletic fields) in the vicinity of unsuitable landing areas. Rescue helicopter services should take advantages of the transitional provisions of JAR-OPS 3 for hospital heliports.

To provide emergency assistance in situations where human life and health are endangered, rescue helicopters will, in the future, continue to be able to fly to the heliports that are available today.

Practical implications in summary

The introduction of harmonized aviation law throughout Europe will have a pronounced impact on the commercial transport of persons by helicopter. In the field of air rescue, moreover, it will result in sweeping changes and higher safety standards. New flight procedures during take-off and landing in the Performance Classes 1 and 2 urgently require a critical evaluation of the procedures followed to date. In the future, helicopters will no longer be able to use all of the hospital landing sites in service today. A critical risk assessment should be conducted at all older heliports. JAR-OPS 3 is a

bisherigen Verfahren unumgänglich. Nicht alle bisher genutzten Landemöglichkeiten an Krankenhäusern können auch zukünftig angeflogen werden. Im Sinne einer Risikoabschätzung sind alte Landemöglichkeiten kritisch zu prüfen. JAR-OPS 3 ist eine Vorschrift, die mehr als fünf Jahrzehnte unterschiedlicher Entwicklungen von nationalem Luftrecht für ein vereintes Europa zusammenfasst.

Schon heute hat JAR-OPS 3 den Flugsicherheitsstandard für Flugbetrieb mit zivilen Hubschraubern in Europa wesentlich verbessert.

standard combining more than five decades of non-uniform development of national aviation law for a united Europe. Today JAR-OPS 3 has already brought about substantial improvements in the safety standards for flight operations with civillian helicopters in Europe.

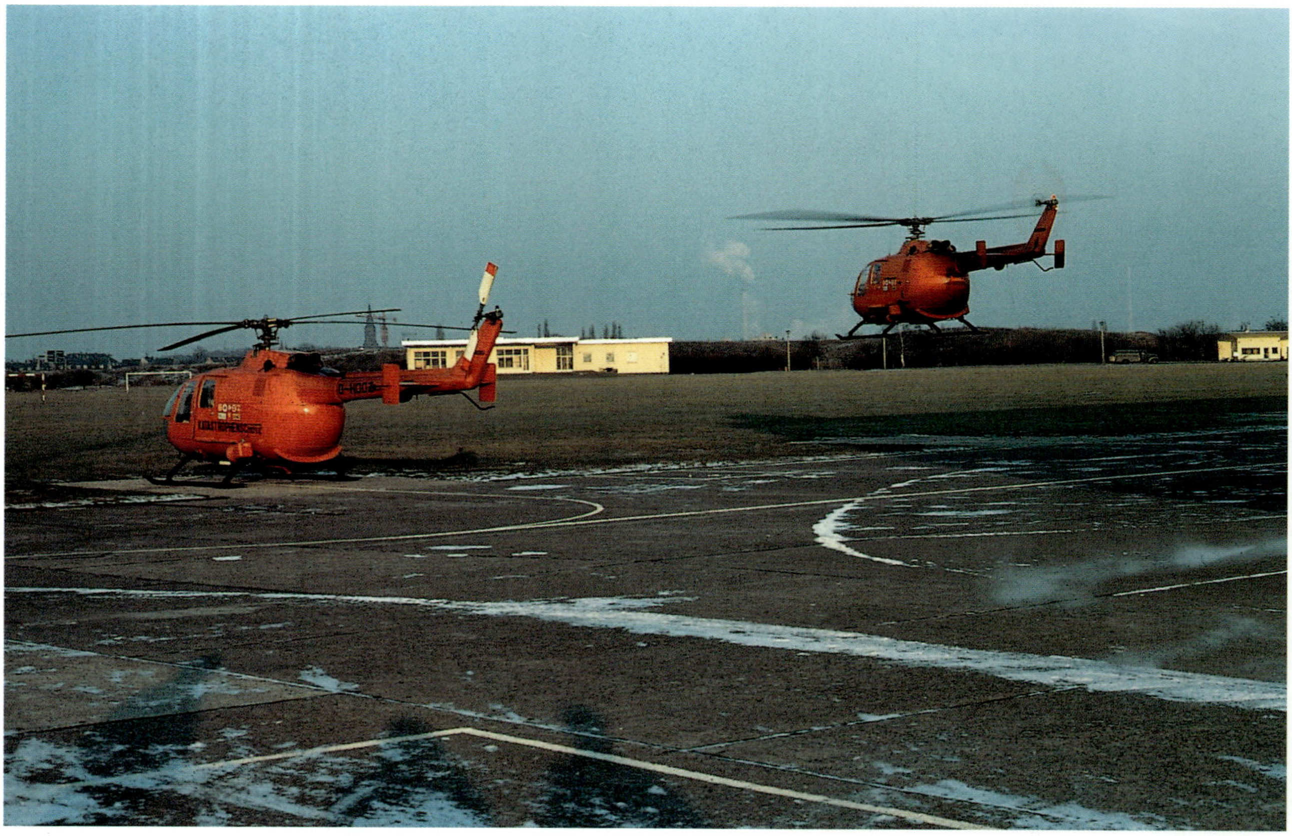

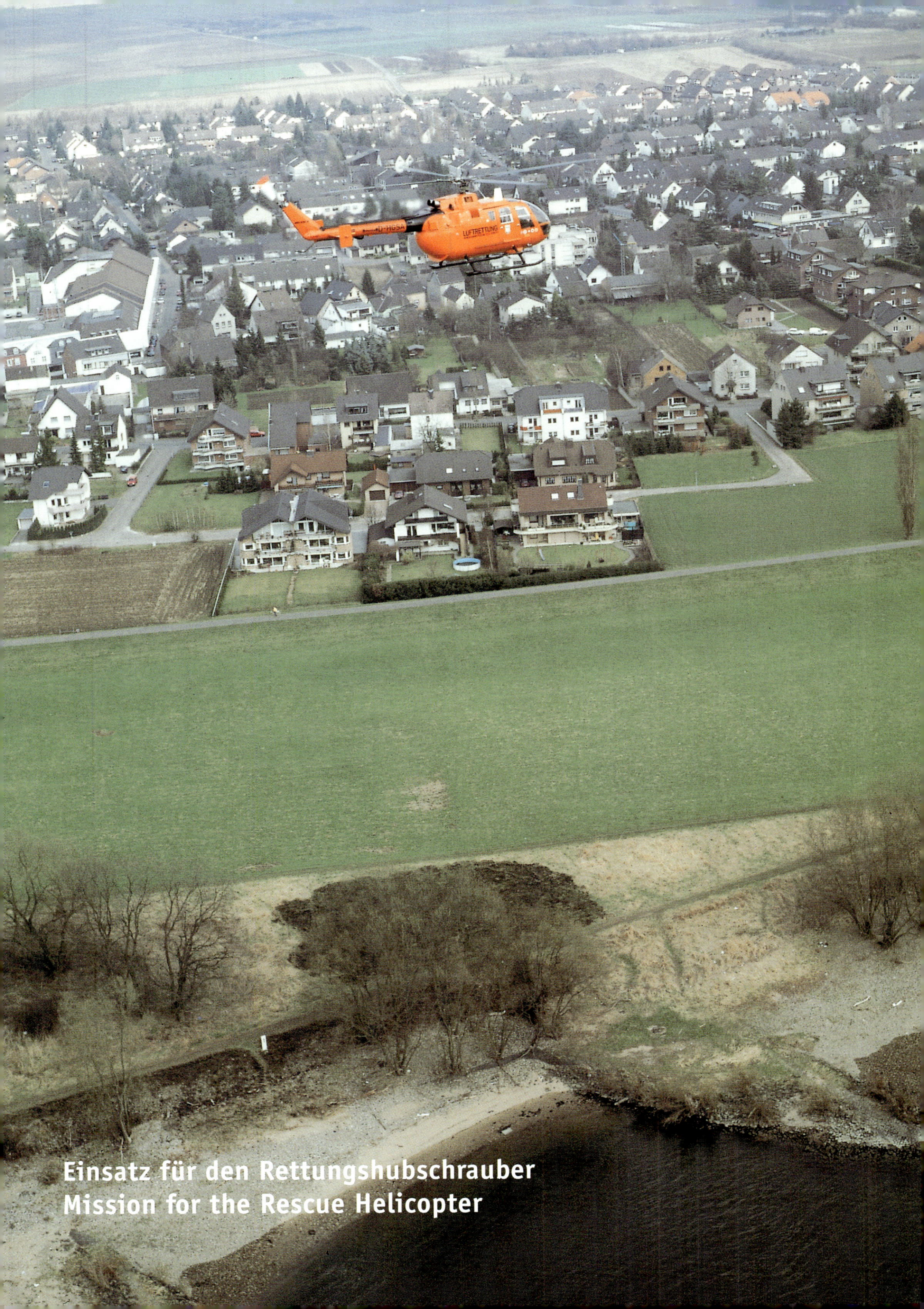

Einsatz für den Rettungshubschrauber
Mission for the Rescue Helicopter

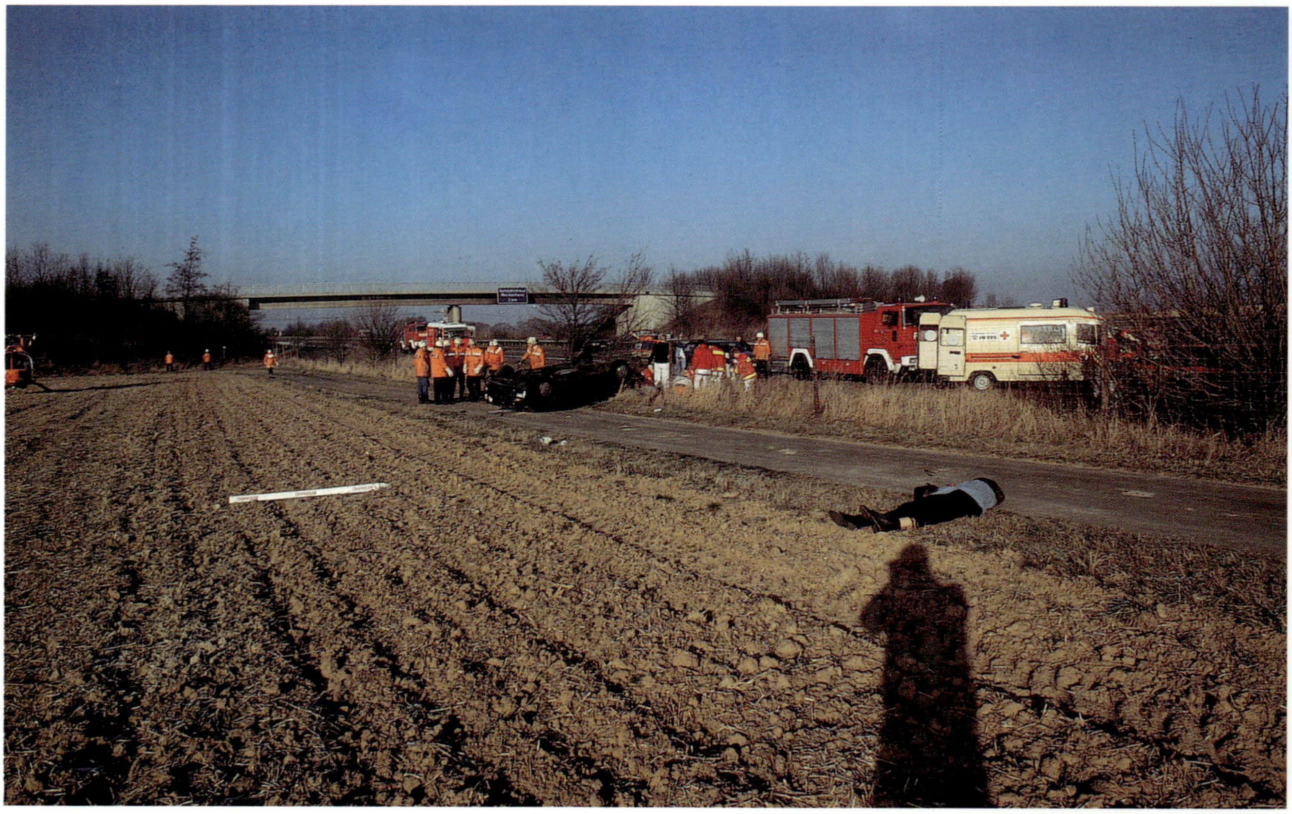

PKW überschlagen, Personen eingeklemmt.

Im Anflug auf die Einsatzstelle kommen weitere Erklärungen. Eine Person ist aus dem Fahrzeug geschleudert worden. Weitere Erklärungen vom bodengebundenen Notarzt. Zwei Personen sind bereits tot. Weitere Rückmeldung: Dritte Person ist schwer verletzt, müsste in die Neurochirurgie transportiert werden.

An automobile has turned over; several persons are trapped inside.

During the approach, the crew receives additional information. One person has been thrown out of the vehicle. An additional bulletin from the physician with emergency & rescue certification on the ground: two people are already dead. Another report: a third person has serious injuries and had to be transported to a hospital with a neurosurgery department.

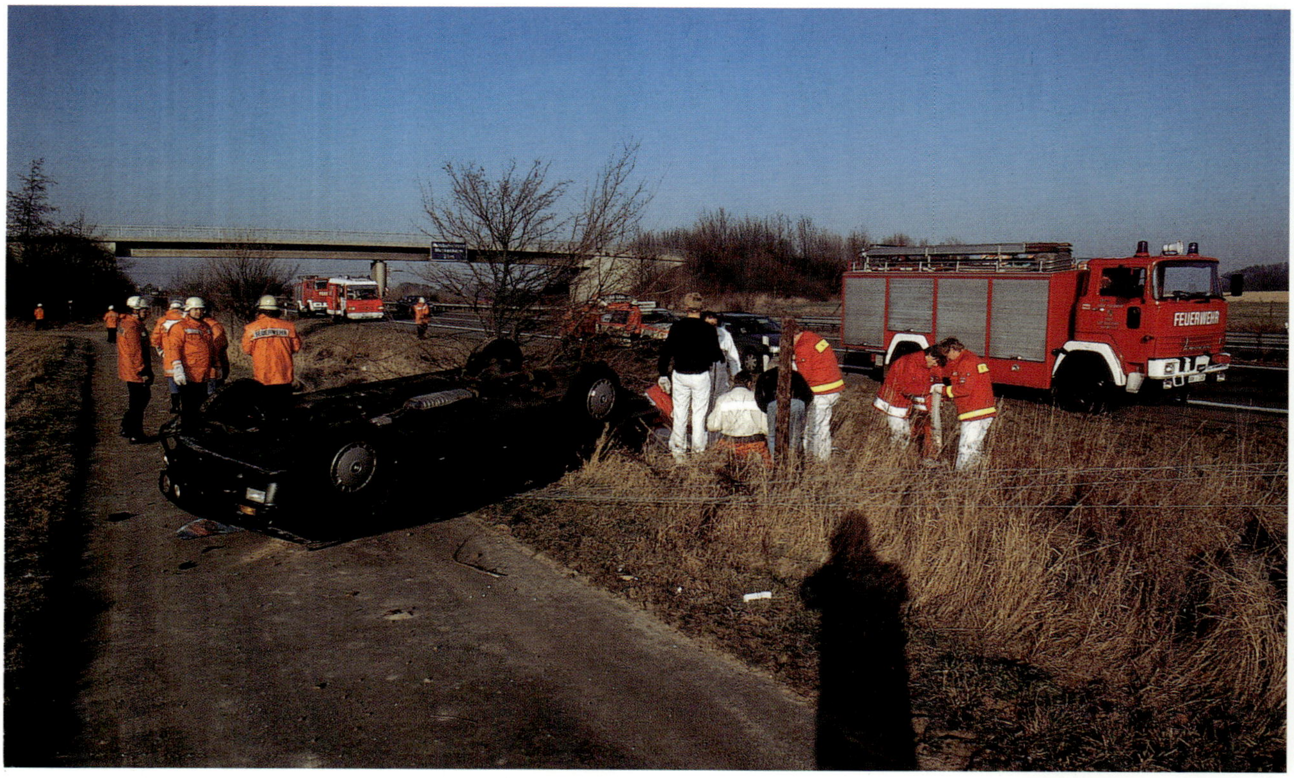

Einsatz für den Rettungshubschrauber
Mission for the Rescue Helicopter

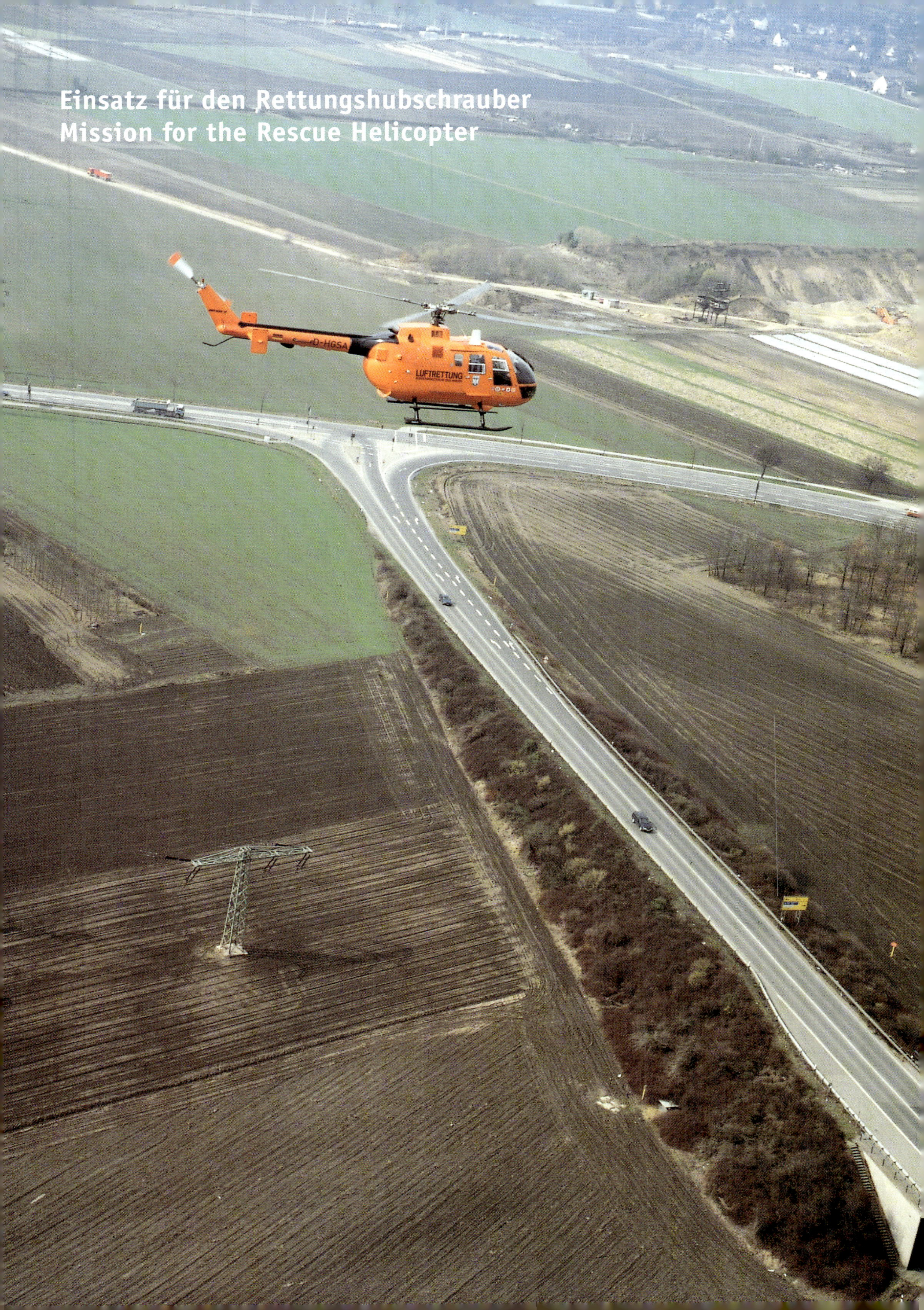

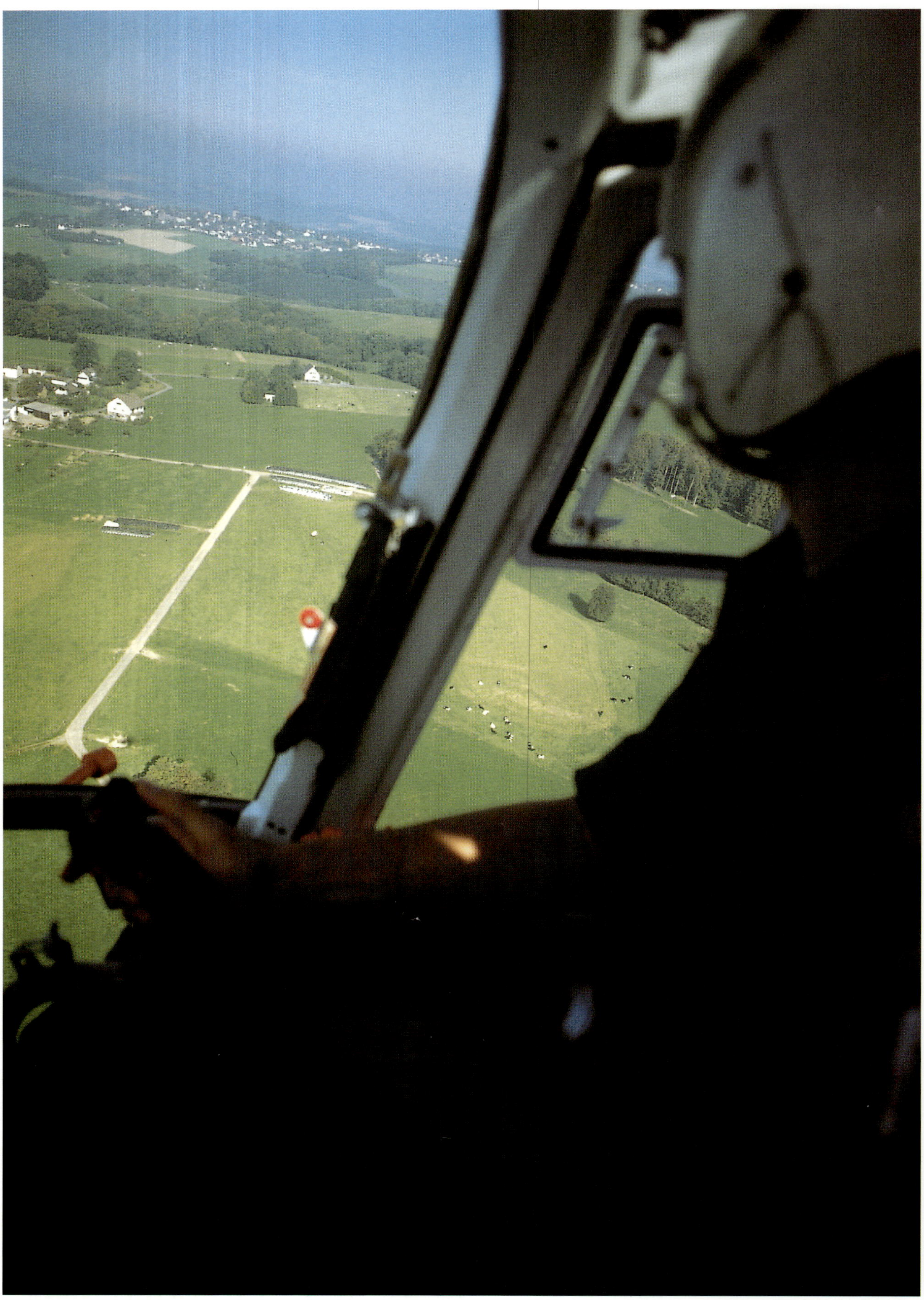

Im Anflug auf die Einsatzstelle der Blick zur Pilotenseite des Cockpits hinaus.

The view from the cockpit on the pilot's side during the approach to the accident site.

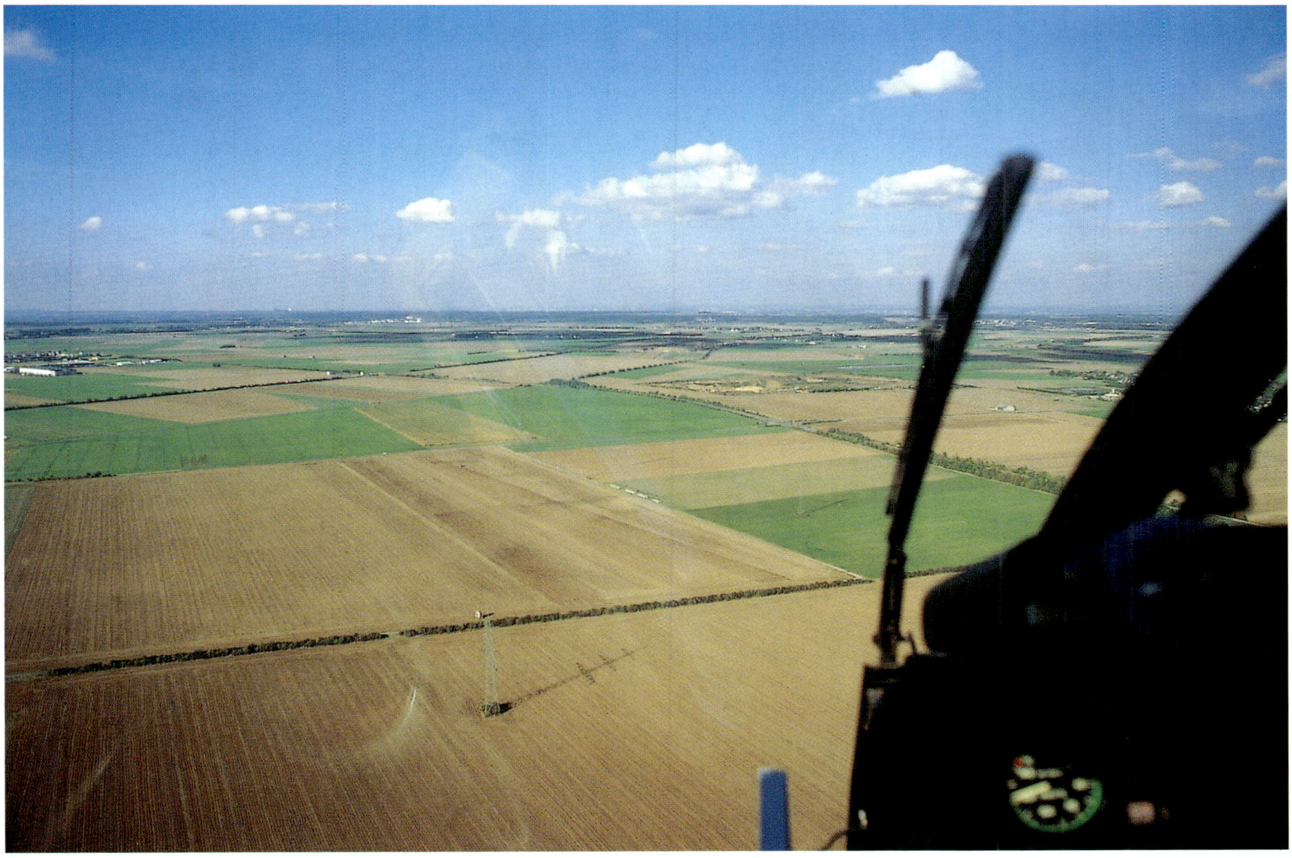

Im Anflug auf die Einsatzstelle der Blick aus der Rettungsassistentensicht.

The view from the cockpit on the paramedic's side during the approach to the accident site.

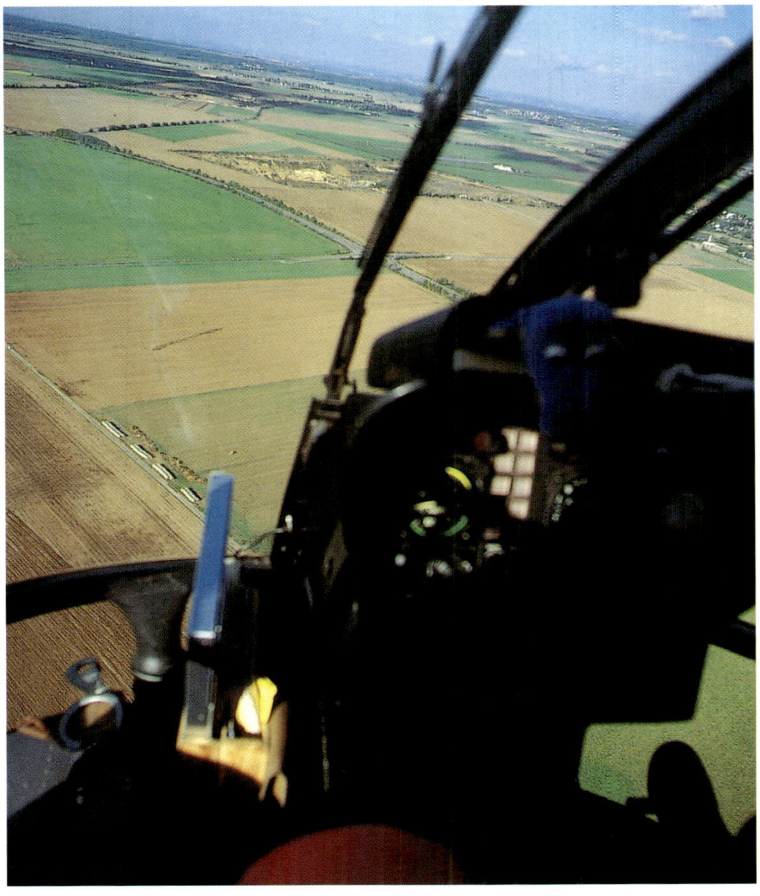

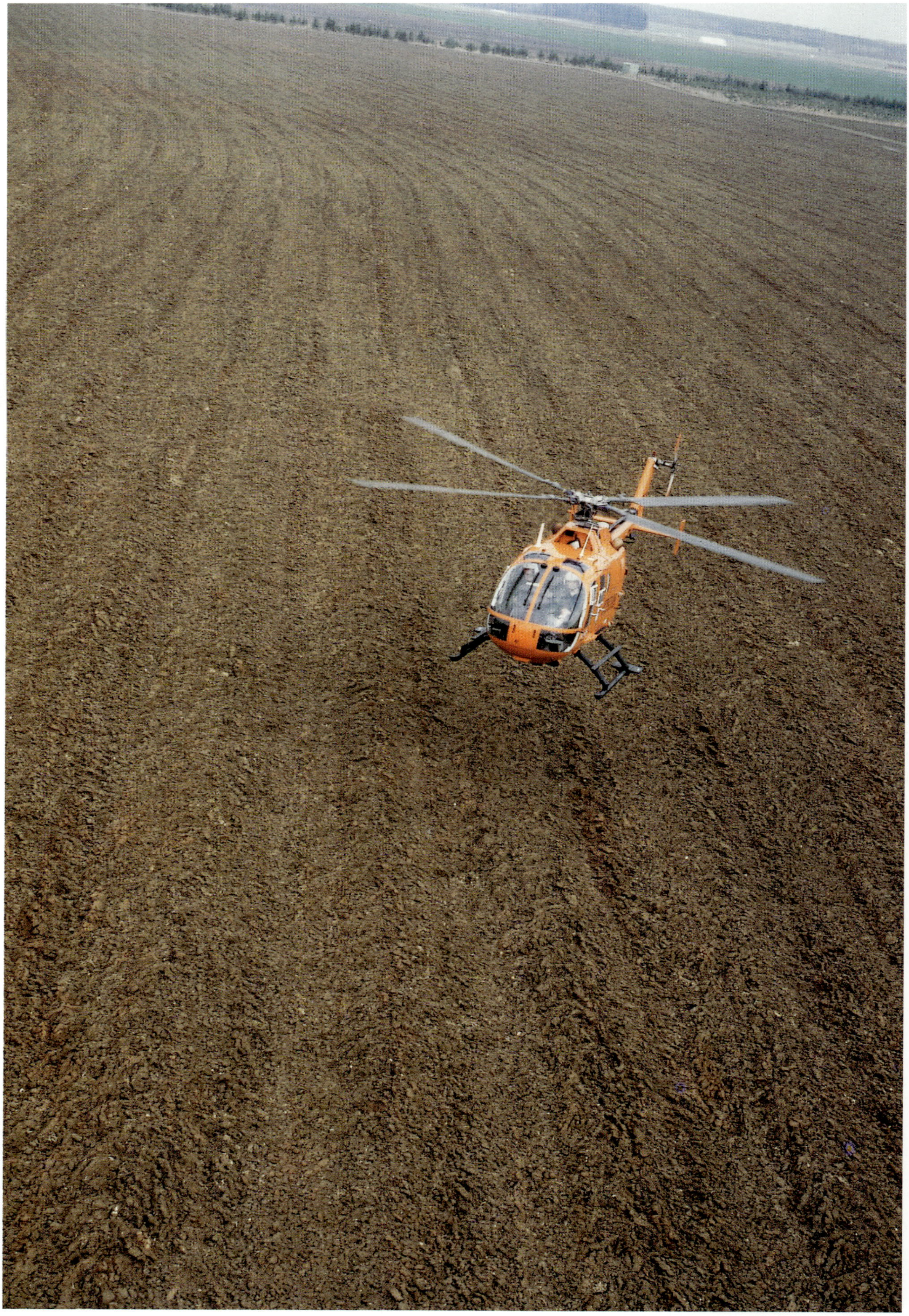

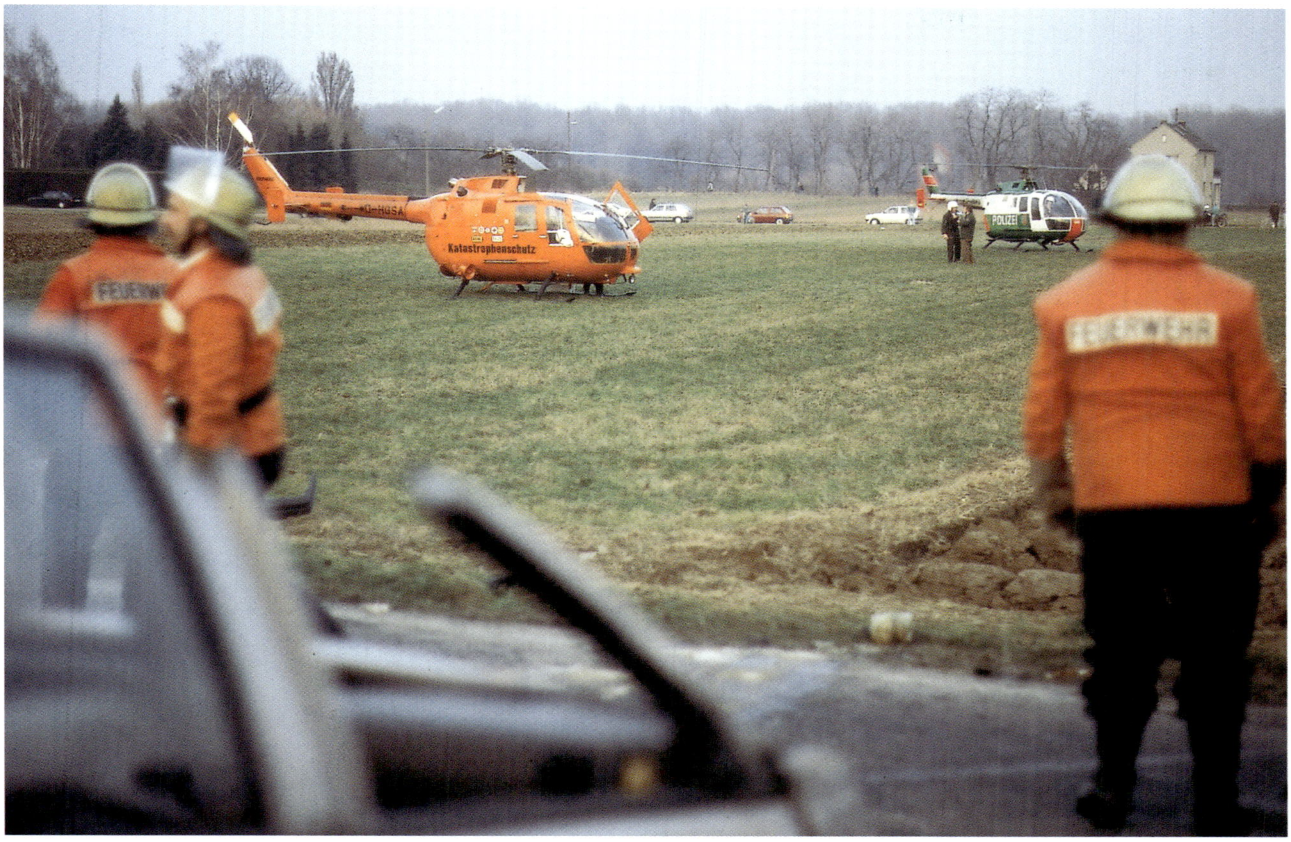

Ein PKW ist mit einem anderen zusammengestoßen. Two cars have collided.

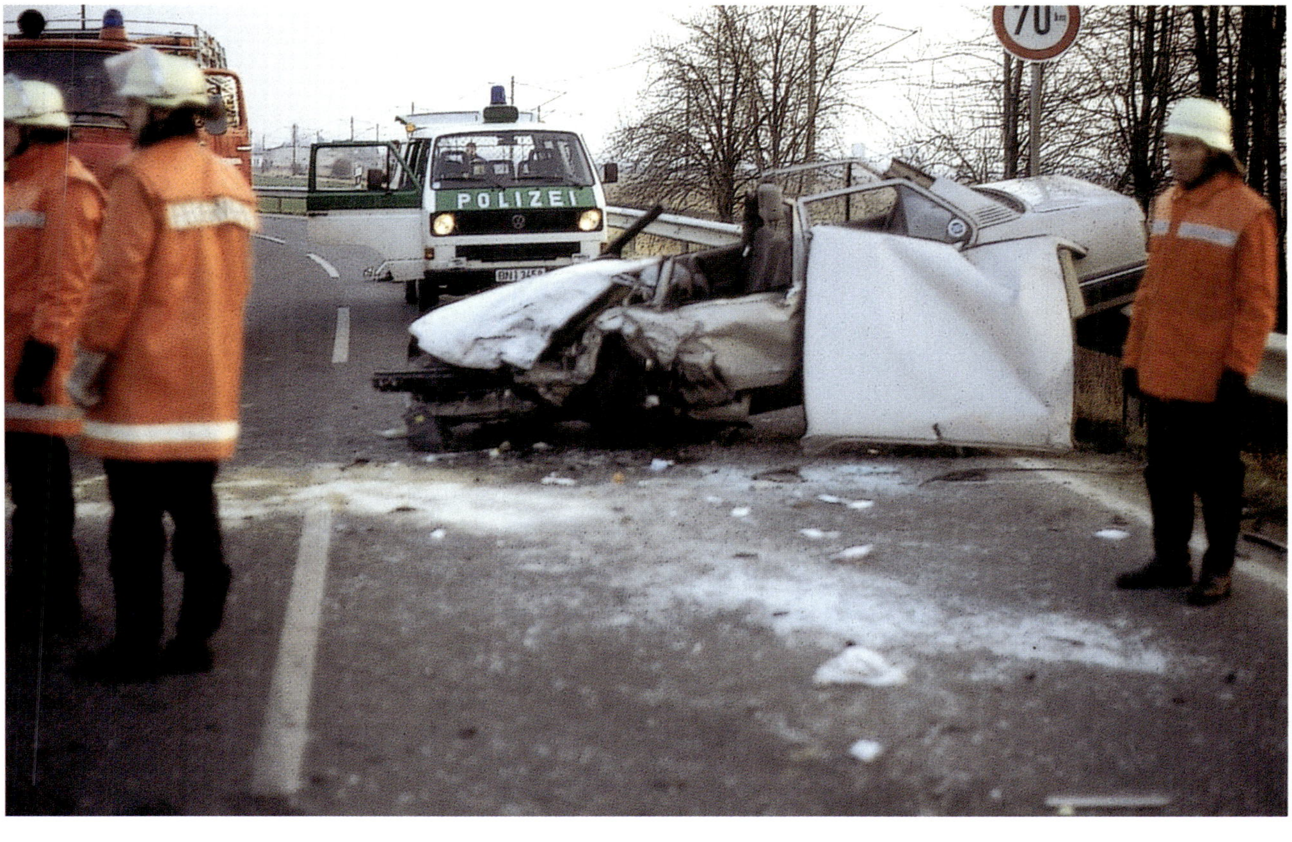

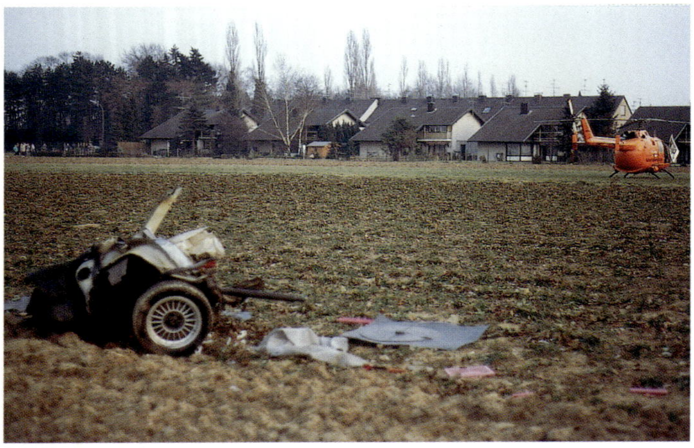

Die Gewalt war so stark, dass der PKW auseinandergerissen wurde.

The force of the impact has ripped the car apart.

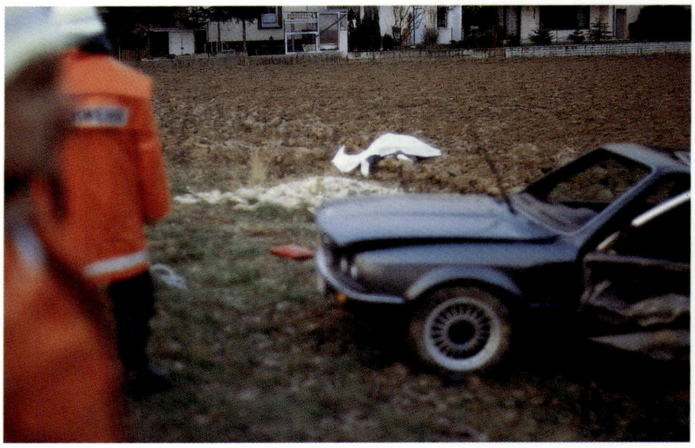

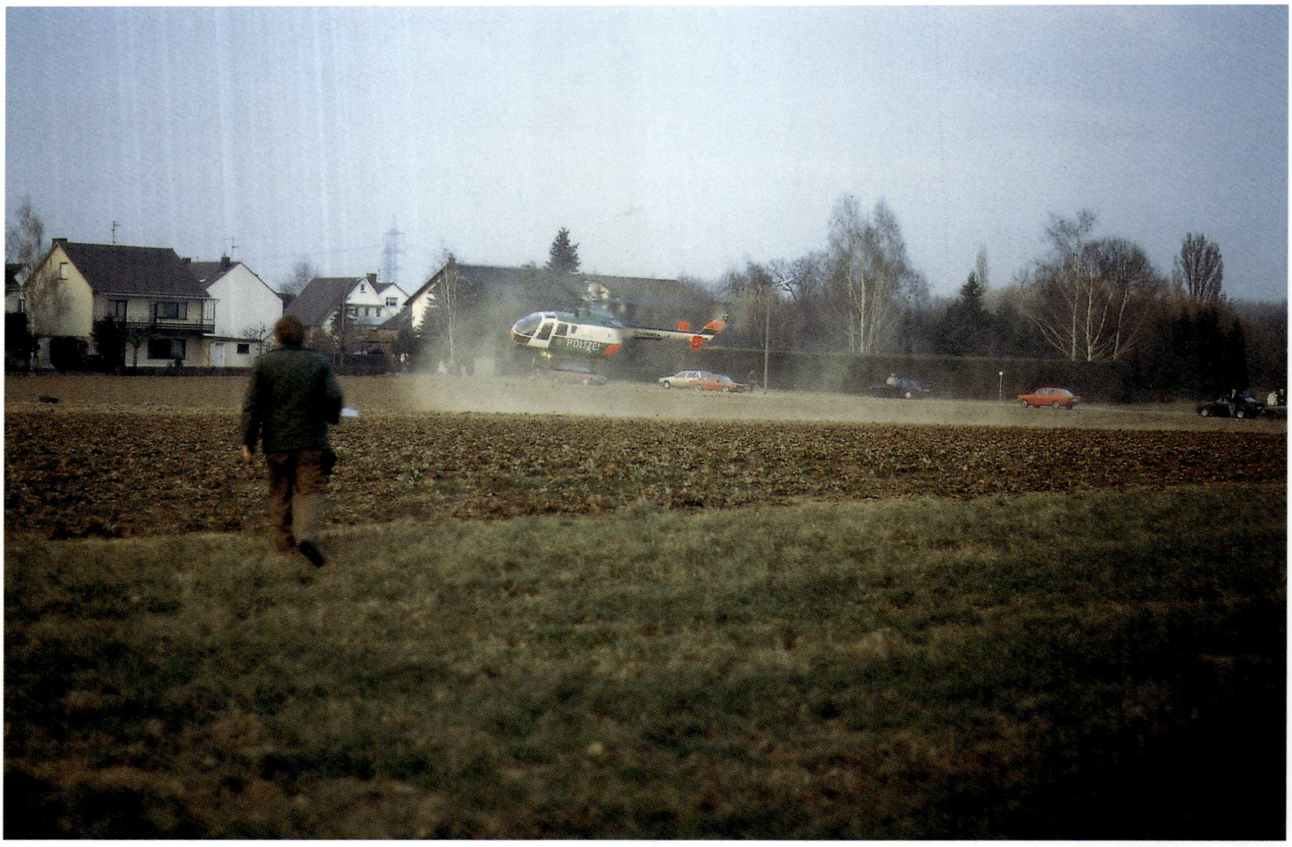

Ein Polizeihubschrauber, der bei der Suche geholfen hat, landet ebenfalls.

A police helicopter which assisted in the search touches down, too.

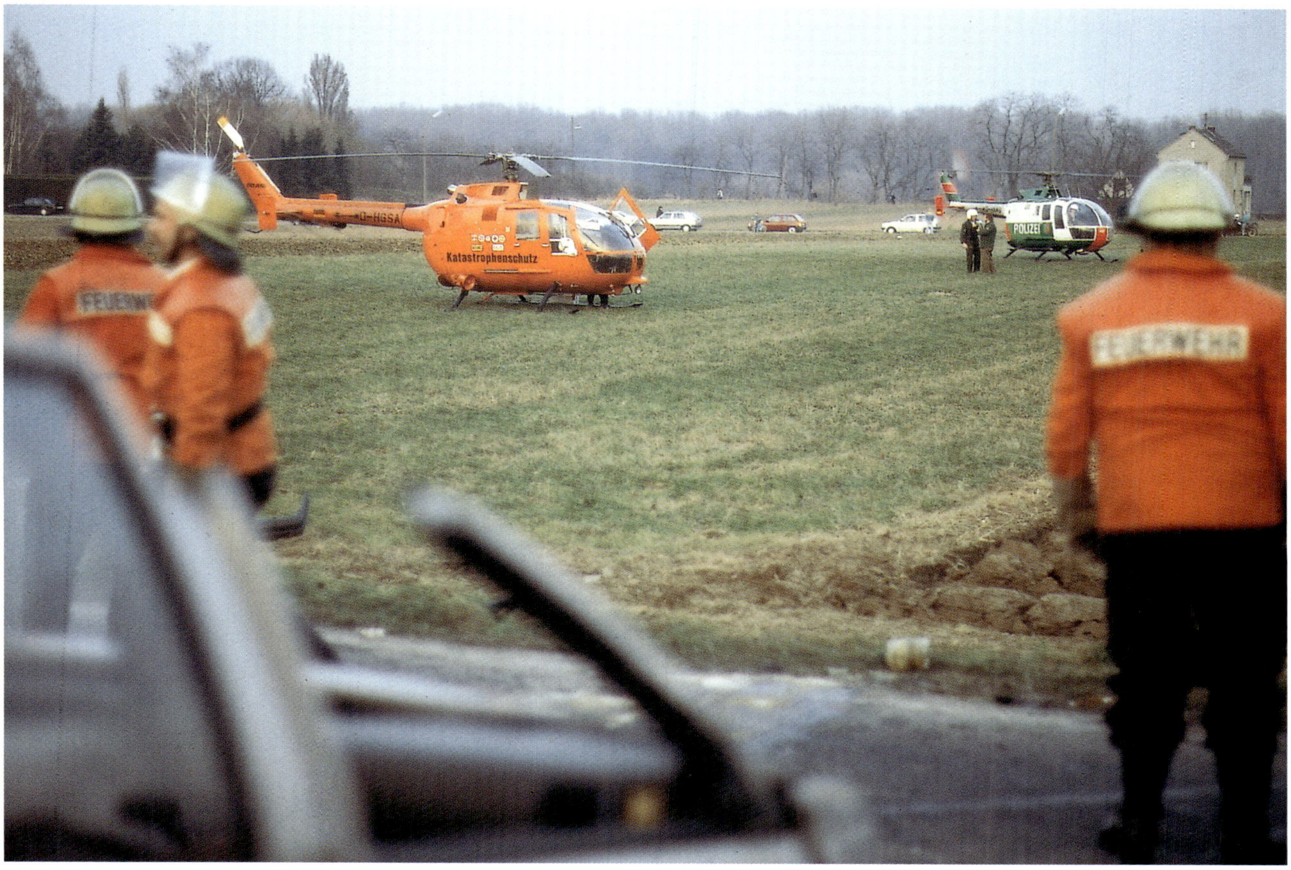

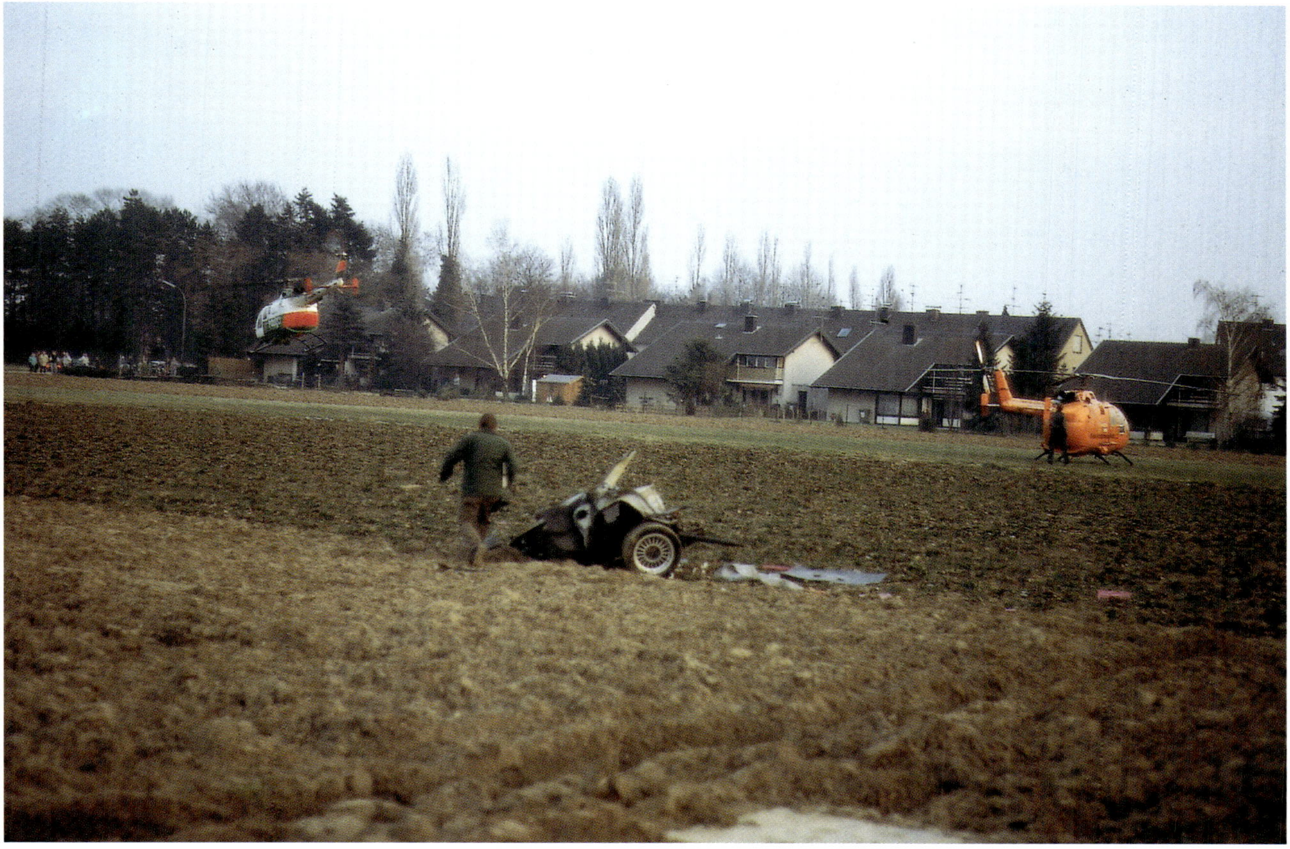

Der Polizeihubschrauber und kurze Zeit später der Rettungshubschrauber starten.

The police helicopter takes off, followed shortly afterwards by the rescue helicopter.

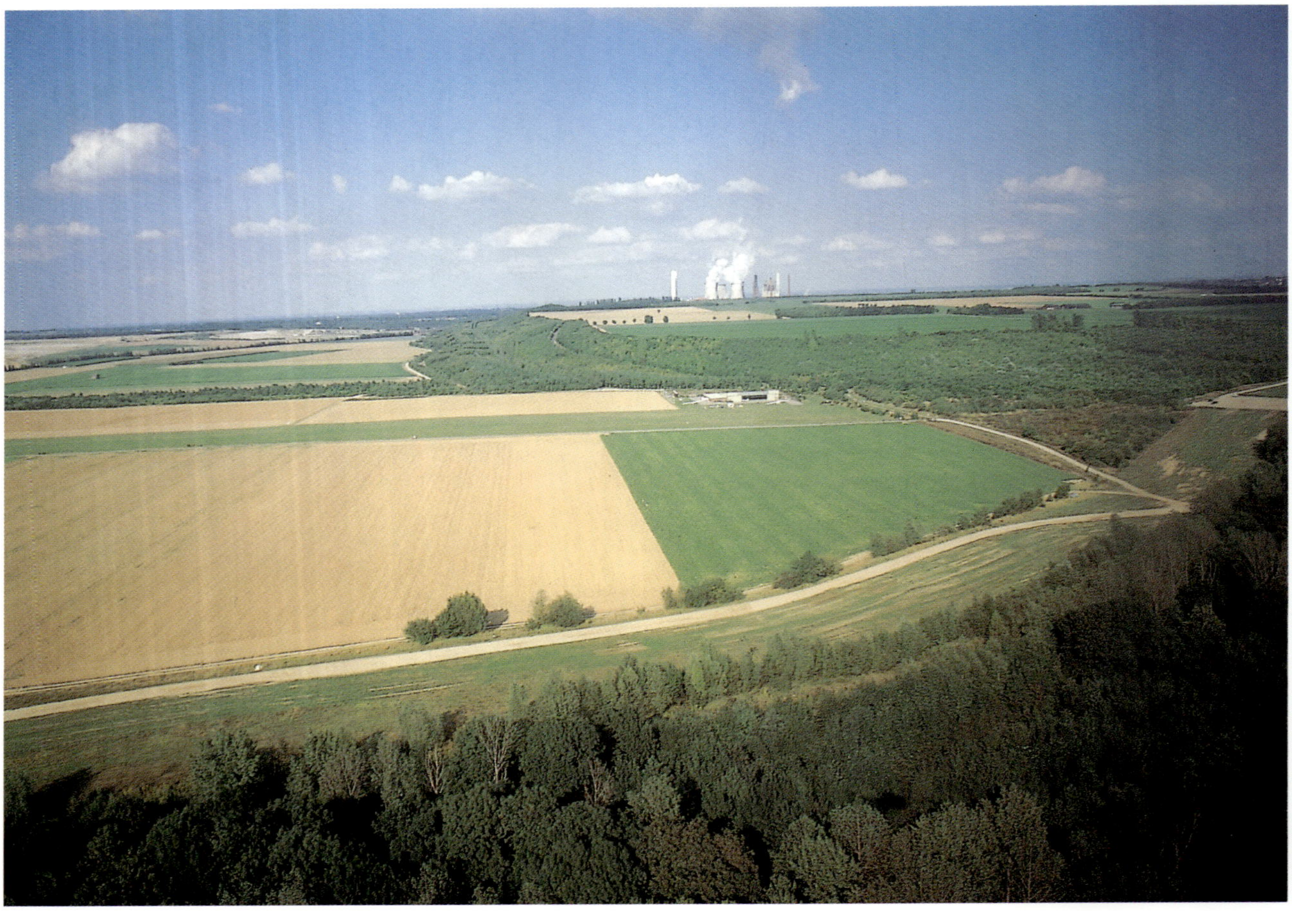

Auf dem Rückflug zur Station.

On the way back to base.

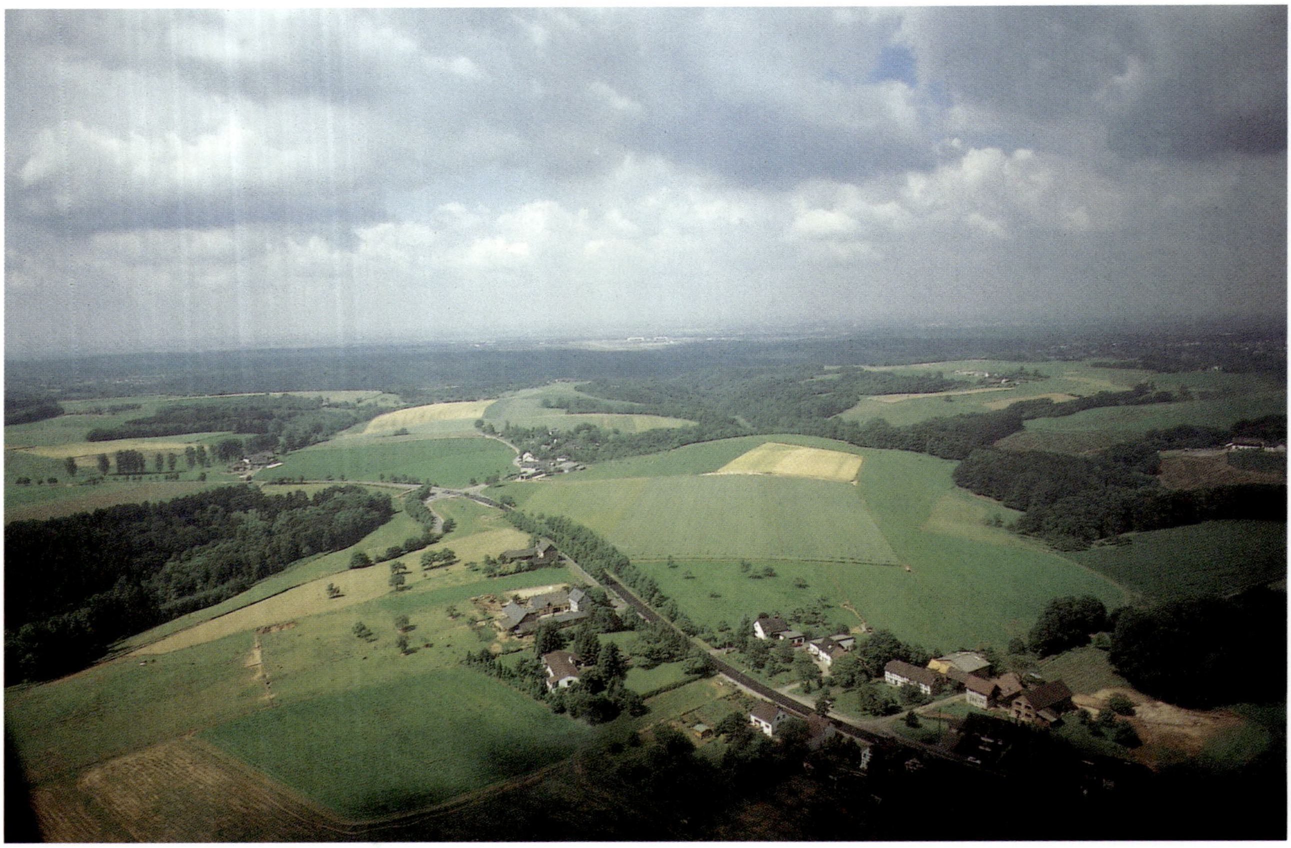

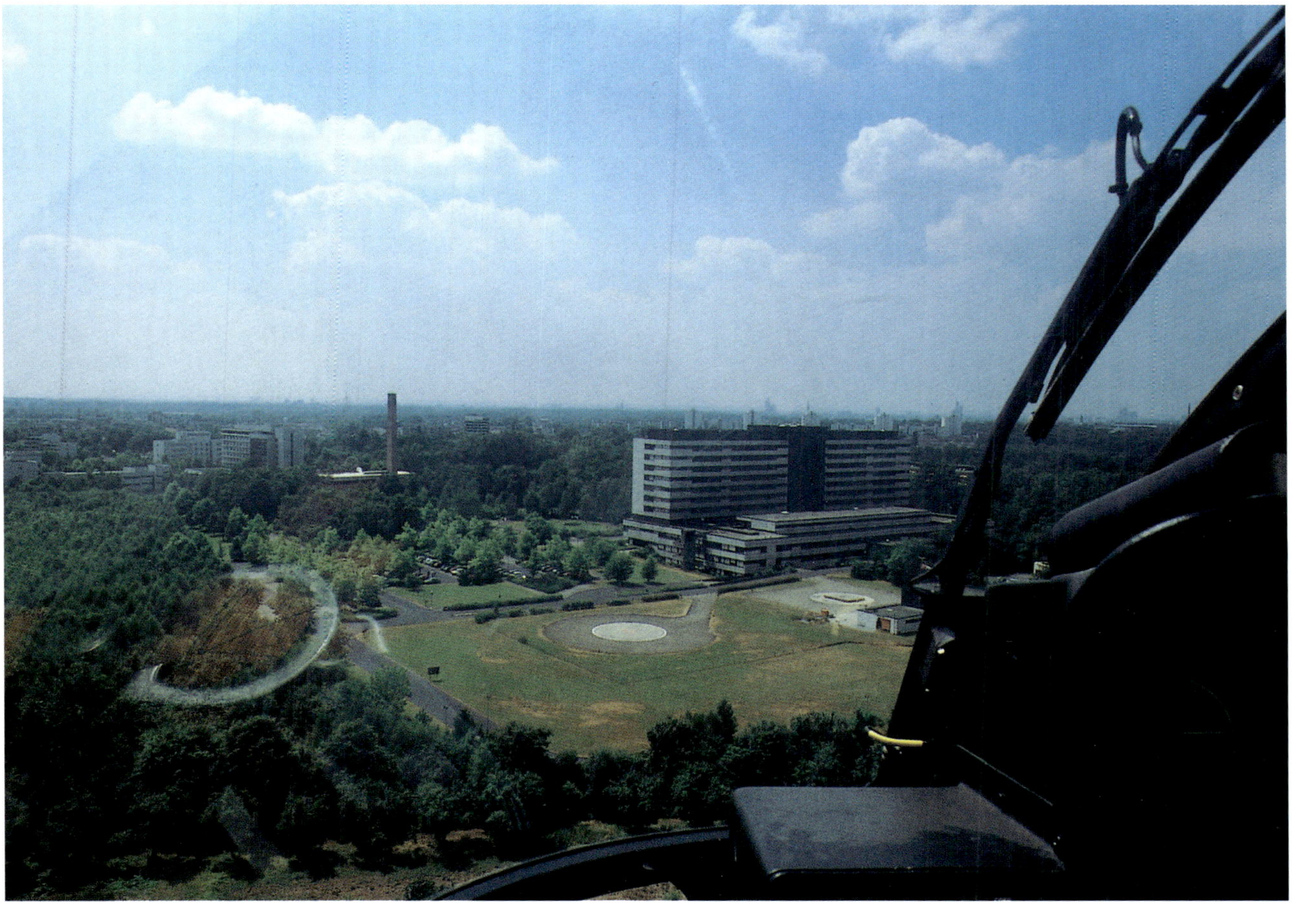

Neuer Einsatz ohne Landung auf der Station zu einem Notarztwagen, der einen Patienten für einen Hubschraubertransport vorbereitet hat.

Before it reaches its base, however, the rescue helicopter is sent on a new mission to a rescue ambulance, where a physician with emergency & rescue certification has prepared a patient for transport by rescue helicopter.

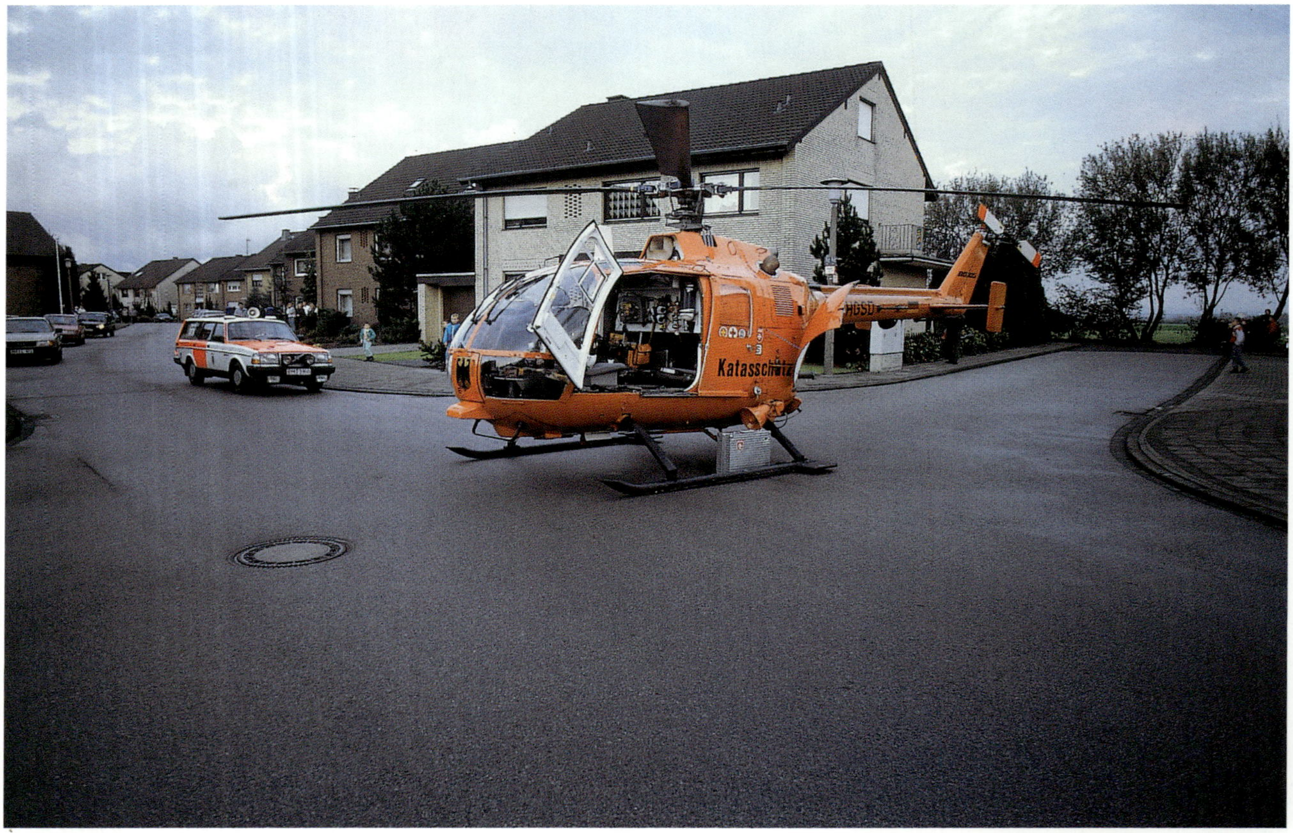

Der Rettungshubschrauber übernimmt den Patienten.

The rescue helicopter picks up the patient.

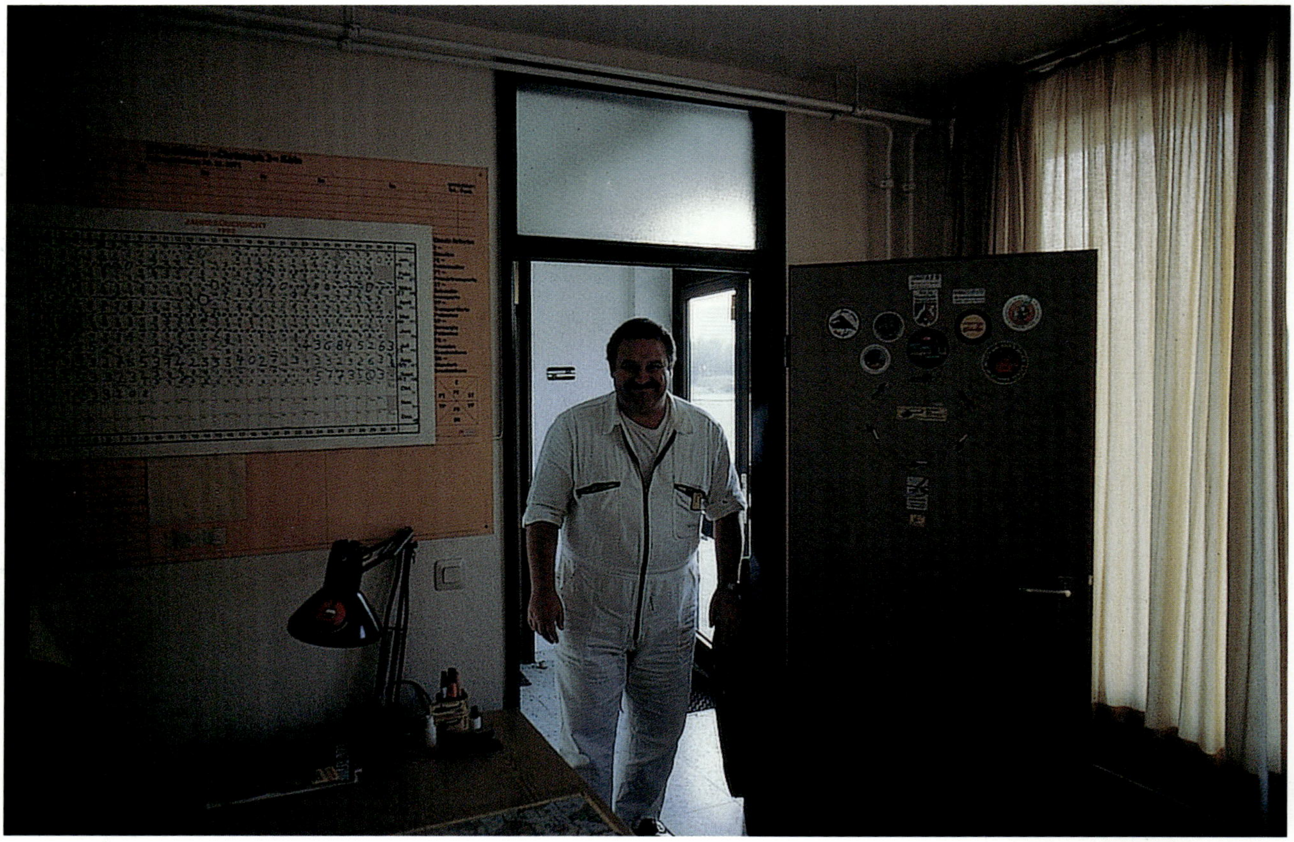

Rückkehr zur Station. Die Tasse Kaffee wartet.

Return to base. Five minutes for a cup of coffee.

Einsatz für den Rettungshubschrauber
Mission for the Rescue Helicopter

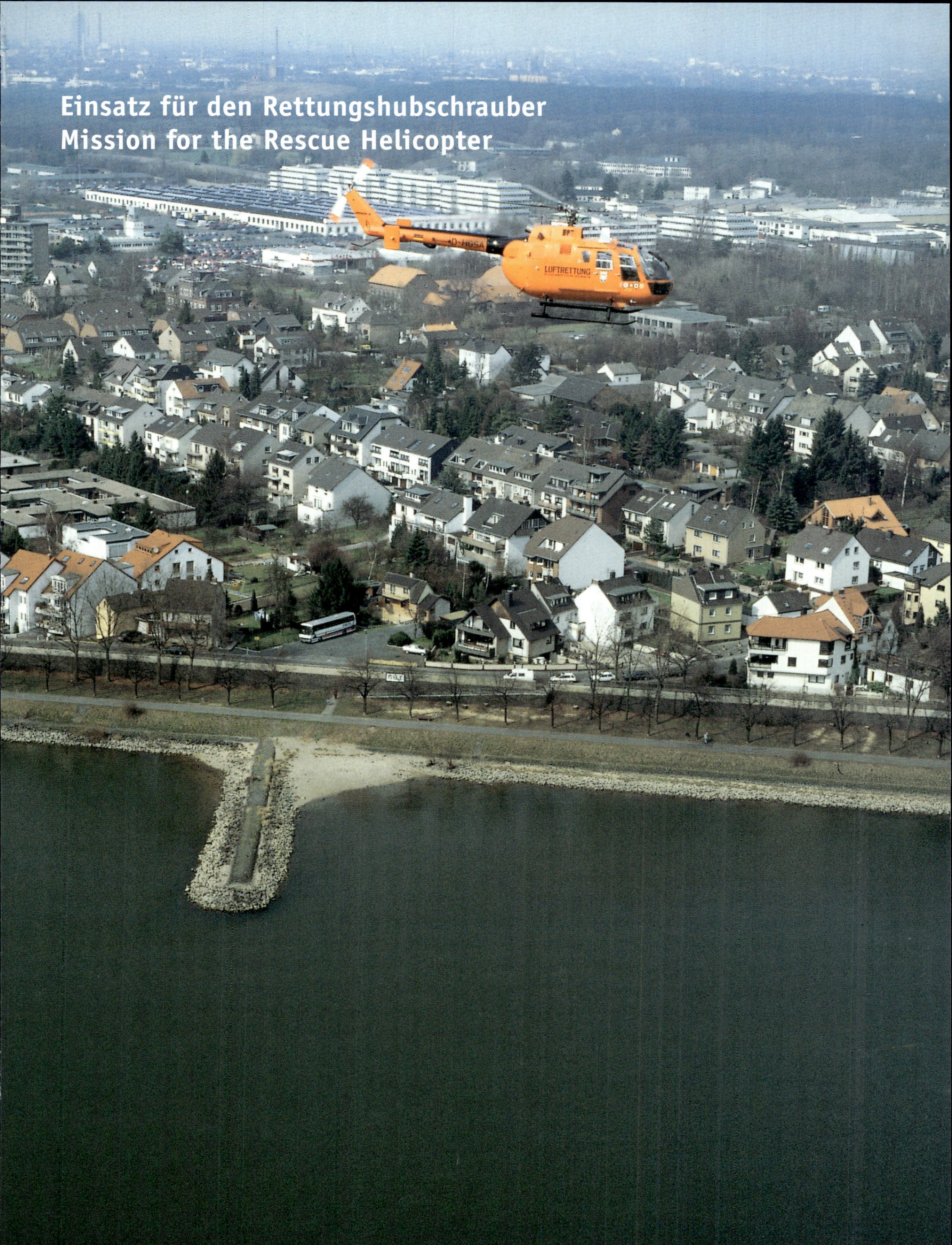

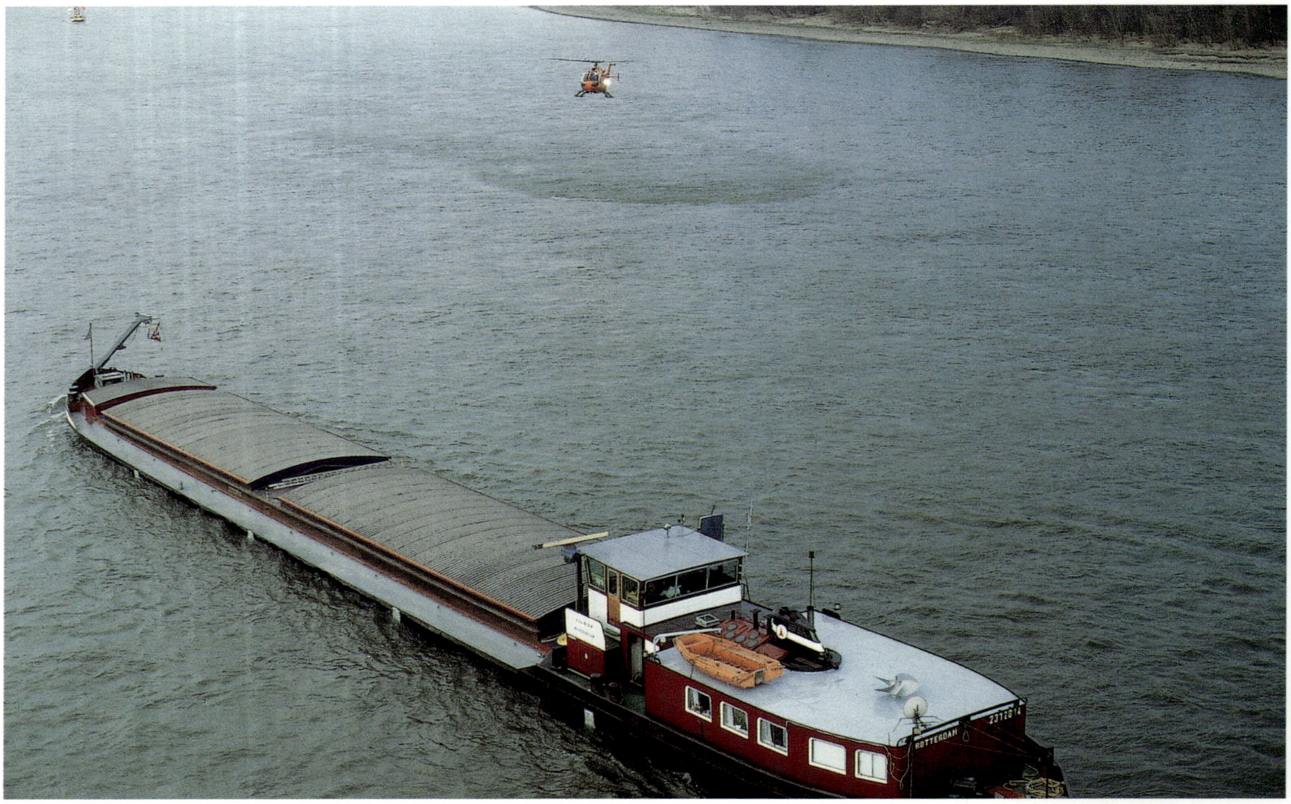

Auf einem Rheinschiff hat die Schiffersfrau Wehen verspürt, die in regelmäßigen Abständen seit einiger Zeit wiederkehrend sind.

Aboard a Rhine barge, the captain's wife has gone into labor; the labor pains are now coming at regular intervals.

Augenblicke

Anforderung von einer entfernten Leitstelle. Drei schwerstverletzte Kinder in einem Haus. Mehrere Notärzte unterwegs. Während des Fluges hören wir: Erster Rettungshubschrauber gelandet. Weitere Rückmeldungen: Drei Kinder von Familienangehörigem schwerstverletzt. Erstes Kind wahrscheinlich tot. Weitere Rückmeldung: Zweites Kind wahrscheinlich auch tot. Weitere Rückmeldung: Die Mutter hat sich die Pulsadern aufgeschnitten und wird mit dem Rettungswagen in die Klinik gefahren. Wir landen. Der koordinierende Notarzt weist uns Kind 3 zu. Kind 3 schwer verletzt, aber noch Lebenszeichen. Die Entscheidung unter allen Ärzten, wir sollen das Kind in die Uniklinik fliegen. Wir tragen das Kind aus dem Haus. Das Kind auf der Trage, der Vater vor der Tür. Polizist: „Soll ich den Vater wegschicken?" Antwort: „Nein, ist doch sein Kind." Der Vater begleitet sein Kind zum Hubschrauber. Wir laden das Kind ein. Flug zur Uniklinik unkompliziert. Nach zwei Wochen Rückfrage. „Wie geht es dem Kind?" „Gestern gestorben".

Snapshots

Request for assistance from a distant Coordination Center. Three seriously injured children in a house. Several physicians with emergency & rescue certification are already heading toward the scene. During the flight we are informed that the first rescue helicopter, sent by an adjoining district, has already landed. Additional reports come in: the first child is probably dead ..... the second child is probably dead, too. .... the mother has slit her wrists and is being taken to the hospital in a rescue ambulance. We touch down. The physician with emergency & rescue certification coordinating the rescue activities assigns child no. 3 to us. Child no. 3 is severely injured but still alive. The unanimous decision of all the doctors on the scene is that we should transport the child to the university hospital. We carry the child out of the house on a stretcher. The father is standing in front of the door. A policeman asks: "Shall I send the father away?" Answer: "No, it is his child." The father accompanies the child to the helicopter. We load the child into the helicopter. The flight to the university hospital is without incident. Two weeks later we inquire how the child is doing. Answer: "It died yesterday".

Augenblicke

Frisörsalon. Innenstadt. Wendehammer. Im Landeanflug wird ein Motorrad durch den Abstrahl umgeworfen. Im Frisörsalon alte Dame. Frage: „Wie geht es Ihnen?“ Antwort. „Hauen Sie ab.“ „Gott sei Dank. Es geht Ihnen gut.“ „Hauen Sie ab, sonst hole ich die Polizei.“ Der Frisör: „Sie hat die Augen verdreht und ist im Stuhl zusammengesackt. Wirklich.“ Die alte Dame: „Ein letztes Mal. Hauen Sie ab, sonst hole ich die Polizei. Da bin ich nämlich gut bekannt.“ Der Arzt: „Können wir Sie denn wenigstens nach Hause bringen.“ Die Dame: „Das könnte Ihnen wohl so passen, dann wissen Sie ja, wo ich wohne. Hauen Sie jetzt endlich ab oder soll ich es Ihnen auf lateinisch sagen.“ Wir gehen raus. Der Pilot klärt die Schadensmeldung wegen des Motorrades. Wir schauen immer mal wieder in den Salon, die alte Dame hat sich ganz offensichtlich erholt. Es dauert noch eine Weile, bis alle Schadensmeldungen hin und her ausgetauscht worden sind. Ein letzter Blick auf die alte Dame. Es geht ihr gut. Rückflug. Wir hauen ab.

Snapshots

Hairdresser's salon in a downtown area. We land in a turning area. During the landing approach, the rotor wash knocks over a motorcycle. We find our patient, an elderly lady who is reportedly unconscious, in a hairdresser's salon. Our question: "How are you?" Her answer: "Get lost!" Our friendly reply: "Thank God you're o.k.!" Her response: "F--- off or I'll call the police!" The hairdresser is apologetic: „A few minutes ago her eyes sort of rolled back and she collapsed right here in the chair. Honest!" The elderly lady gives us a last warning: "Get the hell out of here or I am calling the police. They all know me." The doctor: "Can't we at least bring you home?" The woman: "That would suit you just fine. Then you would know where I live. Are you going to leave finally or do I have to give you a written invitation?" We leave finally. The pilot supplies the facts for the damage claim submitted by the motorcycle's owner. We take another peek into the salon: the elderly lady has evidently recovered. It takes some time before the various damage reports are exchanged. A last look to see how the woman is doing. She appears to be doing just fine. Return flight. We leave it finally.

Ein gesunder Junge ist schon geboren. Mutter und Kind werden versorgt.

The woman has already given birth to a healthy baby boy. Mother and child receive medical attention.

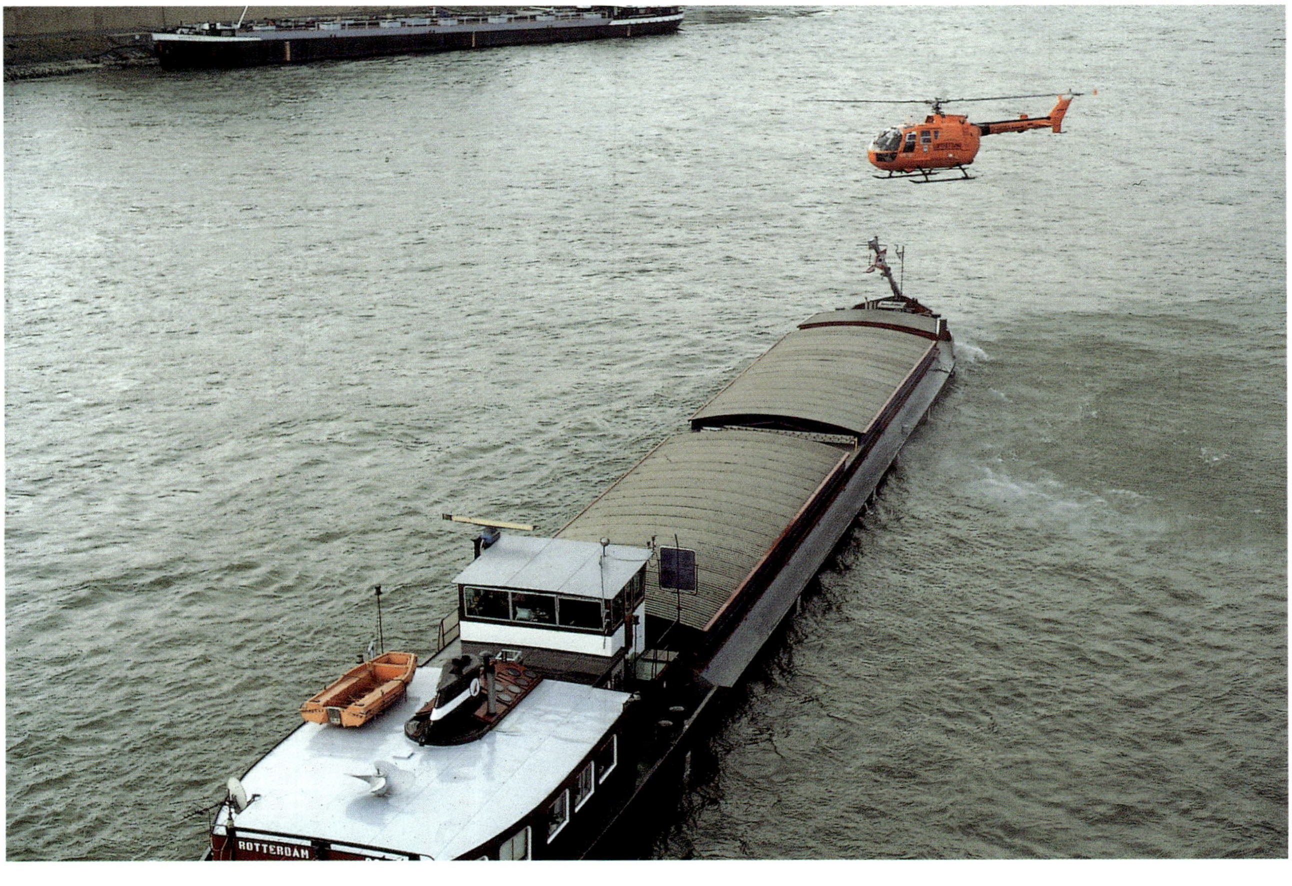

Einsatz für den Rettungshubschrauber
Mission for the Rescue Helicopter

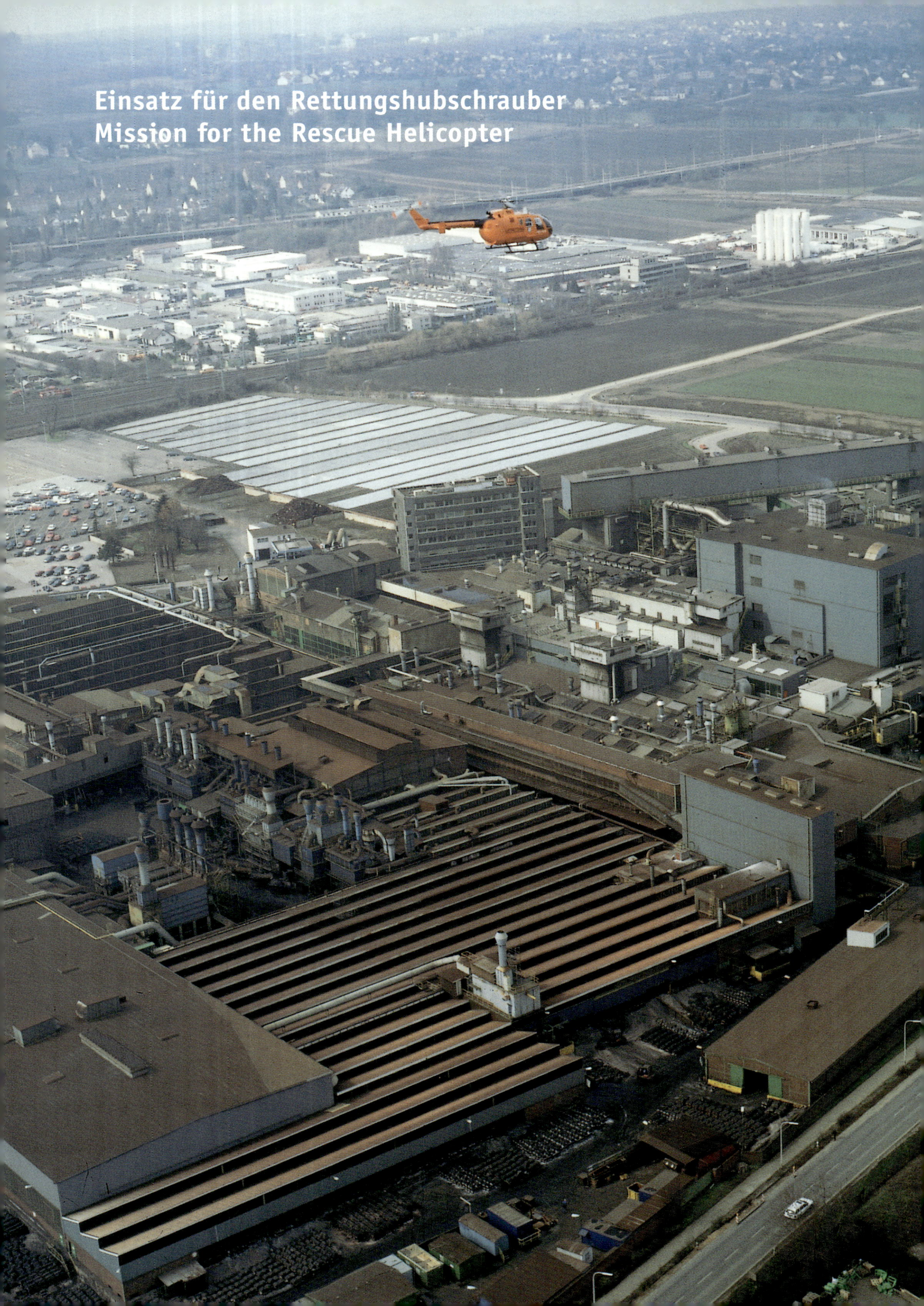

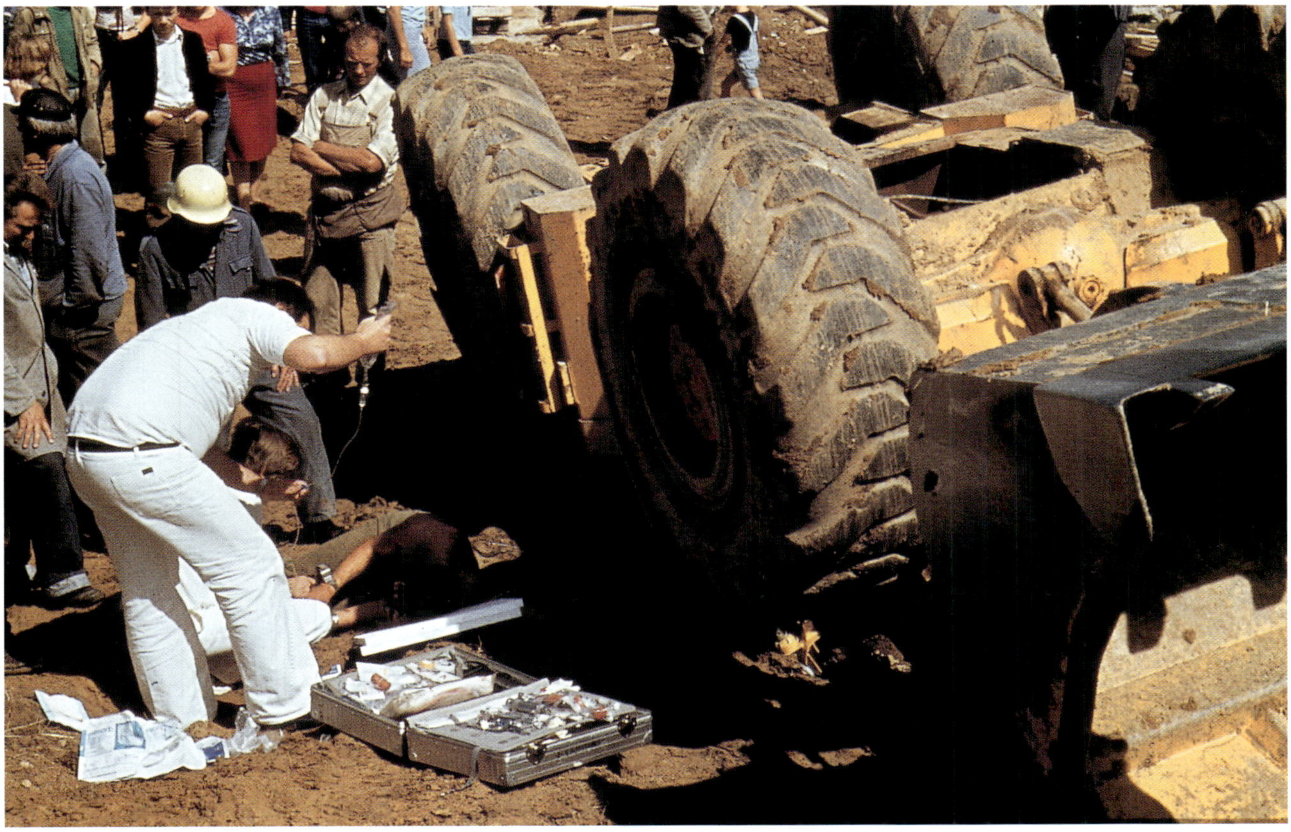

Ein Radlader ist umgekippt und hat den Fahrer unter sich begraben.

On-the-job accident: a tractor-trailer has overturned, pinning the driver underneath it.

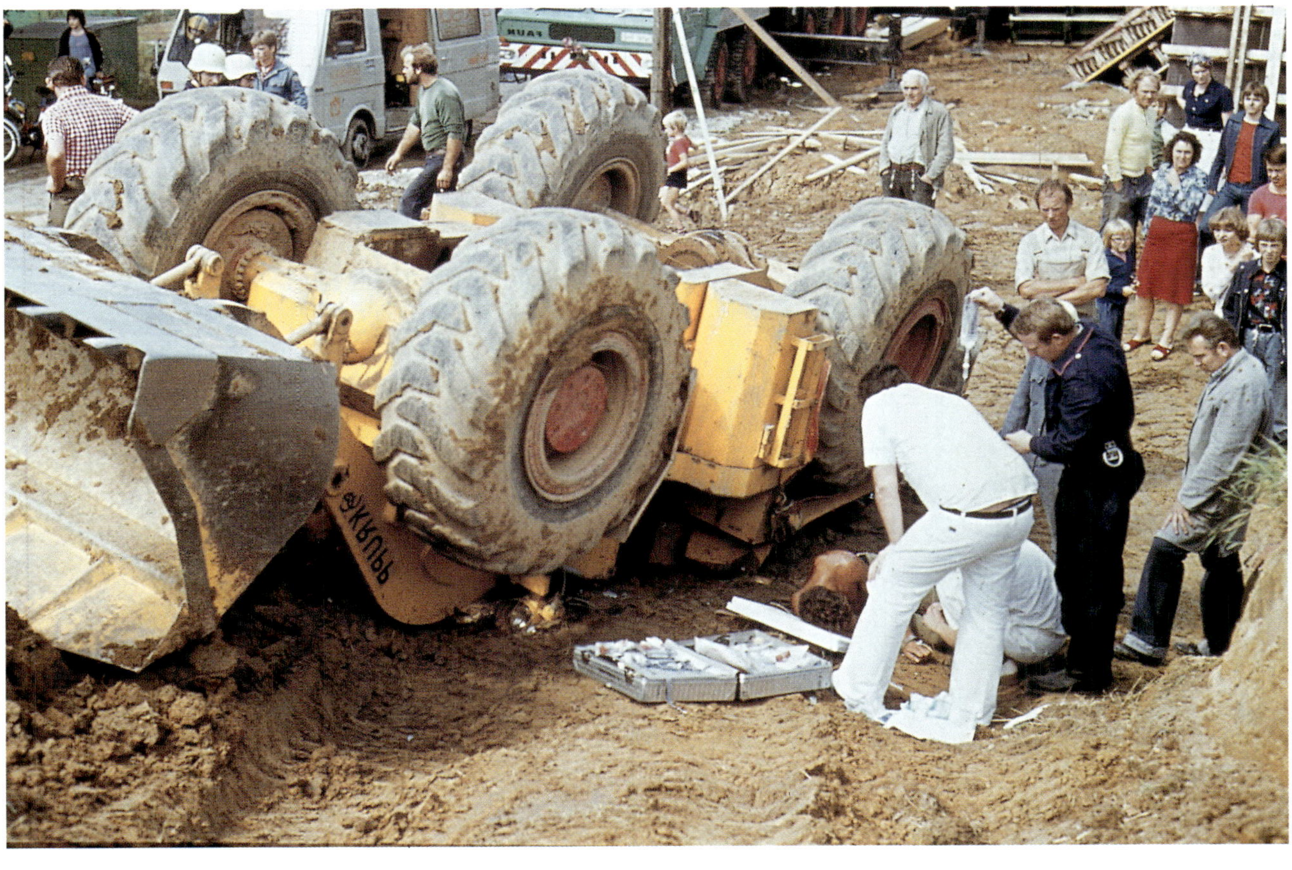

Einsatz für den Rettungshubschrauber
Mission for the Rescue Helicopter

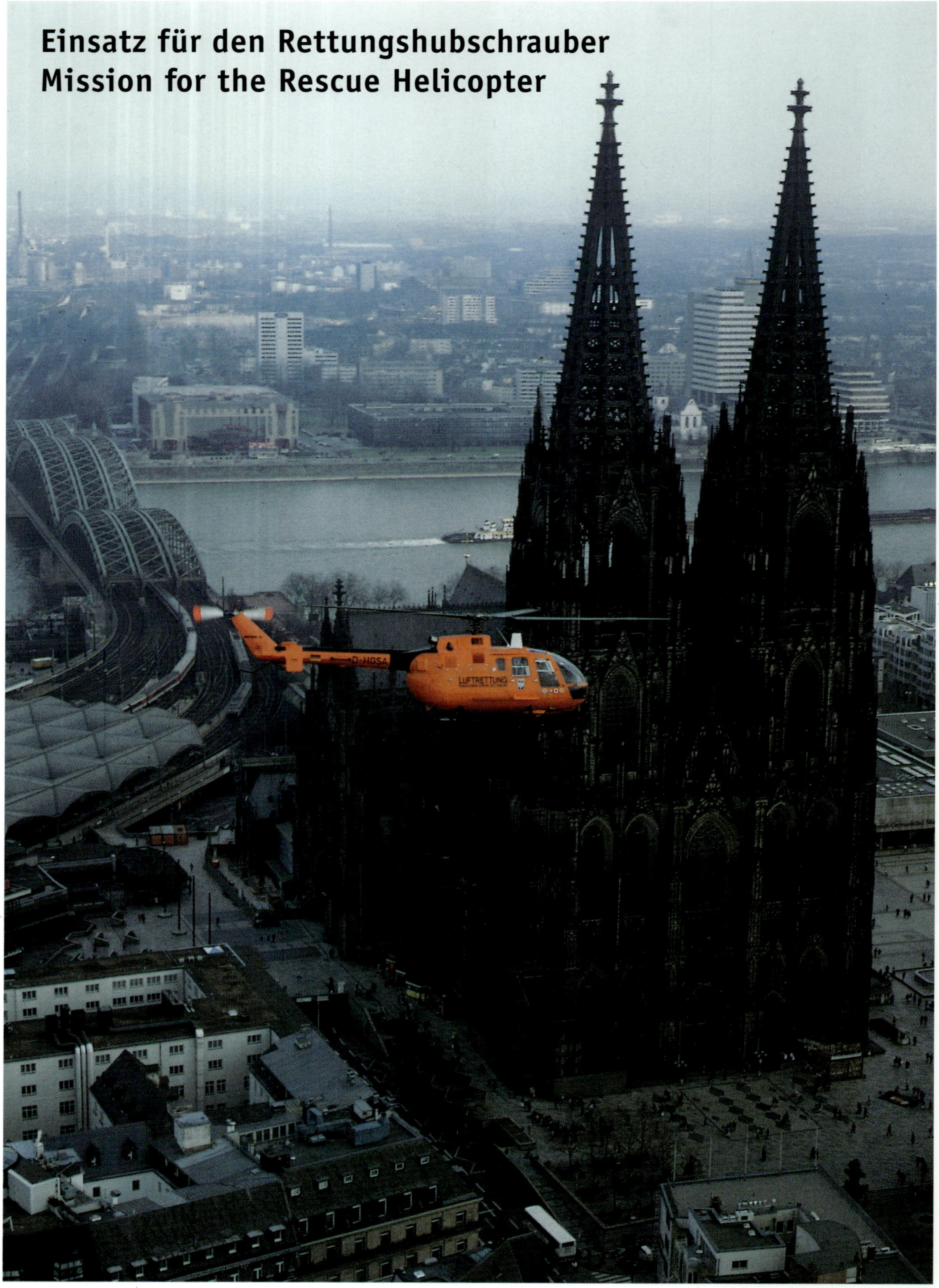

Während der Messe ist ein älterer Herr mit Herzinfarkt zusammengebrochen. Er wird versorgt und ins Krankenhaus gebracht.

During mass an elderly man has collapsed with a heart attack. He is given emergency medical care and transported to a hospital.

Einsatz für den Rettungshubschrauber
Mission for the Rescue Helicopter

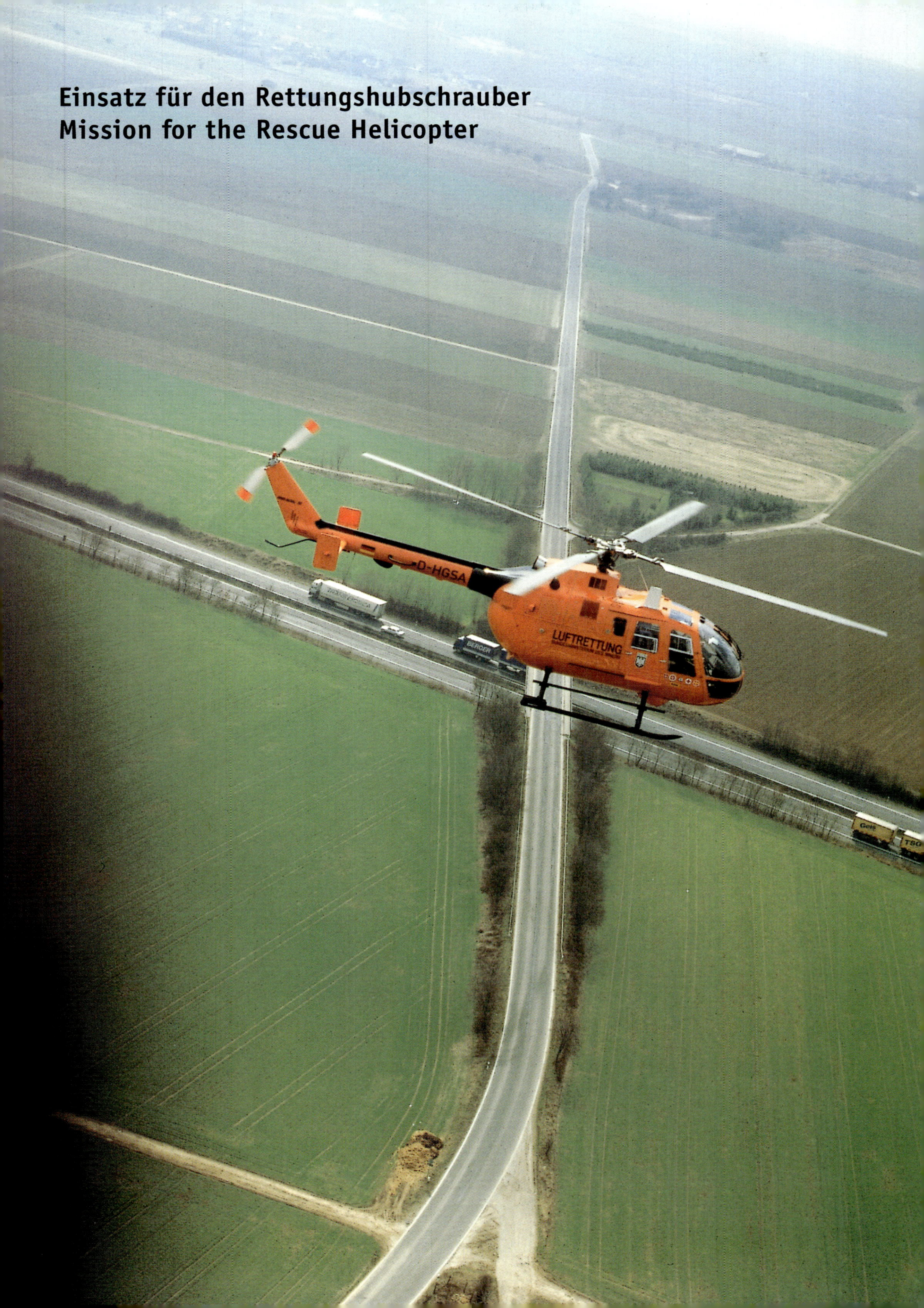

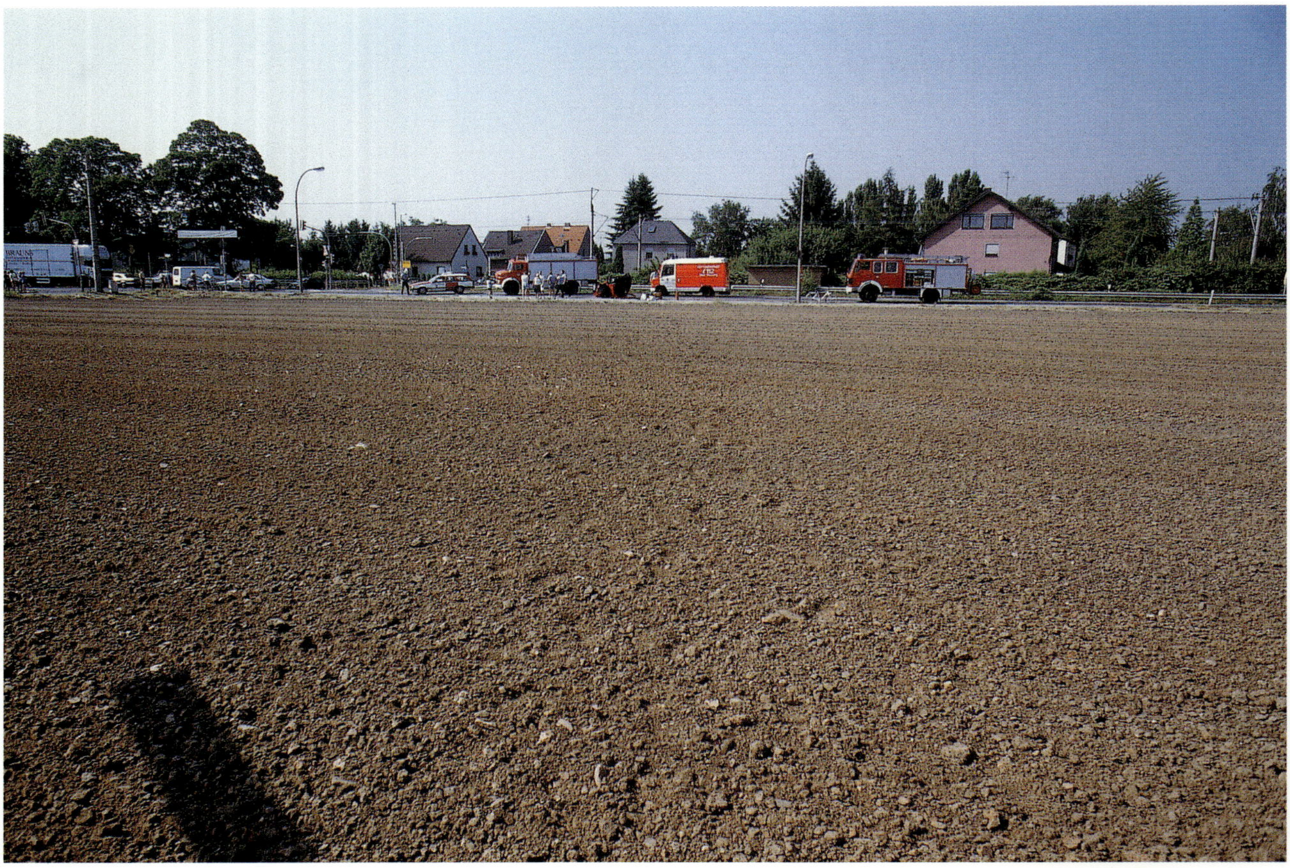

Unfall am Dorfrand. Ein PKW hat sich überschlagen.

An automobile has turned over on the village outskirts.

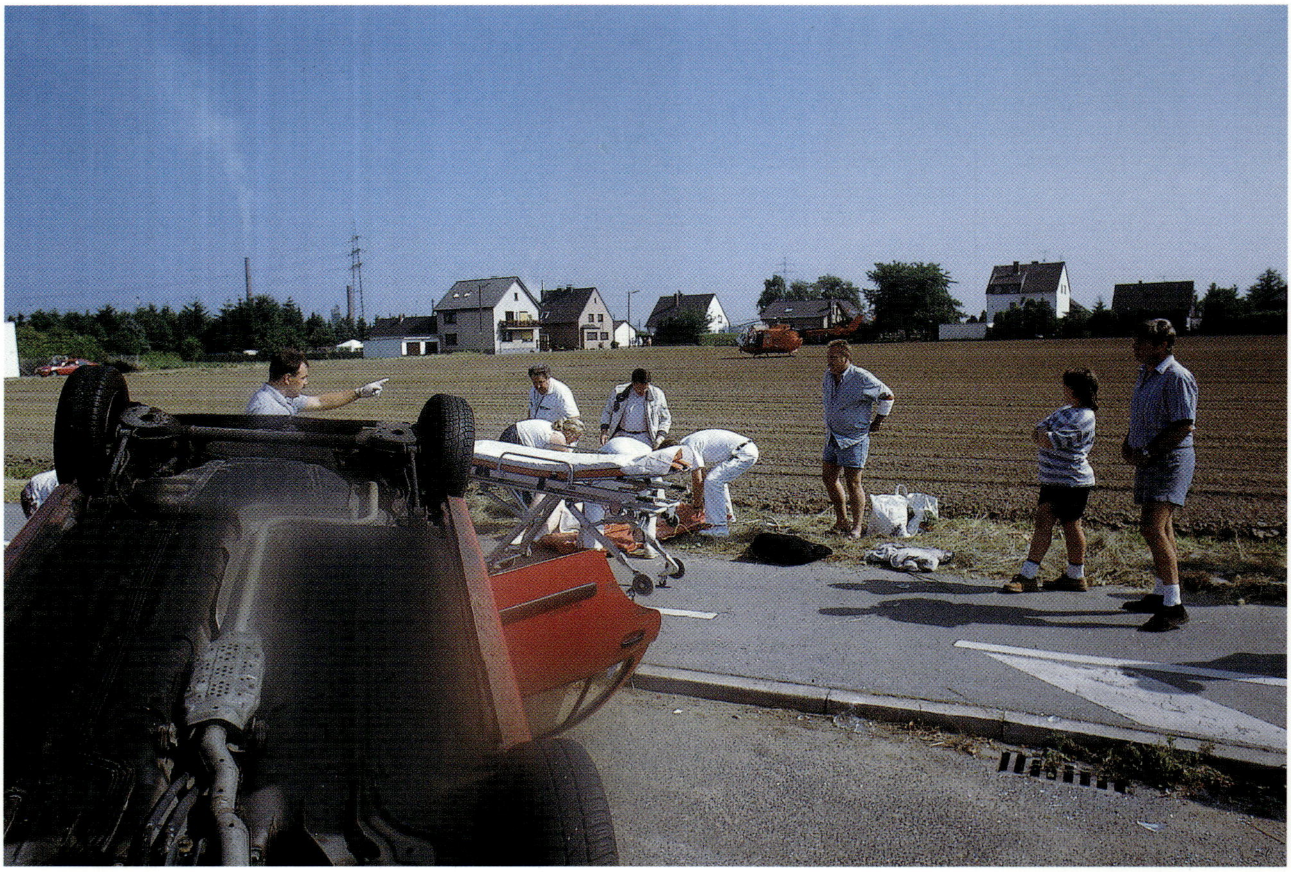

Der Patient wird versorgt.

The patient is given emergency medical care.

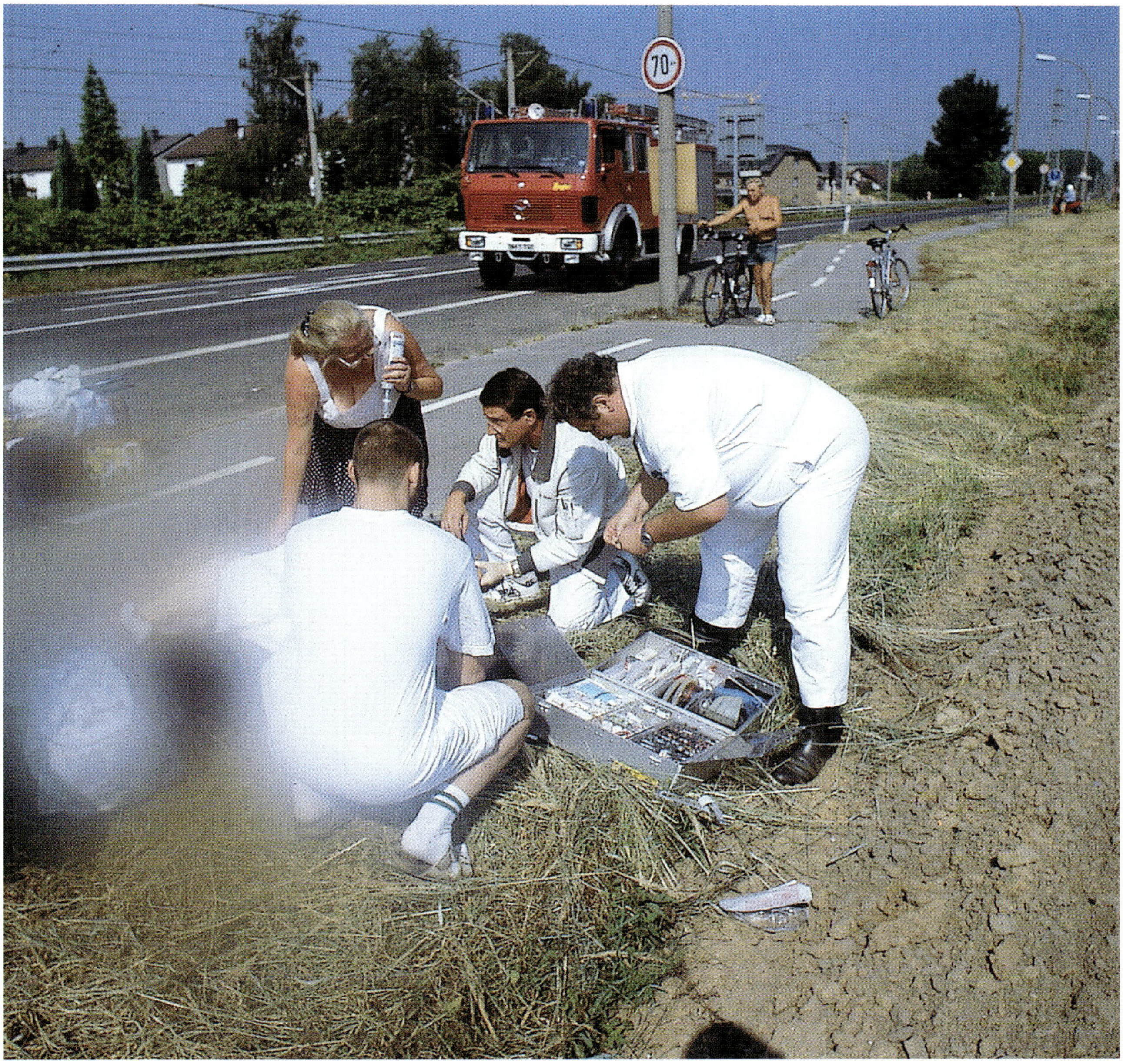

Augenblicke

Silvestermorgen. Ruhige Stimmung. Einsatz zur Schussverletzung. Im Rettungswagen Mann mit Schussverletzung im Kopfbereich. War noch ansprechbar. Wird von uns geflogen. Warum? Während des Spazierganges mit seinem Hund kommt der Nachbar, mit dem er Streitigkeiten hat, sagt ihm noch, wir haben eine Rechnung offen und schießt. Während des Transports stellt ein Polizeikommando den Mann in seinem Haus.

Snapshots

A peaceful morning on New Year's day. Mission to pick up a patient with a gunshot wound. Inside the rescue ambulance we find a man with a gunshot wound in the head but still conscious. We fly him to the hospital. How did it happen? While out walking his dog, the man met a neighbor with whom he had had several serious altercations in the past. The neighbor announced that he had a score to settle and fired. During the transport we hear that the offender has been apprehended by the police inside his own house.

Einsatz für den Rettungshubschrauber
Mission for the Rescue Helicopter

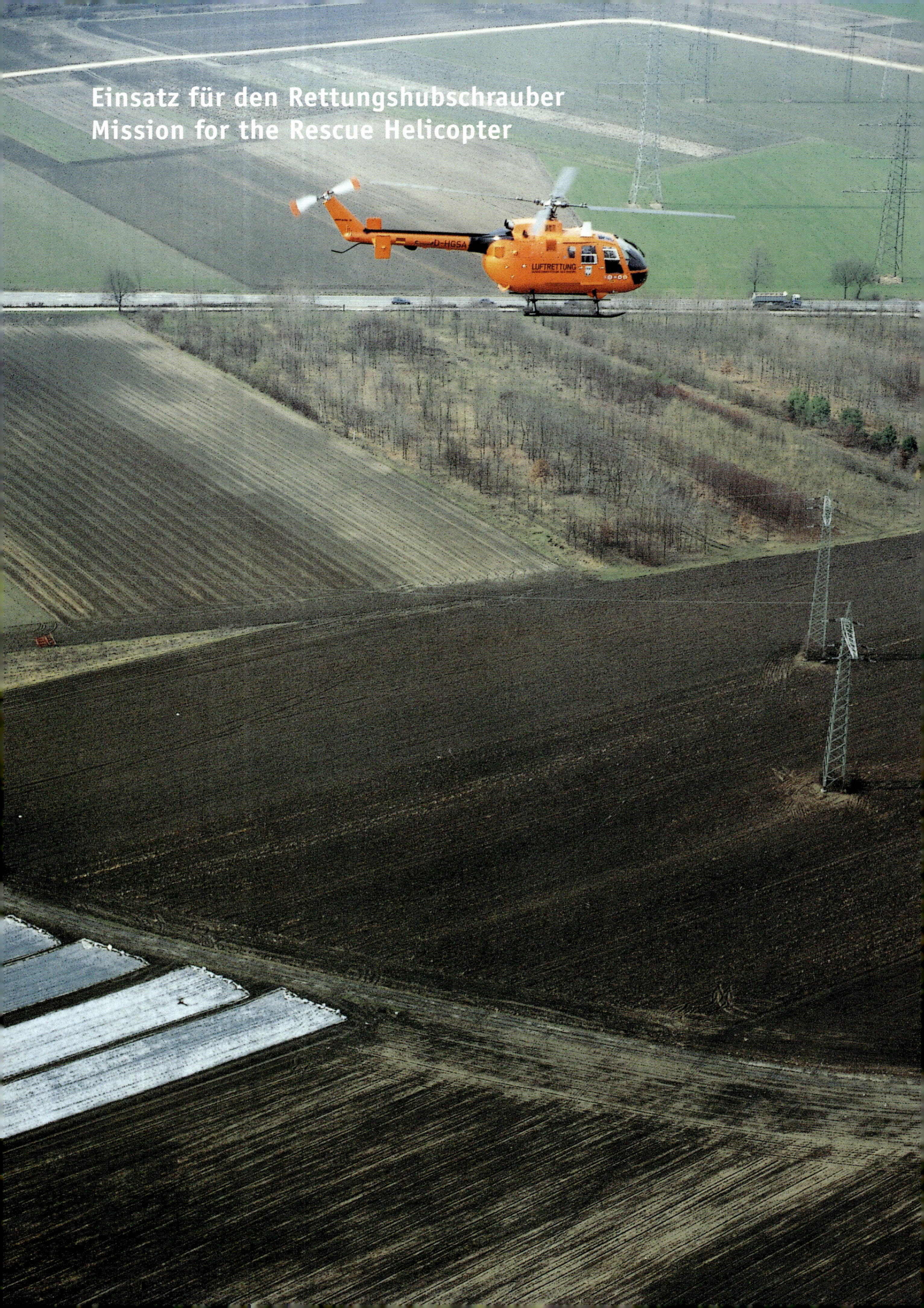

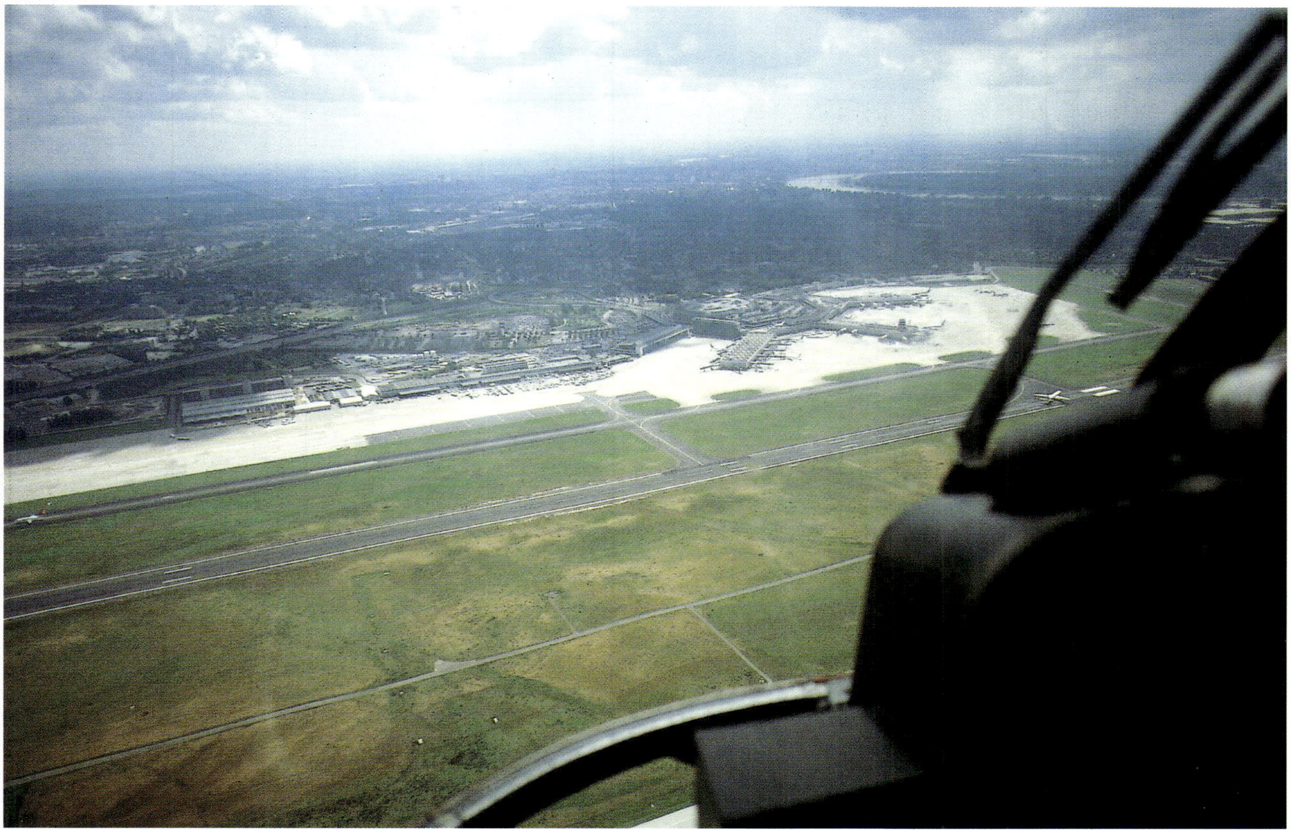

Person im Rhein. Wir fliegen zurück zum Rhein.

Emergency call: person in the Rhine. We fly back to the Rhine.

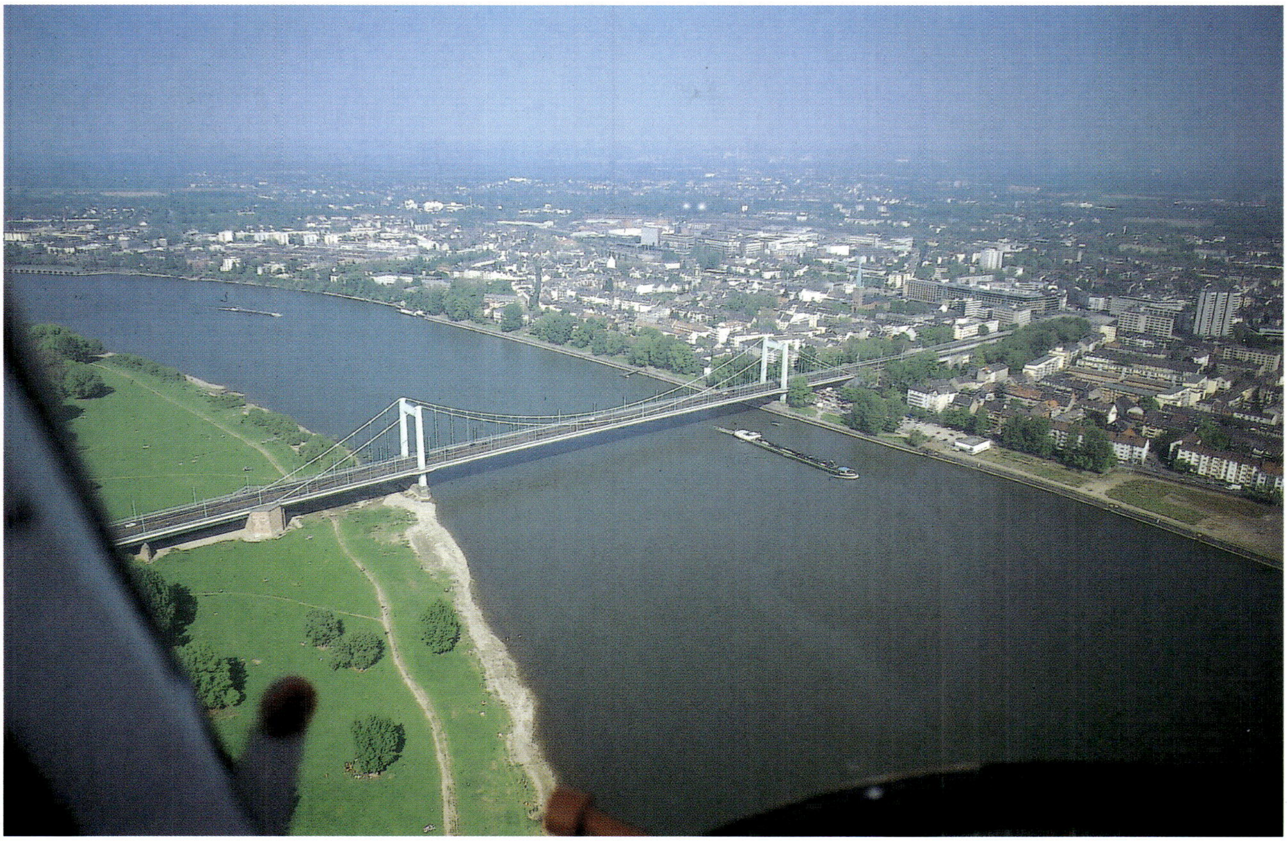

Rhein ist erreicht.

We reach the Rhine.

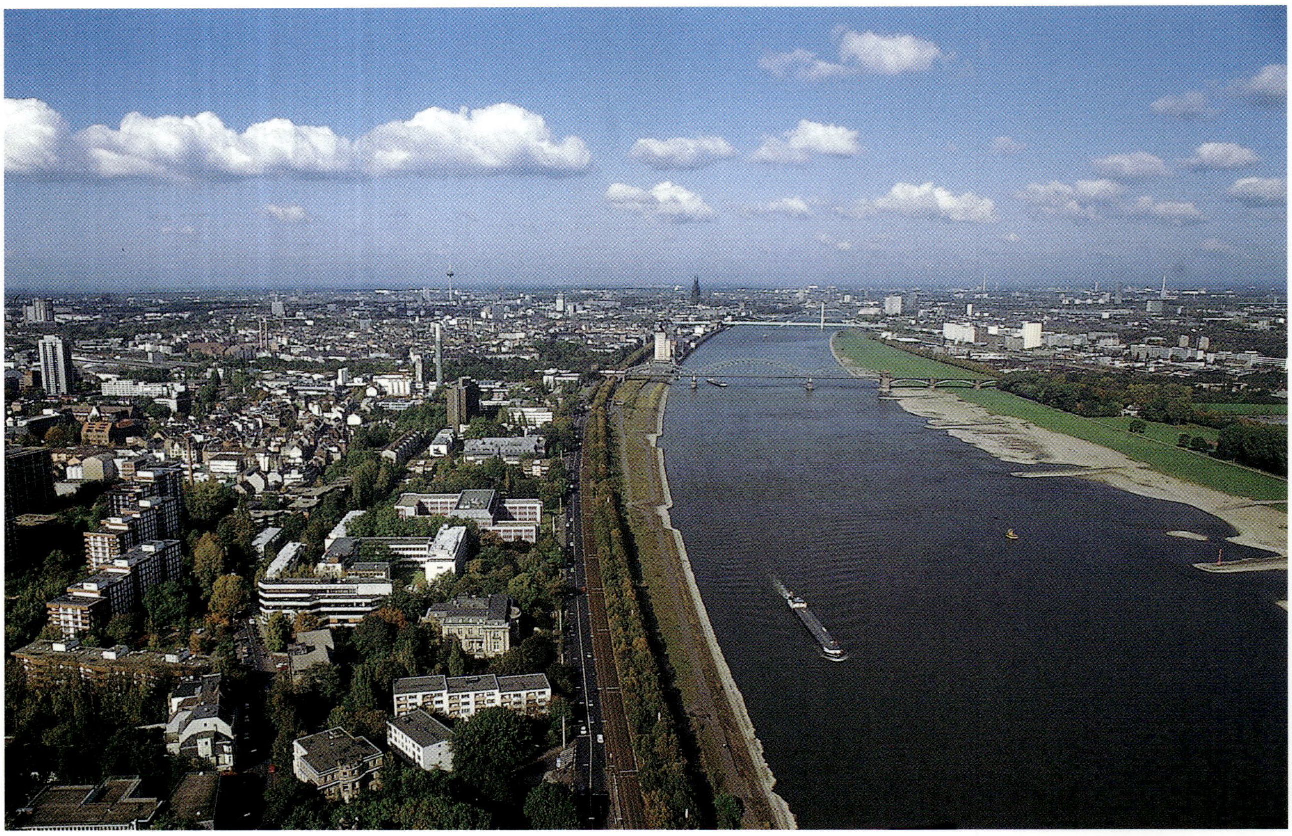

Wir suchen die Stelle, an der die Frau in den Rhein gegangen sein soll.

We look for the spot where the woman is reported to have gone into the Rhine.

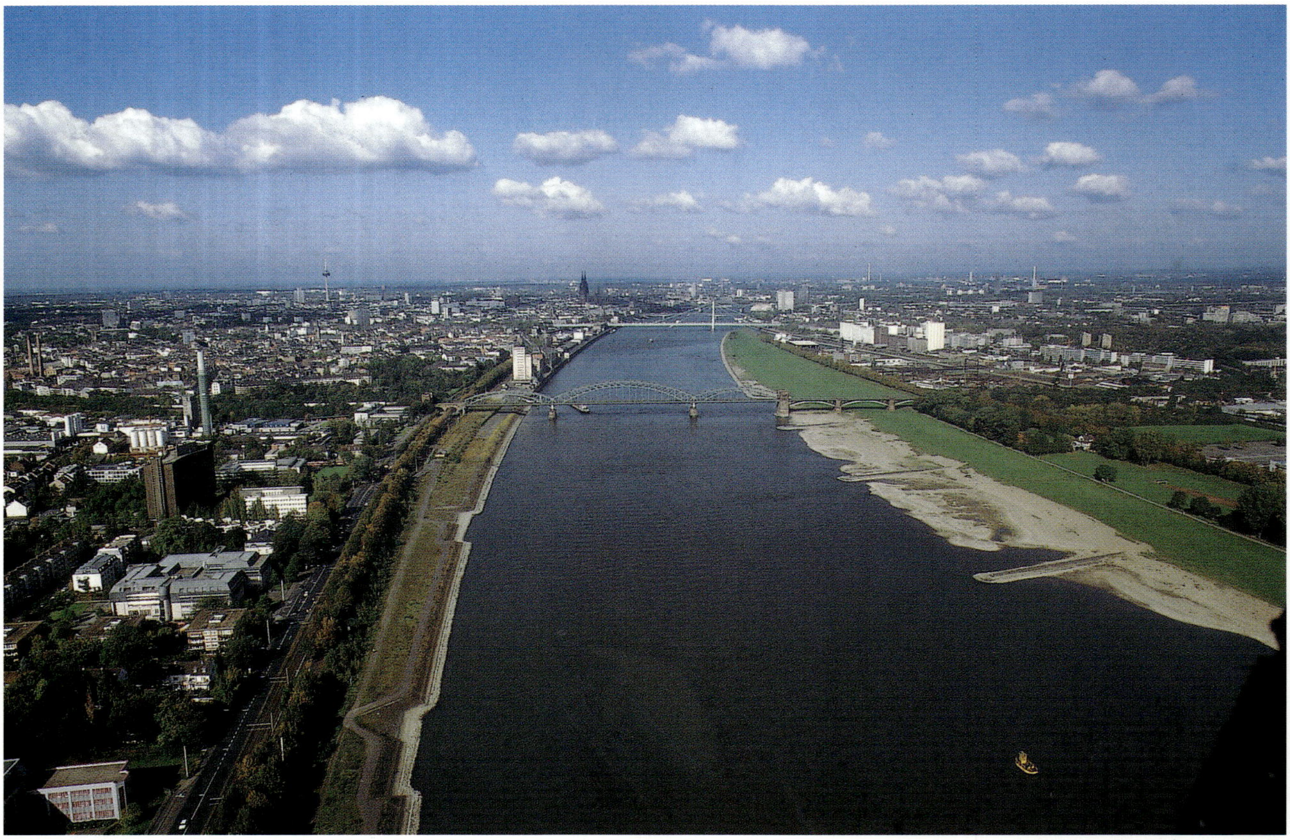

Wir fliegen in Mitte des Rheinstroms. Rückmeldung der Polizei. Frau ist schwimmend unterhalb einer Brücke gesehen worden.

We fly above the middle of the Rhine. The police report that the woman has been sighted swimming underneath a bridge.

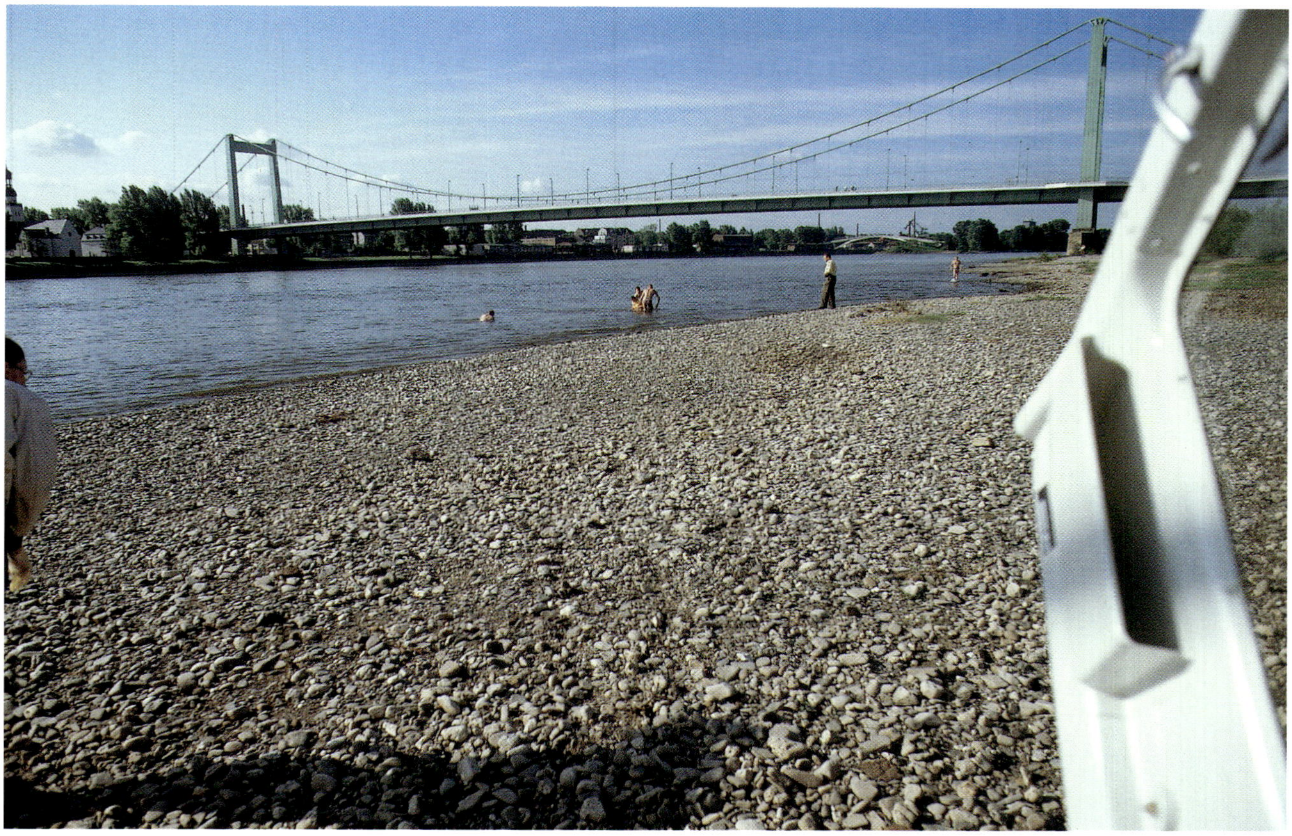

Im Überflug sehen wir, dass drei Streifenwagenbesatzungen ihre Uniform ausziehen und ins februarkalte Rheinwasser schwimmen. Die schwimmende Person wird von den Beamten zur Ufernähe gezogen.

During the flyover, we see three police officers strip off their uniforms and dive into the icy February waters. A police officer pulls the woman to the banks of the Rhine.

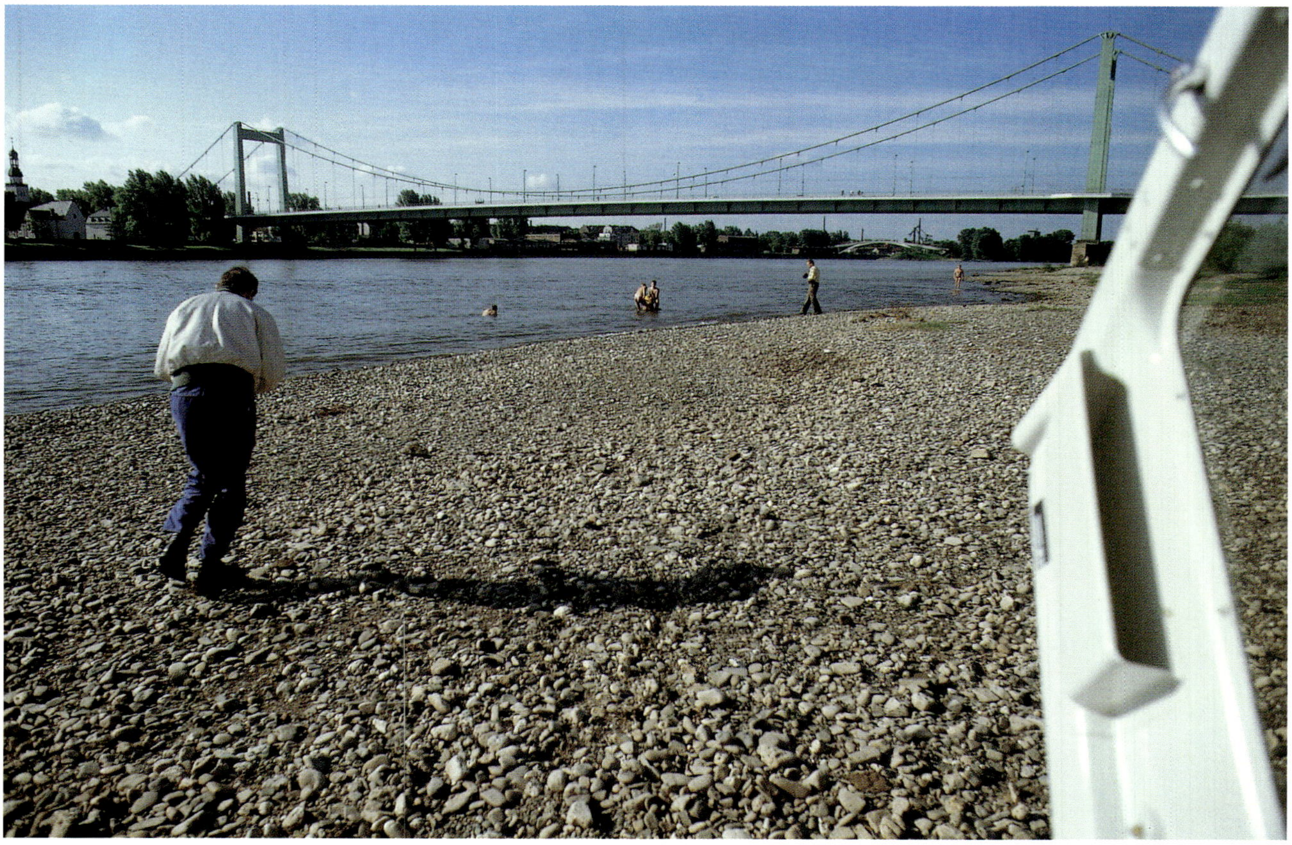

Die Person ist geborgen.

The woman is rescued.

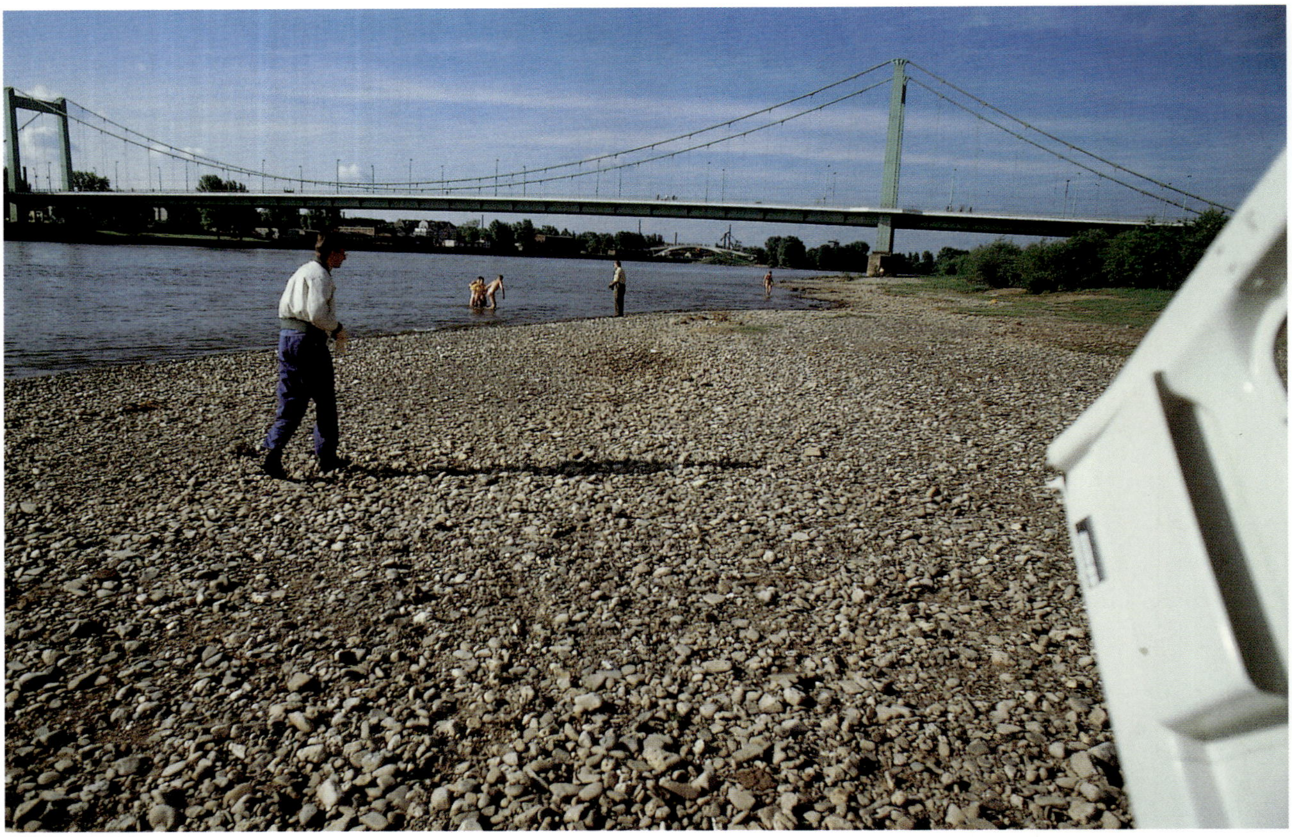

Sie wird zum Ufer gebracht.

She is brought ashore.

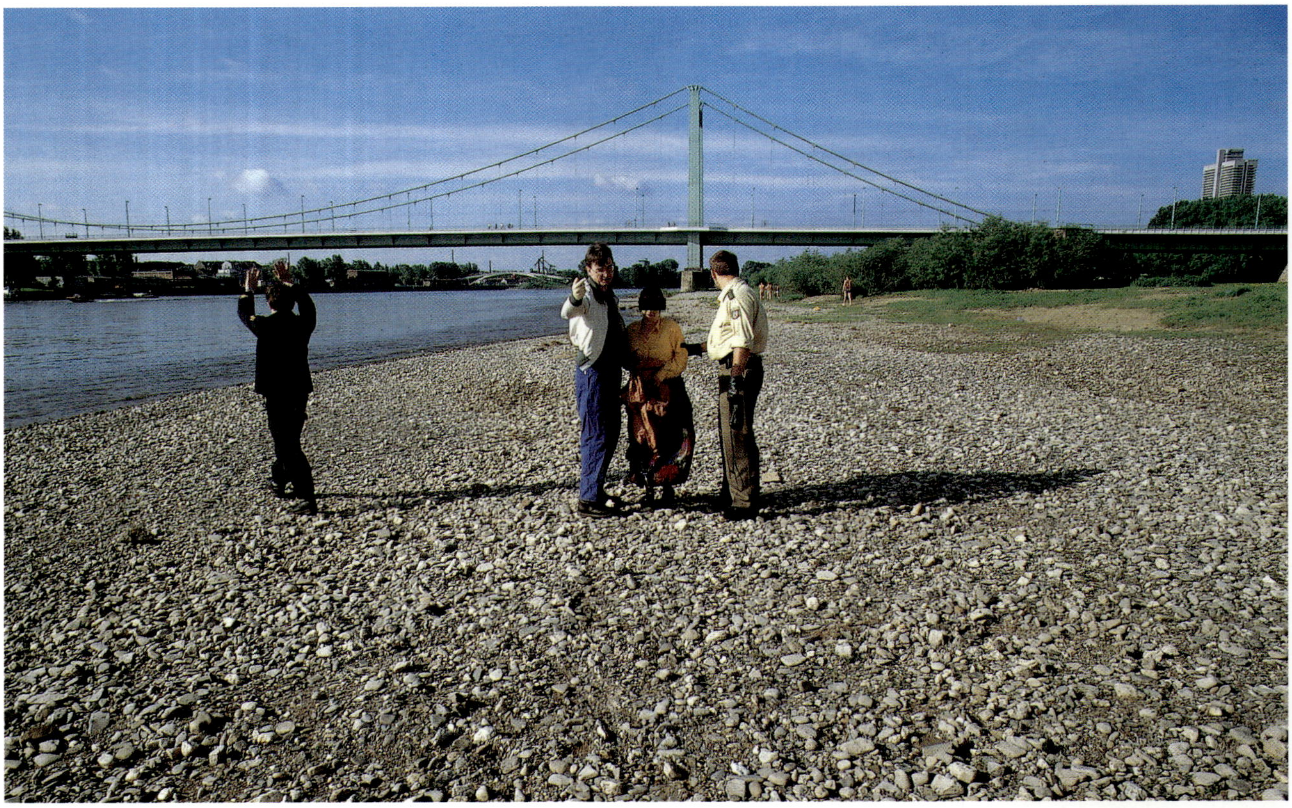

Löschboot und alle weiteren Kräfte können abbrechen.

The fire-fighting boat and all other rescue workers are notified that they can suspend their activities.

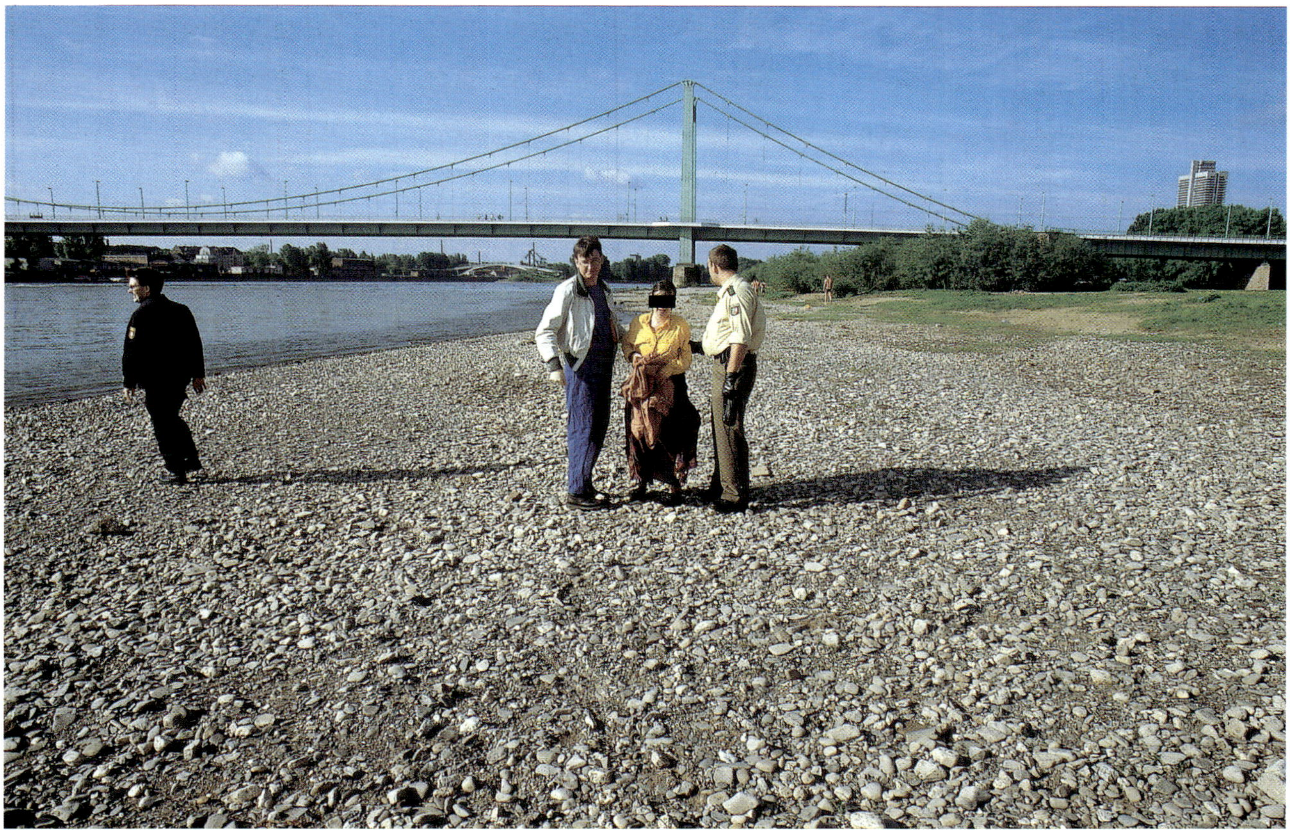

Die Patientin wird ins Krankenhaus verbracht.

The patient is brought to a hospital.

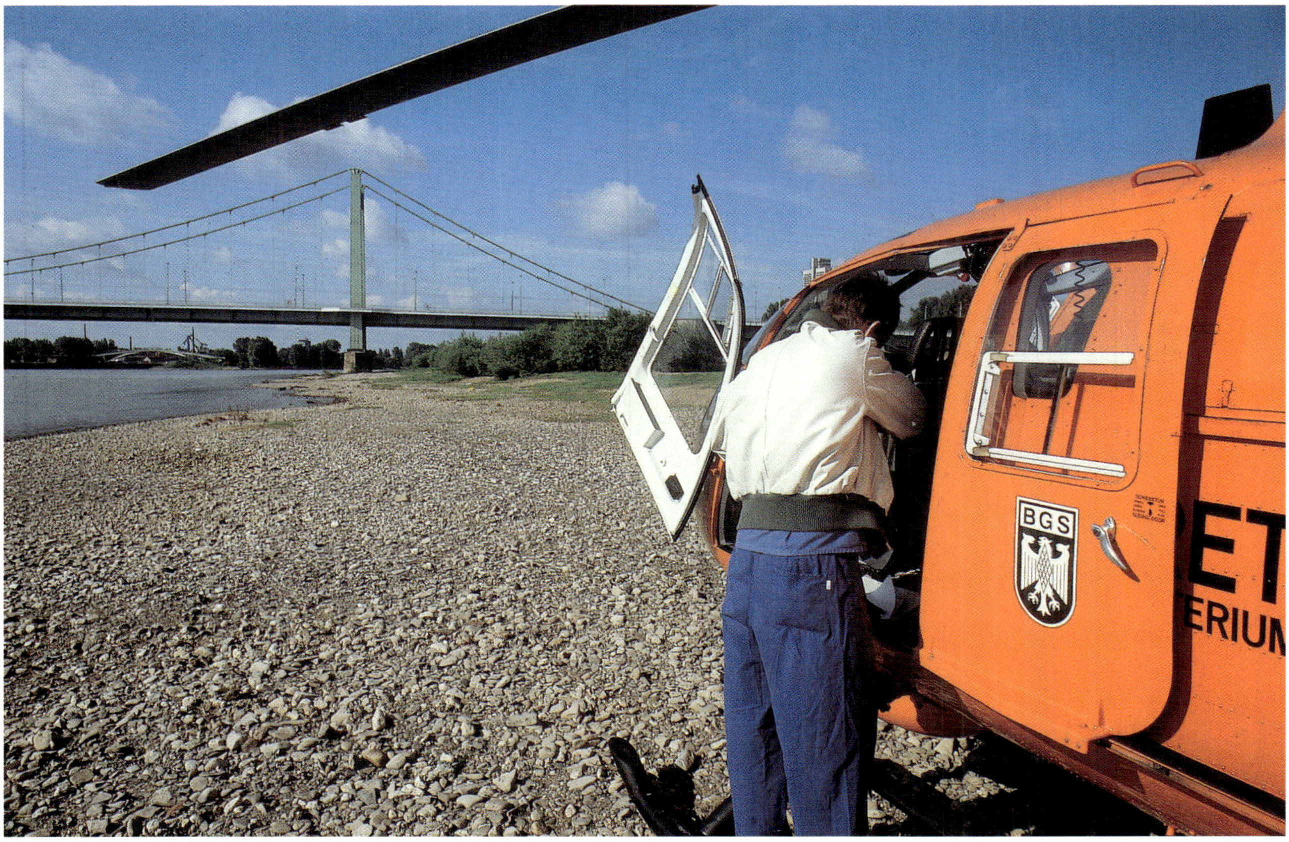

Dokumentation des Einsatzes und Krankenhauseinweisung.

Documentation of the mission and hospital admission.

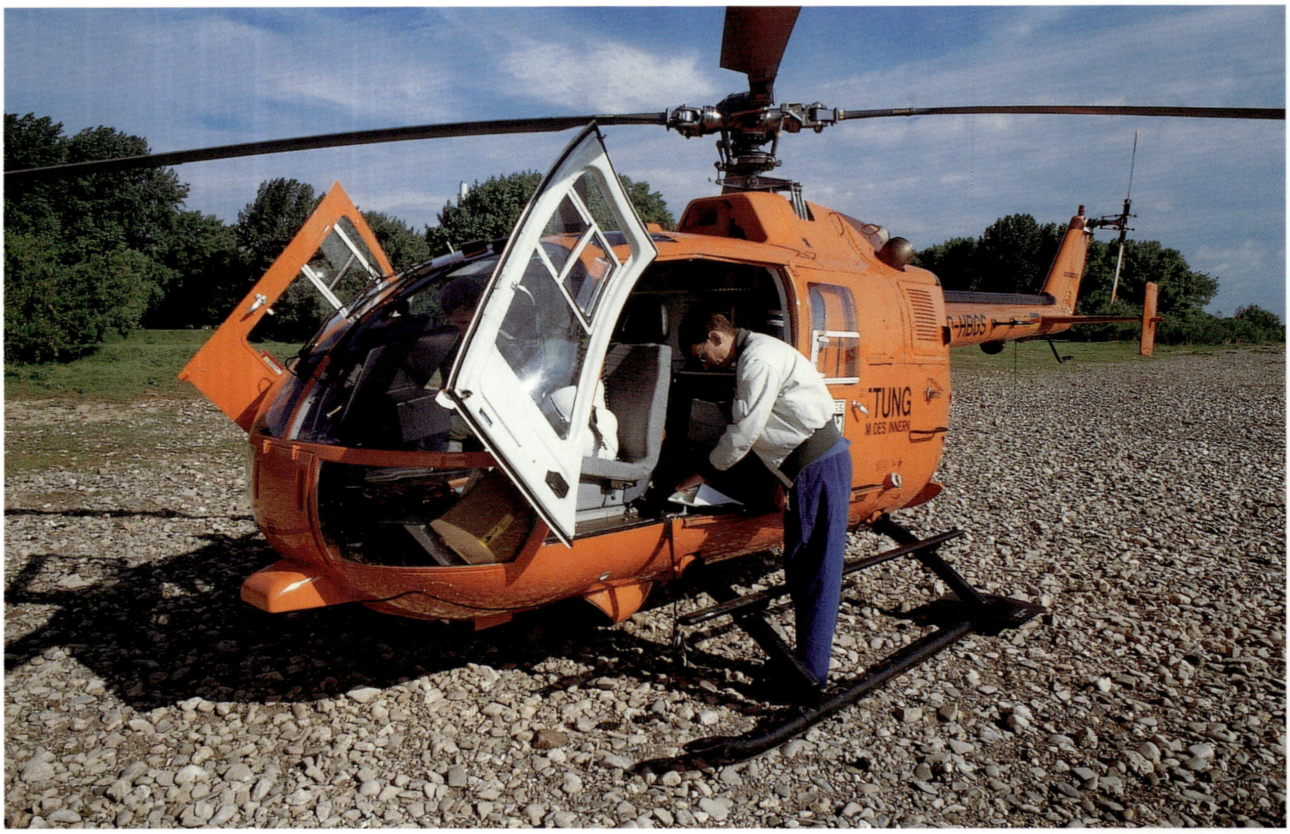

Motiv der Aktion: Liebeskummer.

Motive for the woman's action: problems with her boyfriend.

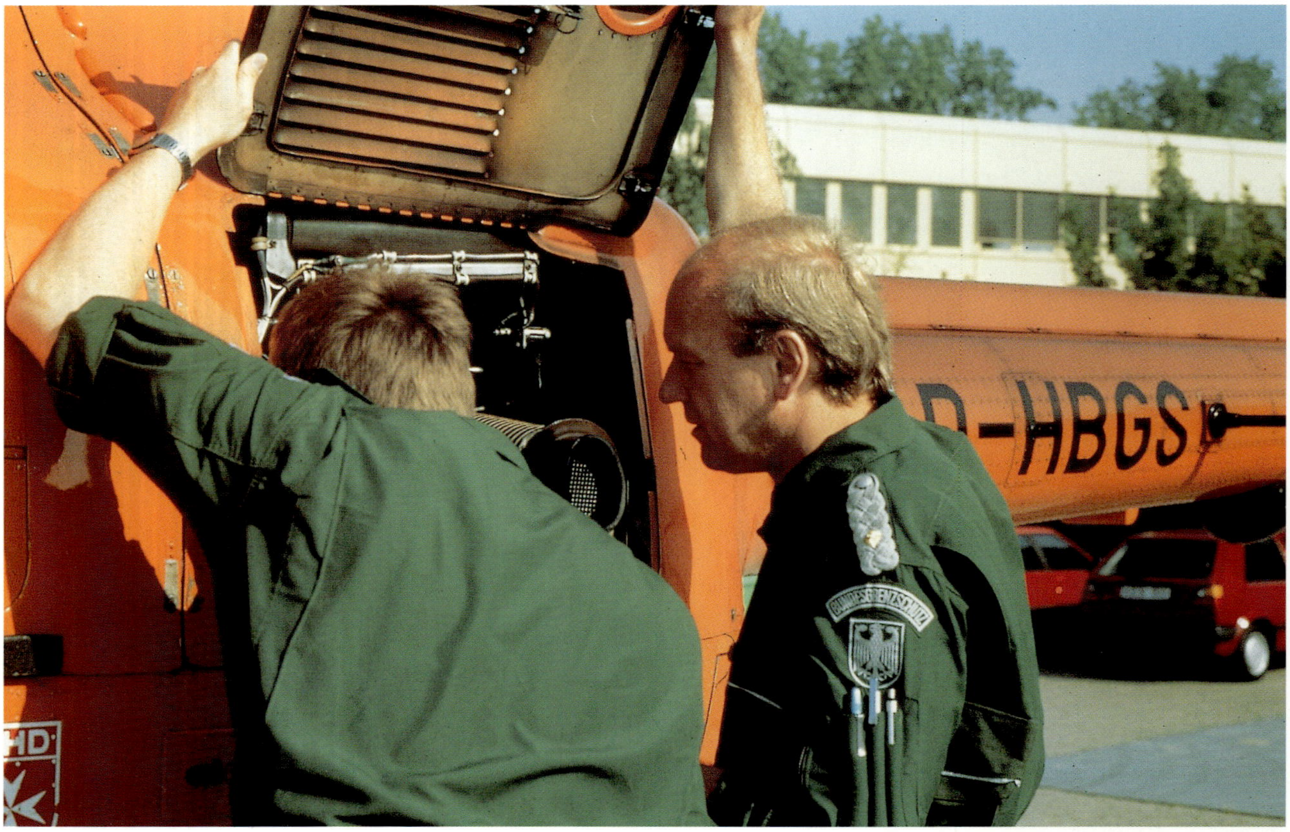

Pilotenwechsel – Übergabe des Hubschraubers

Changing of the guard: the helicopter pilot who is going off duty hands over the aircraft to the pilot who has just come on duty.

Einsatz für den Rettungshubschrauber
Mission for the Rescue Helicopter

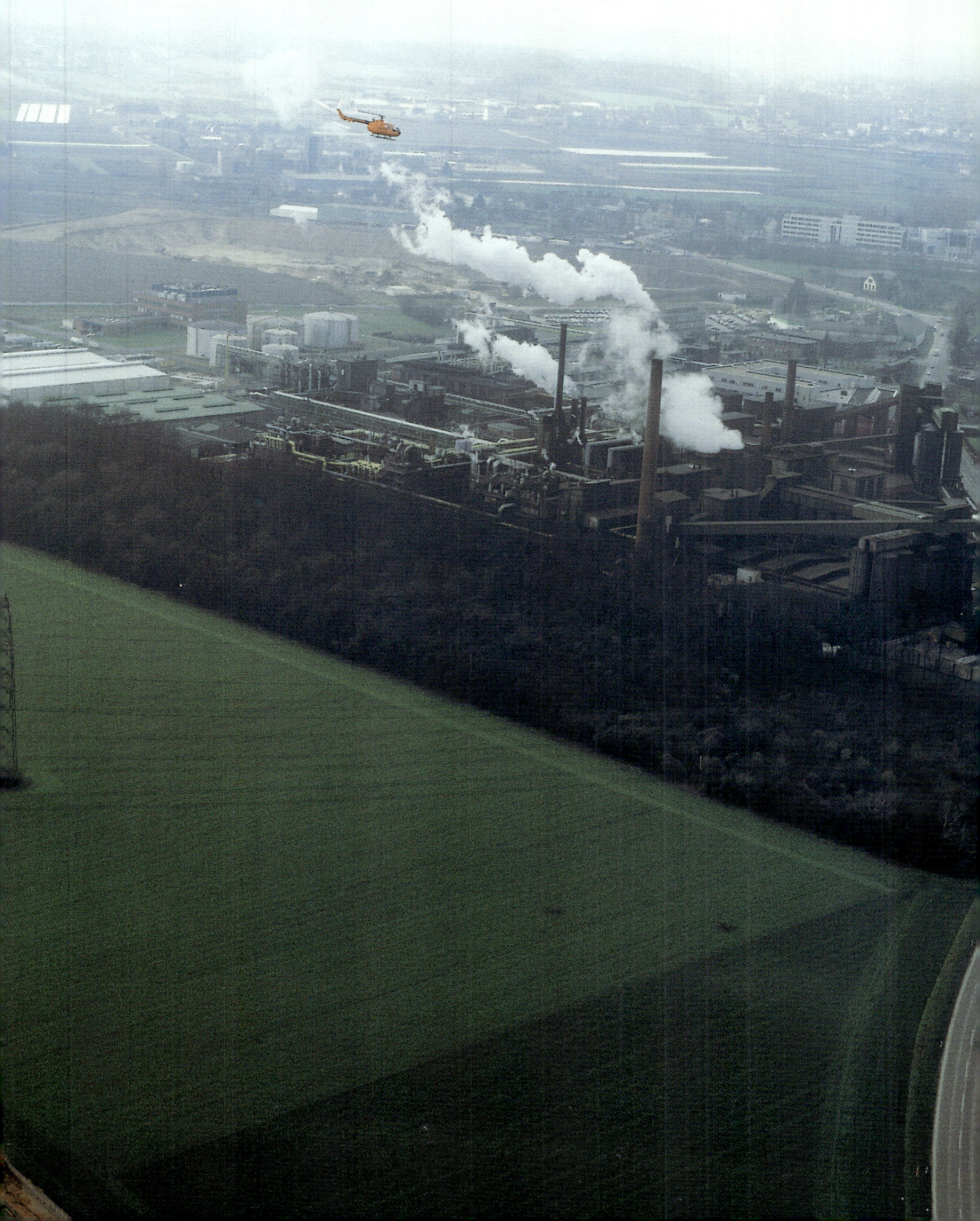

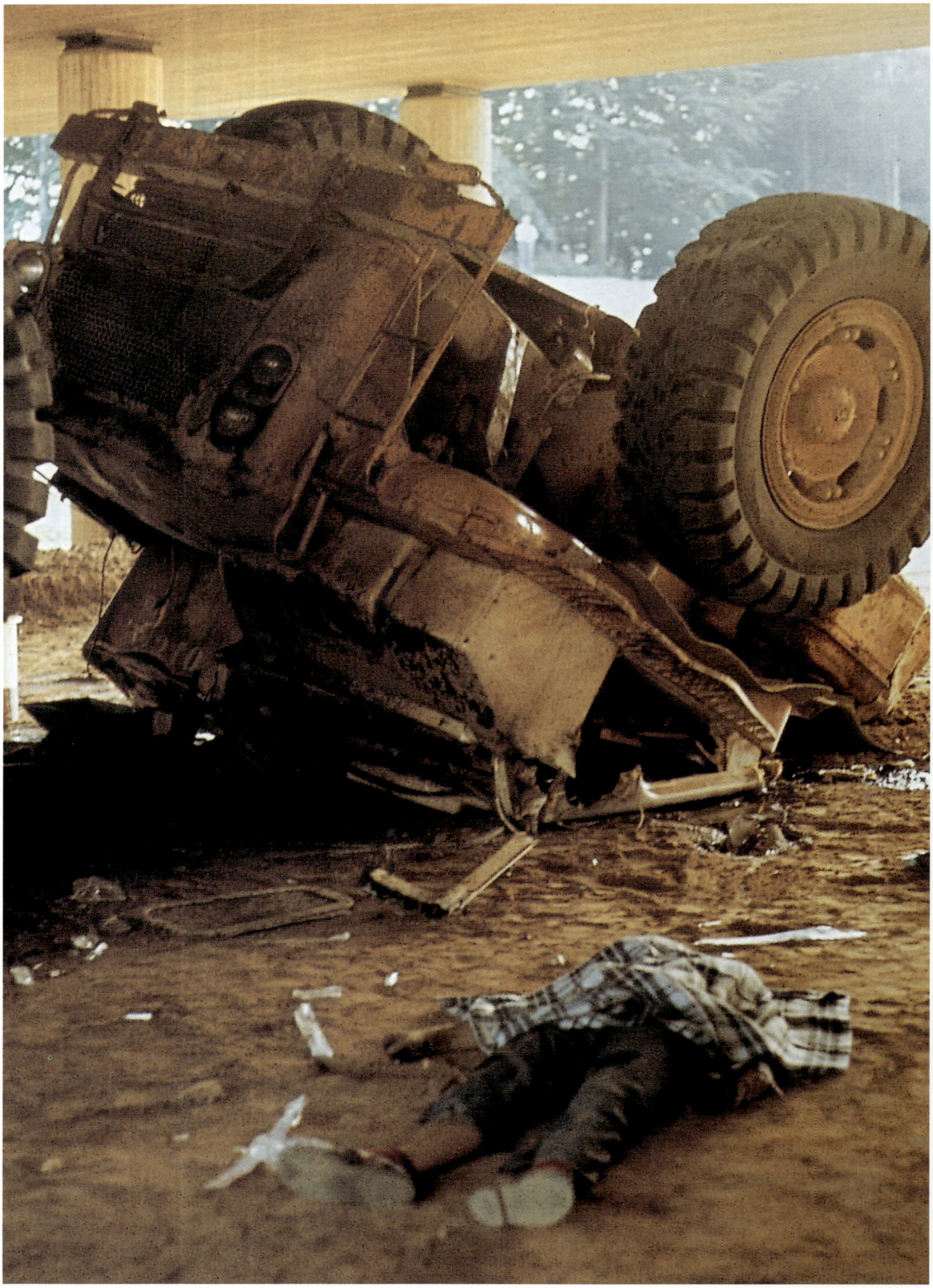

Ein großer Sattelschlepper ist gegen eine Brücke gefahren. Christoph 3 ist nicht mehr erforderlich. Polytrauma. Schädel-Hirn-Trauma. Exitus letalis.

A large tractor-trailer has run into a bridge. Polytrauma: craniocerebral trauma with fatal outcome. Christoph 3 is no longer needed.

Einsatz für den Rettungshubschrauber
Mission for the Rescue Helicopter

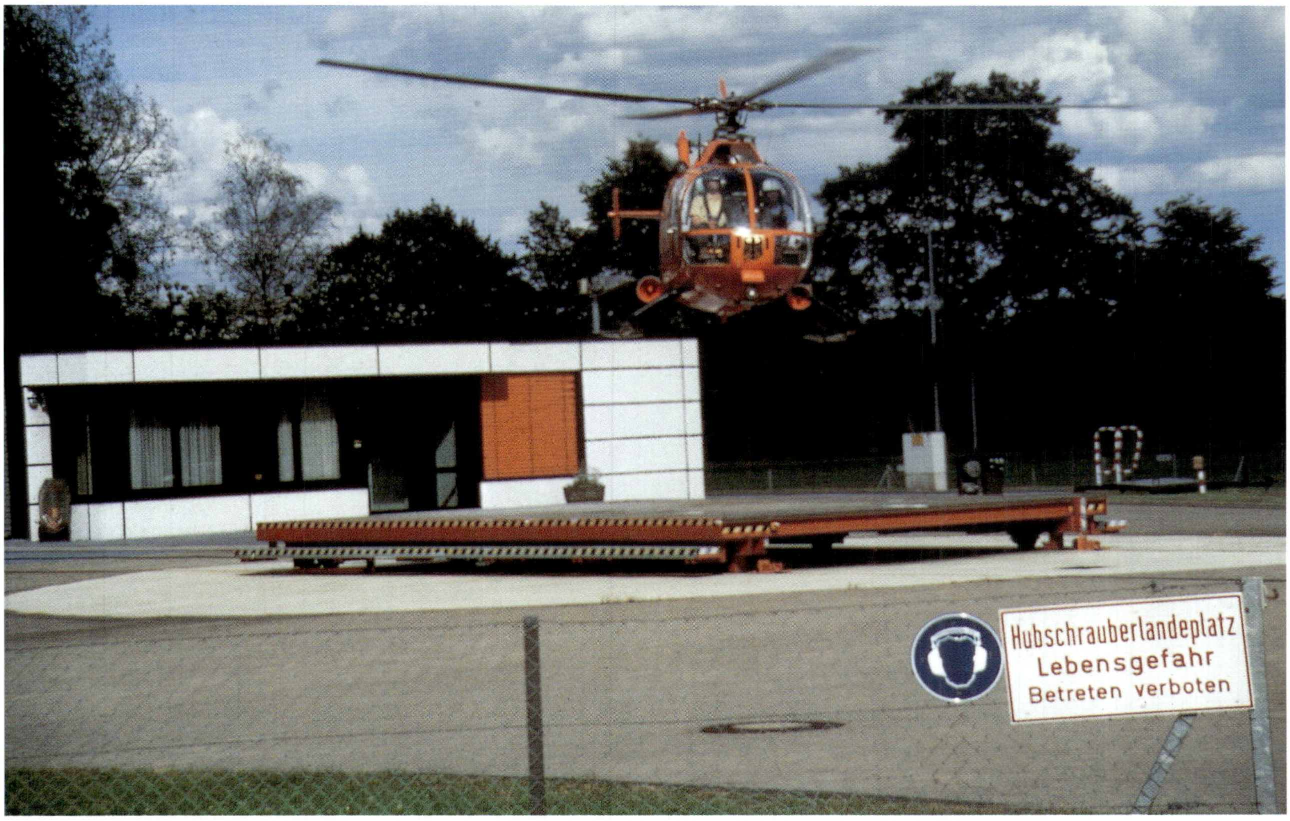

Internistischer Notfall auf der Autobahn.

Ein Gefängnisinsasse hat mehrere Rasierklingen, offene Stecknadeln und andere Nadeln geschluckt. Das Röntgenbild zeigt uns die Anzahl und Lage der einzelnen Nadeln und Rasierklingen.

Die Gefängnisbeamten sagen uns, auf keinen Fall könne der Patient alleine mit uns fliegen. Er müsse bewacht werden. Wir fordern zum Weitertransport ein SAR-Hubschrauber der Bundeswehr an und machen am Sonntagnachmittag auf dem leeren Parkplatz eines Einkaufscentrums den Treffpunkt aus. Der Gefängnisinsasse wird unruhiger. Er hatte vermutlich gehofft, in ein normales Krankenhaus verlegt zu werden.

Medical emergency on the autobahn.

A prison inmate has swallowed several razor blades, tailor's pins and sewing needles. The x-ray shows the number and position of the various pins, needles and razor blades.

The prison guard informs us that the patient cannot fly alone with us under any circumstances; he has to be accompanied by a guard for security reasons. We request a SAR helicopter from the German Airforce for the onward transport. Since it is a Sunday afternoon, we agree to rendezvous on an empty parking lot at a shopping mall. The prison inmate is getting increasingly restless; he had presumably counted on being taken to a normal hospital.

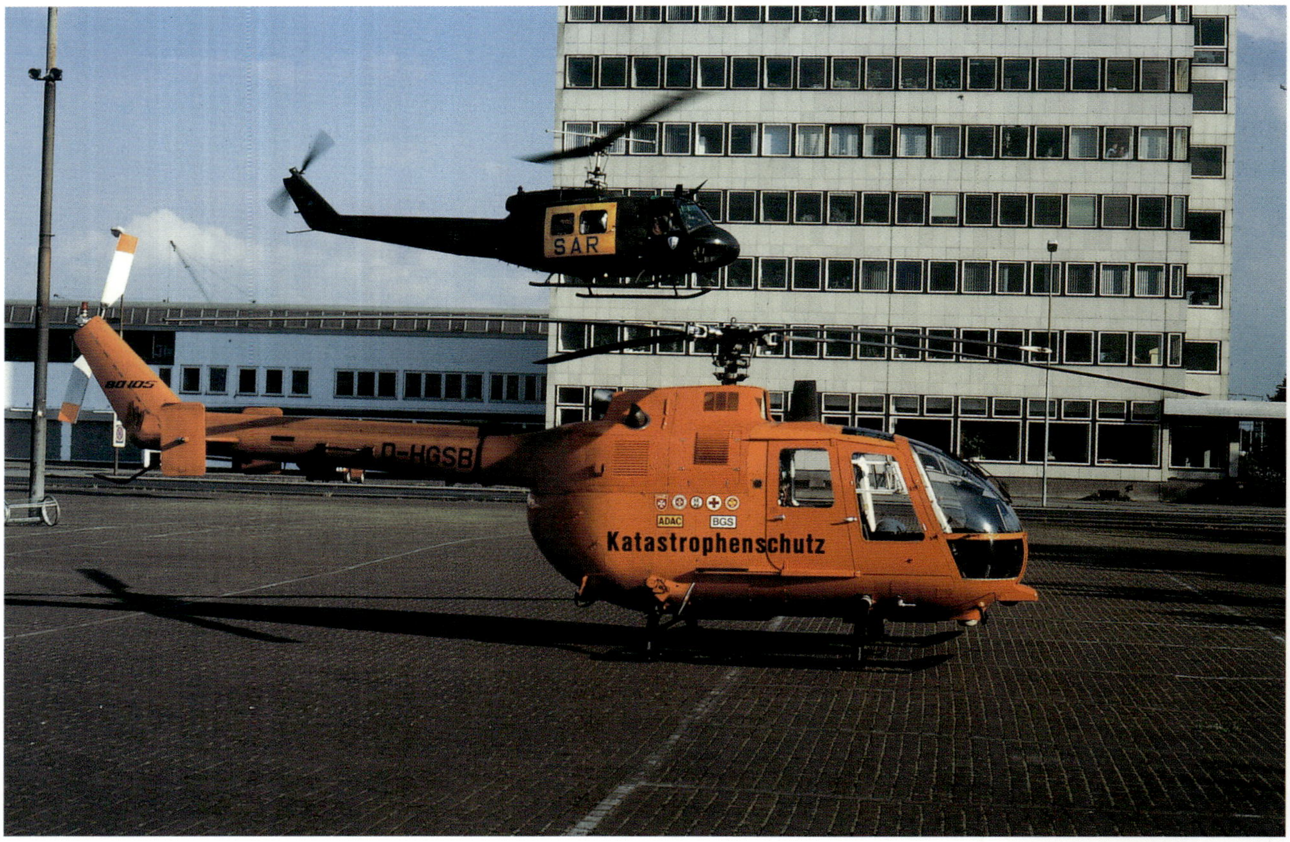

Der SAR-RTH landet.

The SAR rescue helicopter touches down.

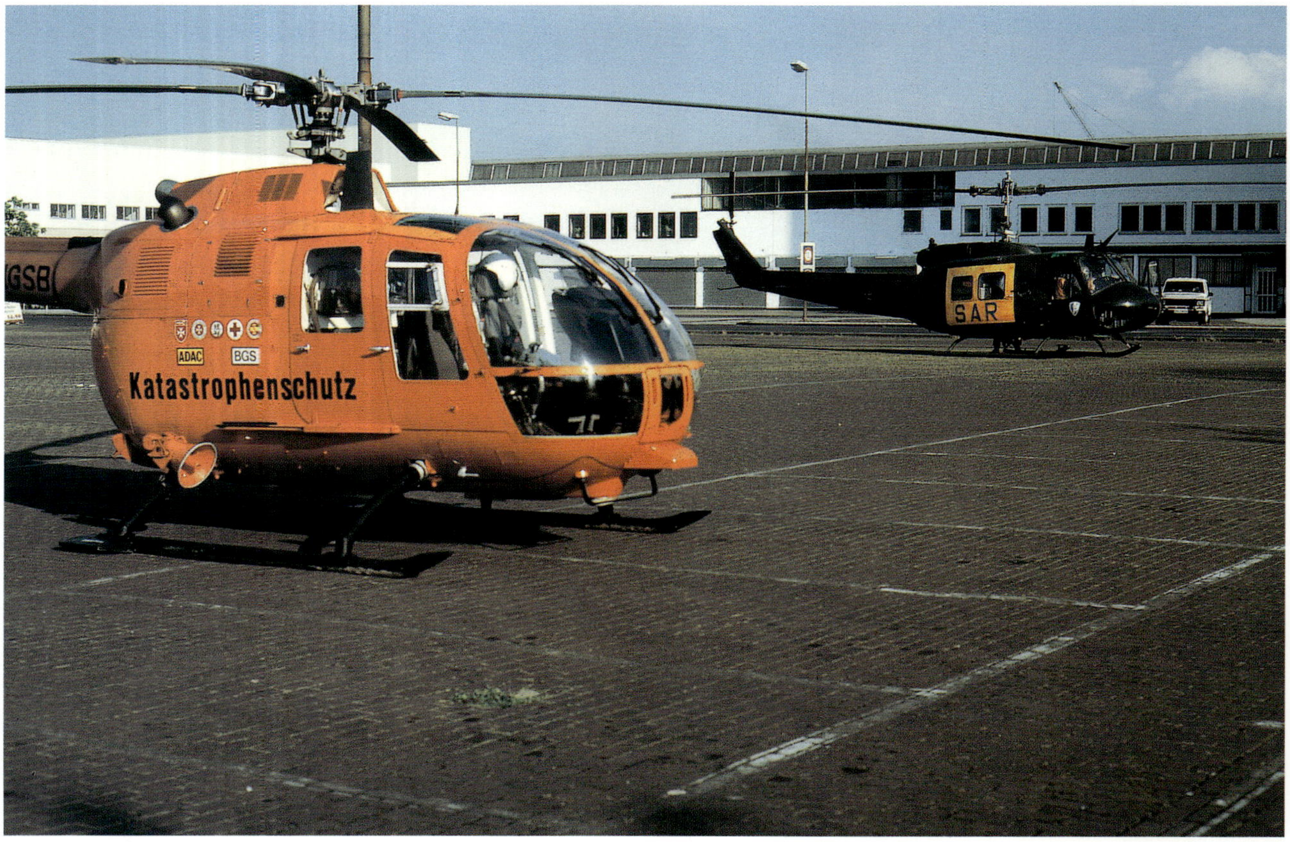

Der Patient wird in der Bundeswehrmaschine von dem Notarzt von Christoph 3 versorgt.

Inside the German Airforce helicopter, a physician with emergency & rescue certification from Christoph 3 administers emergency treatment.

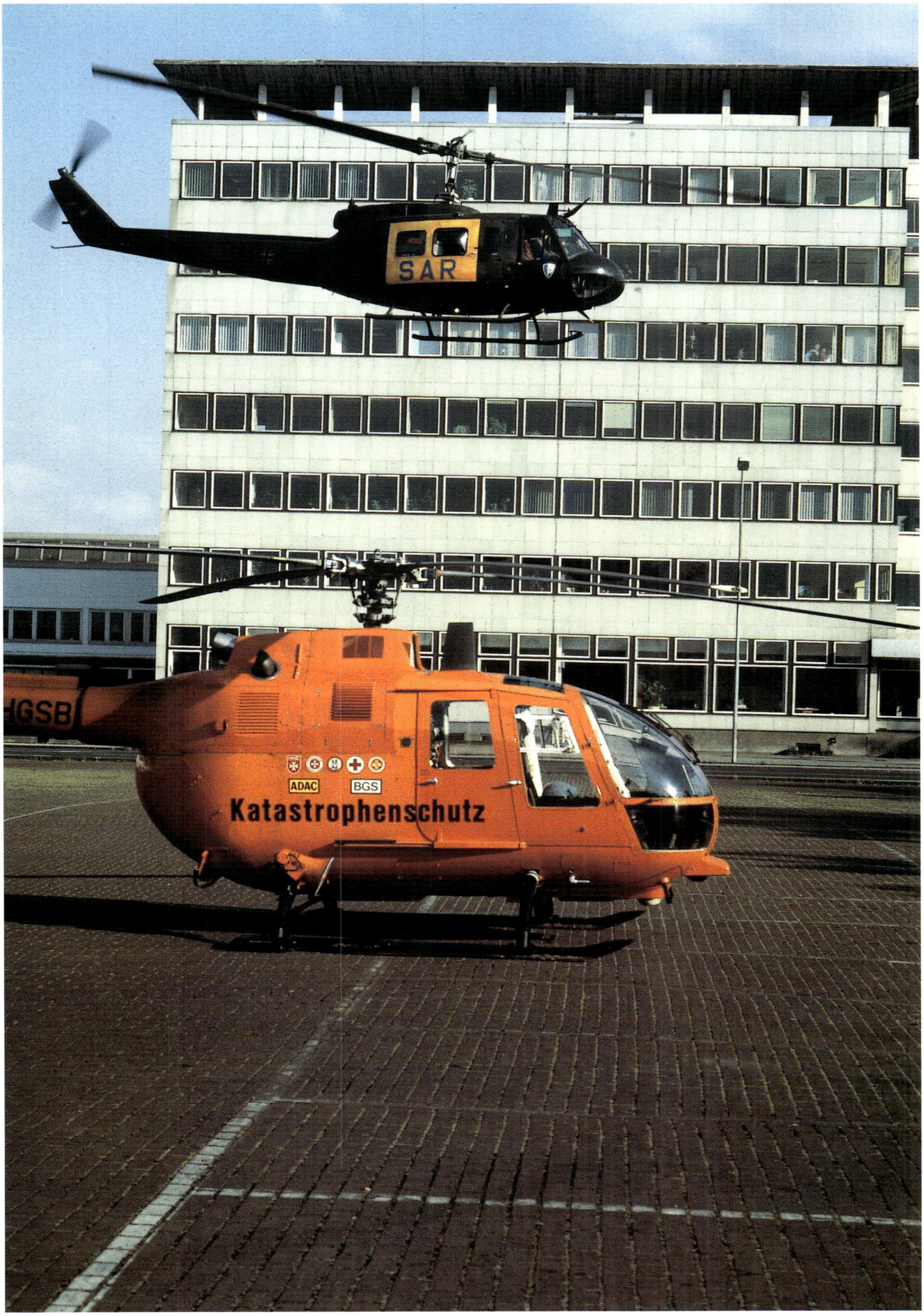

Start. Take-off.

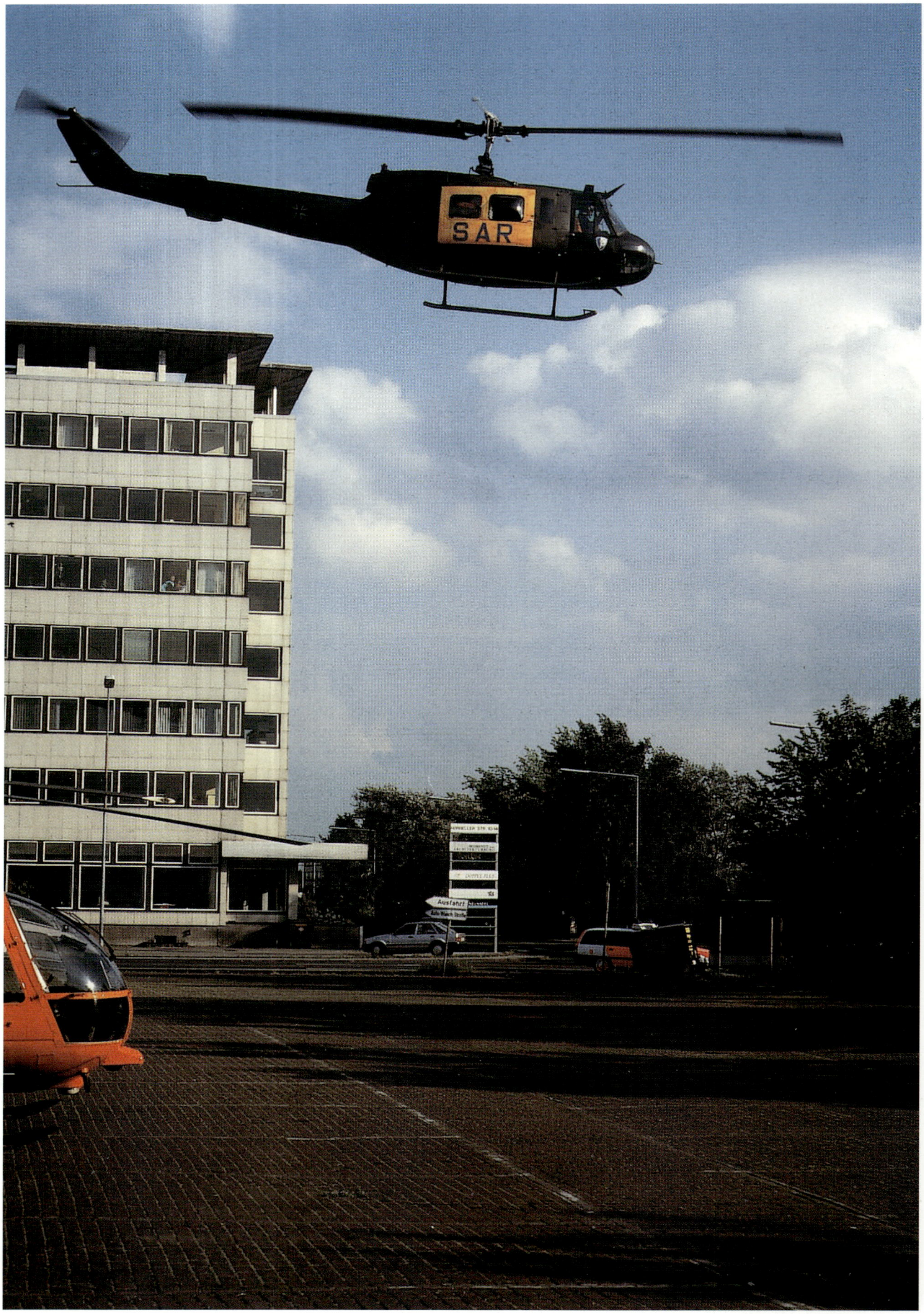

Der Patient wird zum Gefängniskrankenhaus geflogen.

The patient is flown to the prison hospital.

Einsatz für den Rettungshubschrauber
Mission for the Rescue Helicopter

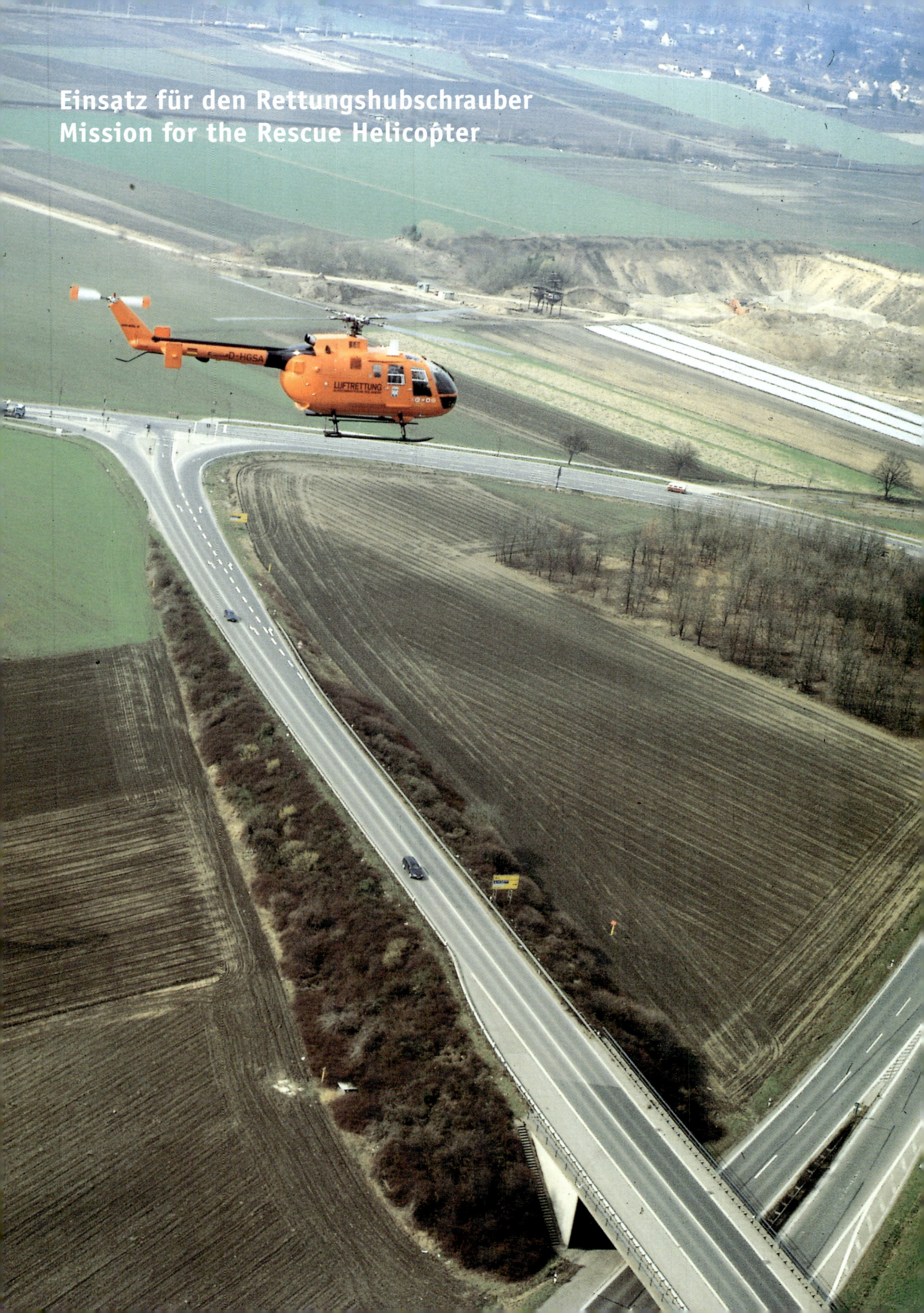

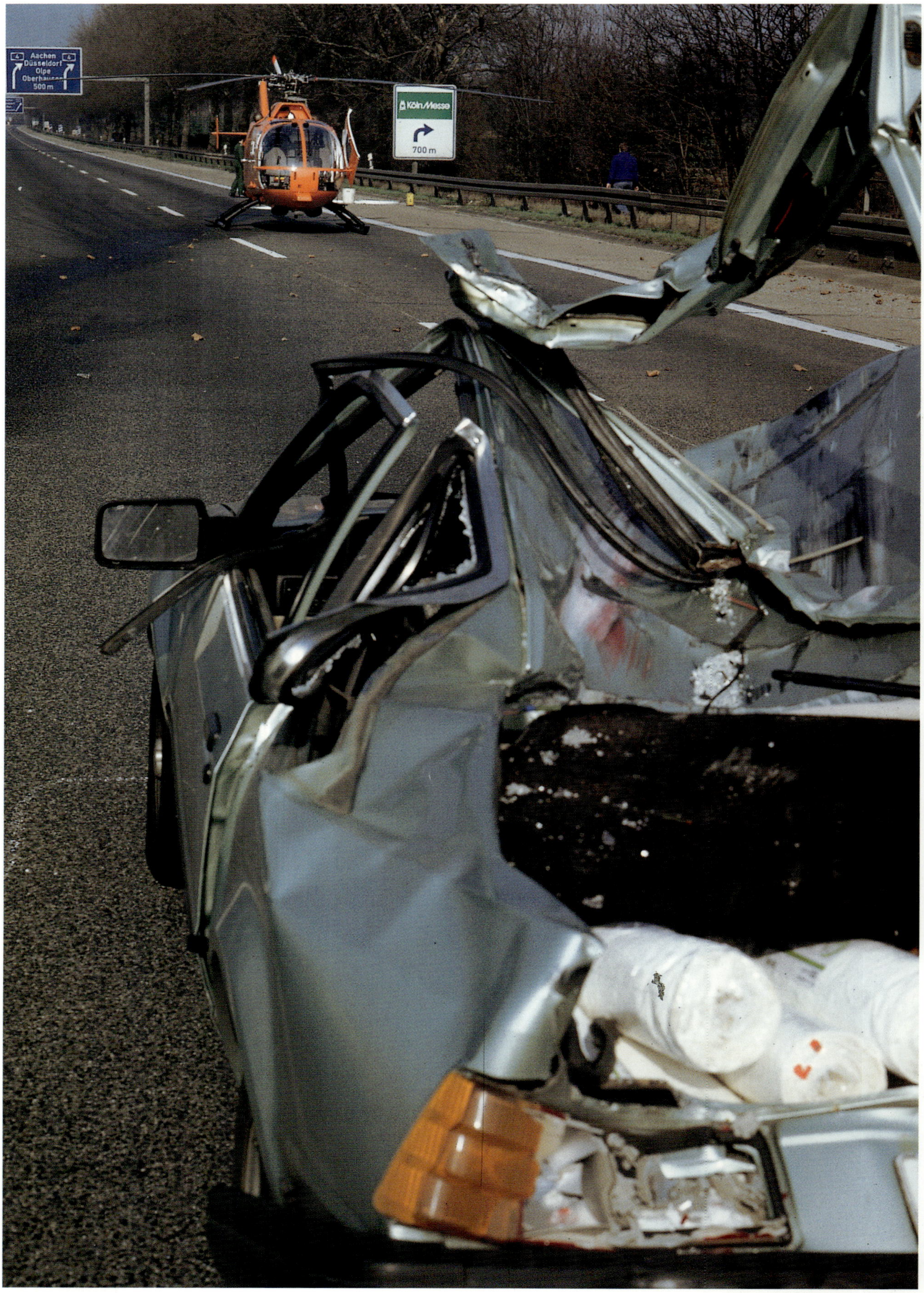

Unfall auf der Autobahn. Motorrad gegen PKW.

Accident on the autobahn: a motorcycle has collided with an automobile.

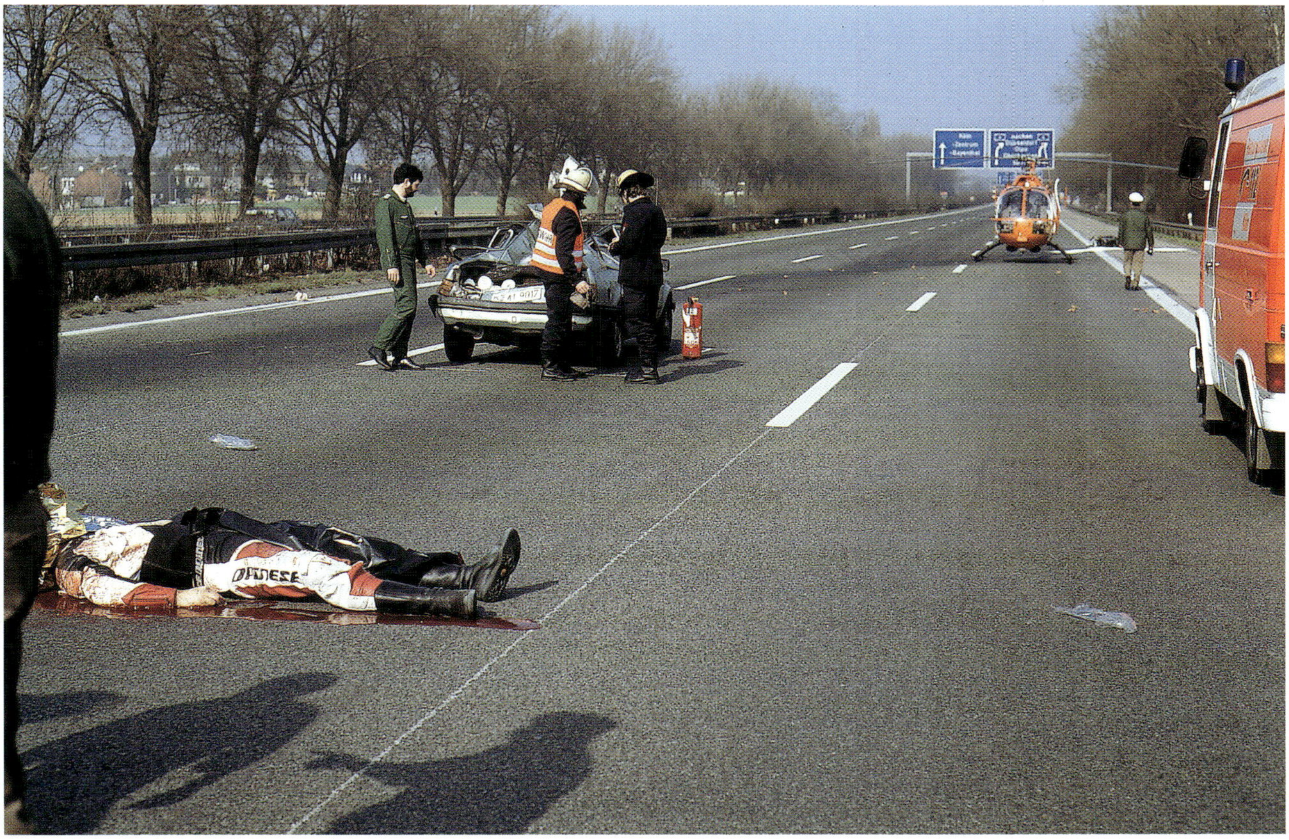

Ein Motorradfahrer ist von hinten auf einen PKW, der die Fahrbahn gewechselt hat, aufgefahren.

A motorcycle has run into an automobile which suddenly pulled into its lane.

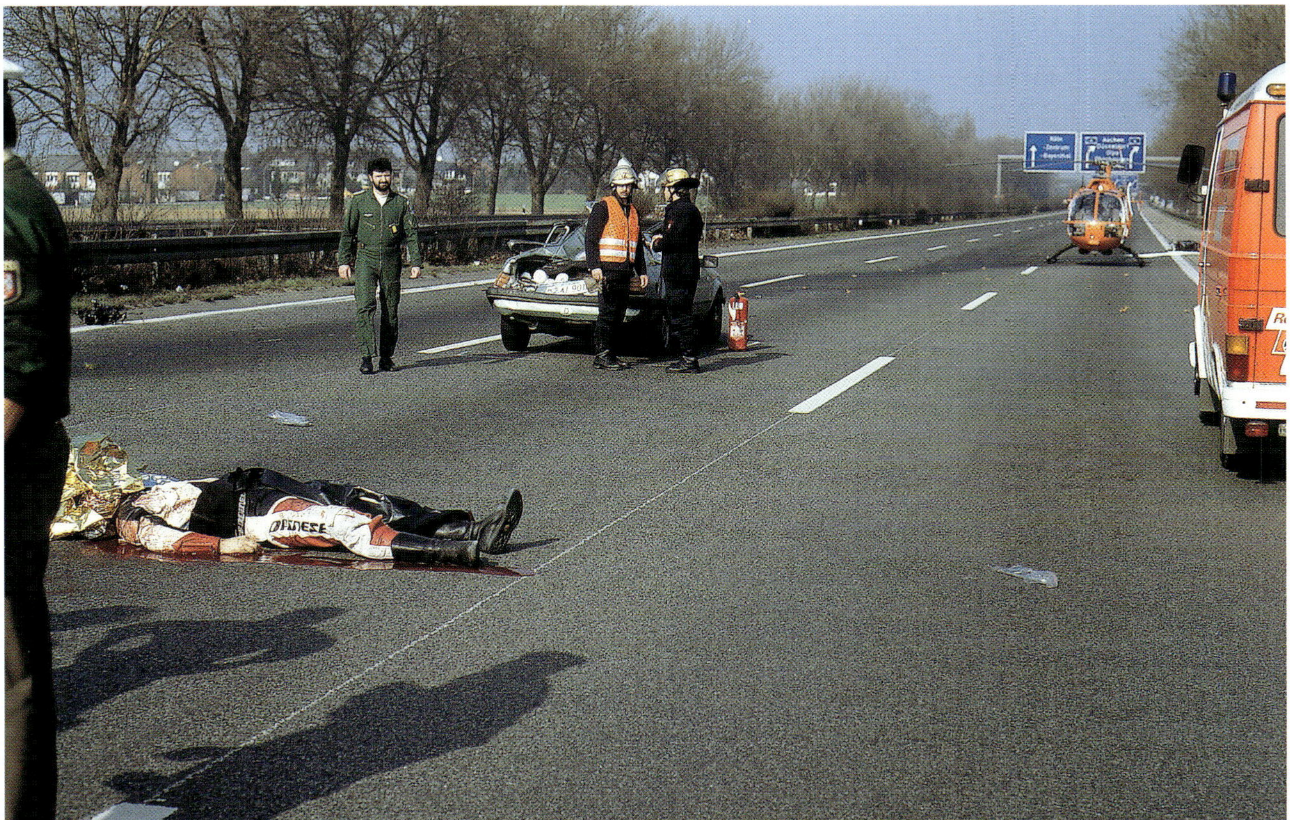

Keine Chance.

No chance of survival.

Augenblicke

Person unter Zug im Bahnhofsbereich. Am Ort junges Mädchen, abgetrenntes Bein in einem großen Plastiksack. Ein junger Mann, der das Bein hält. Das Mädchen ansprechbar. Versorgung. Narkose. Hinter mir ein Knipser. Stört mich. Ich frage: „Presse?“ Antwort: „Kripo“. Gut. Wir laden das Mädchen auf die Trage, bringen es zum Hubschrauber. Der junge Mann mit dem abgetrennten Bein folgt uns. Wir laden das Mädchen ein. Ich frage nach den Personalien. Keiner hat sie. Der junge Mann: „Das Mädchen heißt...... und ist mit mir in der Psychiatrie....“ Wir laden das Bein ein, fliegen das Mädchen zum Krankenhaus.

Snapshots

Person under a train at the railway station. On the scene we find a young girl whose leg has been severed and a young man holding the leg. The young girl is still conscious. We administer medical treatment and anesthesia. I am bothered by someone behind me taking photos. "Press?" I ask. Answer: "No, detective from the Criminal Investigation Squad". In that case . . . We lift the girl onto a stretcher and bring her to the helicopter. The young man carrying the amputated leg follows us. We load the patient into the helicopter. I try to obtain her personal data. No one has them. The young man speaks up: "The girl's name is ....; we are both patients in the psychiatric ward at ..... hospital." We load the leg into the helicopter and fly to the hospital.

Einsatz für den Rettungshubschrauber
Mission for the Rescue Helicopter

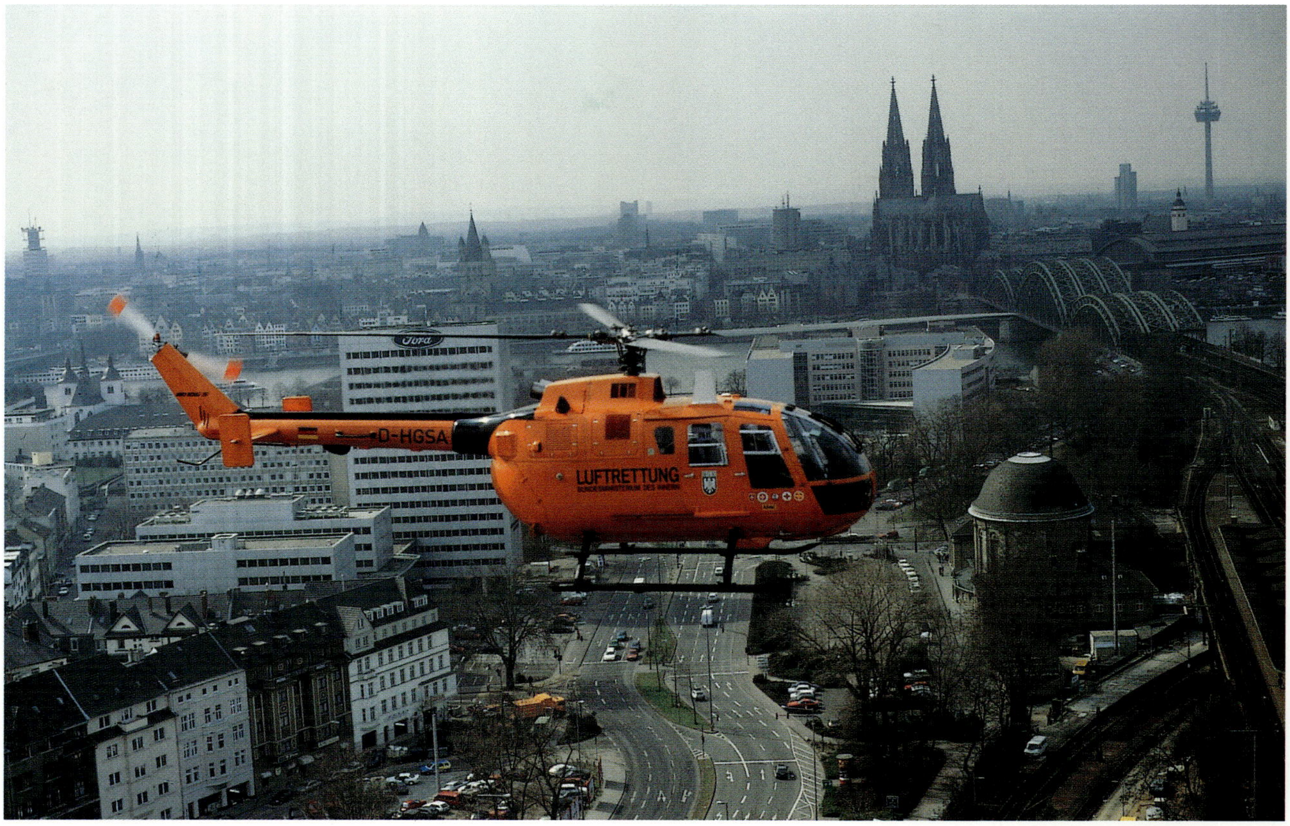

Brennende PKW und eingeklemmte Personen auf der Autobahn.

Major accident on the autobahn, with burning automobiles and people trapped inside their vehicles.

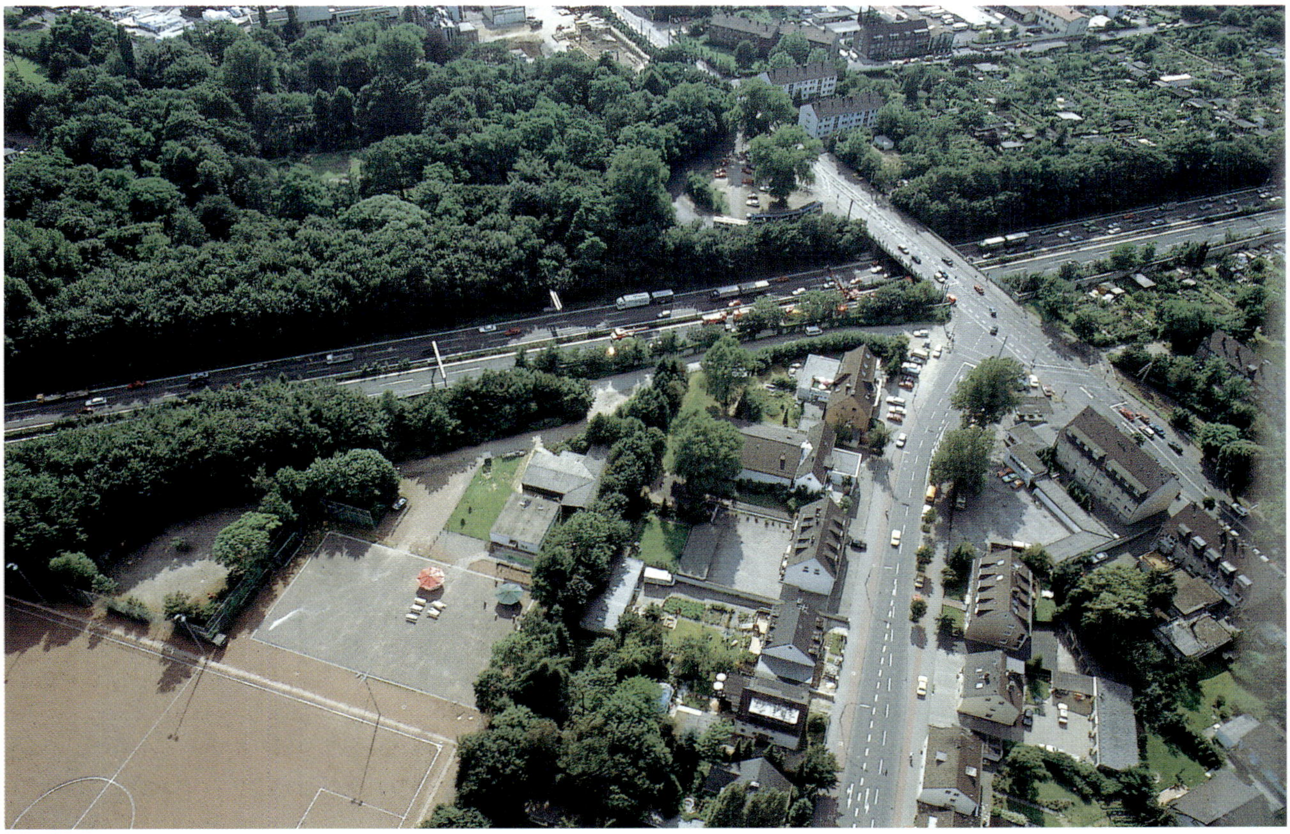

Anflug auf die Einsatzstelle.

Approach to the accident site.

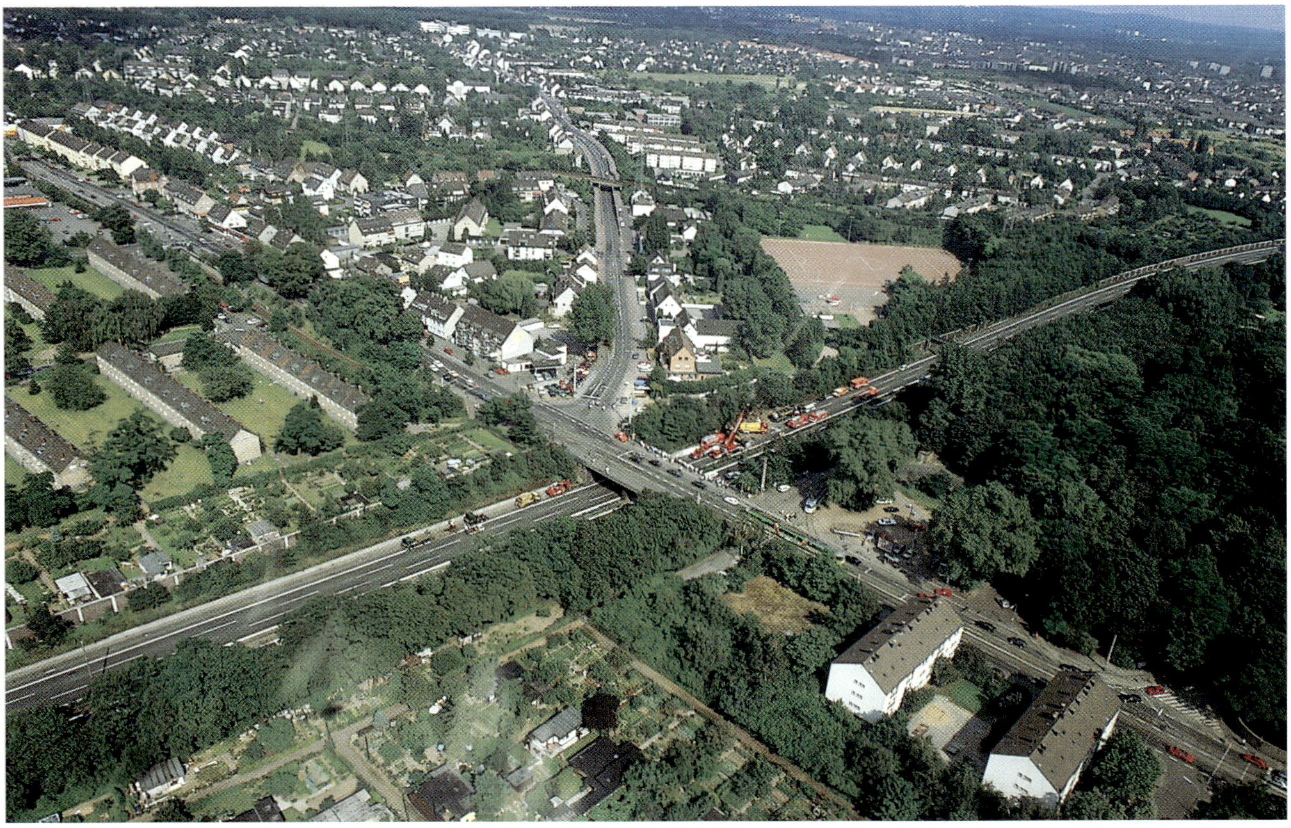

Einsatz für den Rettungshubschrauber
Mission for the Rescue Helicopter

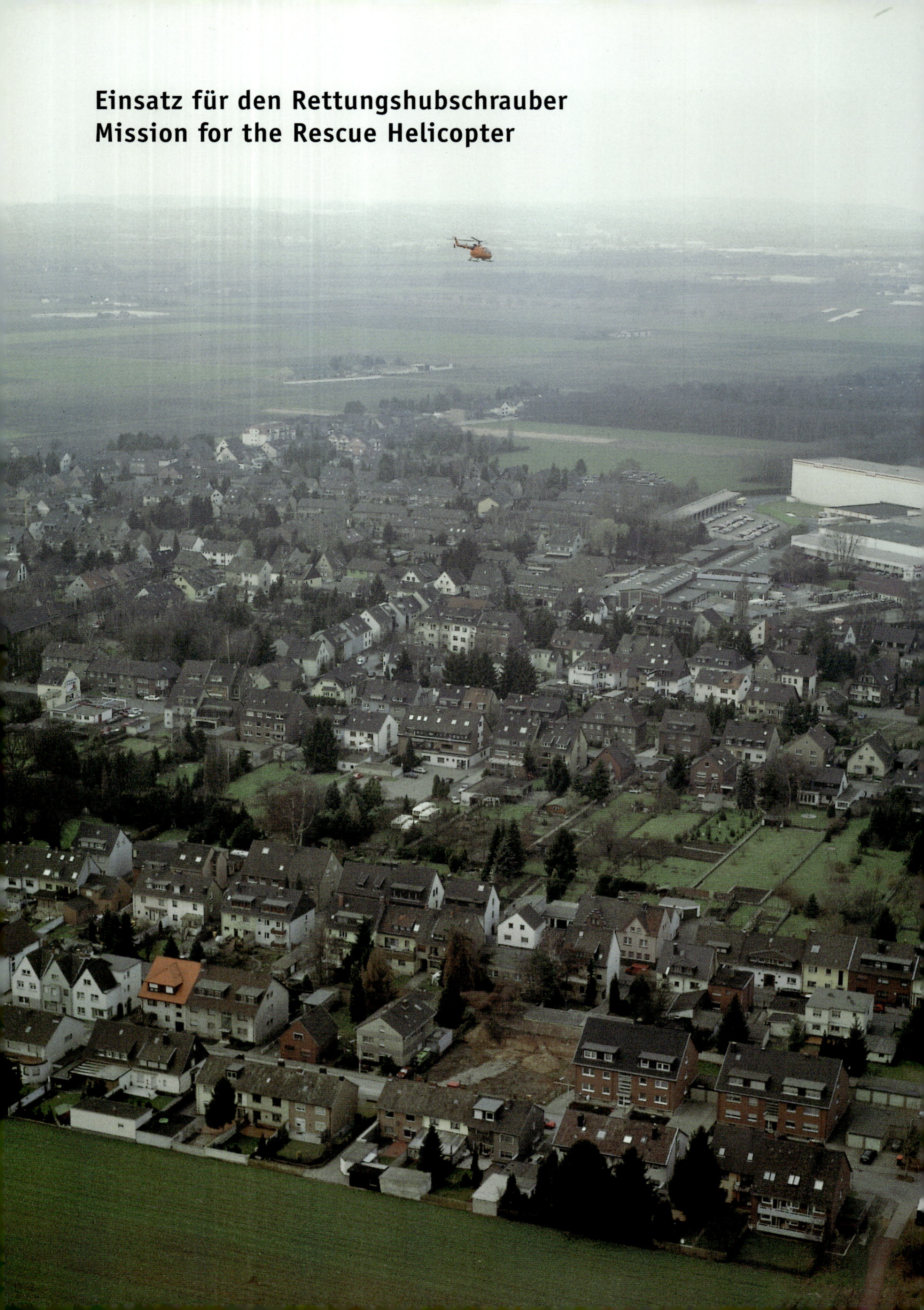

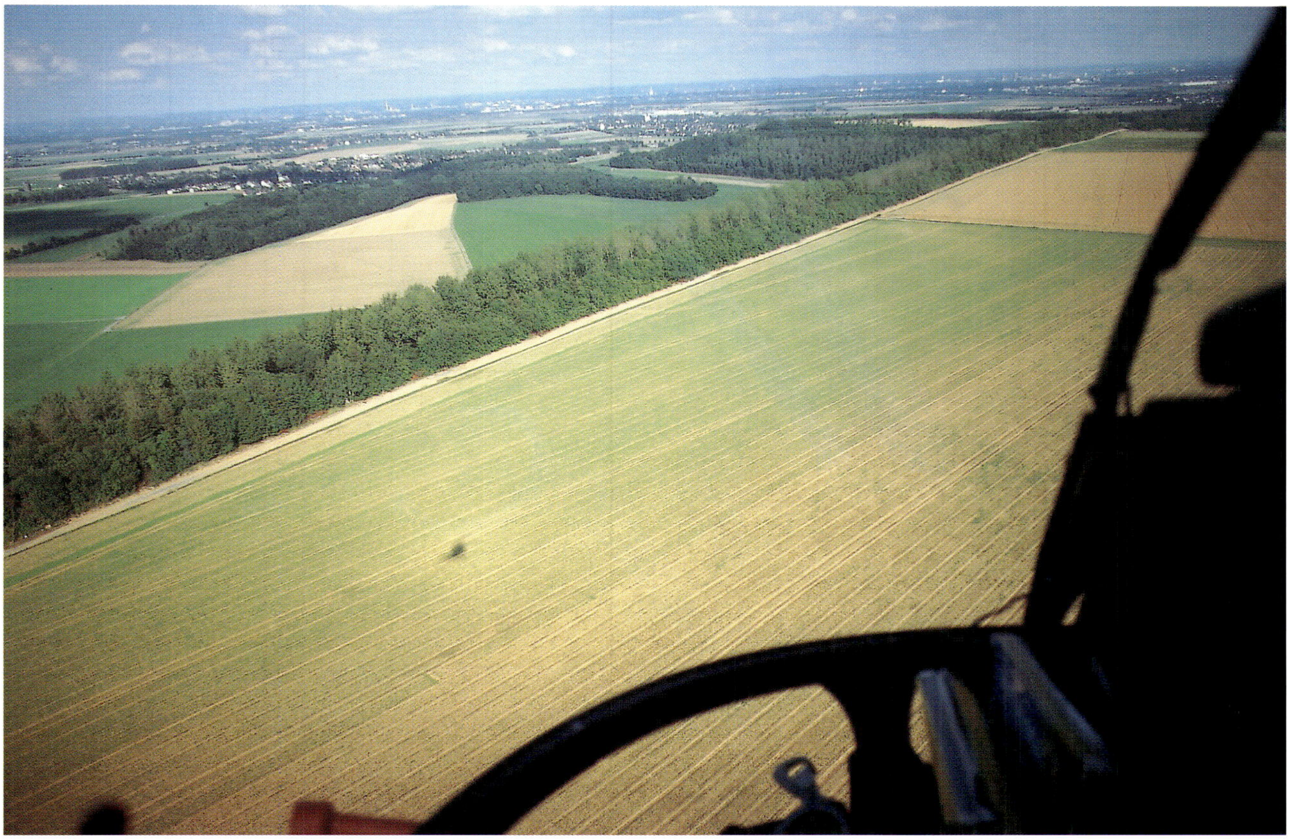

Verkehrsunfall auf der Landstraße. Ein Notarzt fordert zum Transport nach.

Anflug auf die Einsatzstelle.

Motor vehicle accident on a rural road. A physician with emergency & rescue certification calls for transport support.

Approach to the accident site.

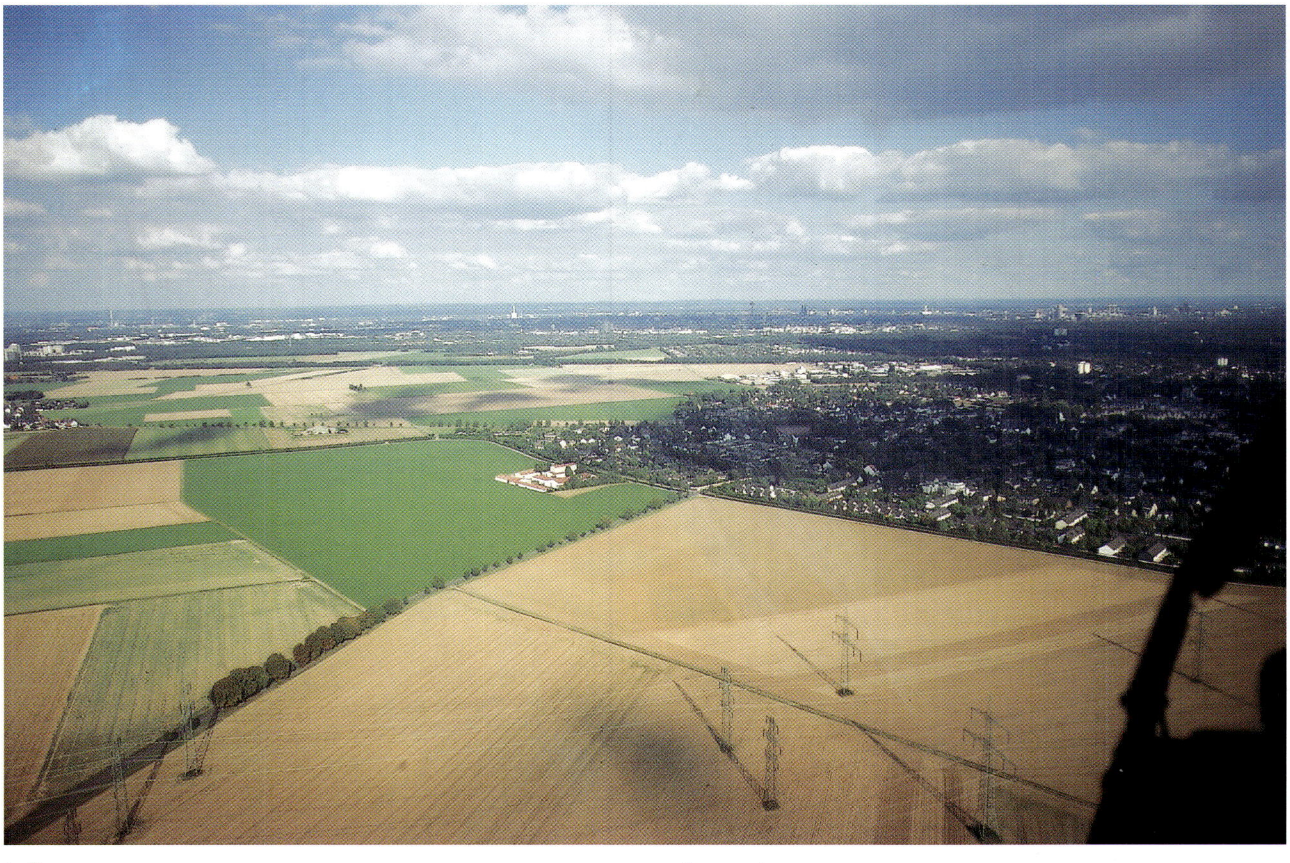

Anflug.

Approach.

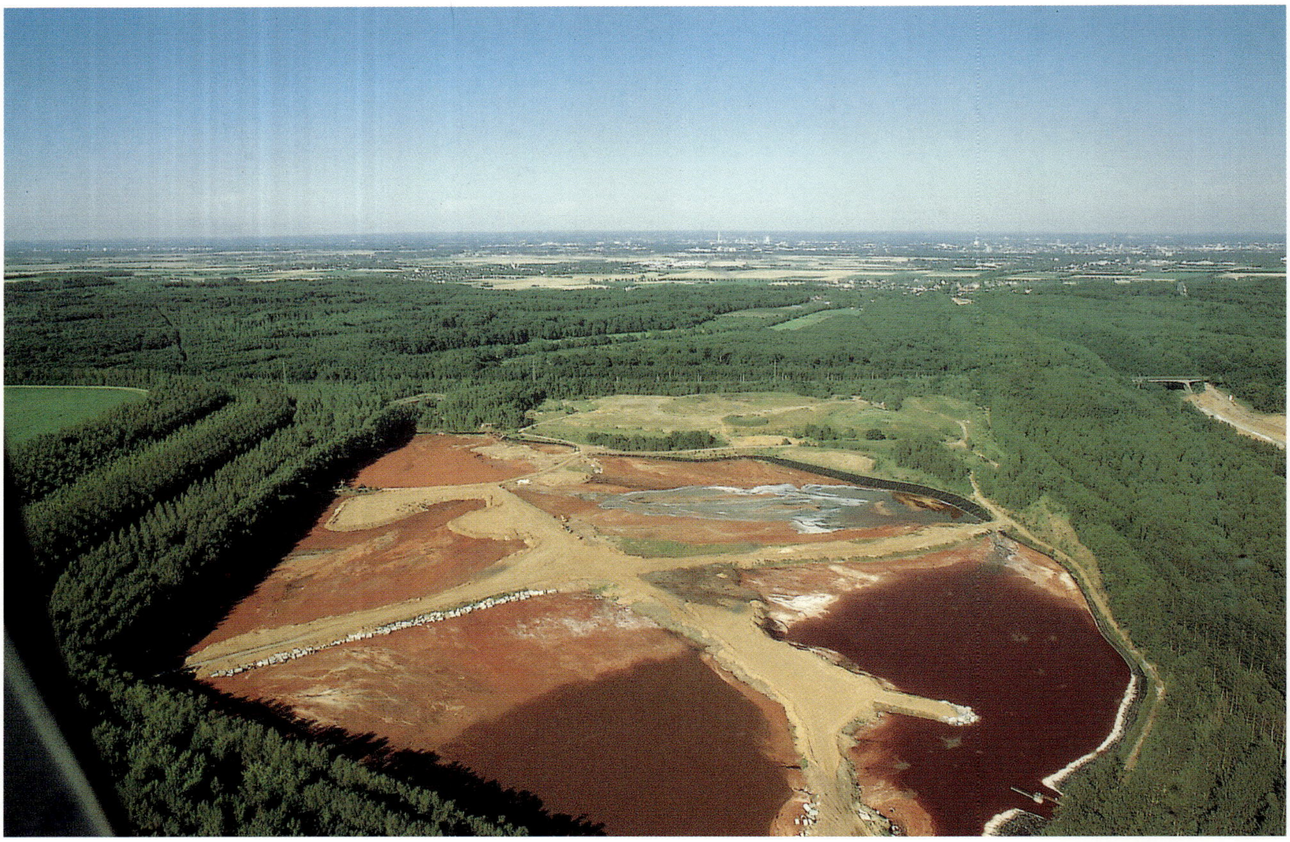

Überflug. Flyover.

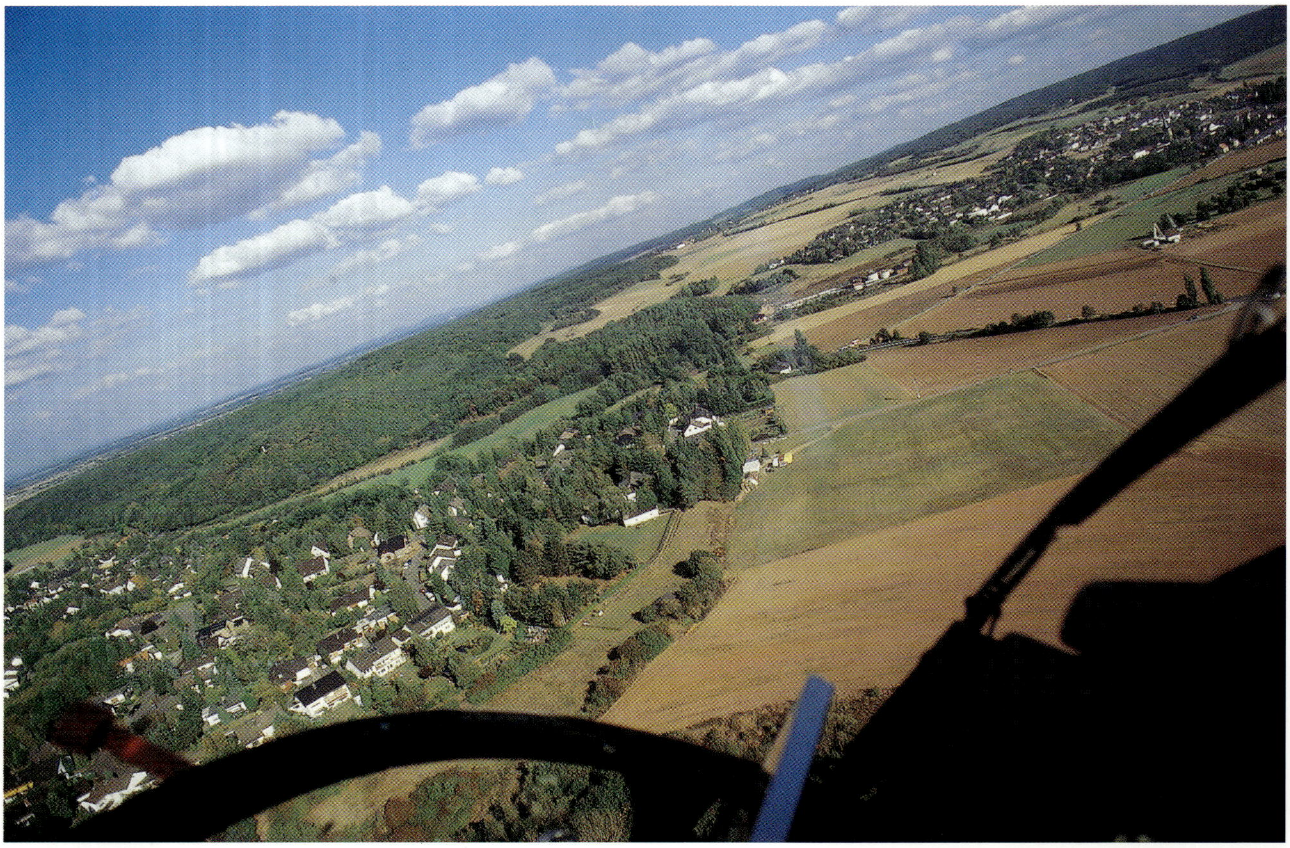

Der Rettungswagen spricht uns an. Er sieht uns und weist uns ein.

The driver of the rescue ambulance spots us. He guides us to the site.

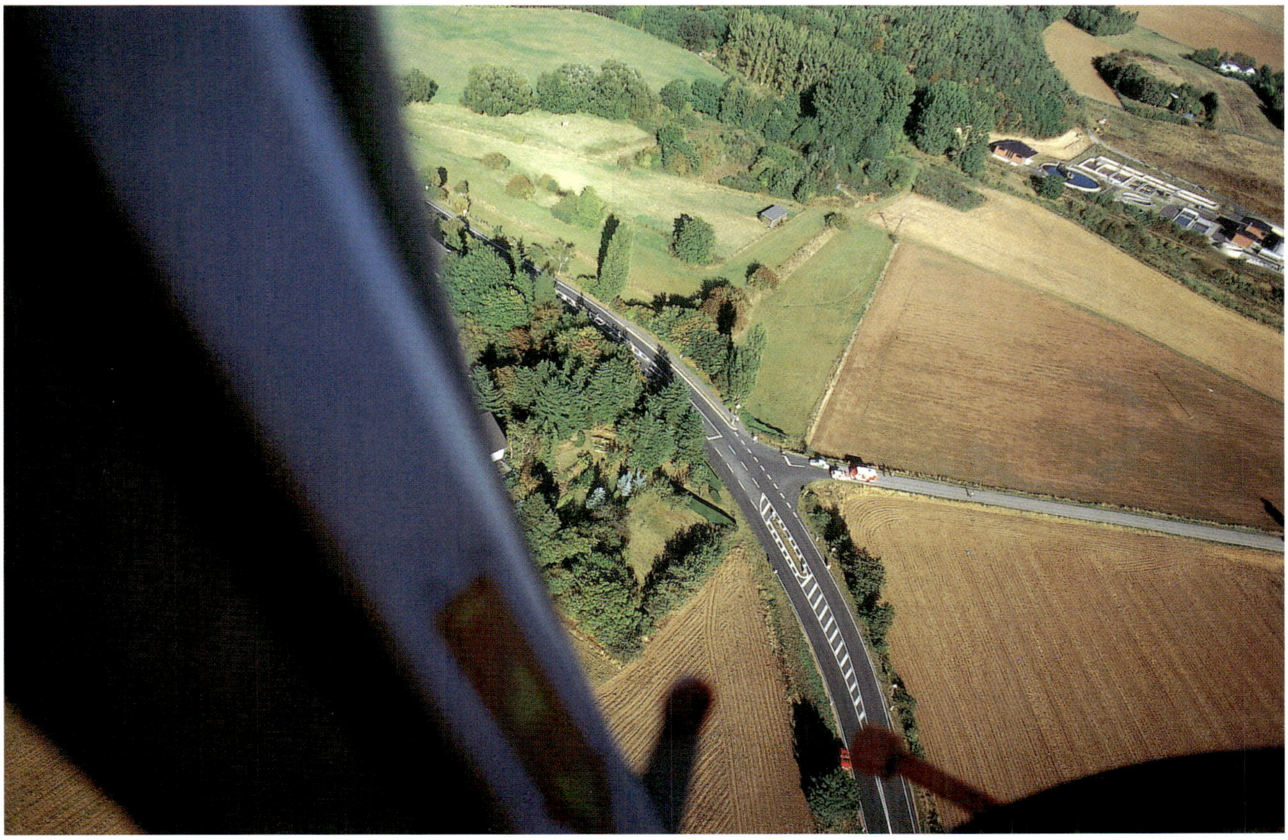

Die Einsatzstelle ist erkannt.

We have identified the accident site.

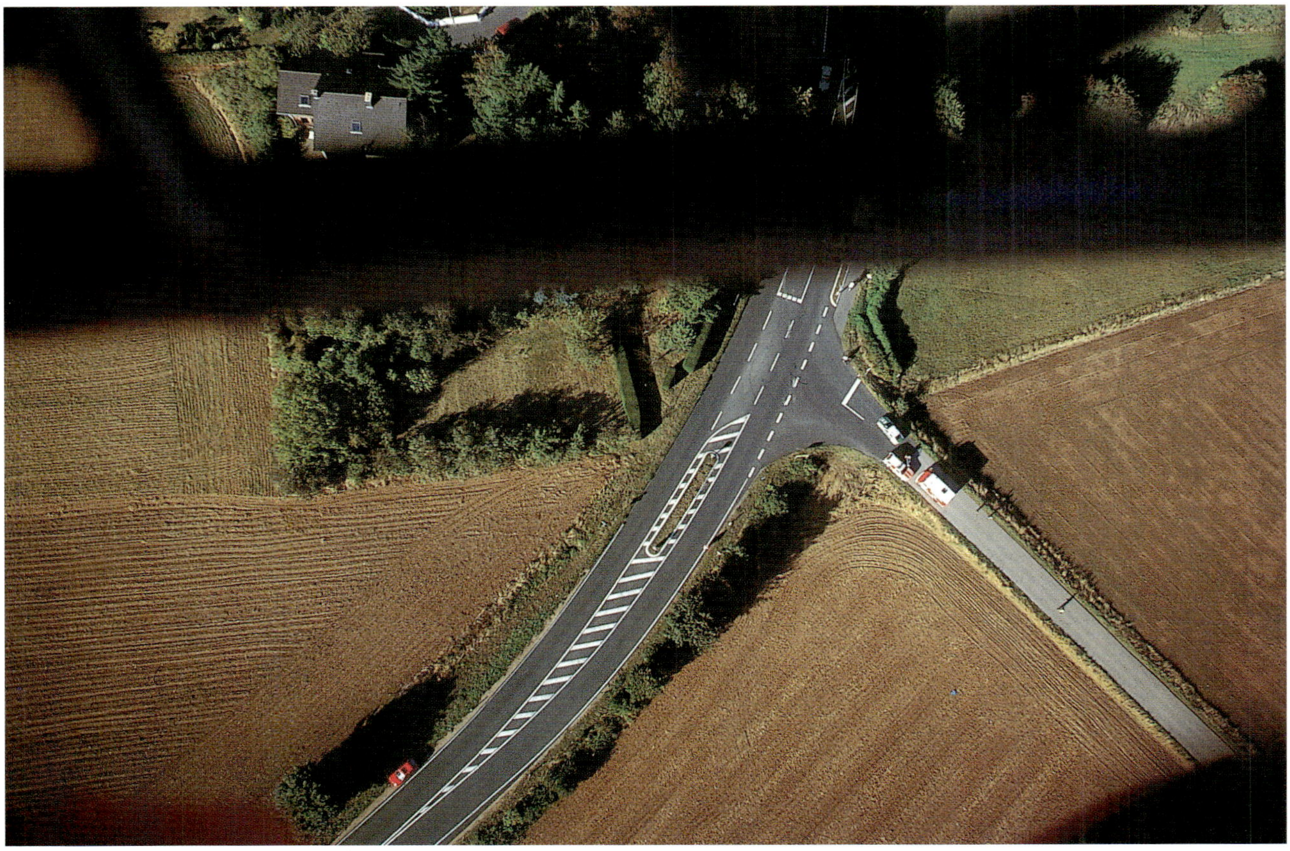

Wir gehen zur Landung.

We prepare to land.

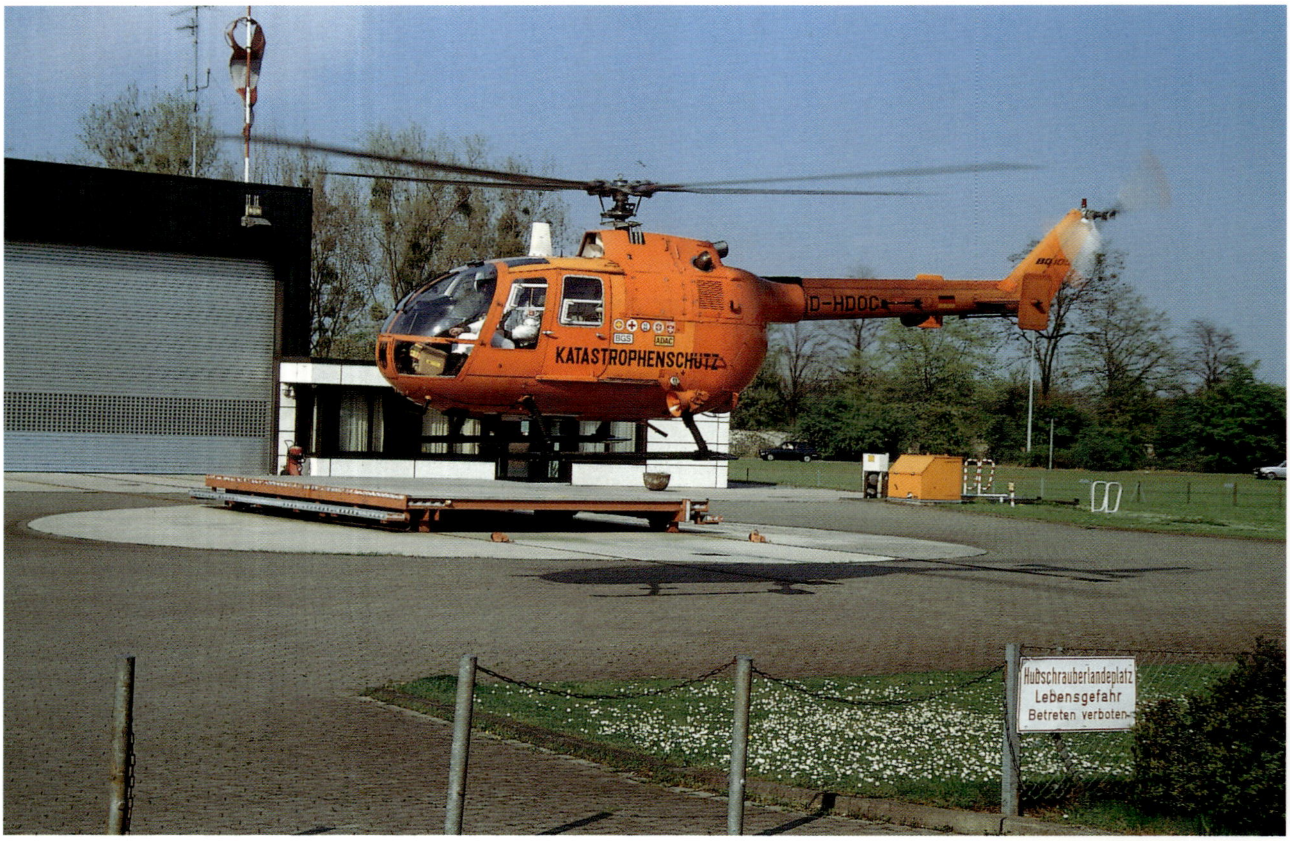

Der Patient wird zum Standortkrankenhaus gebracht.

The patient is taken to the hospital where the helicopter is based.

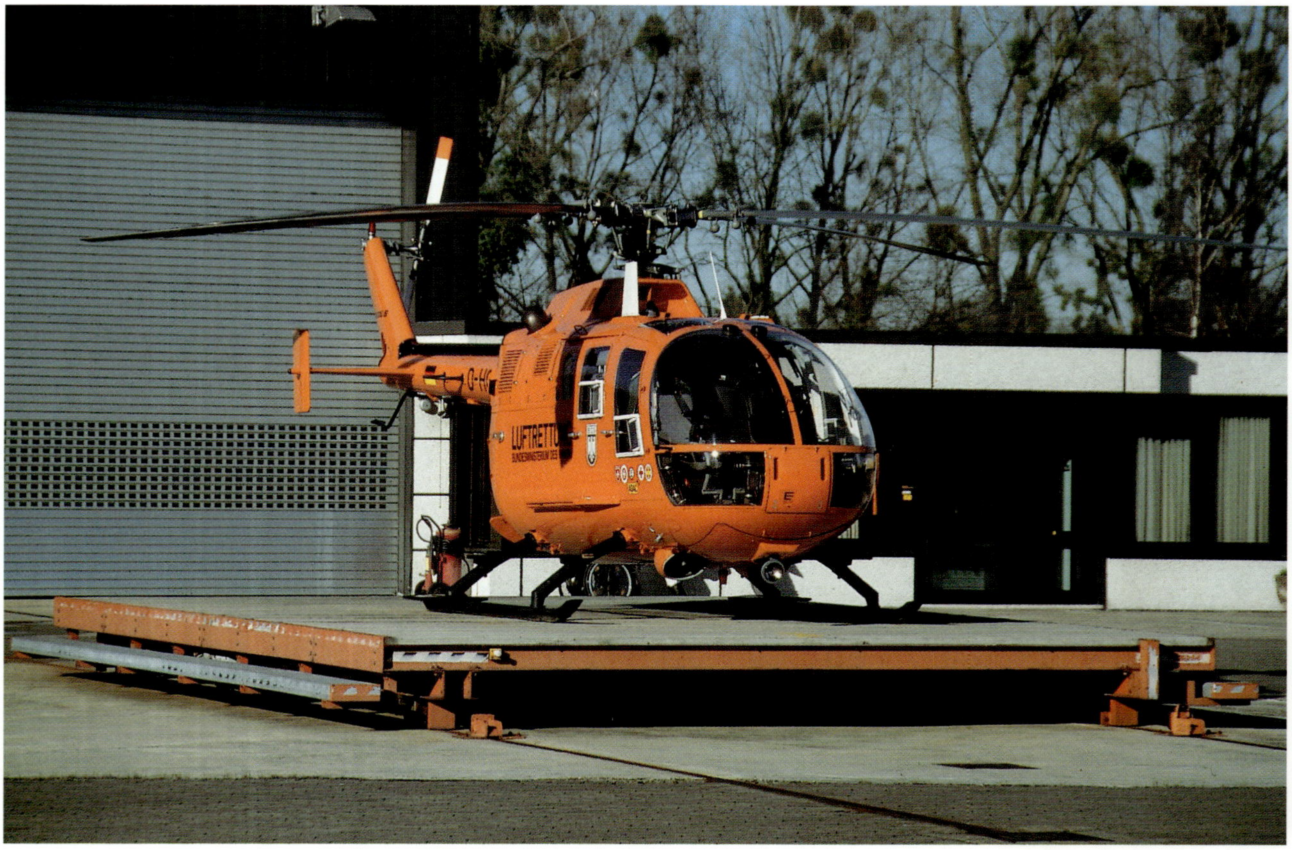

Der Rettungshubschrauber ist wieder einsatzbereit.

The rescue helicopter is ready for a new mission.

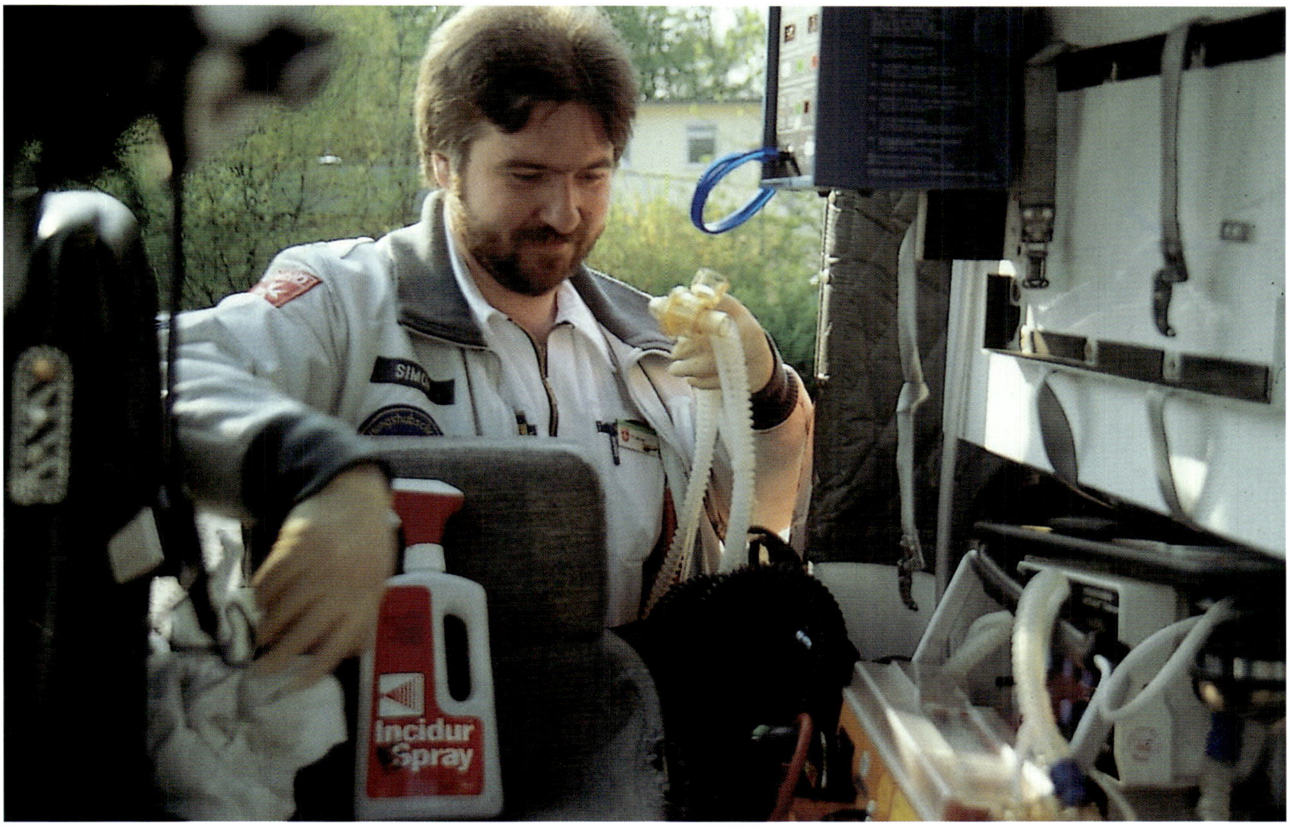

Alltag. Reinigungsarbeiten.

Routine work. Cleaning the helicopter.

Die häufigsten Fragen an der Einsatzstelle
Frequently Asked Questions

Wieviel Minuten nach der Alarmierung ist der Rettungshubschrauber in der Luft?

Spätestens nach zwei Minuten, meistens jedoch nach ca. 90 Sekunden, ist der Hubschrauber nach dem Starten der Triebwerke und Hochfahren aller Systeme, in der Luft.

How many minutes after an emergency call is the rescue helicopter in the air?

After two minutes at the latest – but usually after approx. 90 seconds – the helicopter is airborne. This is the time it needs to start its engines and run up all systems.

Einsatz für den Rettungshubschrauber
Mission for the Rescue Helicopter

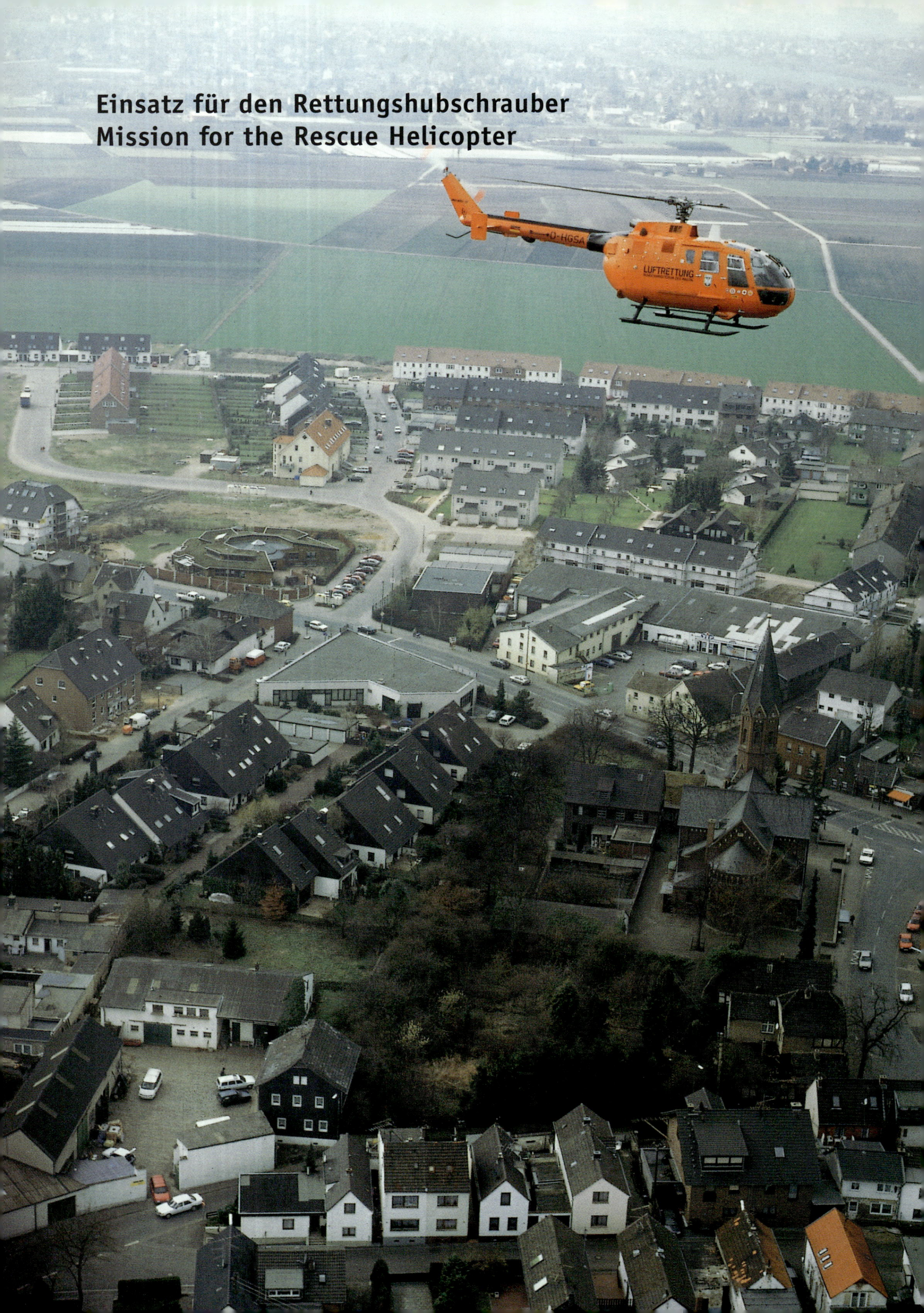

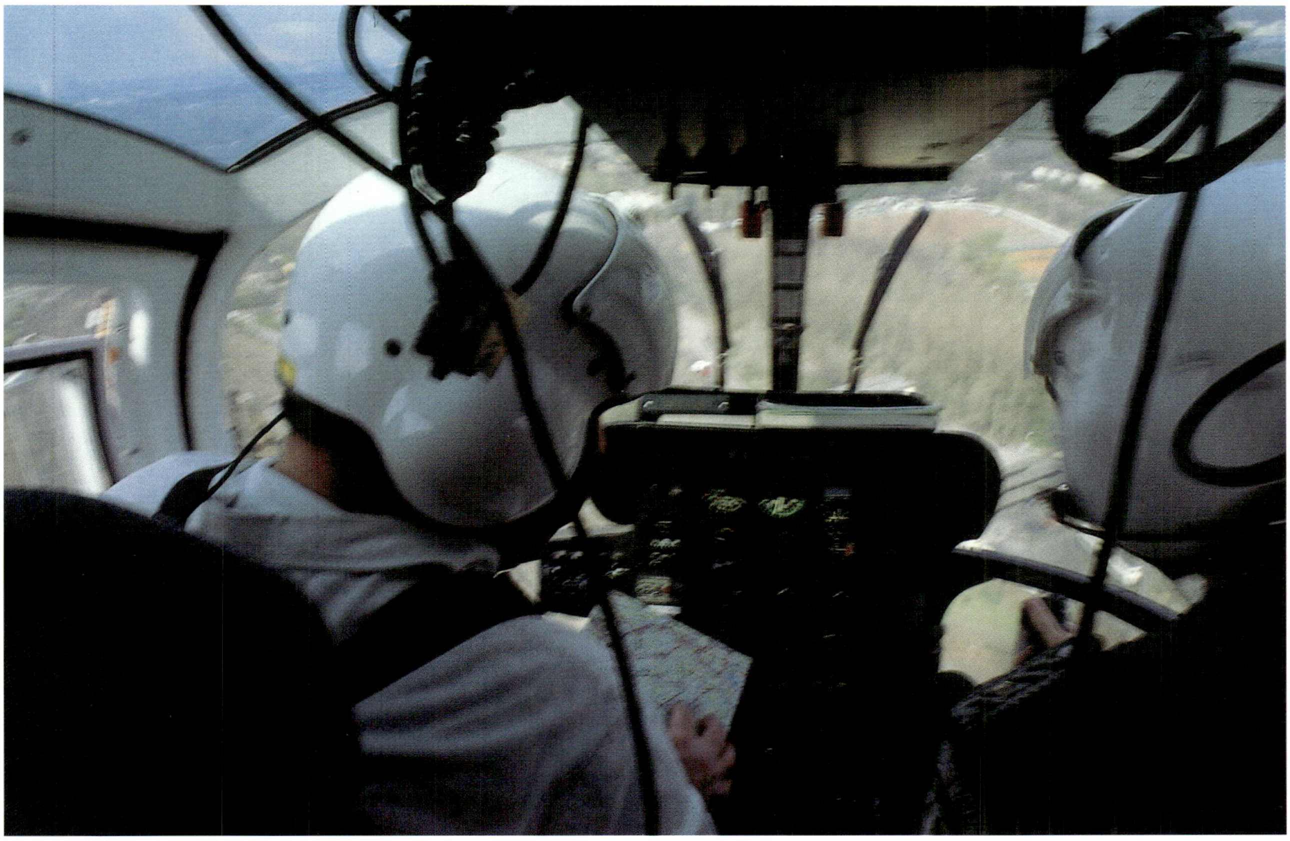

Start und Markieren der Einsatzposition auf der Landkarte.

Take-off and search for the mission coordinates on the map.

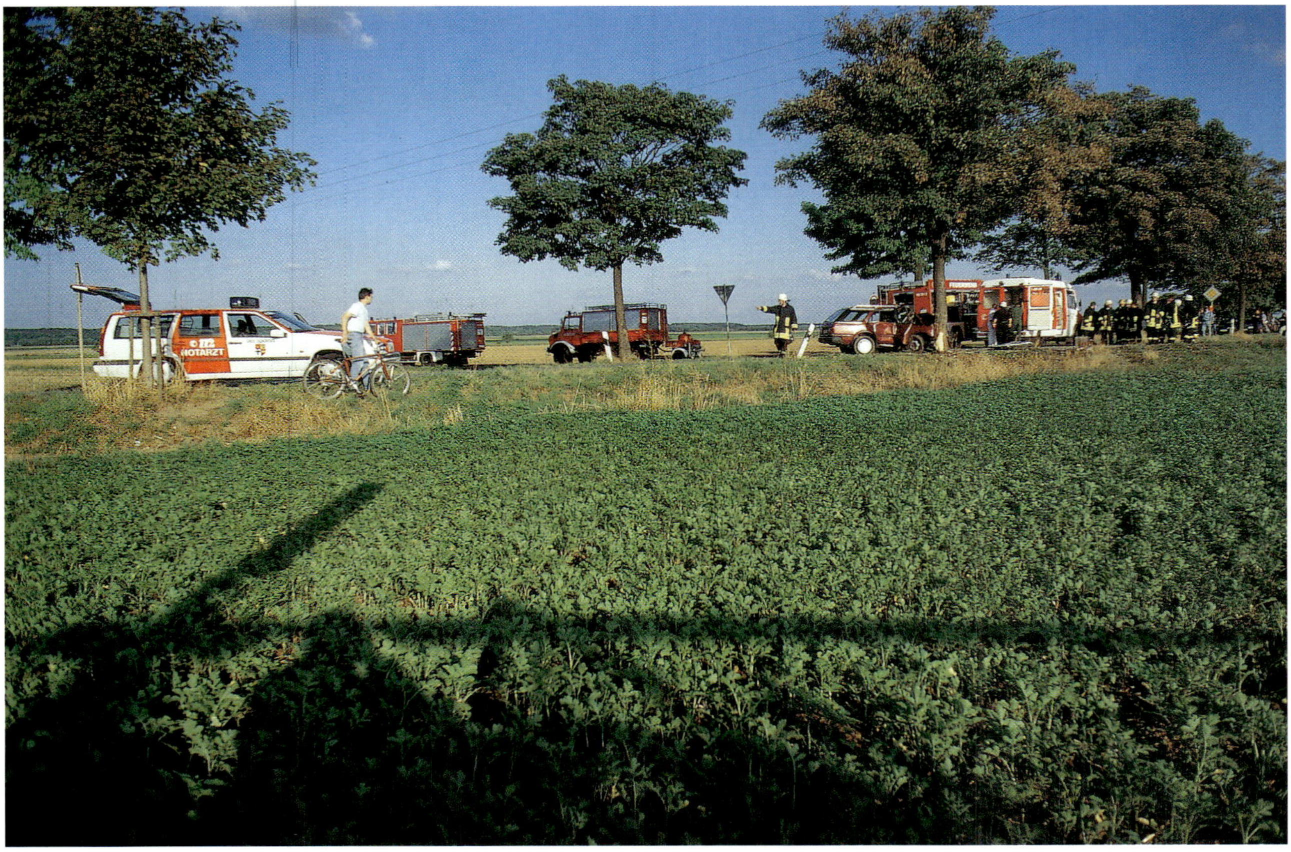

Landung an der Einsatzstelle. PKW gegen PKW. Personen sind eingeklemmt.

Landing at the accident site. Two cars have collided. People are trapped inside.

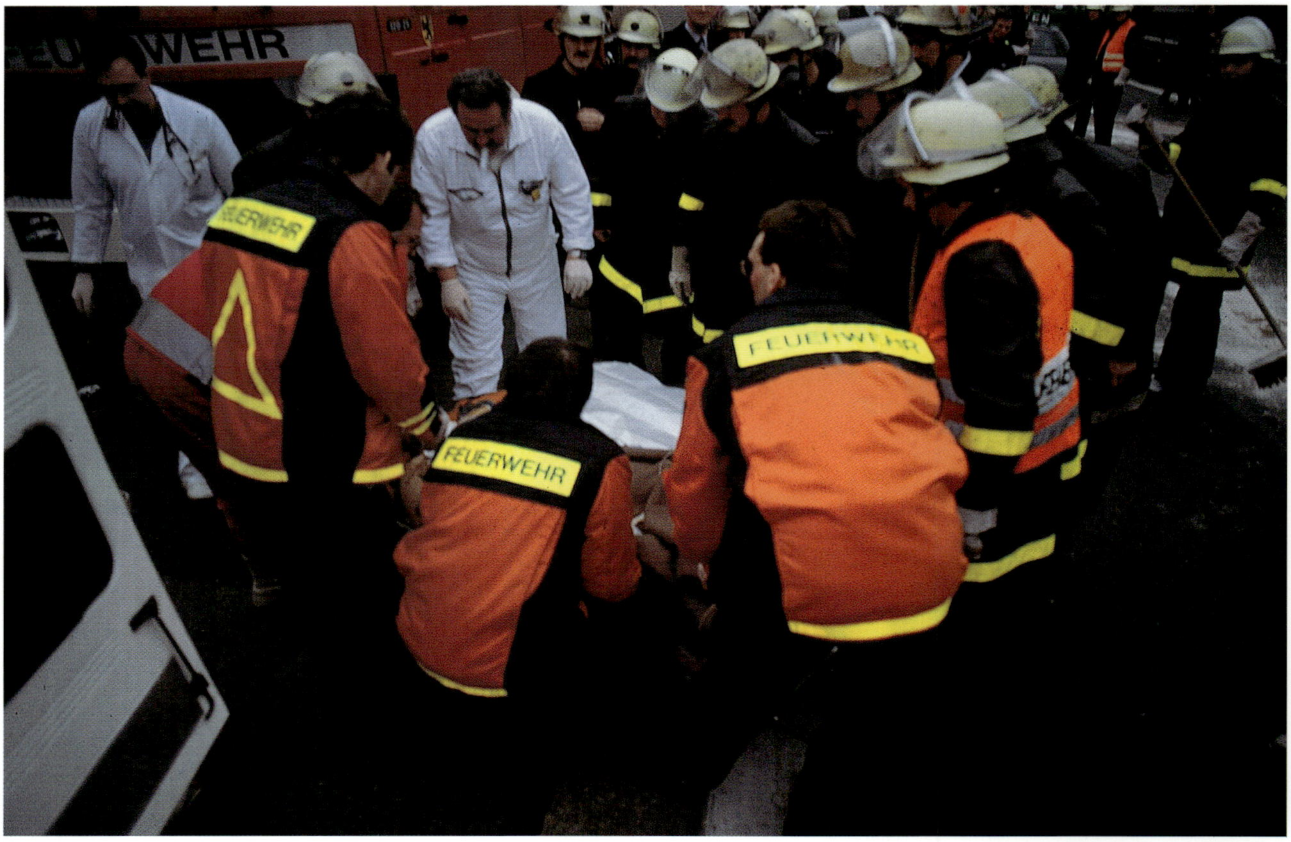

Der Patient wird zum Transport vorbereitet.

The patient is prepared for transport.

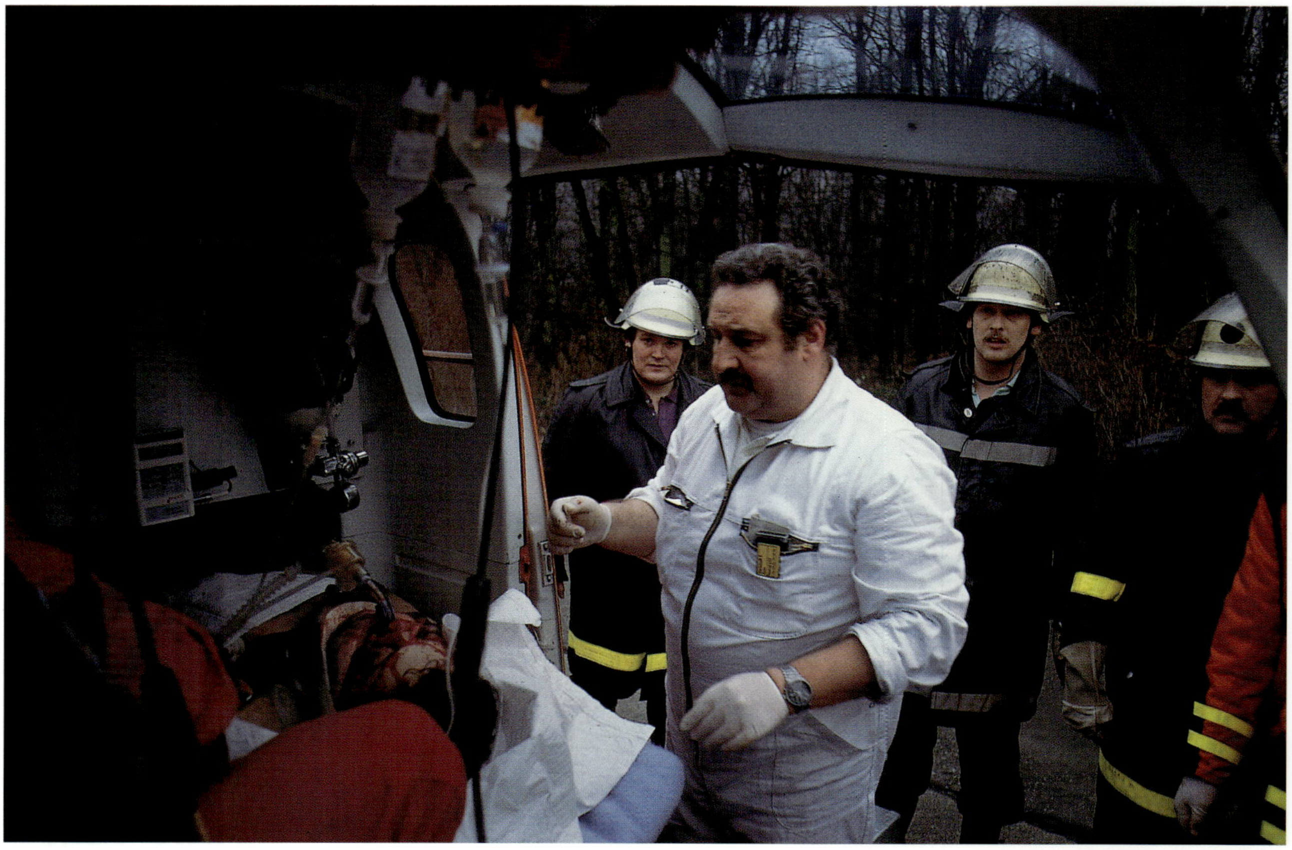

Der Patient ist eingeladen. Er wird beatmet. Flug zur Uni.

The patient is loaded into the helicopter. He receives artificial respiration. Flight to the university hospital.

Einsatz für den Rettungshubschrauber
Mission for the Rescue Helicopter

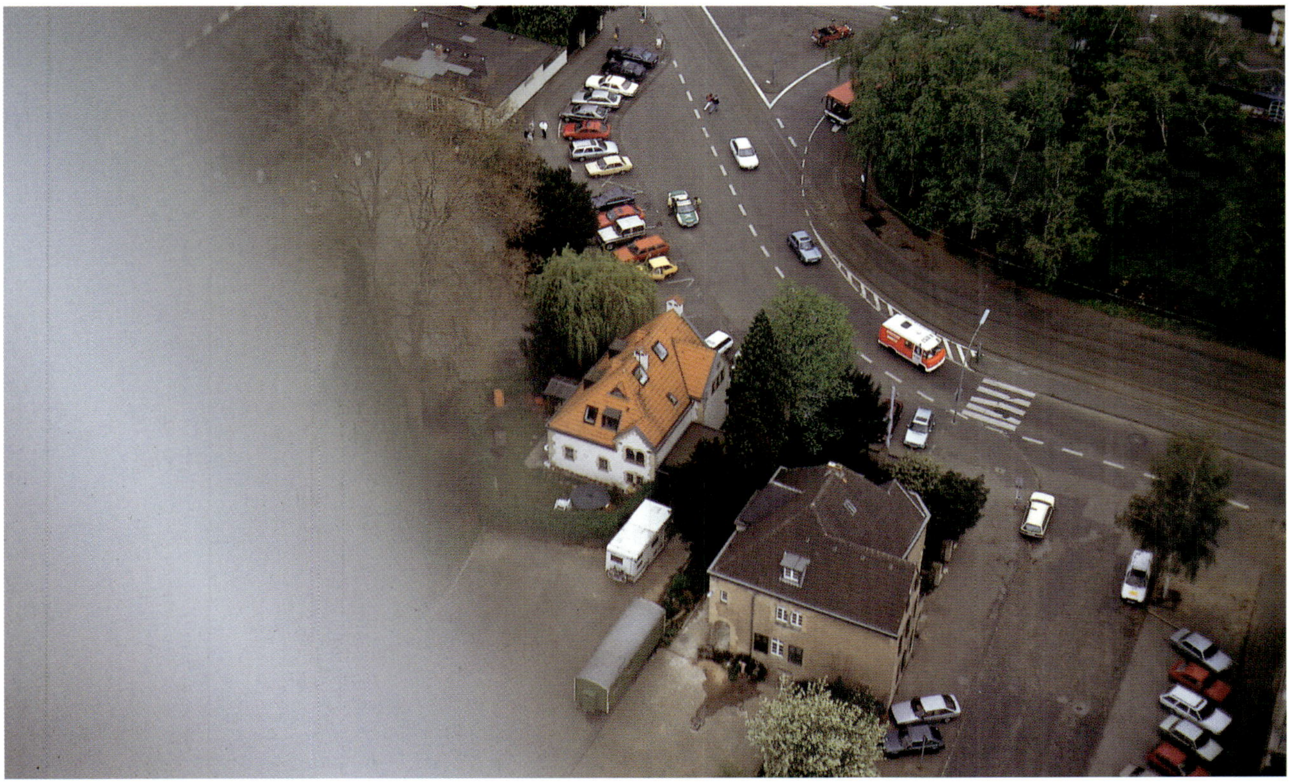

Der Rettungswagen fährt zur Einsatzstelle.

The rescue ambulance drives to the accident site.

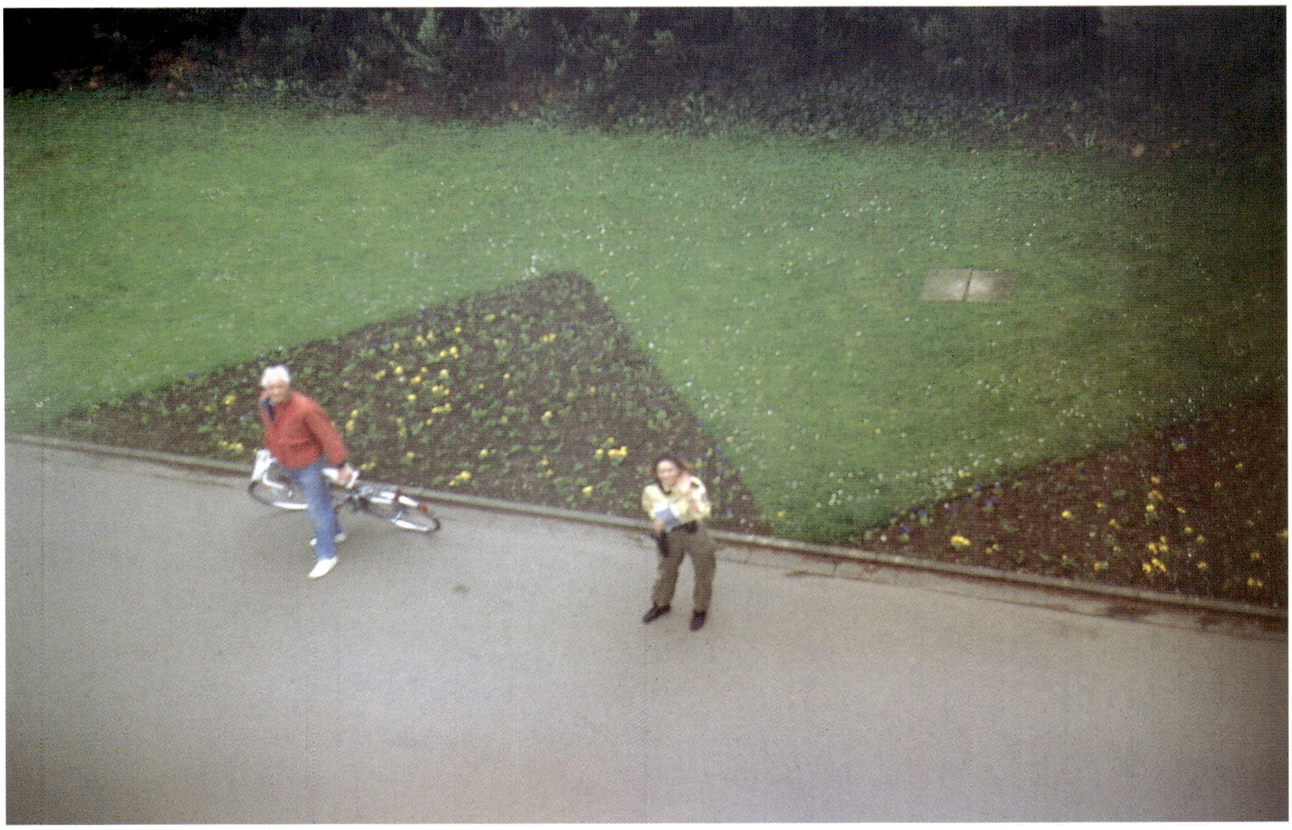

Eine Polizistin weist auf dem Friedhofsgelände ein.

A policewoman guides us onto the cemetery grounds.

Augenblicke

Altenheim. Heißer Sommertag. Eine 90-jährige Patientin ist verstorben. Keine Reanimation. Ich bringe unsere Geräte zurück zum Rettungswagen. Zwei alte Damen: „Hören Sie mal junger Mann. Da spricht einer im Auto. Ist aber keiner drin." Ich: „Das ist ein Funkgerät. Wie ein Telefon. Kann man laut stellen, damit alle mithören." Die Damen: „Kann man mal sehen, was die heute für tolle Erfindungen haben. Ist keiner drin, aber spricht trotzdem einer."

Snapshots

An old people's home on a hot summer day. A 90-year-old woman has just died. No resuscitation measures are mounted. As I carry our equipment back to the rescue ambulance, I am accosted by two elderly ladies: "Listen here, young man, somebody is talking inside the truck but there's nobody inside!" I explain: "That's a radio. It's our telephone. We can turn up the volume so that everyone in the ambulance can listen." The women are delighted: "Amazing, isn't it, the kind of inventions they have today? Nobody in the truck but somebody talking all the same!"

Die häufigsten Fragen an der Einsatzstelle
Frequently Asked Questions

Wer bezahlt den Einsatz des Rettungshubschraubers?

Die insgesamt 51 „Christoph"-Rettungshubschrauber in Deutschland sind ein wesentlicher Bestandteil des Rettungssystems in unserem Land. Und wie der Notarzt oder der Rettungswagen wird auch der RTH von den Krankenkassen und den Trägern des Rettungsdienstes, den Ländern und Kommunen, finanziert.

Who pays for the operation of the rescue helicopters?

The total of 51 "Christoph" rescue helicopters in Germany represent an important constituent of the search and rescue system in this country. Like the physicians with emergency & rescue certification and the rescue ambulances, the rescue helicopters are financed by the health insurance companies and the sponsors of the rescue services, i.e. the states and municipalities.

Einsatz für den Rettungshubschrauber
Mission for the Rescue Helicopter

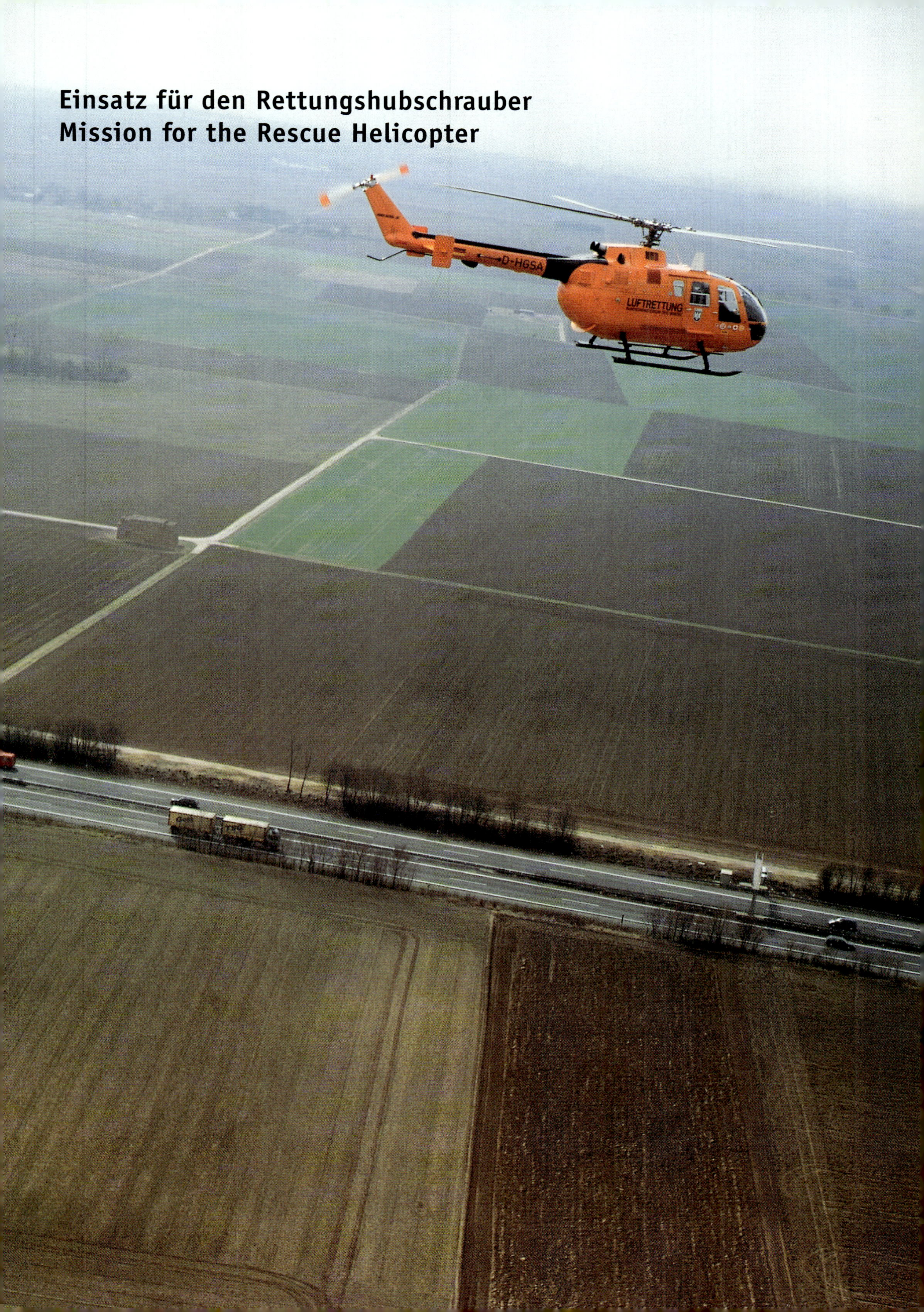

PKW-Unfall auf der Autobahn.
Anflug auf die Einsatzstelle.

Automobile accident on the autobahn.
Approach to the accident site.

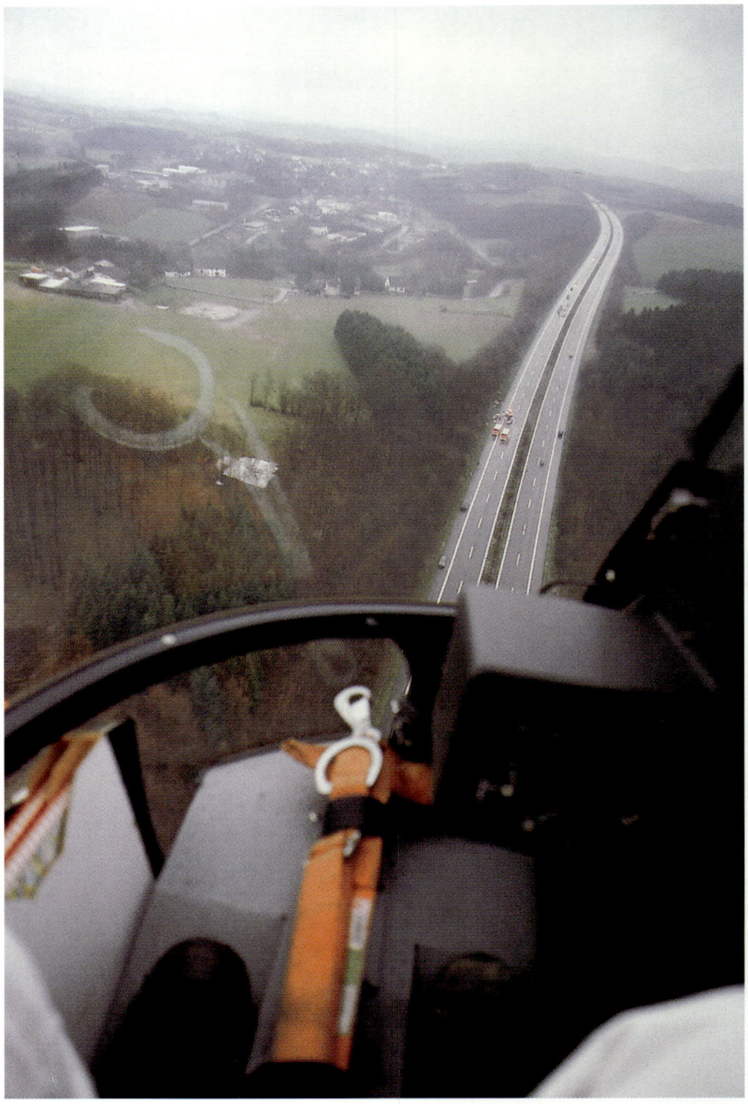

Landung.

Landing.

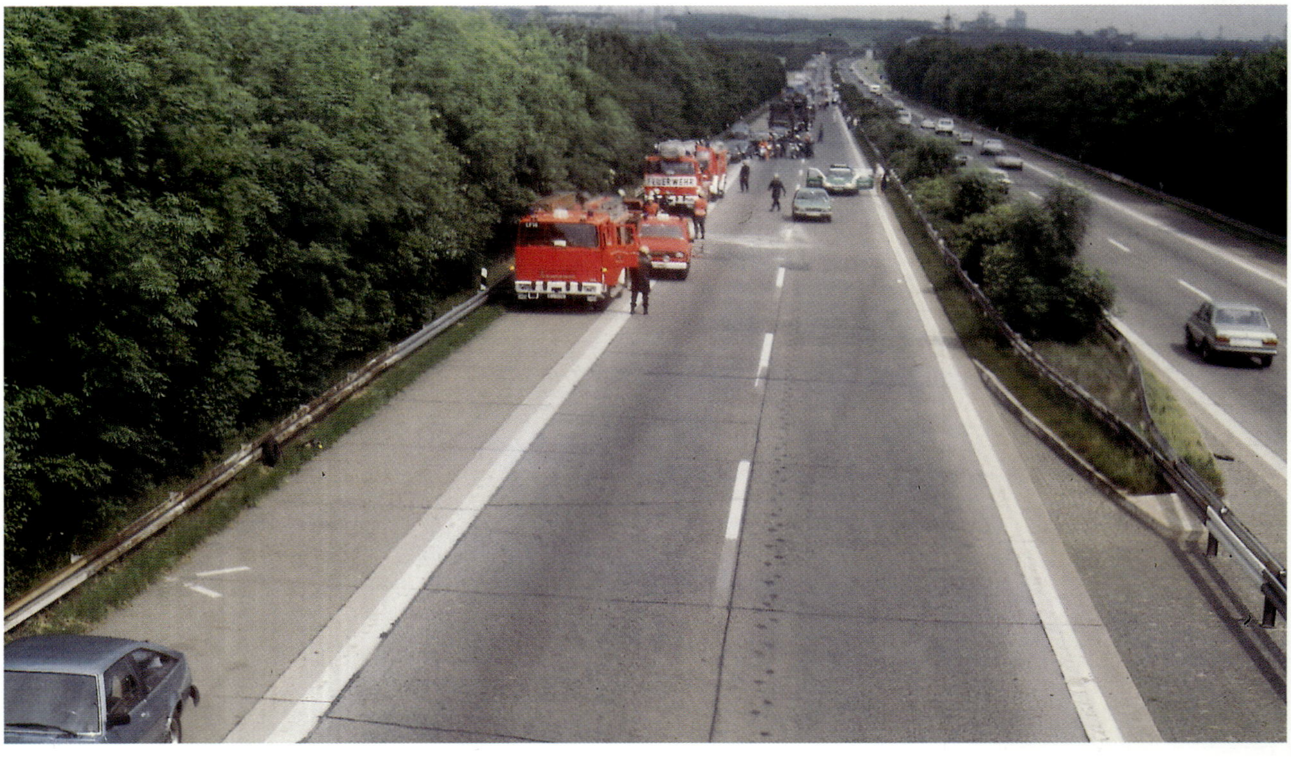

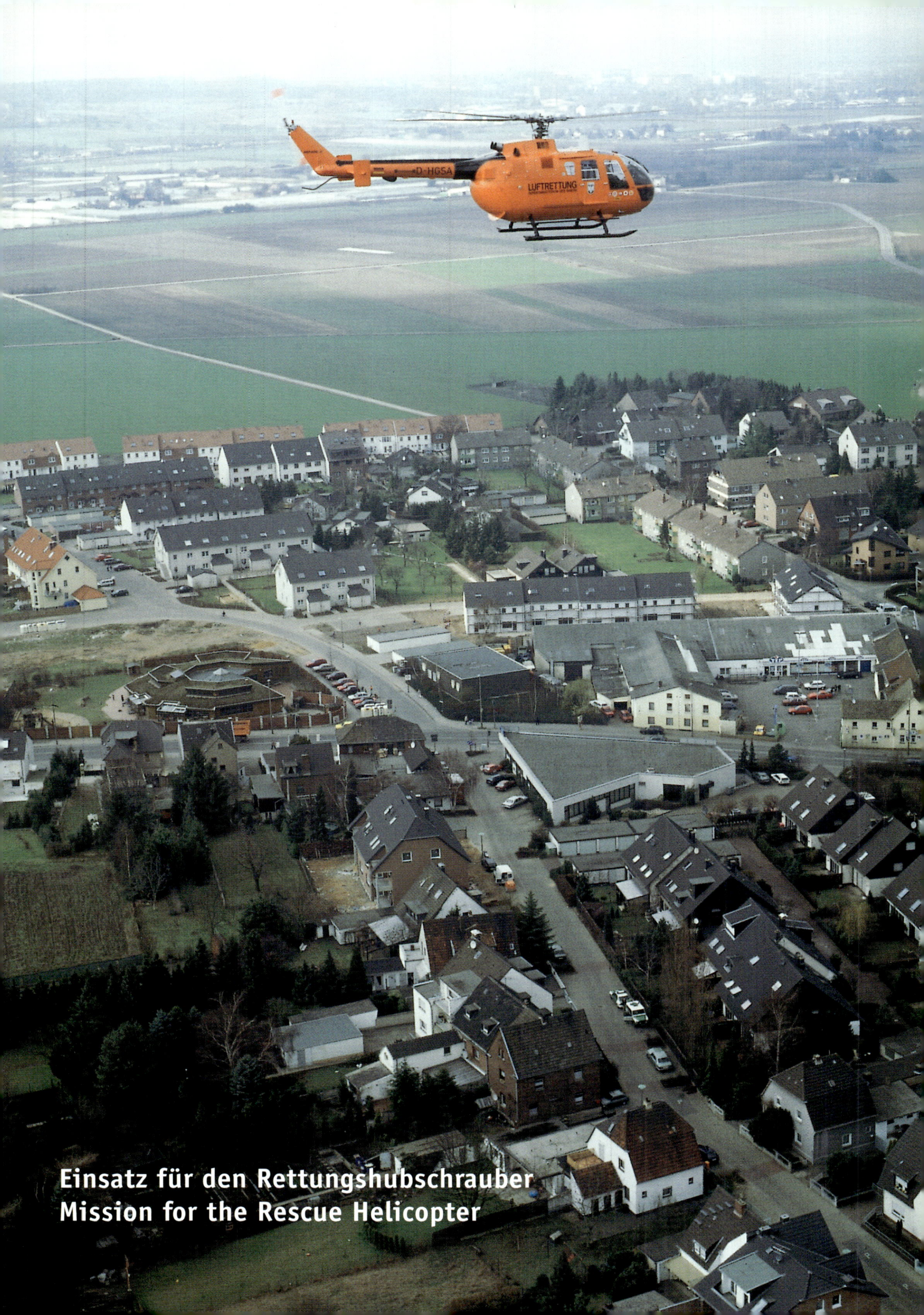

Einsatz für den Rettungshubschrauber
Mission for the Rescue Helicopter

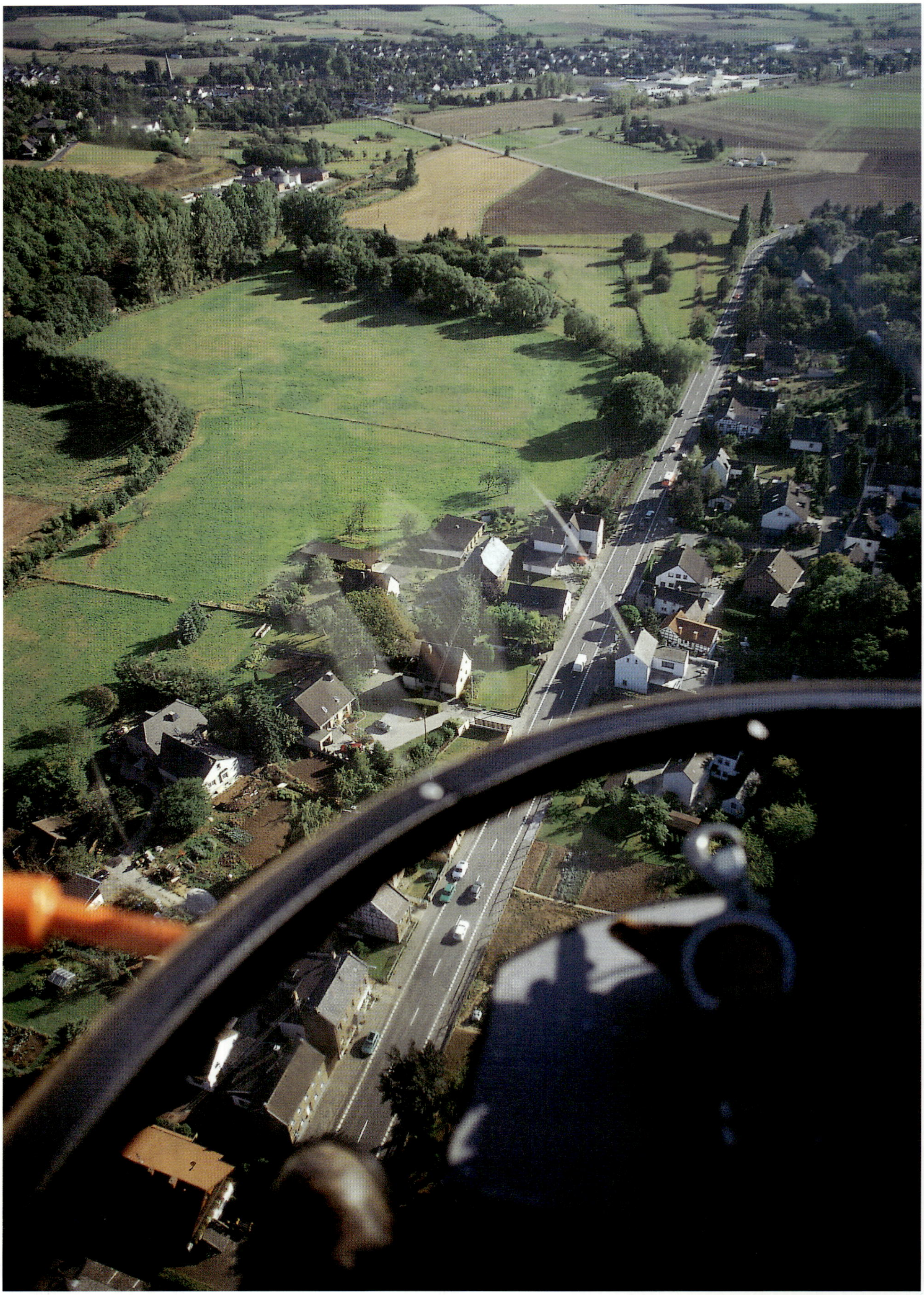

Rettungswagen und Notarzt sind bereits vor Ort.

A rescue ambulance and a physician with emergency & rescue certification are already on the scene.

Einsatz für den Rettungshubschrauber
Mission for the Rescue Helicopter

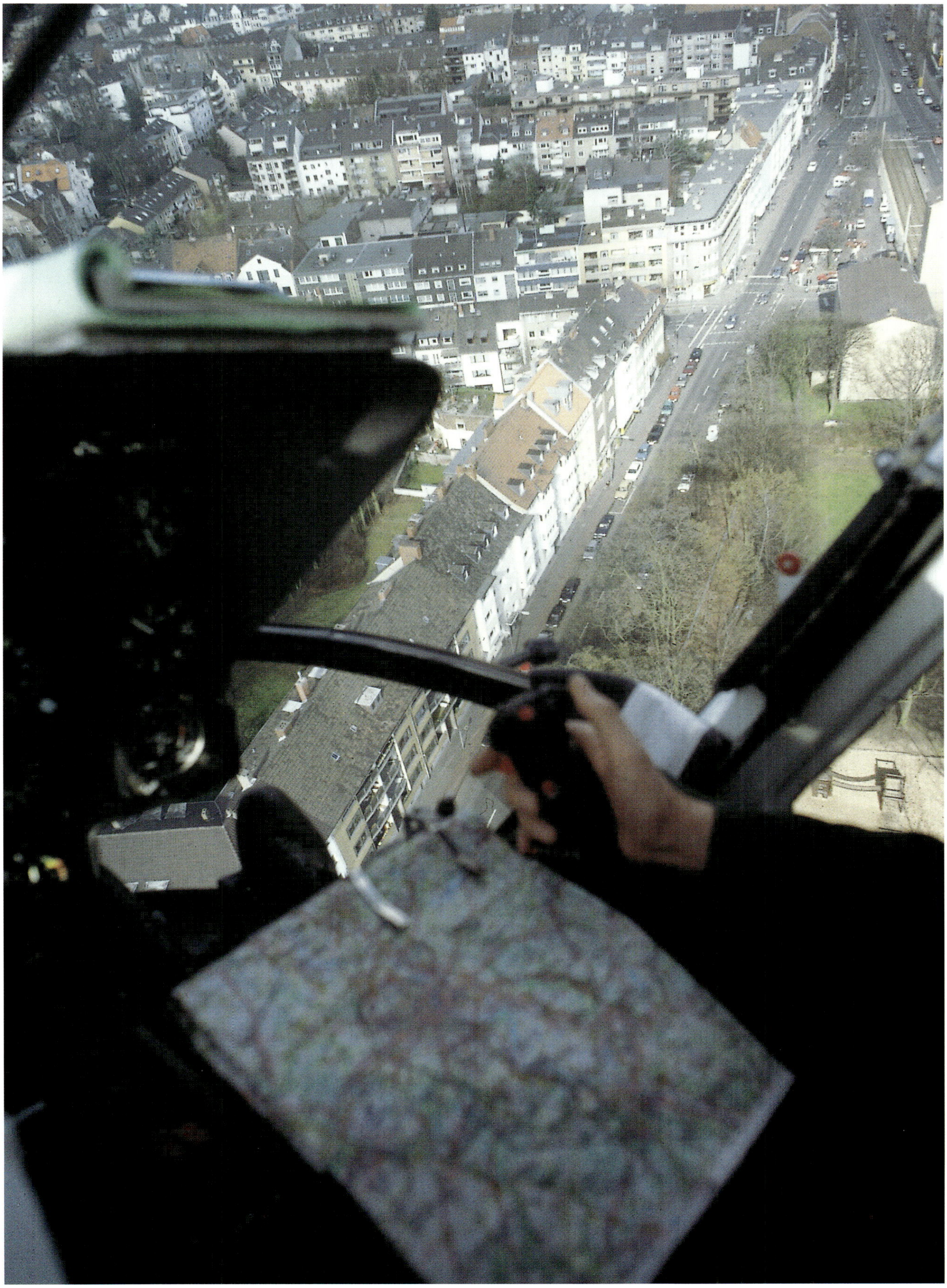

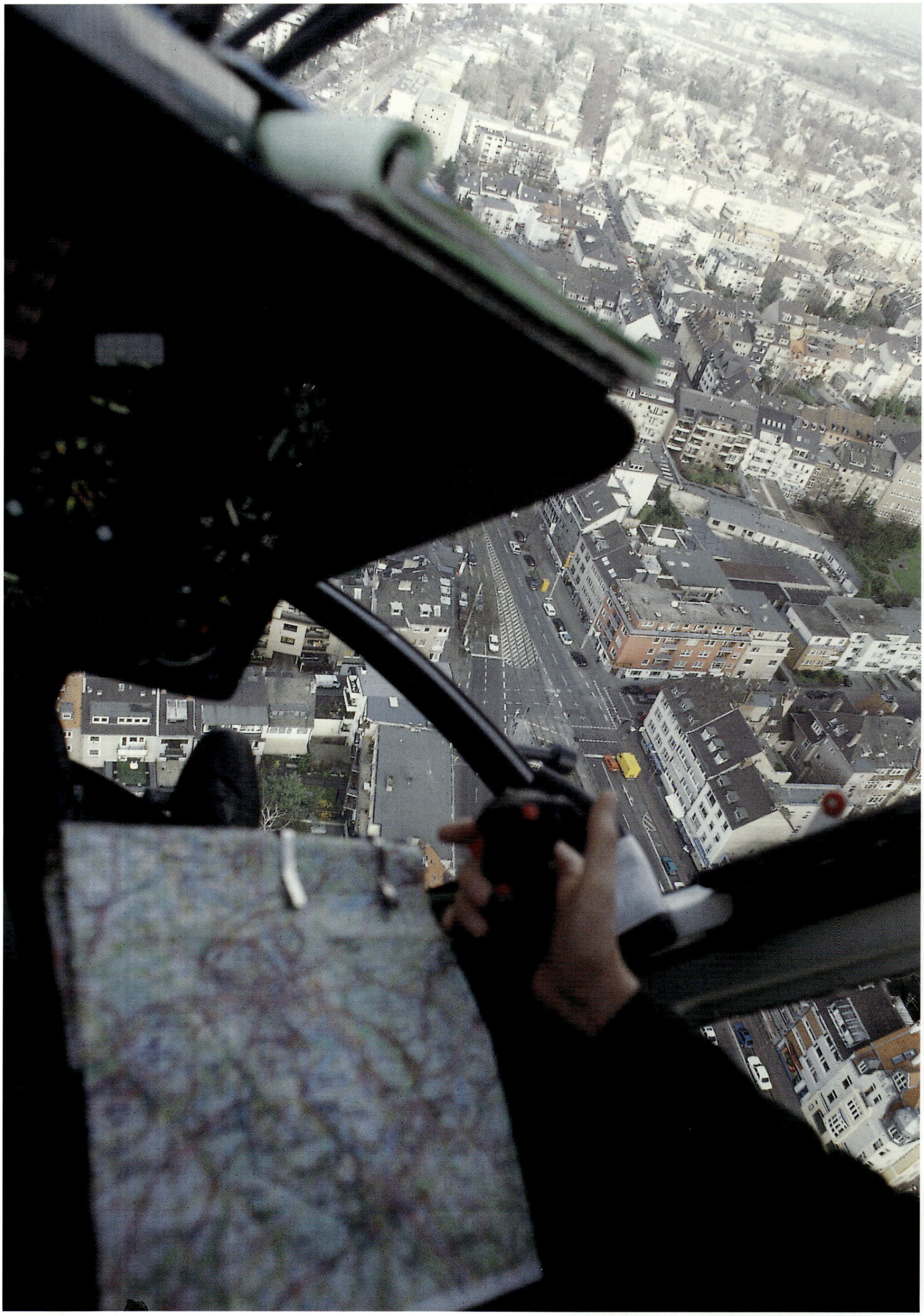

Blick aus dem Cockpit. View from the cockpit.

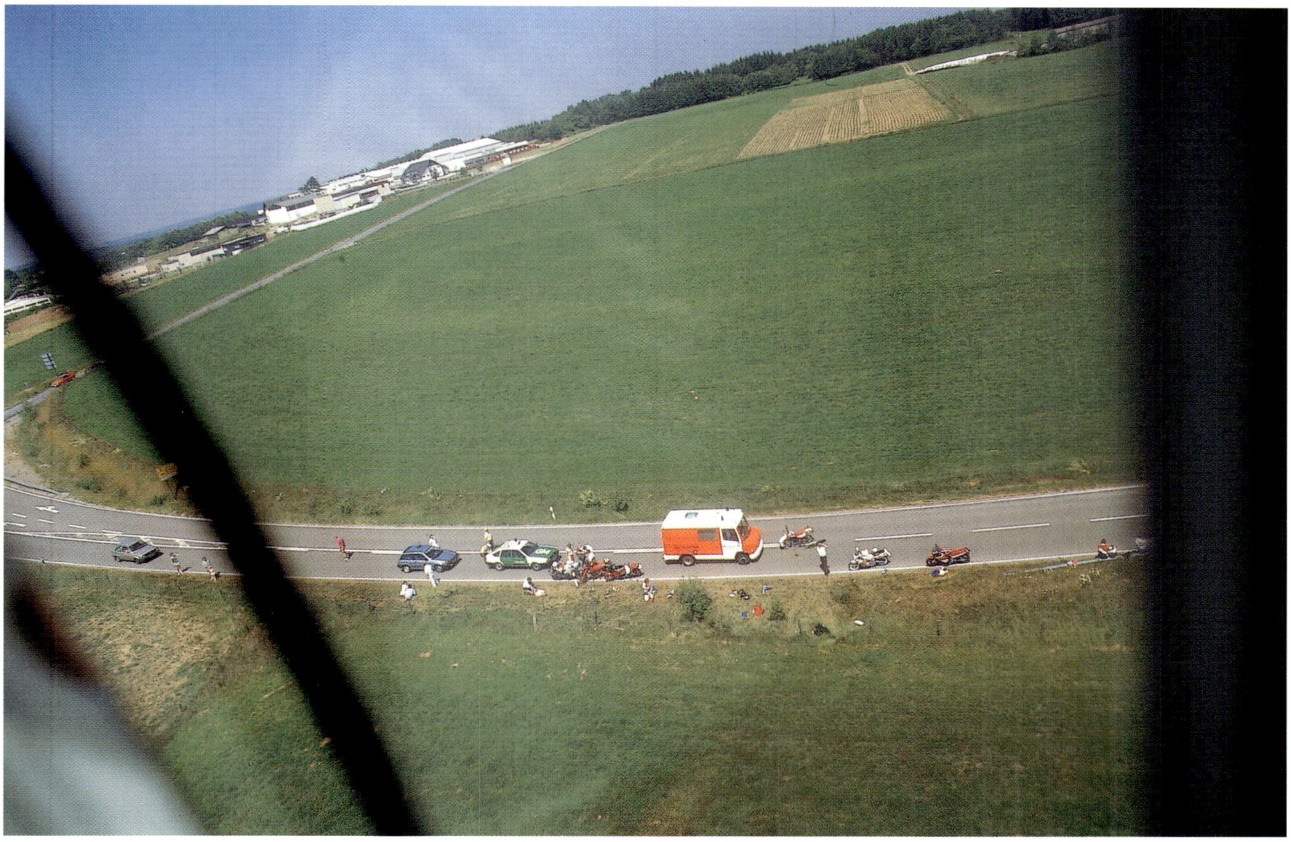

Anflug auf die Einsatzstelle.
Ein Motorradfahrer hat seine Sozia auf dem Motorrad verloren.

Approach to the accident site.
A motorcyclist has lost his pillion passenger.

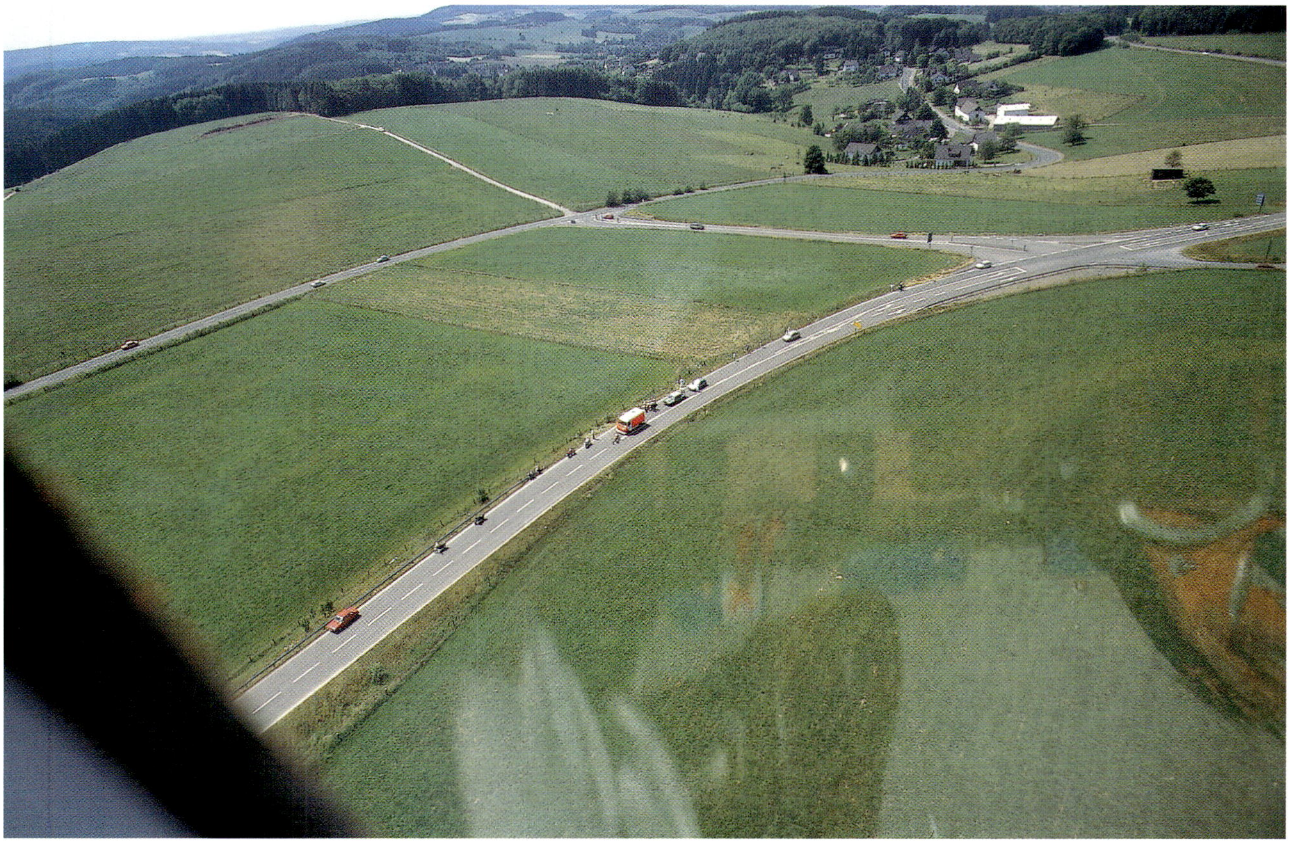

Die häufigsten Fragen an der Einsatzstelle
Frequently Asked Questions

Wie groß muss der Landeplatz für den Rettungshubschrauber sein?

Eine Größe von 35 mal 35 Metern wäre das Optimum. So viel Platz steht jedoch nicht in jedem Falle, besonders nicht in der Stadt, zur Verfügung. Der Pilot entscheidet deshalb nach gründlicher Beurteilung, in die er u.a. die Entfernung zur Notfallstelle, die Bebauung, Hindernisse und die Windsituation miteinbezieht, an welcher Stelle er zur Landung geht.

How much space does a helicopter need to land?

A landing site with the dimensions 35 x 35 meters would be ideal. This amount of space is not always available, however, especially in urban areas. As a result, the pilot decides where to set down after conducting a thorough evaluation of factors such as the distance to the emergency site, the degree of development, obstacles and wind.

Augenblicke

Sozialer Brennpunkt. Sonntagmorgen. Kirchenglocken. Säuglingsreanimation. Im Rettungswagen liegt ein toter Säugling von etwa vier Monaten. Die Mutter schreit und heult: „Ich war's nicht. Ich war's nicht." Ich gehe zurück zum Hubschrauber und hole die Mappe mit den Totenscheinformularen. Auf dem Weg sagen Nachbarn: Das war der Mann, die Schweinebacke. Polizei trifft ein. Der entkleidete Säugling weist über und über Blutergüsse unterschiedlichen Alters auf. Die Polizei wird informiert. Rückflug. Der Leichnam des kleinen Kindes geht in die Gerichtsmedizin.

Snapshots

Sunday morning in a deprived area. Church bells peal in the distance. Futile attempts to resuscitate an infant in the rescue ambulance. The dead infant is about four months old. The mother sobs and screams: "I didn't do it. It wasn't me!" I go back to the helicopter and get the folder with the empty death certificates. On the way back to the ambulance, I hear neighbours saying: it was the husband. The police arrive at the scene. The infant's body is covered with bruises inflicted on different dates. We notify the police and fly back to base. The dead infant is taken to the Dept. of Forensic Medicine.

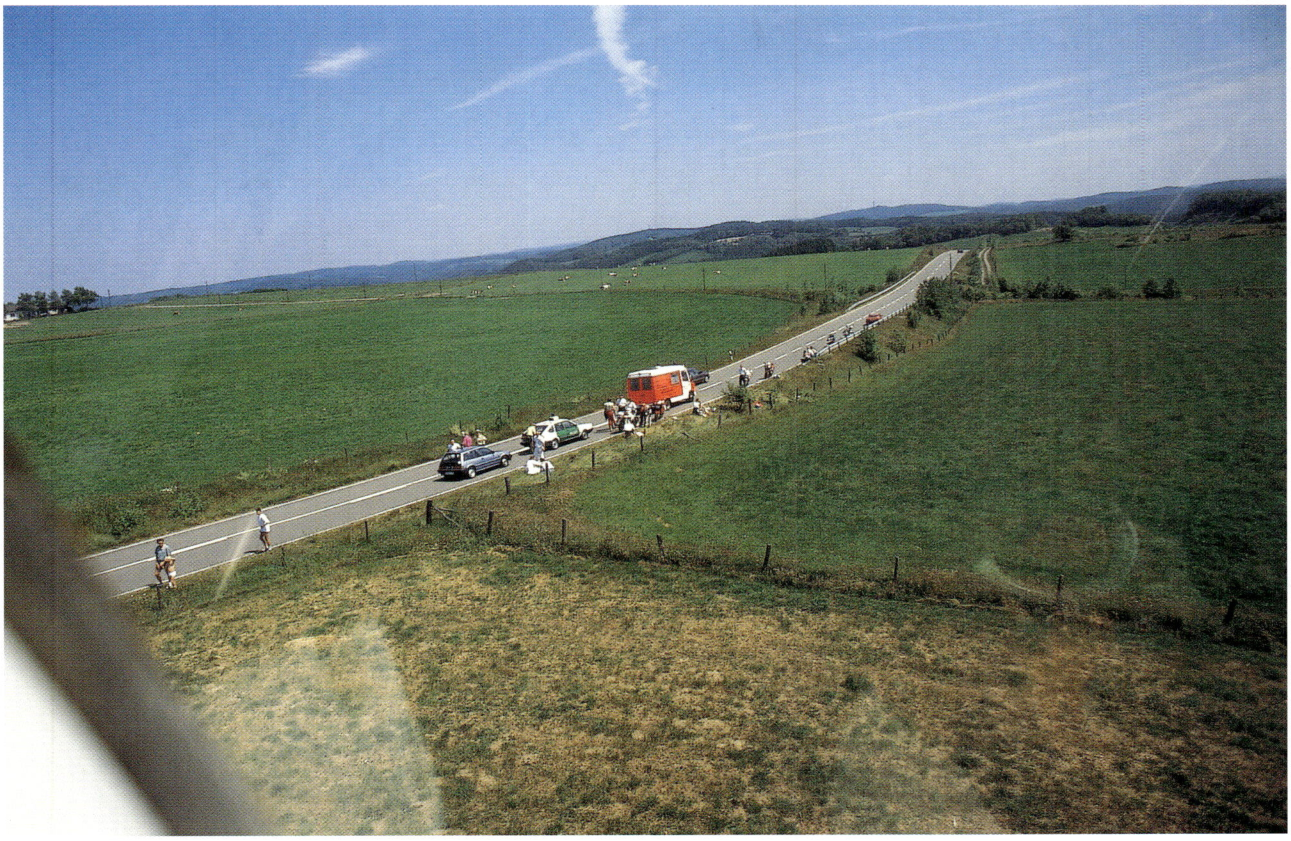

Landeanflug. Approach.

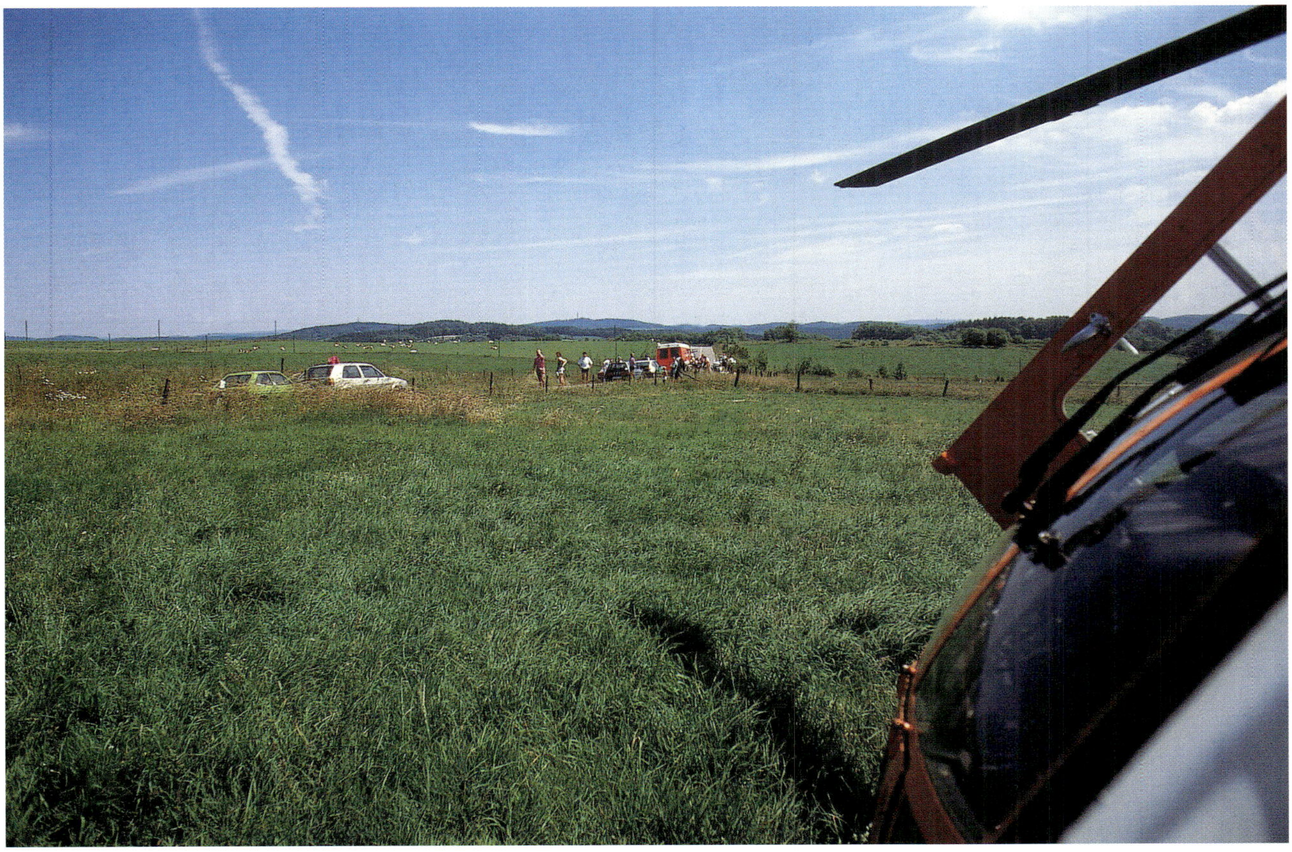

Landung. Landing.

Einsatz für den Rettungshubschrauber
Mission for the Rescue Helicopter

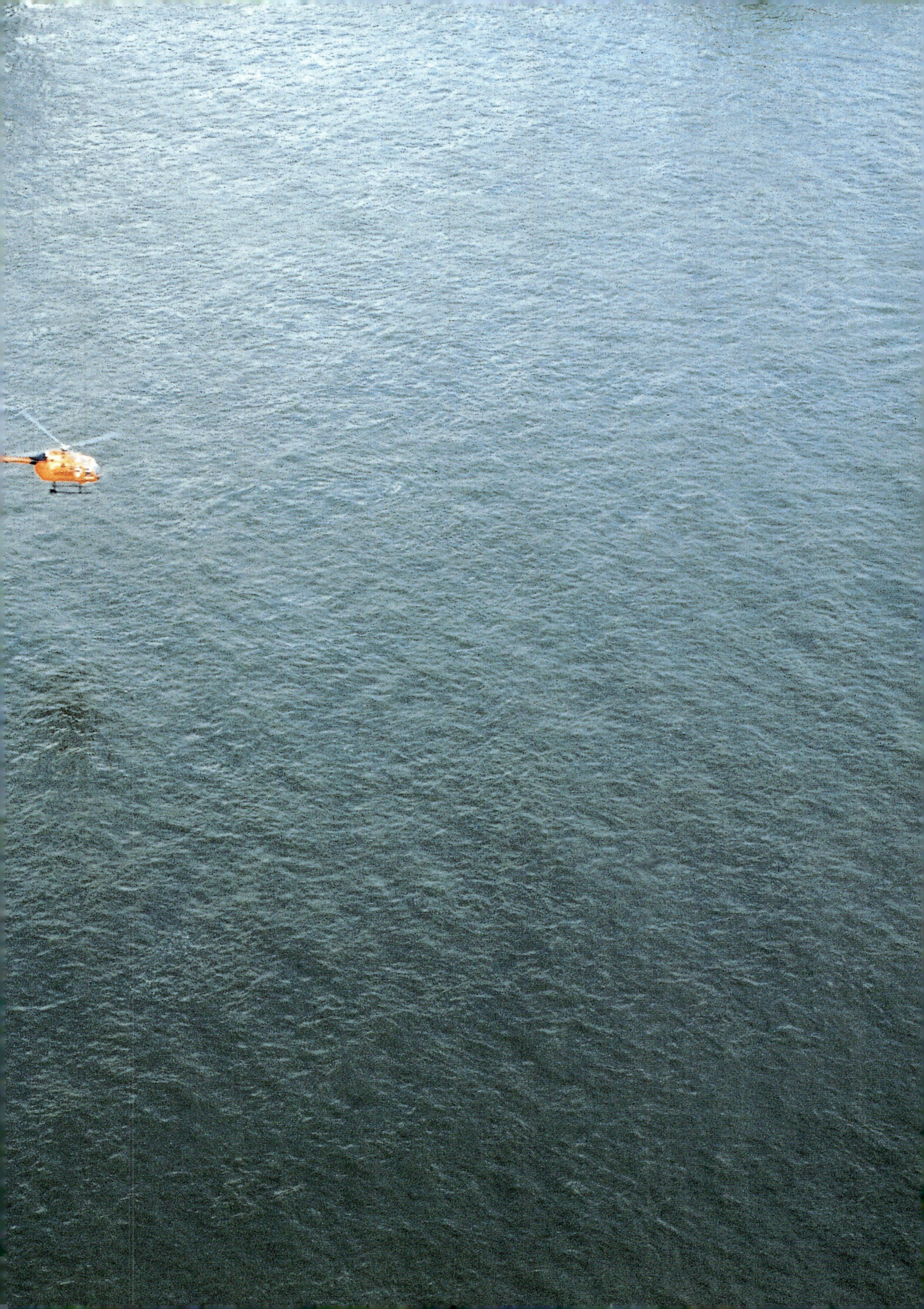

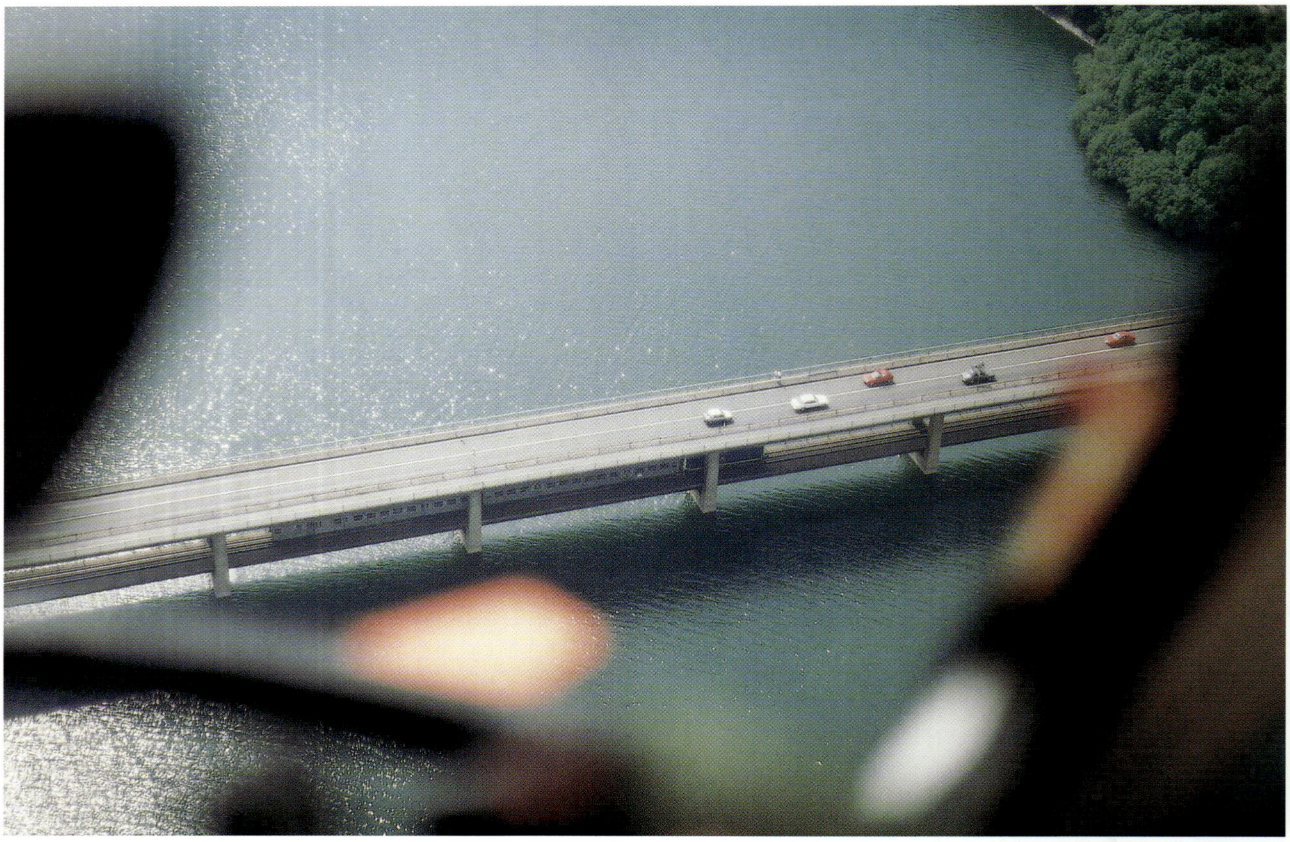

Tauchunfall.
Ein Taucher hat unangeleint die Kontrolle über sich verloren und ist im Badesee abgesackt. Reanimation. Erfolglos.

Diving accident.
At a popular recreational lake, an unlined diver has lost control of the situation. Resuscitation efforts are fruitless.

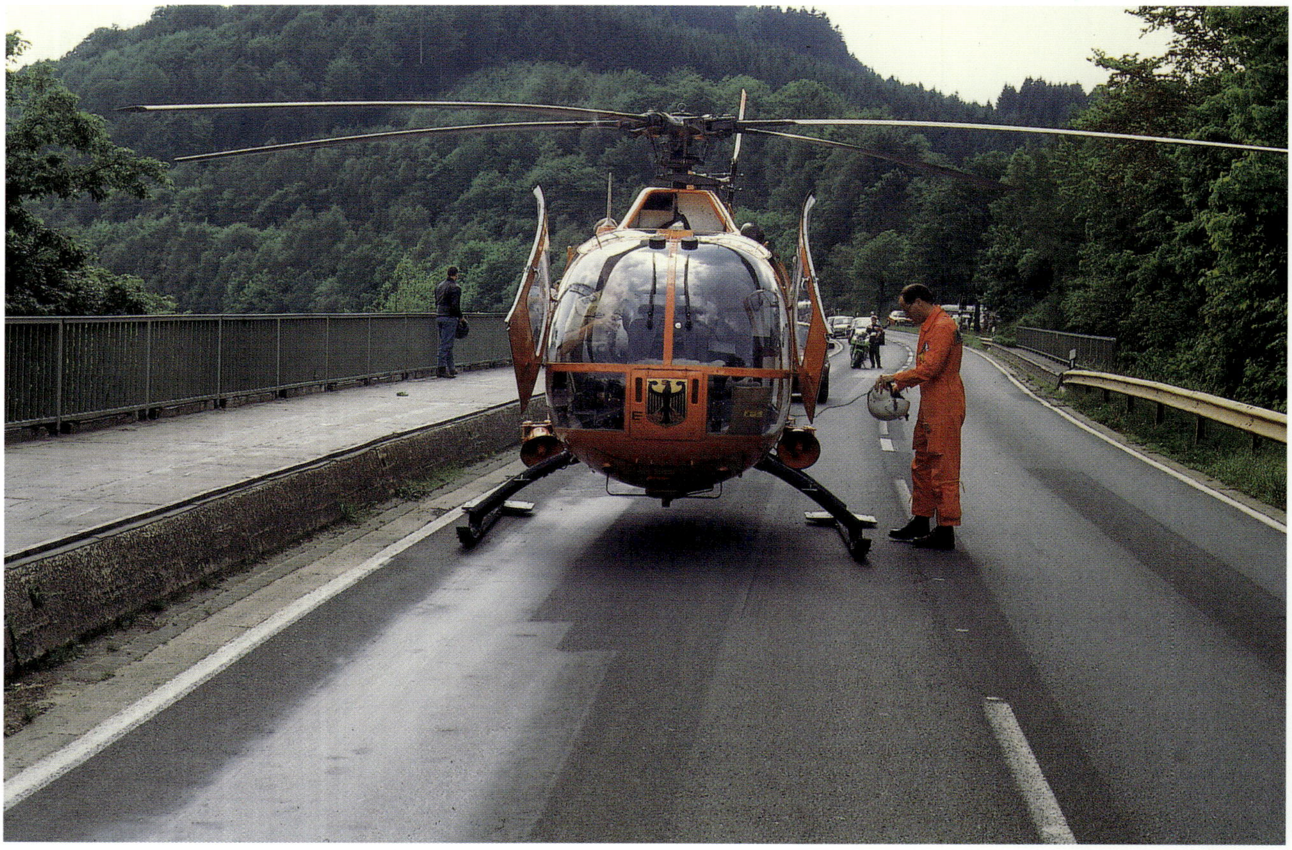

Startvorbereitungen.

Before Take-off.

Einsatz für den Rettungshubschrauber
Mission for the Rescue Helicopter

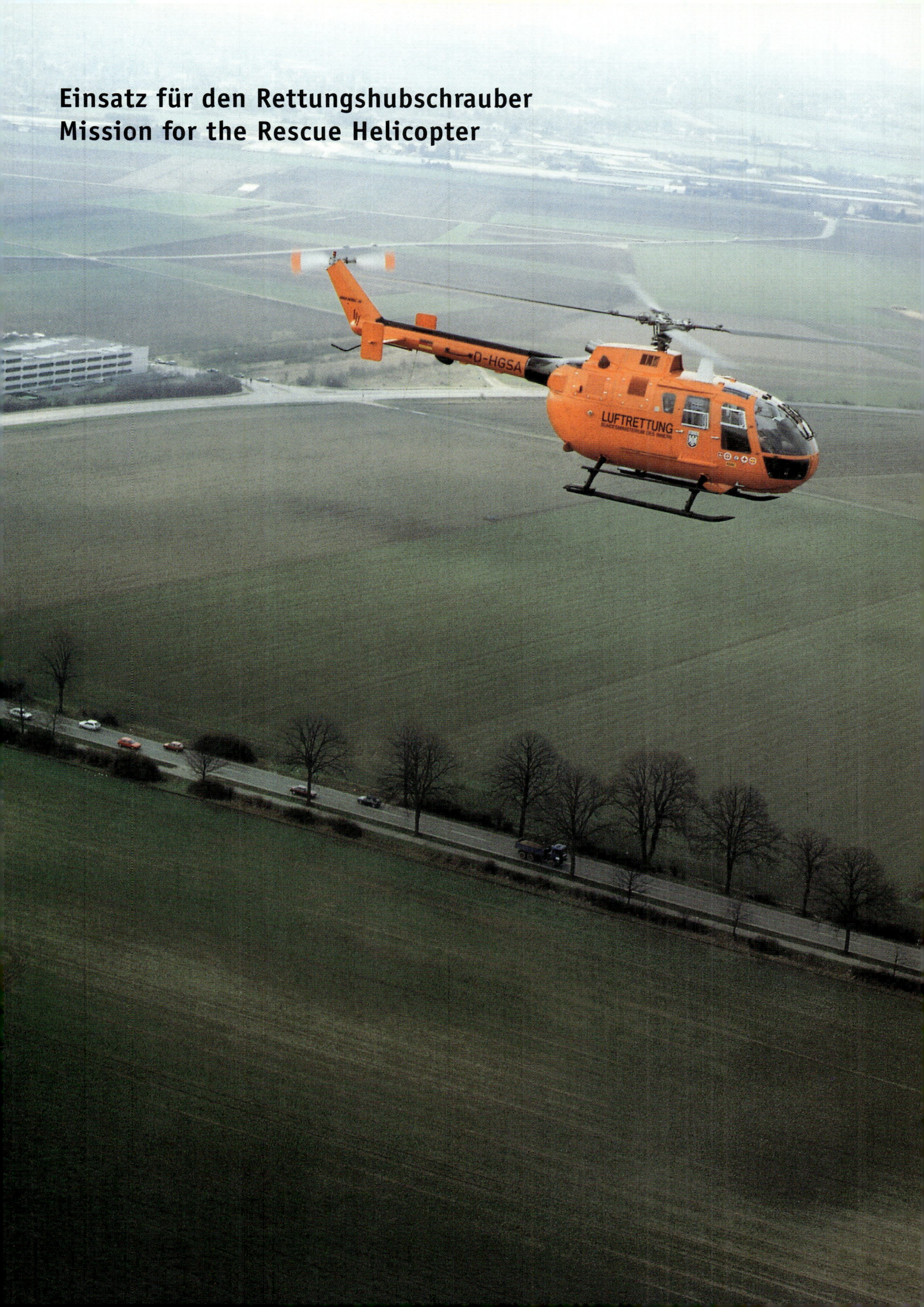

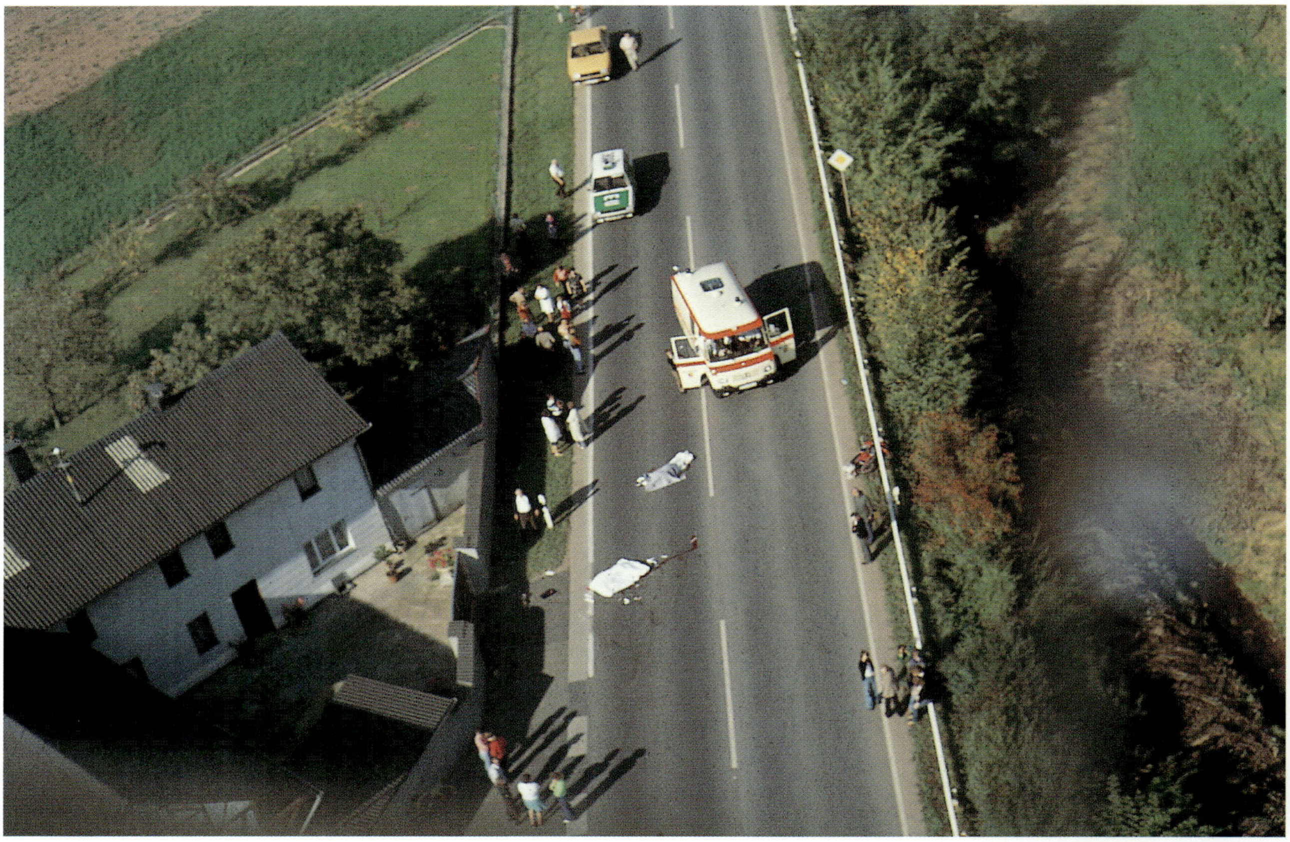

Ein Motorradfahrer ist auf der Landstraße gestürzt. Überflug.

A motorcycle has fallen over on a rural road. Flyover.

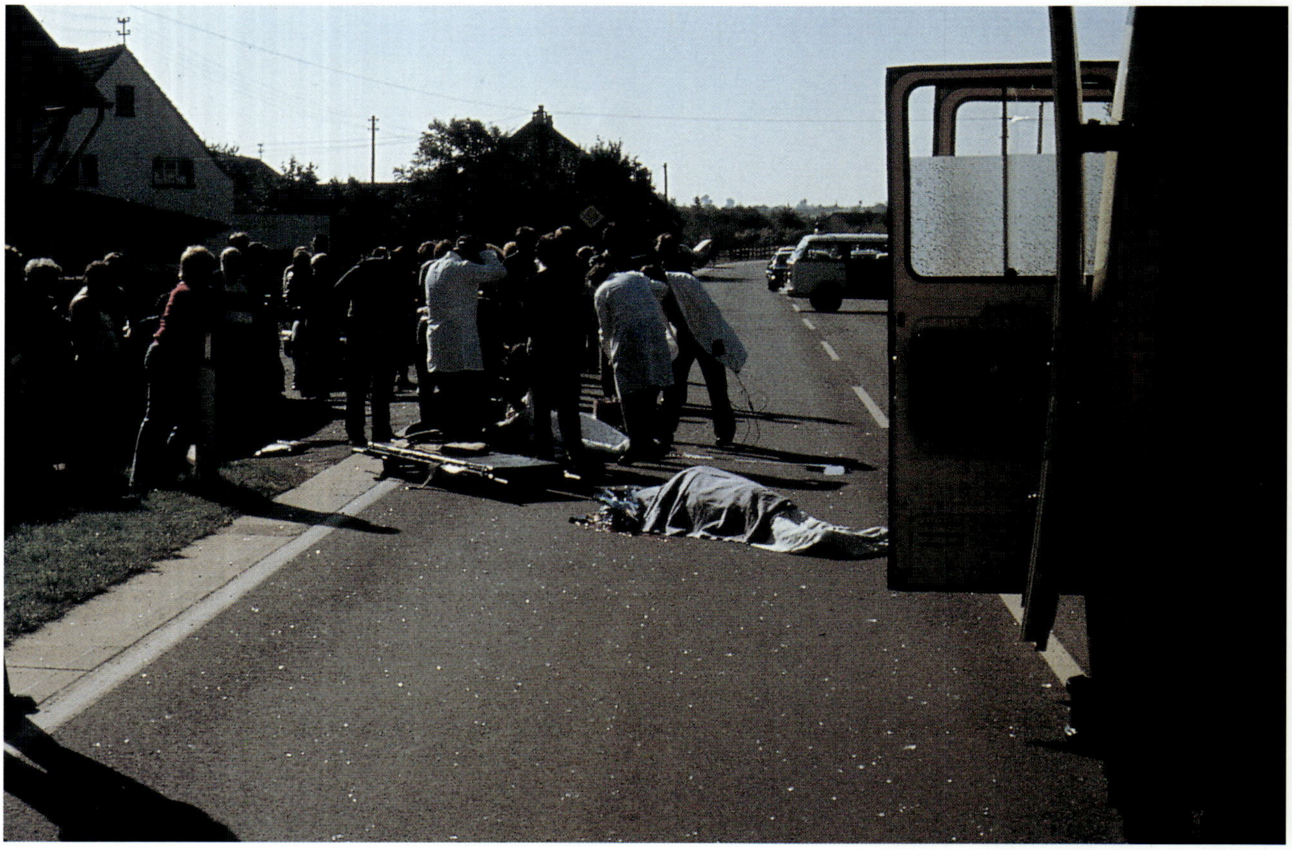

Keine weitere Maßnahmen.

No further measures.

Die Leitstelle der Berufsfeuerwehr Köln, Leitstelle des Rettungshubschraubers Christoph 3

von Klaus Maurer

Zur Koordination eines funktionierenden Rettungssystems bedarf es einer über alle Ressourcen verfügenden Leitstelle. Ihre Aufgabe ist es, an der Schnittstelle zwischen den Hilfeersuchen aus der Bevölkerung und den im Rettungsdienst mitwirkenden Organisationen jeweils das geeignete Einsatzmittel auszuwählen, zu entsenden sowie sicher und schnell an den Einsatzort zu leiten. Während des Einsatzes stellt die Leitstelle die Verbindung zu den Kräften vor Ort sicher, bearbeitet ergänzende Einsatzmittelnachforderungen und sorgt frühzeitig für eine adäquate Unterbringung der Notfallpatienten. Eines der dabei disponierten Rettungsmittel ist der Rettungshubschrauber „Christoph 3".

Nach den einschlägigen Gesetzen des Landes Nordrhein-Westfalen sind die kreisfreien Städte und die Kreise verpflichtet, so genannte „integrierte Leitstellen" zu unterhalten. Zur Gewährleistung einer zentralen Einsatzlenkung und aus Gründen eines wirtschaftlichen Verwaltungshandelns sind die Leitstellen für Feuerschutz, Rettungsdienst und Katastrophenschutz zusammengelegt. Als einheitliche Notrufnummer für alle nichtpolizeilichen Hilfeersuchen ist die Nummer 112 als „Euro-Notruf" flächendeckend aufgeschaltet. Andere, in Deutschland übliche Rufnummern der Rettungsleitstellen (z.B.: 19222) sind in der Regel ebenfalls geschaltet. Der Bürger hat damit, unabhängig vom konkreten Schadensereignis, nur einen Ansprechpartner und muß im Notfall nicht vorselektieren. Da viele Szenarien den kombinierten Einsatz von Feuerwehr und Rettungsdienst erfordern, kann schnell und einheitlich in einem Arbeitsgang alarmiert und über einen gemeinsamen Betriebskanal gesteuert und informiert werden. Unterstützt wird diese Einheitlichkeit durch die umfassende Mitwirkung der Feuerwehren im Rettungsdienst. Doppelstrukturen und Doppelalarmierung werden weit-

The Coordination Center of the Cologne Professional Fire Service Coordination Center for the Rescue Helicopter Christoph 3

by Klaus Maurer

A Coordination Center with access to all available resources is essential for the coordination of a well-functioning rescue system. This Coordination Center serves as the interface between emergency calls made by members of the general public and the organizations involved in rescue operations; the task of the Coordination Center is to choose the most suitable rescue resources and to dispatch them quickly and reliably to the site of the emergency. During the rescue operation, the Coordination Center establishes secure lines of communication to the rescue personnel working on the scene, processes supplementary requests for rescue resources, and finds hospitals willing to accept each of the emergency patients. The rescue helicopter "Christoph 3" is one of the resources dispatched by the Coordination Center.

The pertinent laws of the German state of North Rhine-Westphalia stipulate that the counties, as well as towns and cities which do not belong to any counties, are obliged to maintain "integrated coordination centers". To ensure central coordination of all rescue operations – as well as for reasons of economic public administration – the Coordination Centers of the fire, rescue and disaster services have been merged into a Central Coordination Center. The telephone number "112" has been set up and connected as a „European emergency number" with wide-area coverage for all emergency calls other than police calls. Other numbers commonly used by the Coordination Centers in Germany (e.g. 19222) have also been connected at most locations. The advantage of this system for the citizen requesting assistance is that the caller has only to make one contact and does not have to choose between numbers in an emergency. Many emergency scenarios require the combined deployment of fire service and rescue service personnel. These personnel can be called in quickly and uniformly in a single operation; they

gehend vermieden. Mit dem Einsatz von „First Respondern" (zu medizinischen Notfällen ausrückende Löschfahrzeuge mit dazu erweiterter Ausstattung und qualifiziertem Personal) kann das Therapiefreie Intervall wirksam verkürzt werden. Durch den über die Grenzen der Stadt Köln hinausgehenden Einsatzbereich des Rettungshubschraubers mit einem Radius von ca. 50 km um seinen Standort in Köln Merheim, ist die enge Zusammenarbeit mit den jeweils örtlich zuständigen Leitstellen im Einsatzbereich tägliche Praxis.

Die Leitstelle der Berufsfeuerwehr Köln arbeitet mit Unterstützung eines Einsatzleitrechners. Die an 10 Einsatzleitplätzen arbeitenden Disponenten werden durch modernste Technik unterstützt. Der Rechner verfügt über eine Orts-, Straßen- und Objektdatei die hilft, die Einsatzstelle eindeutig zu identifizieren. Den Einsatzkräften stehen gleichzeitig Anfahrthinweise zur Verfügung. Die mit der Alarmierung ausgedruckten Koordinaten des Einsatzortes stehen so auch dem Rettungshubschrauber zur Verfügung. Auf Grundlage der geschilderten Notfallsituation wählt der Disponent ein diesem Ereignis angemessenes Einsatzstichwort(1) aus. Die Festlegung des Einsatzstichwortes verbindet der Einsatzleitrechner mit einer vorab programmierten Kombination der nun erforderlichen Einsatzmittel, den so genannten Einsatzmittelketten. In einem letzten Arbeitsschritt vergleicht der Rechner den Alarmierungsvorschlag der örtlich zuständigen Rettungsmittel mit deren tatsächlicher Verfügbarkeit und stellt so einen Einsatzvorschlag zusammen. So würde der Disponent beispielsweise bei Schilderung von Krankheitssymptomen, die einen Herzinfarkt vermuten lassen, einen Rettungswagen und einen Notarzt alarmieren. Ist der örtlich zuständige bodengebundene Notarzt bereits im Einsatz, wird sofort der Rettungshubschrauber vorgeschlagen und alarmiert. Unterstützt wird das Alarmierungsverfahren durch ein digitales System der Funkalarmierung und ein Funkmeldesystem (FMS), daß den jeweiligen Betriebsstatus aller Einsatzmittel überträgt, verwaltet und anzeigt.

Alle im Bereich des Brandschutzes und des Rettungsdienstes mitwirkenden Einrichtungen und Organisationen sind mit der Leitstelle entweder über Funk, Direktleitung oder Telefon verbunden. Immer sind redundante Alarmierungsmöglichkeiten vorhanden um bei Ausfall einzelner Techniken keine Verzögerungen zu verursachen.

can then be given the necessary instructions and information over a joint operating channel. This uniform structure is supported by the comprehensive participation of the fire services in rescue activities. Duplicate structures and double emergency notification are thus largely avoided. The interval between an accident and the first medical care can be effectively shortened by sending out „first responders" (e.g. fire-fighting vehicles with an expanded range of equipment and qualified personnel) to medical emergencies. Since the rescue helicopter operates within a radius of approx. 50 km of its base in Cologne-Mehrheim – and thus covers a territory extending beyond the boundaries of the City of Cologne – close collaboration with local Coordination Centers is part of its daily routine.

The Coordination Center of the Cologne Professional Fire Service is assisted in its work by an operations host computer. At their individual computer workstations, the 10 dispatchers have access to state-of-the-art technology. The host computer contains town, street and property directories enabling the dispatchers to pinpoint the emergency site quickly; simultaneously, the rescue personnel are supplied with directions to the emergency site. The printout of the site coordinates is therefore made available to the rescue helicopter as well. On the basis of the caller's description of the emergency situation, the dispatcher selects an appropriate mission key word. The input of the mission key word causes the host computer to select the appropriate rescue resources and output a „rescue resource chain". In a last step, the computer checks the availability of the resources in this chain and draws up a mission recommendation. For example, a dispatcher who has received a call describing symptoms suggesting a heart attack will notify a rescue ambulance and a physician with emergency & rescue certification. If the physician with emergency & rescue certification on duty on the ground locally is already on a mission, the dispatcher immediately recommends the rescue helicopter and then notifies it. The emergency notification system is supported by a digital radio emergency notification system and a radio signaling system which transmits, manages and displays the operating status of all rescue resources.

All of the institutions and organizations participating in the activities of the fire and rescue services are connected to the

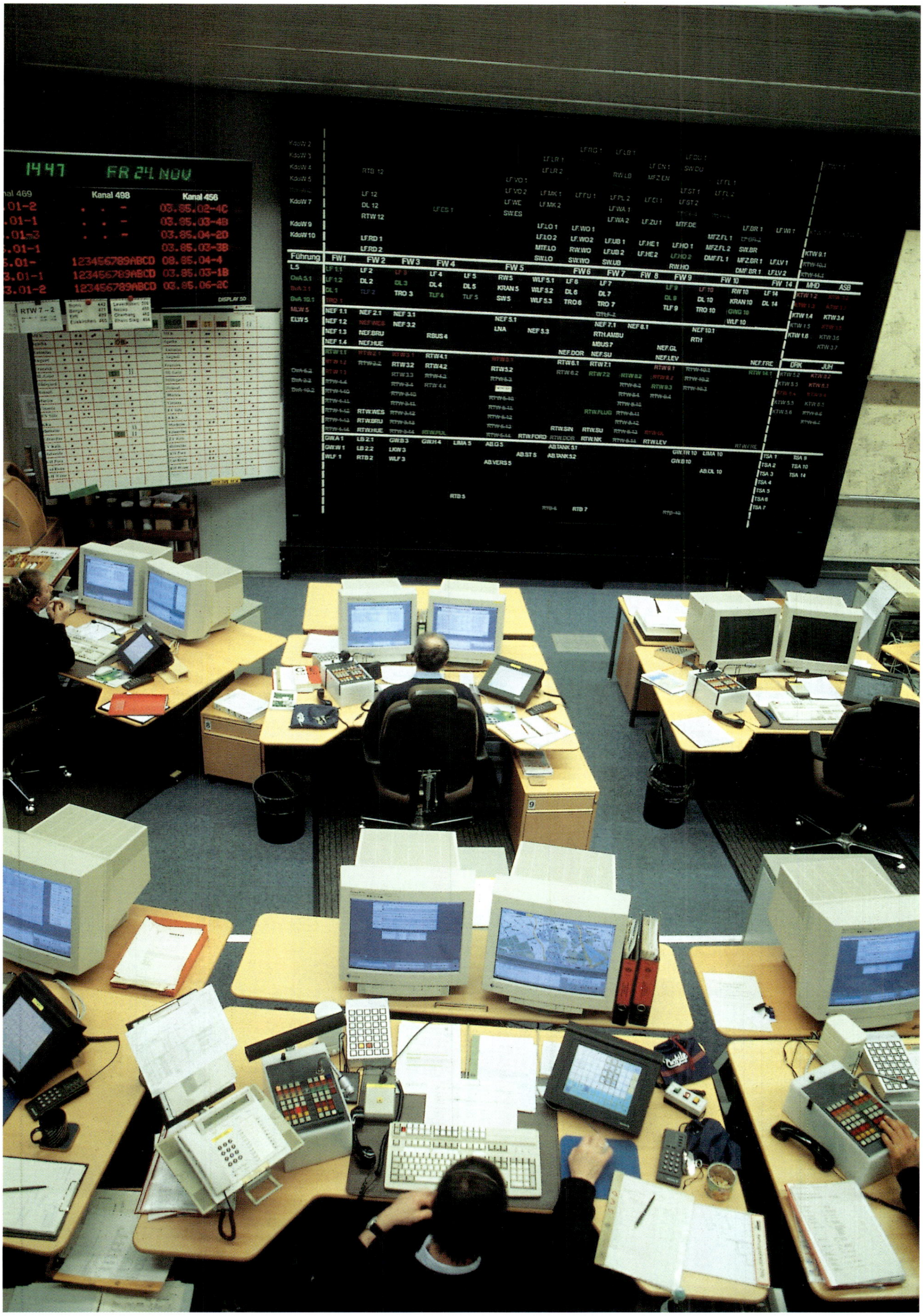

Die Leitstelle.

Coordination Center.

Eine weitere Aufgabe der Leitstelle ist die Bereitstellung eines zentralen Krankenbettennachweises. Dazu melden die 17 in der Notfallversorgung mitwirkenden Krankenhäuser bei der Leitstelle, wenn eine oder mehrere Fachstationen des Hauses (z.B. Intensivstationen) oder besondere, notfallmedizinisch relevante Einrichtungen der Diagnostik oder Therapie (OP-Bereich, CT oder Beatmungsplätze) belegt sind oder anderweitig nicht zur Verfügung stehen. So ist sichergestellt, daß bereits während der Erstversorgung von Notfallpatienten vor Ort die definitive Unterbringung vorbereitet wird. Dies gilt insbesondere für schwerverbrannte oder polytraumatisierte Patienten, für deren Versorgung nur wenige Fachabteilungen geeignet sind.

Alle in der Leitstelle arbeitenden Disponenten sind selbst langjährig erfahrene Rettungsassistenten und Gruppenführer der Feuerwehr, die sich nach einer umfangreichen Fachweiterbildung auf diese Aufgabe spezialisiert haben. Sie versehen ihre Arbeit im 24-Stunden-Dienst, um rund um die Uhr an allen Tagen des Jahres eine maximale Hilfe auch bei Großschadensfällen zu gewährleisten.

Technisch und organisatorisch ist die Leitstelle der Berufsfeuerwehr Köln auf einem aktuellen Stand. Dennoch lassen sich perspektivisch einige zukünftige Entwicklungen andeuten:

Es ist heute der Nachweis zu erbringen, daß die wenigen vorhandenen Mittel auch optimal und vereinbarungsgemäß eingesetzt werden. Damit erfährt die Qualität der erbrachten Leistungen große Bedeutung. Dies gilt aber nicht nur für die zum Betrieb der Leitstellen aufzubringenden Mittel, sondern insbesondere auch für die Qualität der Disposition. Ziel und nachgewiesene Qualität muß es sein, möglichst häufig adäquat zu disponieren, da jede Überdimensionierung der Einsatzmittelketten unnötig Geld kostet und diese Fahrzeuge dem übrigen Einsatzgeschehen entzogen werden, eine Unterdimensionierung zu Nachforderungen und erhöhten Schäden führt.

Ein ganz wesentliches Leistungsmerkmal einer integrierten Leitstelle ist die Integration der Arztrufzentrale des ärztlichen Bereitschaftsdienstes der Kassenärztlichen Vereinigungen. Hier lassen sich durch die Integration weitere Synergismen erschließen.

Auch neue Techniken ermöglichen die Übernahme bzw. die Entwicklung neuer Strategien.

Coordination Center by radio, direct line or telephone. There are always redundant emergency notification channels available so that there will be no delays in the event of a failure of individual systems.

An additional task of the Coordination Center is to prepare a central list of available hospital beds. For this purpose, the 17 hospitals which participate in the emergency care program notify the Coordination Center whenever one or more specialized diagnostic or therapeutic facilities required for the provision of emergency medical care (e.g. Dept. of Surgery, CT or respiratory equipment) are occupied or not available for any reason. This ensures that, during the provision of the initial medical care, definitive plans can already be made for transporting the patient to a hospital. This is especially important for patients with severe burns or polytrauma, since only a few specialized hospital departments have the facilities necessary for the care of these patients.

All of the dispatchers working in the Coordination Center are experienced paramedics or heads of fire-fighting units who worked at these jobs for a number of years before receiving extensive further training preparing them for the role of dispatcher. The dispatchers work in shifts around the clock to provide maximum assistance 365 days a year to even in teh event of major.

Both the technical infrastructure and organization of the Coordination Center of the Cologne Professional Fire Service are state of the art. Nevertheless, several future developments can be hinted at here:

Today rescue organizations have to demonstrate that they use the available resources optimally and in conformance with contractual agreements. In this context, the quality of the services provided is of great importance. This applies, in particular, to the quality of the dispatching work as well as to the quality of the personnel and equipment required for the operation of the Coordination Center. To achieve high-quality dispatching, the Coordination Center must dispatch personnel and equipment in a manner commensurate with the emergency at hand in as many cases as possible. This is vital since over-dimensioning of the rescue resource chain results in unnecessary costs; moreover, vehicles dispatched unnecessarily are not available for other missions.

Neue Techniken zur Disposition sind GPS (Global Positioning System), ISDN (Integrated Services Digital Network), Funkmeldesysteme (FMS), Datenfunk, digitale Funktechniken in Verbindung mit digitalen Sprachspeichern und digitaler Funkalarmierung sowie Fernwirk- und Regeltechniken. GPS kommt zum Einsatz als Navigationshilfe und zur Umsetzung einer „Erstes-Fahrzeug-Strategie“. Die Koordinaten der Einsatzstelle werden einer Datenbank entnommen und dem Einsatzmittel mitgeteilt. In der Luftrettung kann es durch die automatische Erkennung des Notfallorts zu einer Verkürzung der Anflugzeiten kommen. Weitere Verbesserungen lassen sich durch den Einsatz von Geoinformationssystemen (digitalisierte Stadtkarte mit Zusatzinformationen) erreichen.

Neben der schnellen und angemessenen Disposition aller Einsatzmittel ist es Aufgabe der Leitstelle, den Einsatz des Rettungshubschraubers auch über die Stadtgrenzen hinaus zu verfolgen, um damit zur Sicherheit des Flugbetriebs beizutragen.

Underdimensioning, on the other hand, leads to additional demands and increased damage.

A central performance feature of an integrated Coordination Center is the incorporation of the Medical Emergency Line that is part of the on-call duty system run by the Association of Physicians Registered with the Statutory Health Insurance Companies. Additional synergies can be achieved in this area by further integration.

Furthermore, new technologies open up possibilities for pursuing or developing sophisticated strategies. The new technologies available for dispatching include: GPS (Global Positioning System), ISDN (Integrated Services Digital Network), paging (FMS), radio data transmission, digital radio technologies in connection with digital voice mail, digital radio emergency notification, and remote control and I&C. GPS is employed as a navigation aid and to implement a “first responder strategy”. Here the coordinates of the emergency site are taken from a databank and transmitted to the rescue personnel. During air rescue operations, this automatic pinpointing of the emergency site can result in a shortening of the flight time to the scene of the emergency. Additional improvements can be achieved by the use of geographic information systems (e.g. digitized city maps containing additional data).

In addition to dispatching all rescue resources quickly and appropriately, the tasks of the Coordination Center include tracking the rescue helicopter even beyond the city boundaries as a contribution to the safety of air rescue operations.

---

(1) **Einsatzstichworte für den RTH im Einsatzleitrechner**

Unfall: Die Kategorie fasst sowohl lebensbedrohliche Erkrankungen, als auch traumatische Unfälle, Verbrennungen etc. in einem Begriff zusammen.

Unfall 1:
Akutes Geschehen ohne Notarztindikation.

Unfall 2: Notarztindikation
Eine lebensbedrohlich verletzte oder erkrankte Person.

Unfall 3: Notarztindikation
2 bis 3 lebensbedrohlich verletzte oder erkrankte Personen.

Unfall 4: Notarztindikation
4 bis 8 lebensbedrohlich verletzte oder erkrankte Personen.

Unfall 5: Notarztindikation
9 bis 24 lebensbedrohlich verletzte oder erkrankte Personen.

ManV: Notarztindikation
Massenanfall von Verletzten, mehr als 24 Personen.

P-Wasser: Notarztindikation
Person im Wasser. Der RTH wird zur Suche der Person(en), zur Bergung und zur Versorgung eingesetzt.

Gebäudeeinsturz: Notarztindikation
Flugzeugabsturz: Notarztindikation
Notlandung: Notarztindikation
Schiffsunglück: Notarztindikation

(1) **Mission Key Words in the Host Computer**

Accident:
This category comprises both life-threatening diseases and traumatic injuries (fractures, lacerations, 3rd degree burns, etc.)

Accident 1:
Acute incident which does not require a physician with emergency & rescue certification.

Accident 2:
A person with a life-threatening injury or disease requiring immediate assistance from a physician with emergency & rescue certification.

Accident 3:
A number of persons (2-3) with life-threatening injuries or diseases requiring immediate assistance from a physician with emergency & rescue certification.

Accident 4:
A number of persons (4-8) with life-threatening injuries or diseases requiring immediate assistance from a physician with emergency & rescue certification.

Accident 5:
A number of persons (9-24) with life-threatening injuries or diseases require immediate assistance from a physician with emergency & rescue certification.

MassI:
A large number of persons, i.e. more than 24, requiring immediate attention from a physician.

P-water:
Person in the water. The rescue helicopter is sent on a search-and-rescue mission to find, rescue and provide emergency medical care to the person.

Collapsed building, Airplane crash,
Emergency landing, Accident on the Rhine

Einsatz für den Rettungshubschrauber
Mission for the Rescue Helicopter

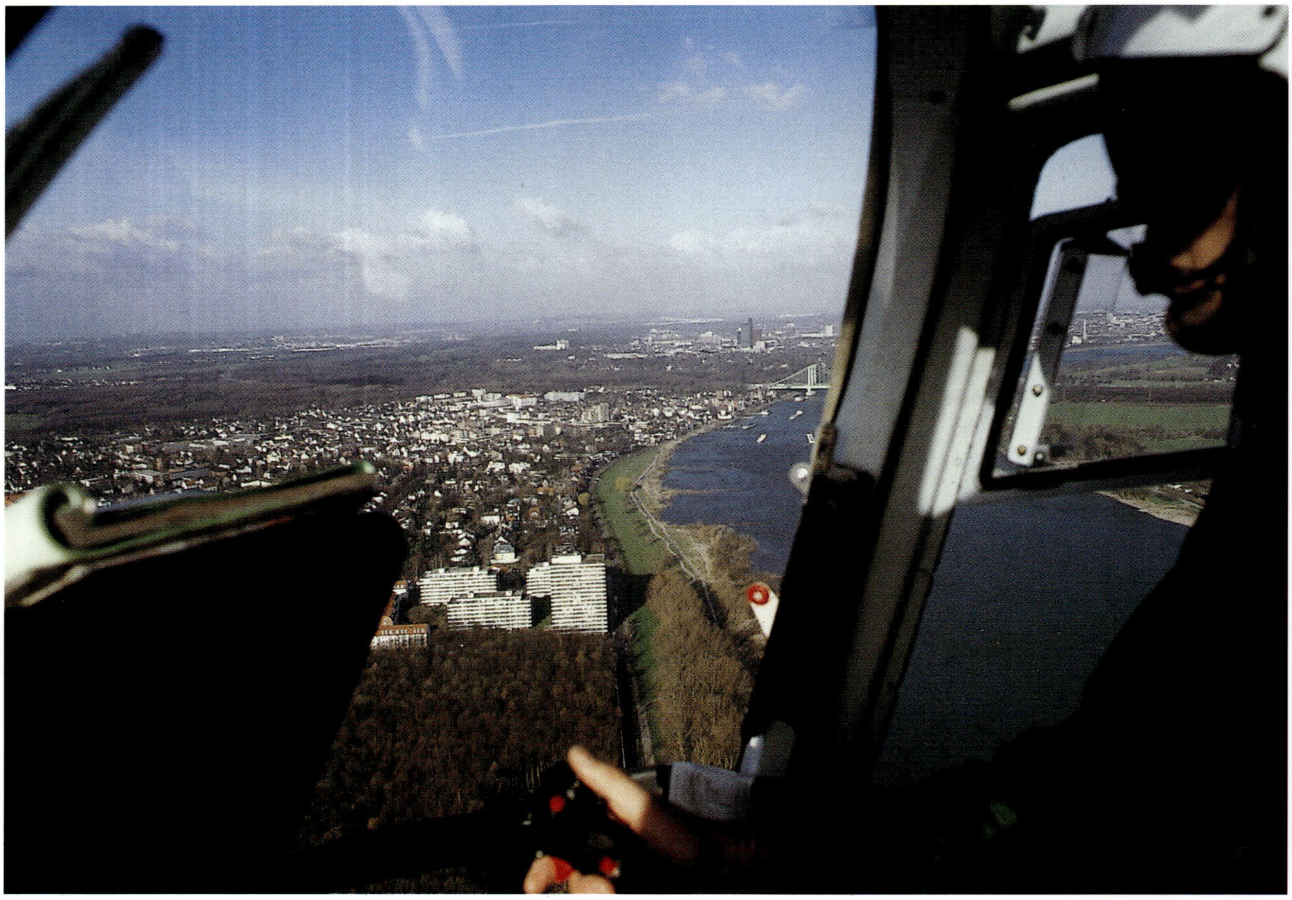

Person im Rhein.

Person in the Rhine.

Augenblicke

Sportler. Radprofi. Im Wohnzimmer Hunderte von Pokalen. Wiederbelebung. Radsportler durchtrainiert. Hat seine Runden gedreht und dann mit seinem Sohn noch einen Waldlauf gemacht. Unter der Dusche bricht er zusammen. Leblos. Wiederbelebung erfolglos. Rückflug.

Snapshots

Emergency call to the house of a well-known professional cyclist. Hundreds of trophies are displayed prominently in the living room. Resuscitation. The cyclist was reportedly in excellent physical shape. He had cycled a few laps and then gone jogging in the woods with his son. While in the shower afterwards, he suddenly collapsed. Resuscitation efforts are fruitless. Return flight.

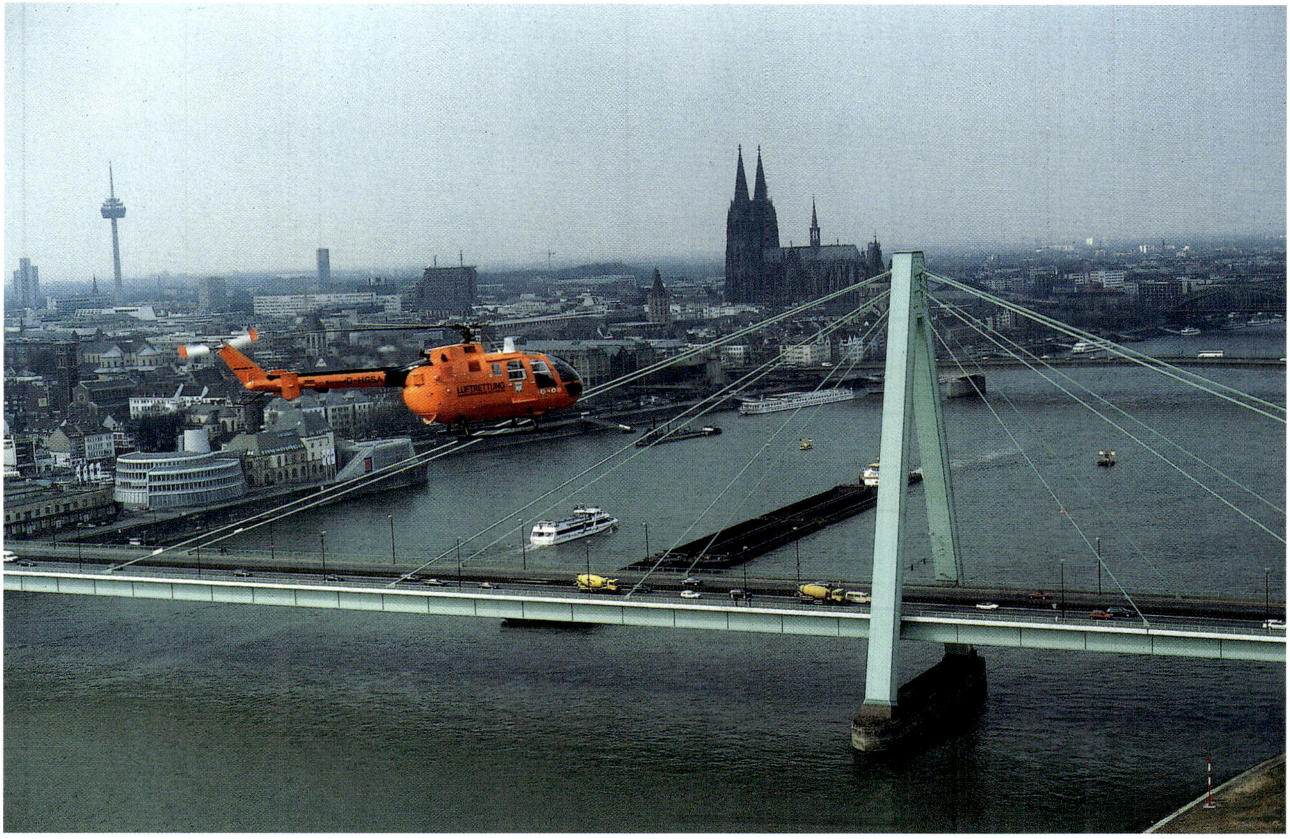

Wir fliegen auf die Einsatzstelle zu.

We fly to the accident site.

Die häufigsten Fragen an der Einsatzstelle
Frequently Asked Questions

Wie wird der Rettungshubschrauber (RTH) alarmiert?

Wie jedes Rettungsmittel wir der RTH über die bekannten Notrufnummern 110 oder 112 (in manchen Bundesländern auch über die 19 222) alamiert. Die zuständige Leitstelle beurteilt anhand der Meldung die Schwere des Notfalls und setzt, wenn erforderlich, den „fliegenden Notarztwagen" RTH ein.

How are emergency calls sent to the rescue helicopter (RH)?

Like every other rescue resource, the rescue helicopter can be requested via the known emergency numbers 110 and 112 (and in some German states over the number 19 222). The responsible Coordination Center assesses the severity of the emergency on the basis of the call; if necessary, it dispatches the "flying rescue ambulance with a physician with emergency & rescue certification aboard" to the scene.

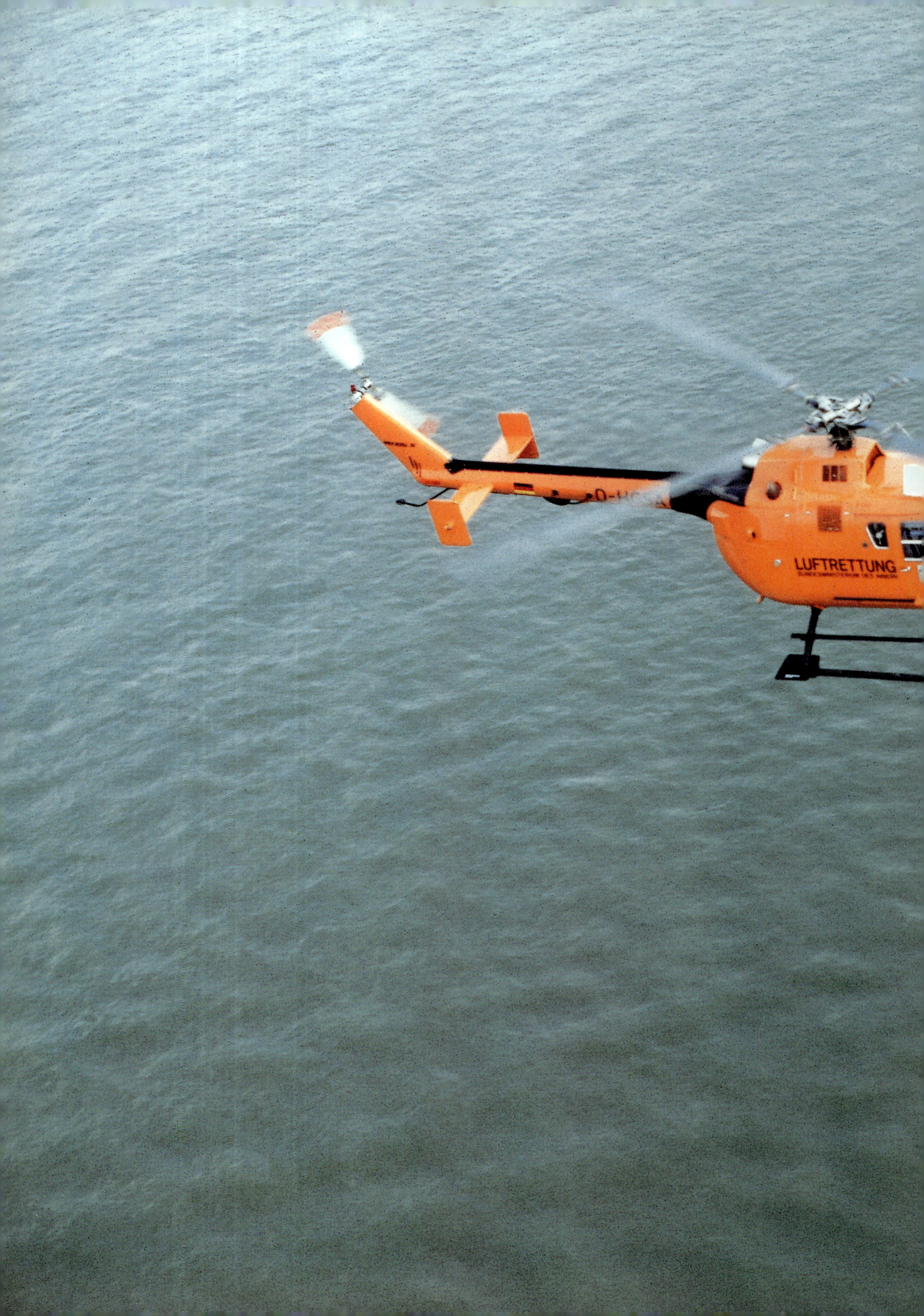
LUFTRETTUNG

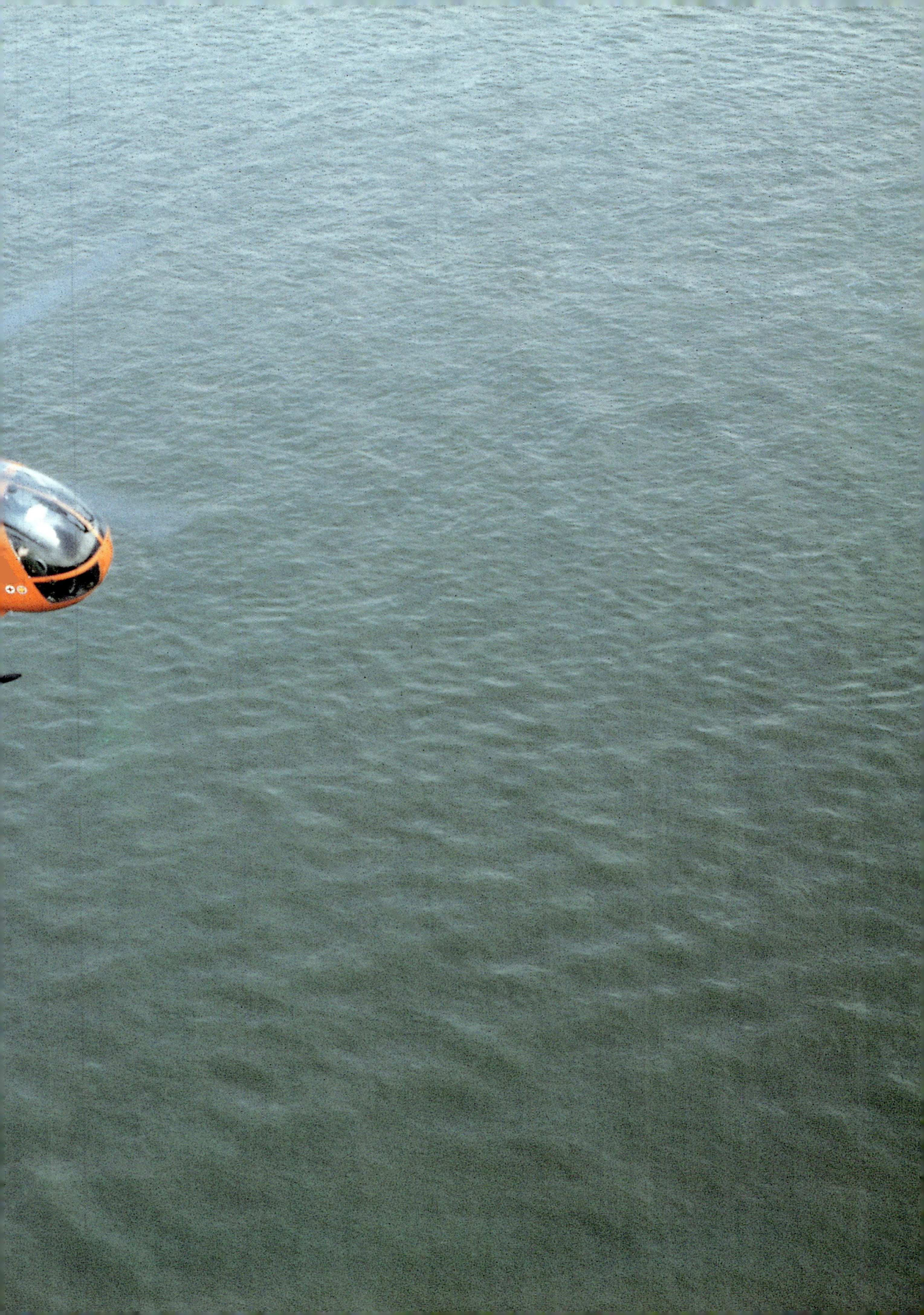

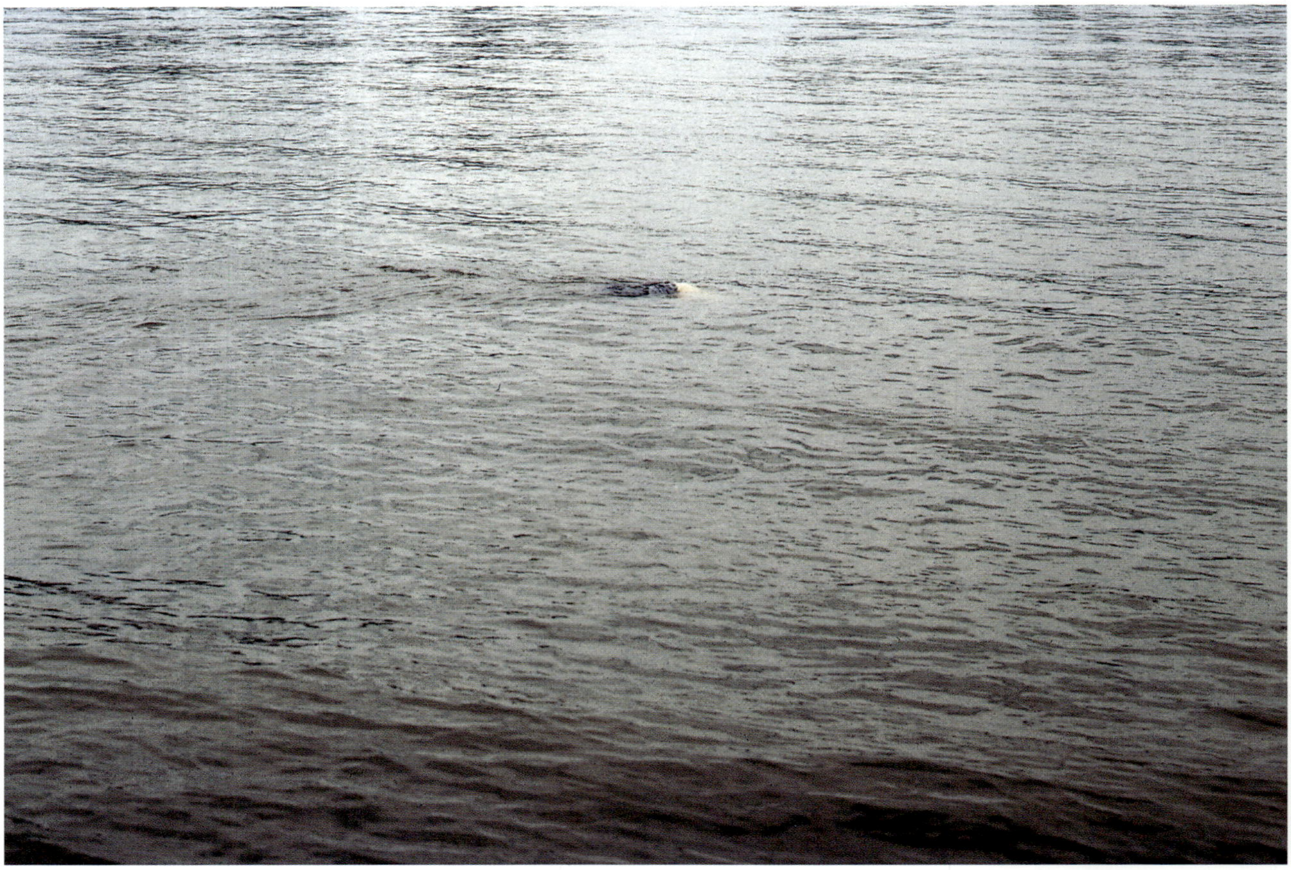

Die Person ist zu sehen.

The person is in sight.

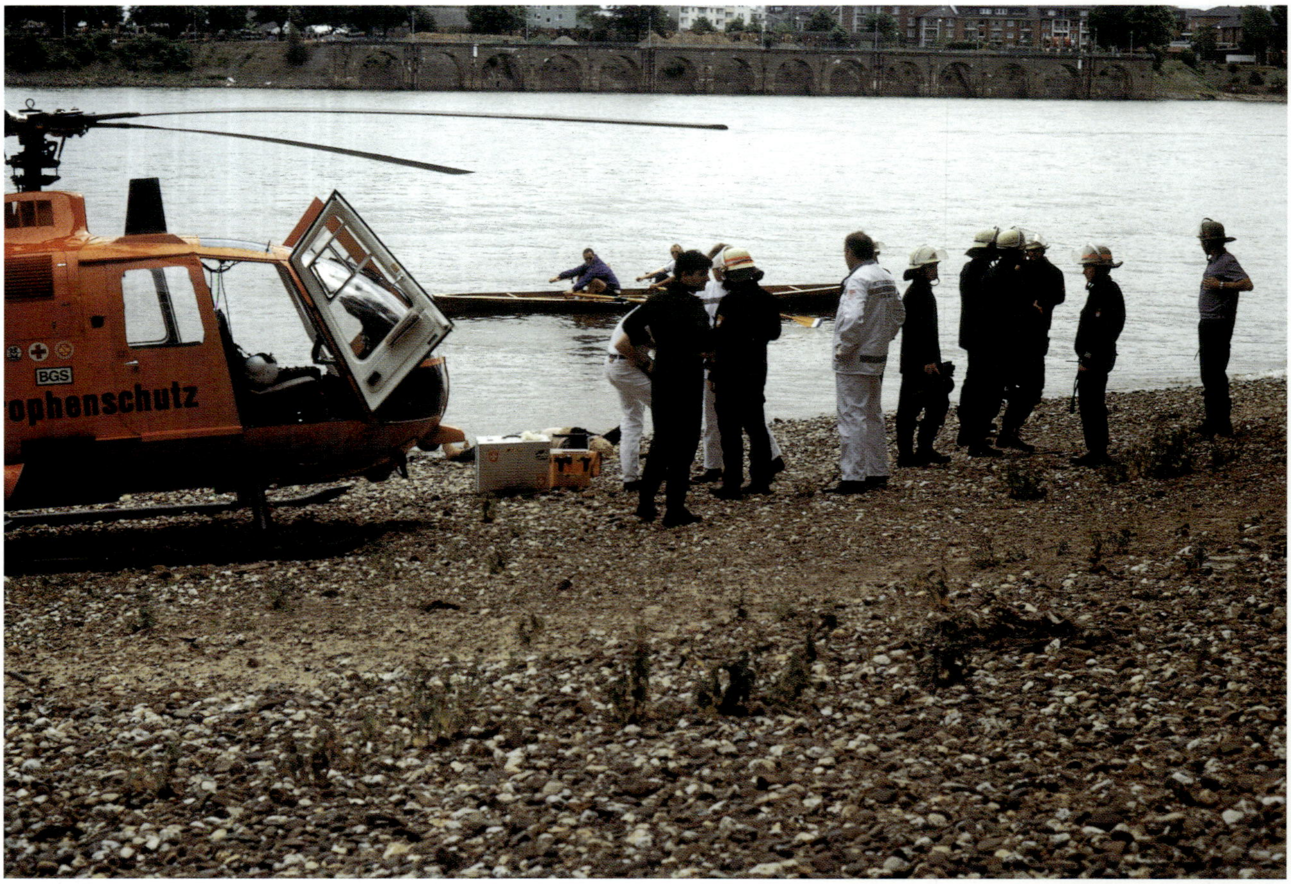

Die Leitstelle meldet, dass zwei Ruderer die Person ausgemacht haben.

The Coordination Center reports that two rowers have sighted the person.

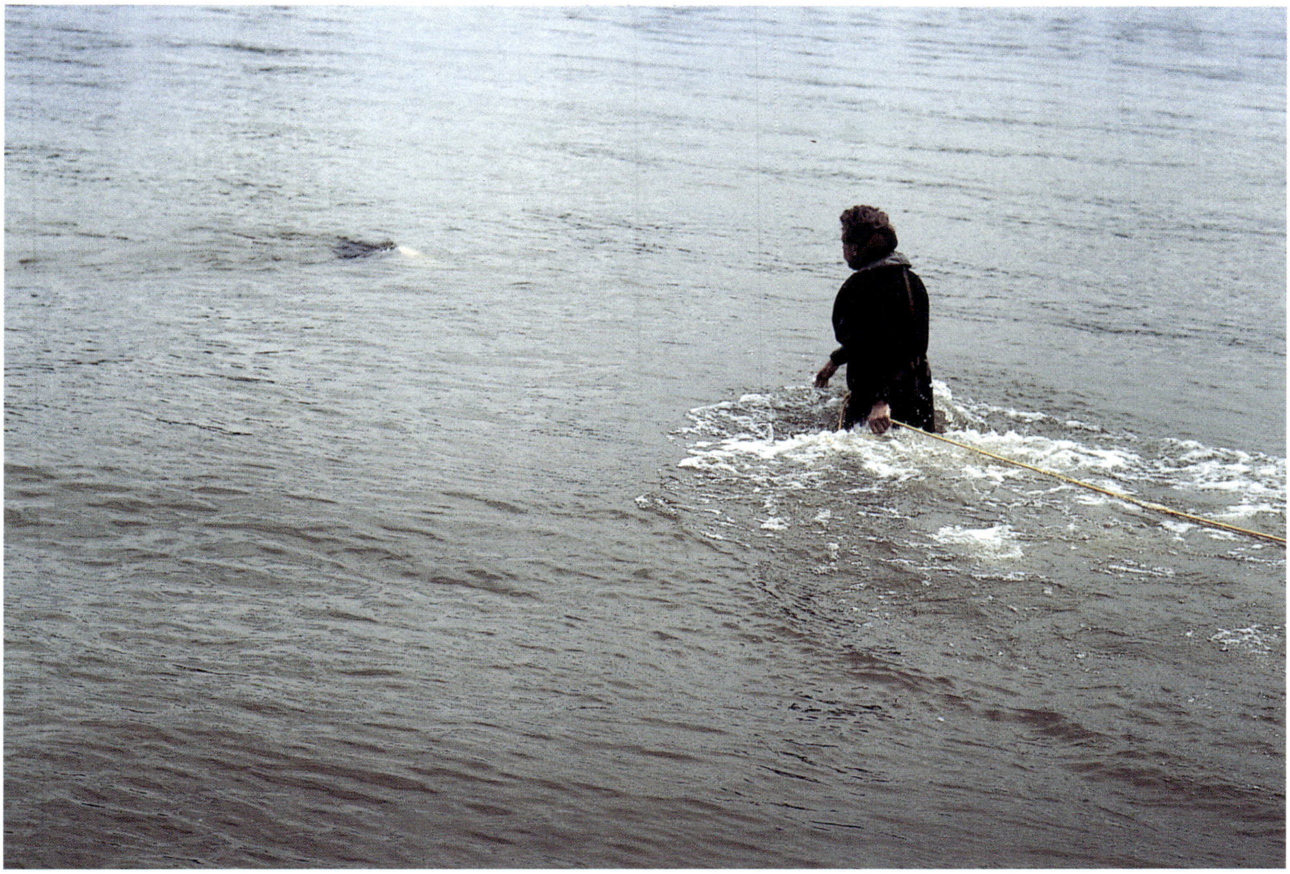

Ein angeleinter Taucher der Feuerwehr birgt die Person.

A lined fire service diver recovers the body.

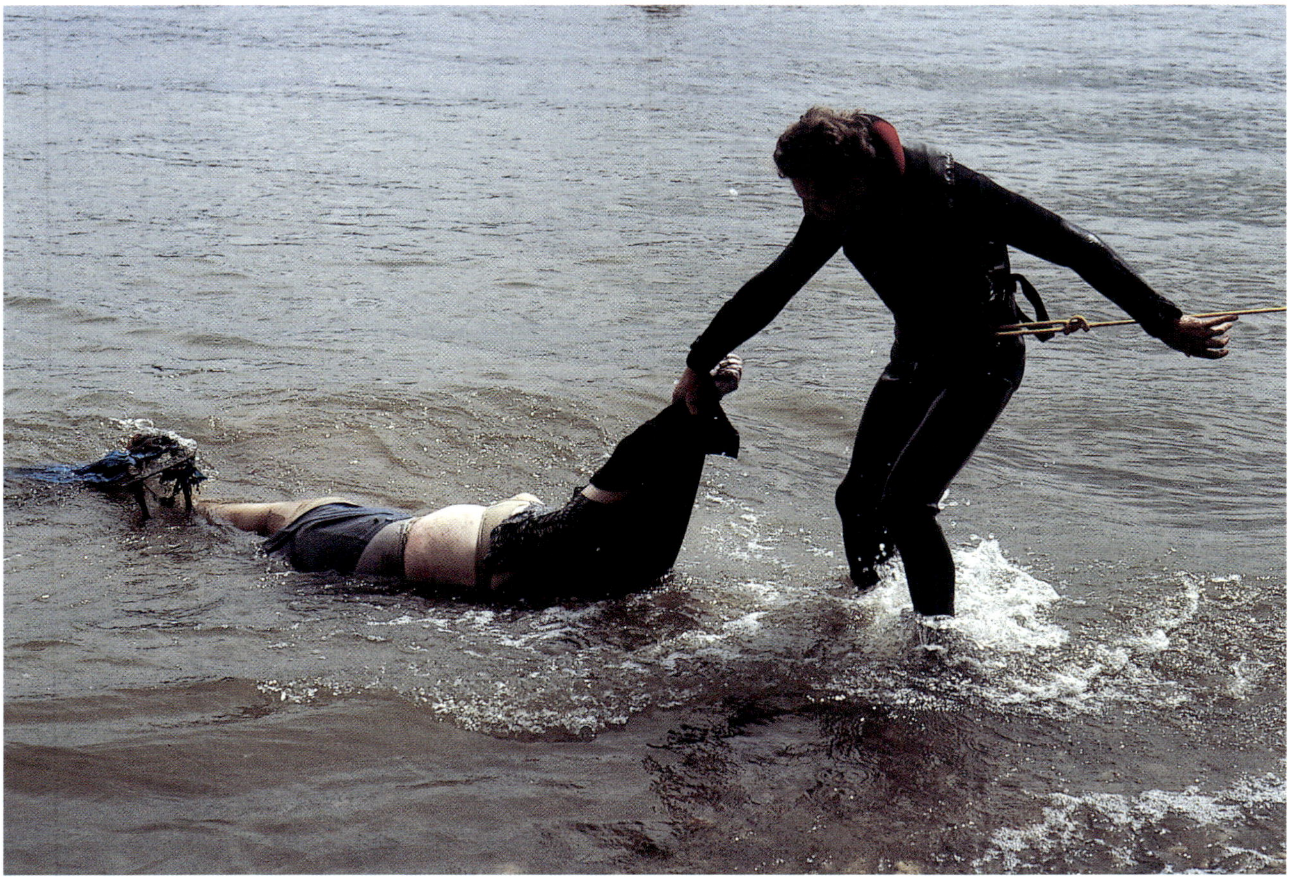

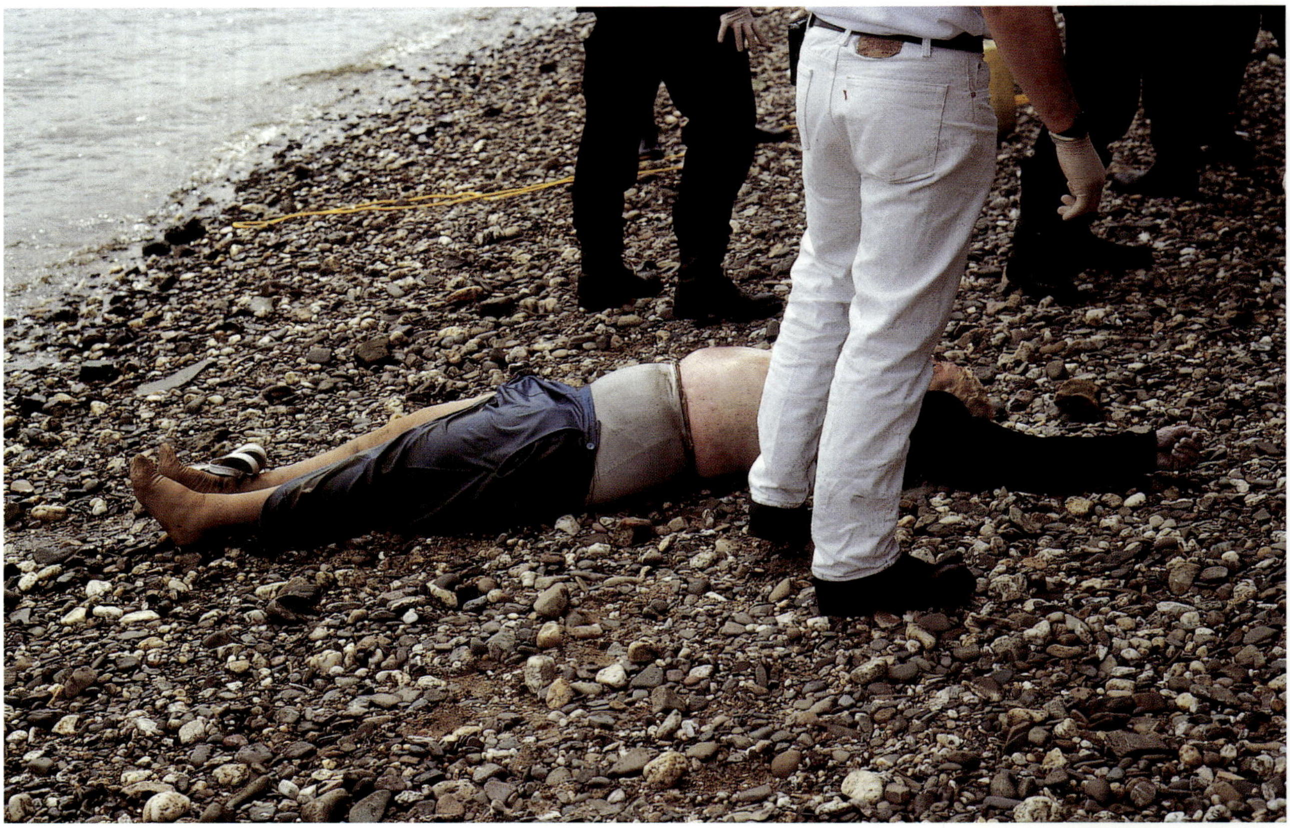

Die Person hat offensichtlich schon mehrere Tage im Rhein getrieben und ist nur dadurch aufgehalten worden, dass sie mit dem Fuß in einem Einkaufswagen, der im Strom lag, hängengeblieben ist.

The body has obviously been floating in the Rhine for several days. It would have floated farther had its leg not got caught in a shopping cart in the river bed.

Augenblicke

Soziale Brennpunkt. Kinderspielplatz. Sandkasten. Kein einziges Kind, aber viele Alkoholisierte. Einer hat Gesichtsverletzungen, Nasenbluten. Die am wenigsten alkoholisierte Frau kümmert sich um ihn. Wenige Sekunden später erkennbar nicht der Ehemann. Ehemann sitzt alkoholisiert auf einer der Bänke. Gruppe aufgebracht. Patient schnell einladen in den Rettungswagen. Türe zu. Junge Frau fährt mit. Nicht der Ehemann. Gesichtsverletzungen.

Snapshots

Emergency call to a deprived area. There is a playground with a sandbox but not a single child in sight. Instead, we see a large group of obviously inebriated people. One of them has facial injuries; his nose is bleeding. A woman who appears to be the most sober person in the group attends to him. Several seconds later it is obvious that she is not his wife. Her own husband is drunk on a nearby bench. The group is up in arms. We load the patient into the ambulance quickly and close the doors. The young woman accompanies the man who is not her husband. We treat his facial injuries.

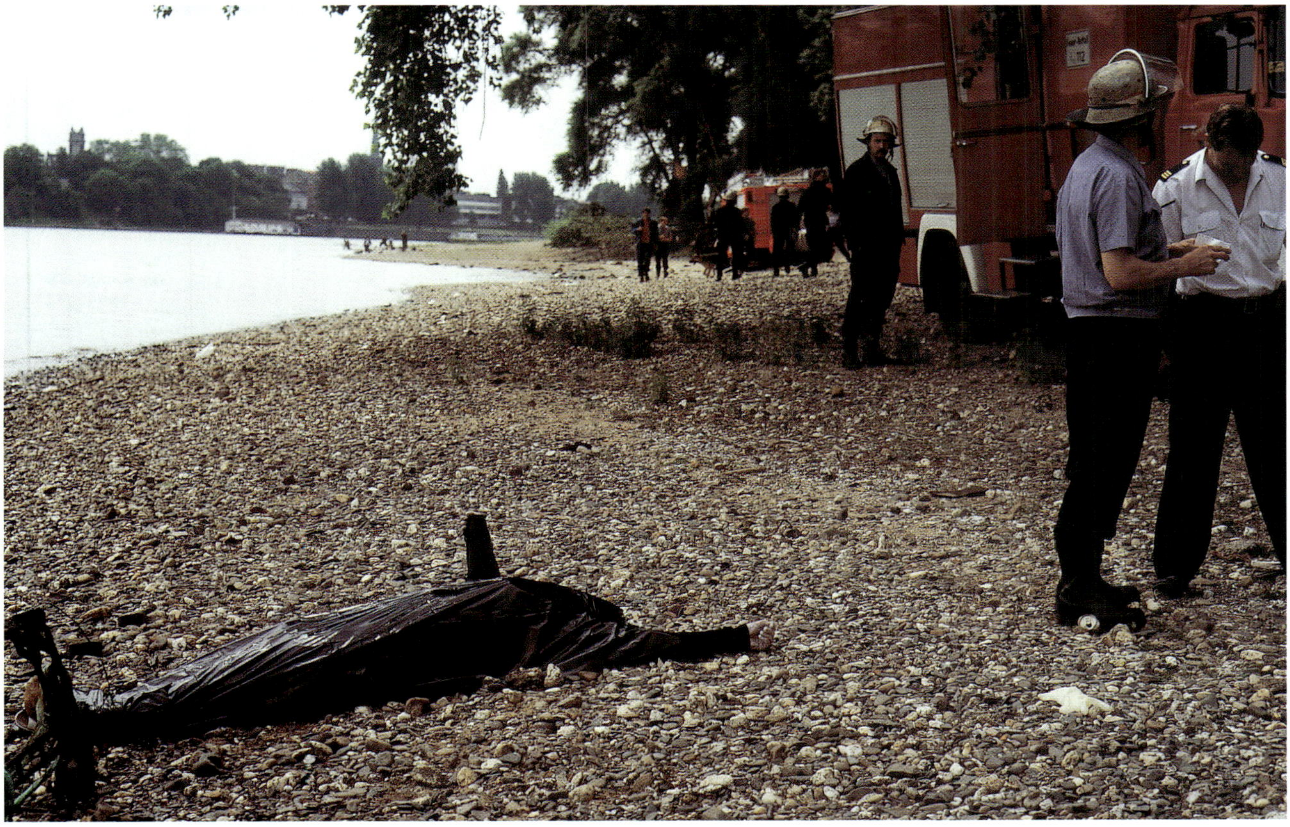

Die Einsatzstelle wird an die Polizei übergeben.

The accident site is turned over to the police.

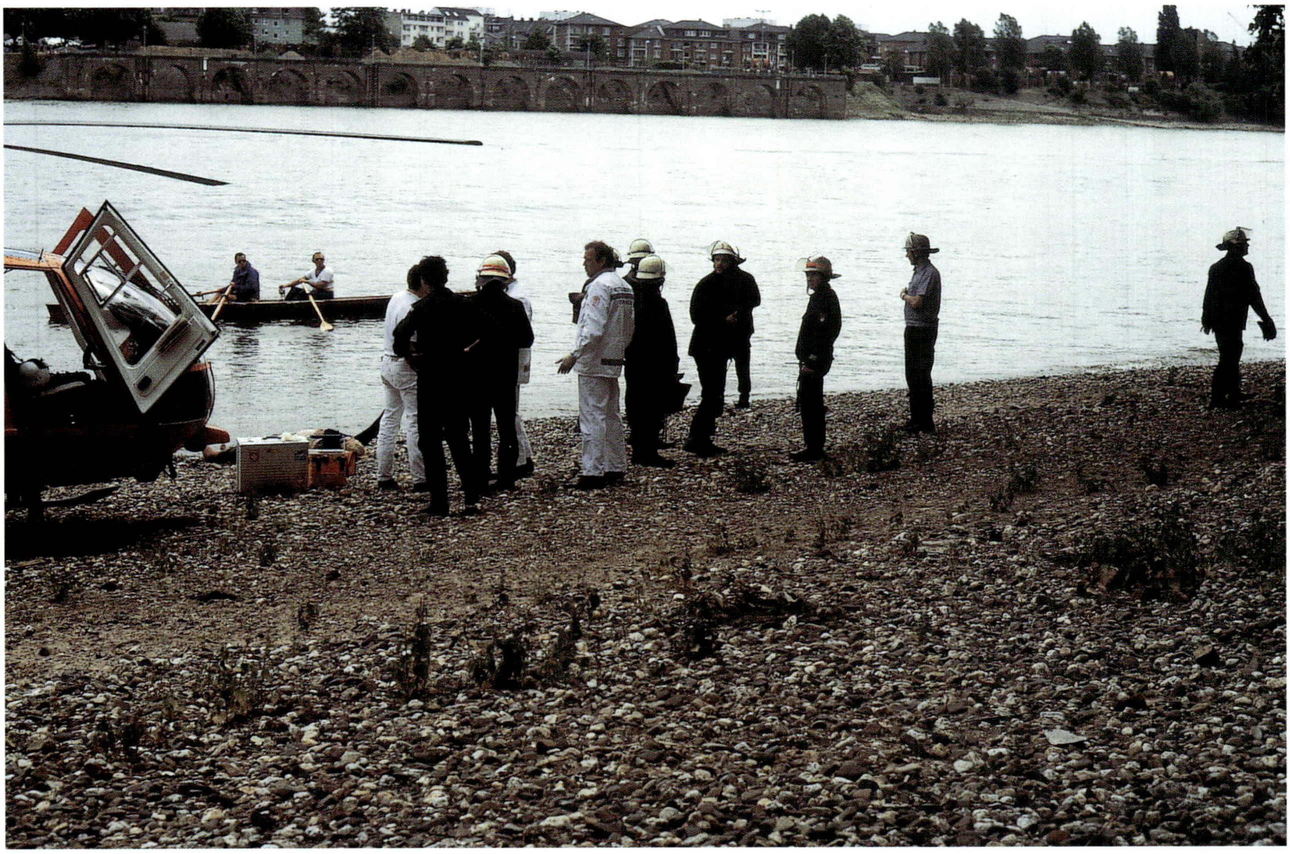

Die Piloten der BGS-Fliegergruppe in Hangelar.
The Pilots of the BGS-Aviation group in Hangelar.

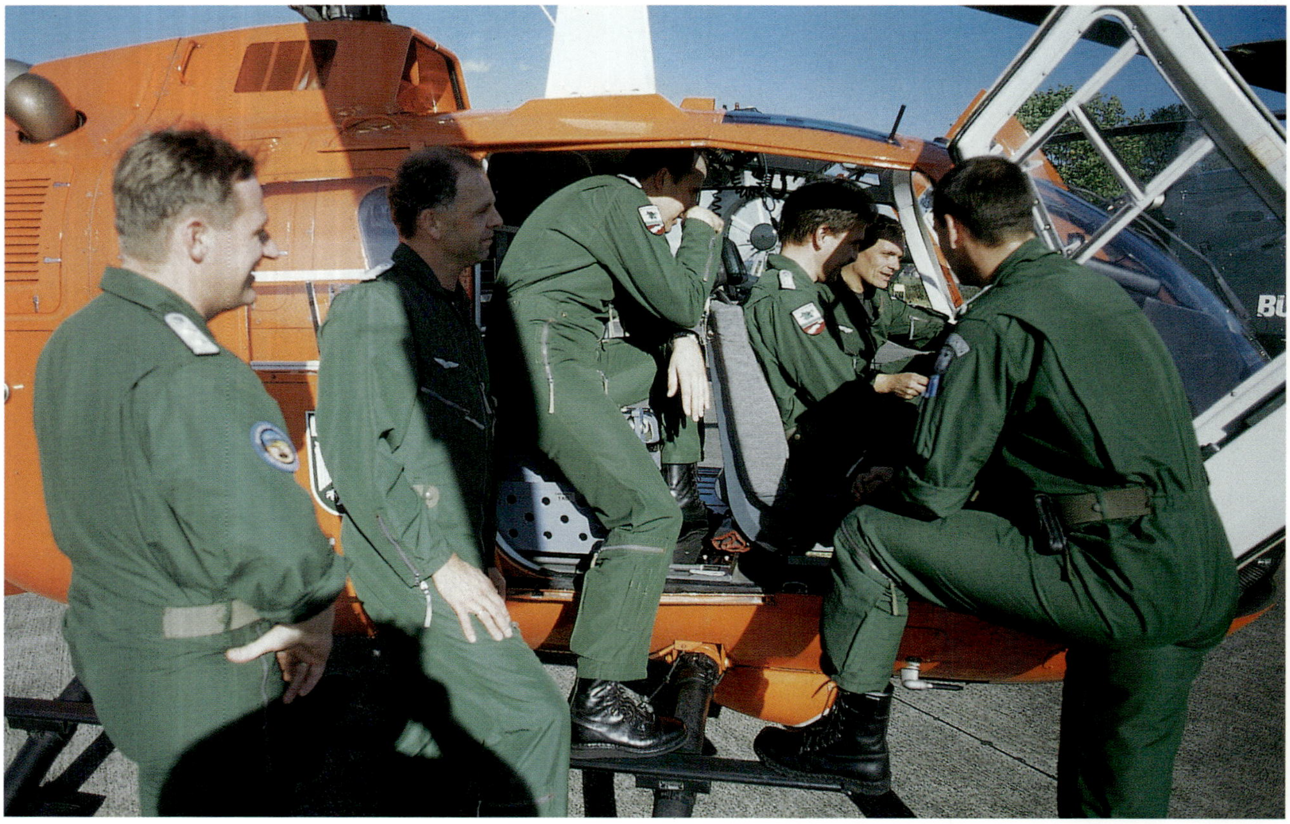

Cockpiteinweisung.

Pilots of the German Federal Border Police receiving cockpit instruction.

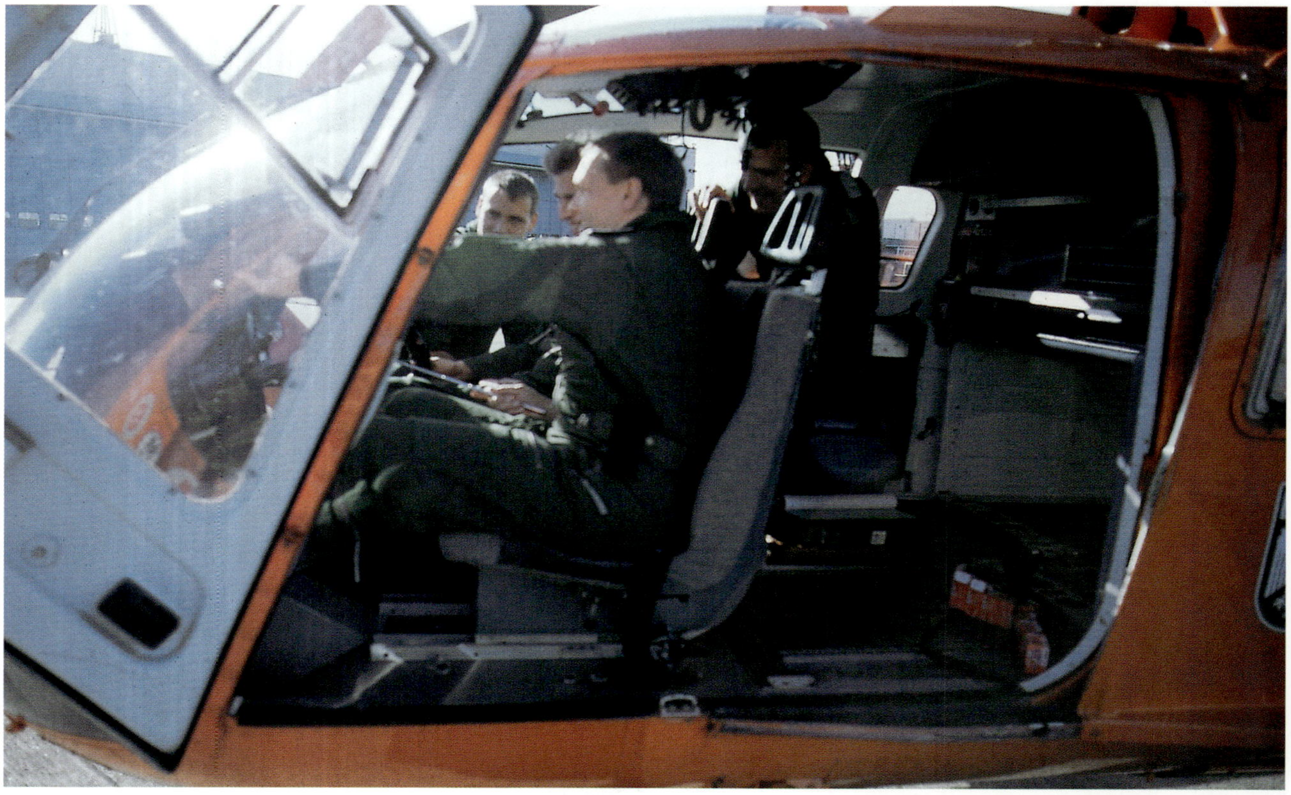

Ein Fluglehrer der Luftfahrerschule der Bundesgrenzschutz Fliegergruppe erklärt das Instrumenten-Panel einer BO 105 CBS-5.

A flight instructor from the Aviation School of the German Federal Border Police explains the instrument panel of the BO-105 CB-5.

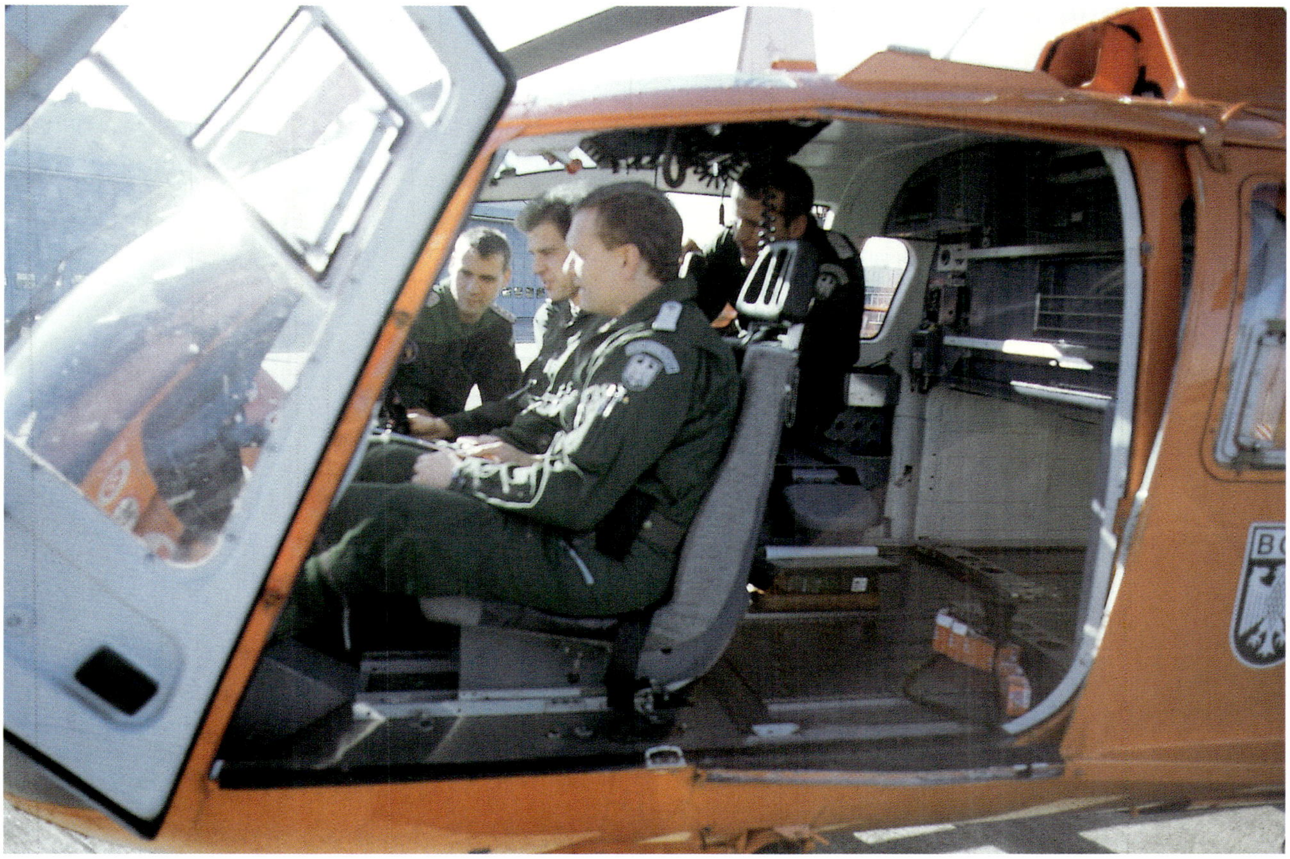

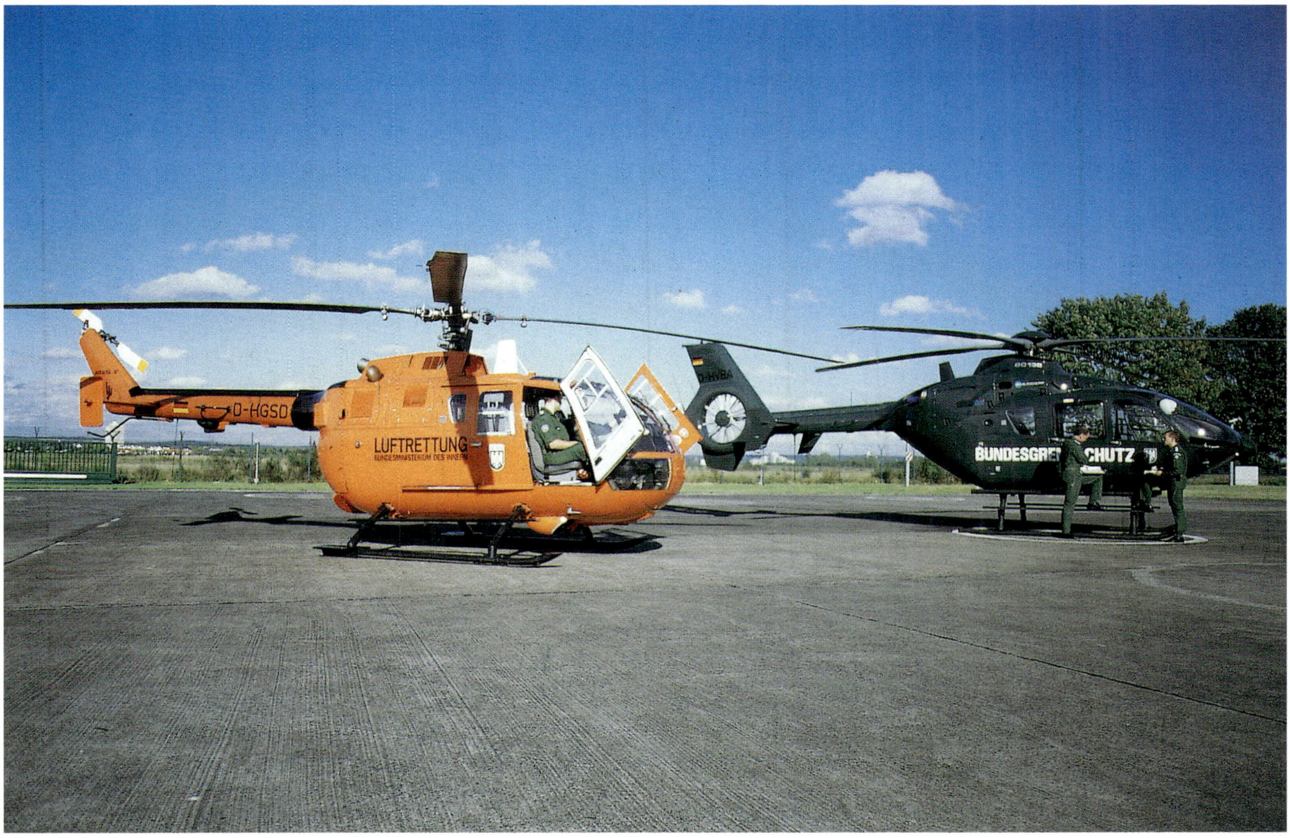

Die BO 105 und einer der möglichen Nachfolgekandidaten, die EC 135. Beim Bundesgrenzschutz wird sie seit September 2000 geflogen.

The BO 105 CBS and its possible successor, the EC 135. The German Federal Border Police have been flying the EC 135 since September 2000.

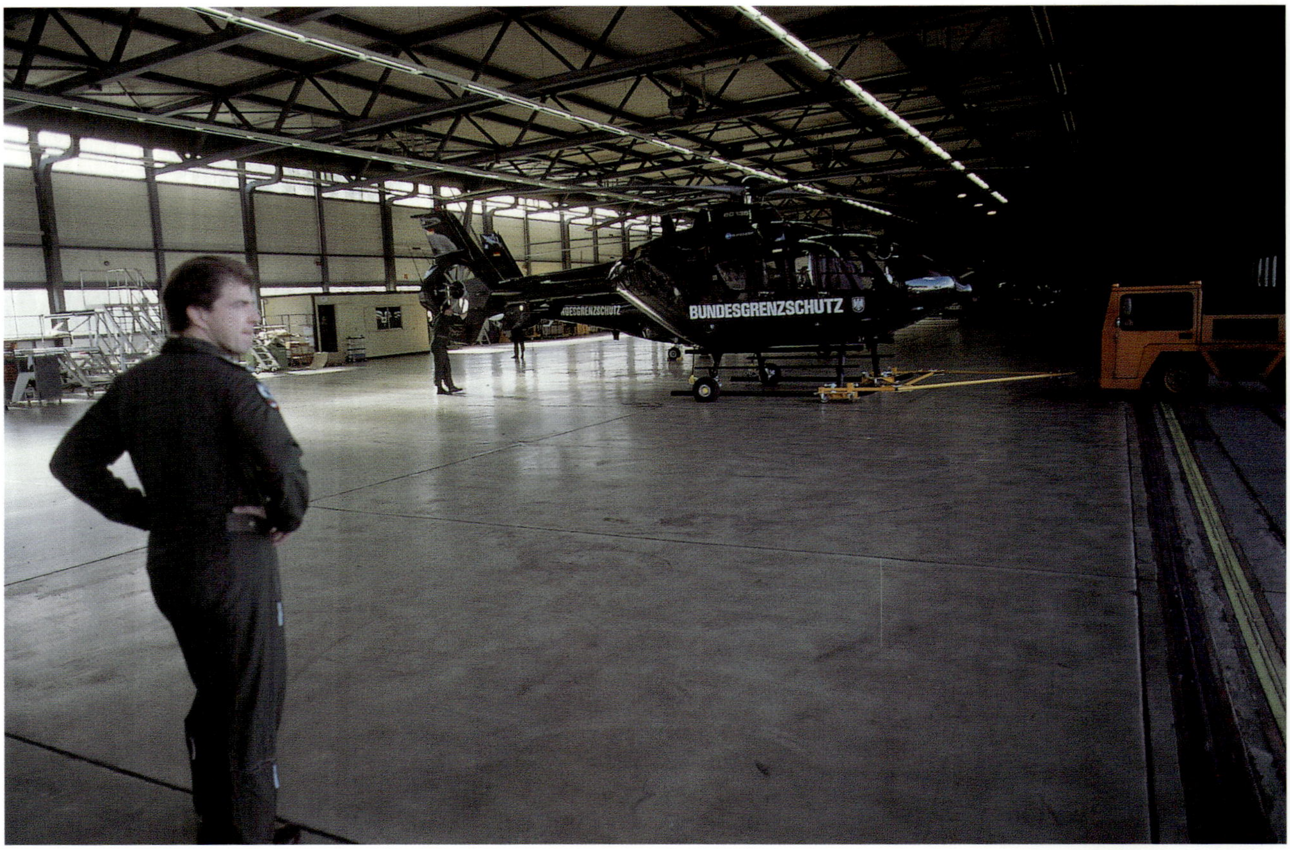

Blick in eine der Abstellhallen der BGS-Fliegerstaffel West in Sankt-Augustin Hangelar.

View inside one of the hangars of the German Federal Border Police – Aviation Squadron West – in St. Augustin-Hangelar.

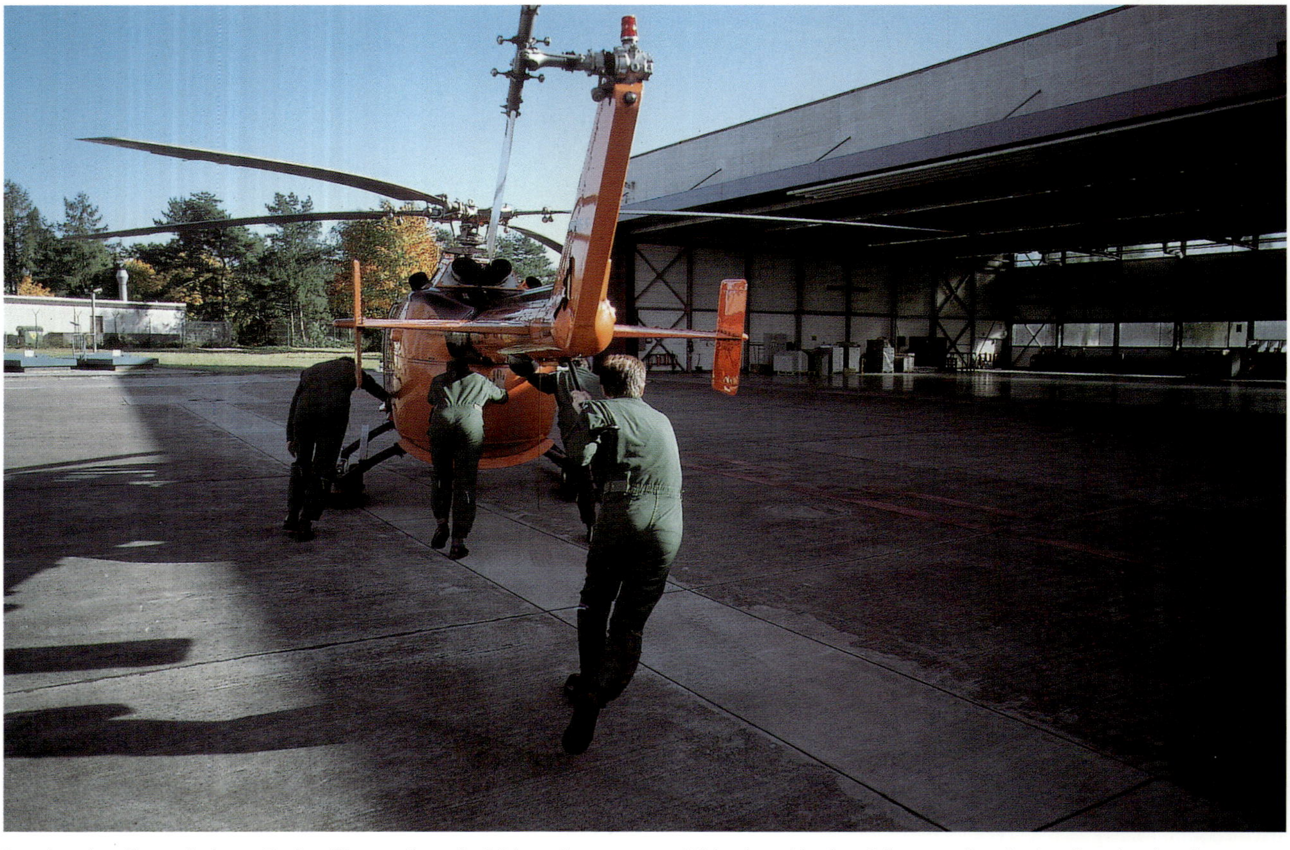

Durch schnellmontierbare Hydraulikgestelle mit Rädern kann man den RTH in alle Richtungen rollen.

With the aid of quick-mounting hydraulic wheels, the rescue helicopters can be moved in all direktions by muscle power.

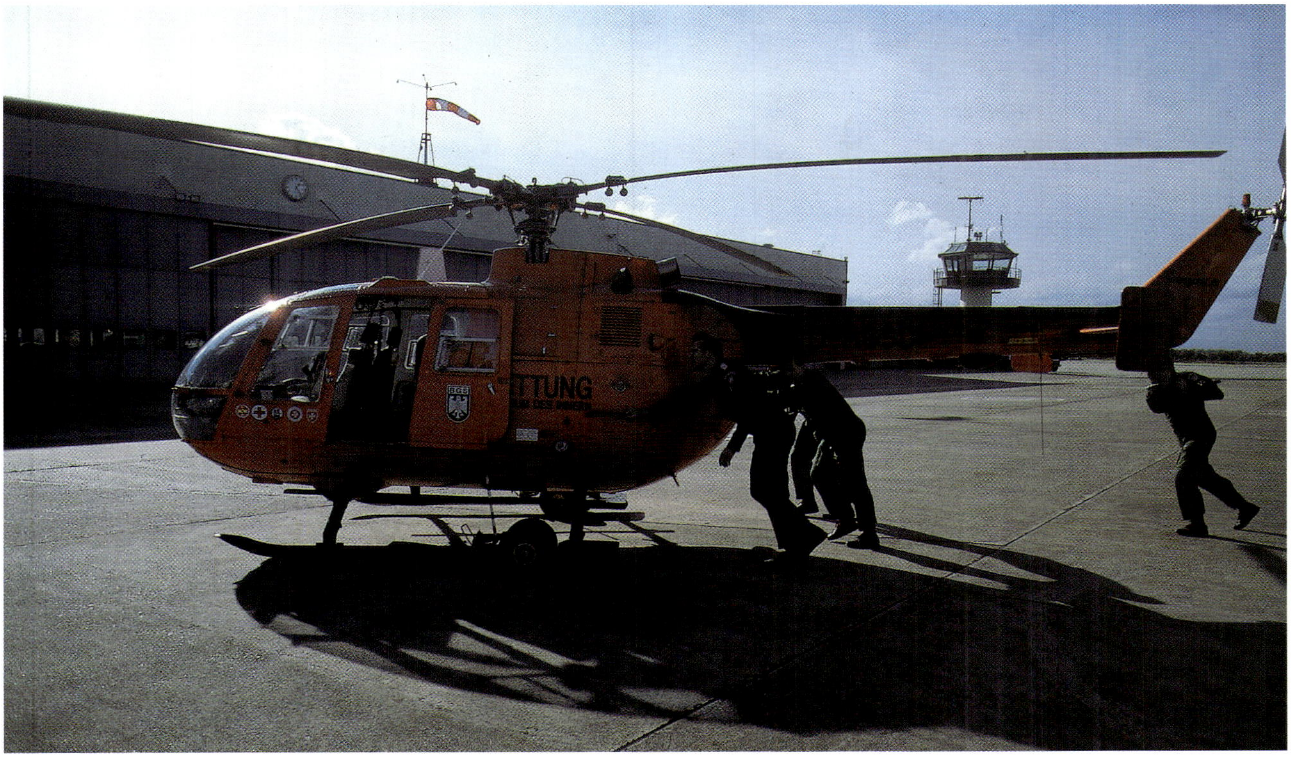

Die häufigsten Fragen an der Einsatzstelle
Frequently Asked Questions

Seit wann ist der Hubschraubertyp BO 105 im Luftrettungsdienst?

Der Hubschrauber MBB (Messerschmidt-Bölkow-Blohm) BO 105 ist seit Beginn der Luftrettung in Deutschland im Jahre 1970, am 01. November des Jahres wurde Christoph 1 in München durch den ADAC in Dienst gestellt, der meisteingesetzte Hubschraubertyp. Am 17. Februar 1967 flog der erste Prototyp des damals revolutionären Hubschraubers mit einem starren Rotorkopfsystem aus Titan, Rotorblättern aus Kunststoff und zwei Turbinentriebwerken.

Die modernste und wohl letzte Version dieses Hubschraubers, EC BO 105 CBS-5, fliegt seit 1996 in 14 von 16 Luftrettungsstationen, die vom Bundesgrenzschutz betrieben werden (In den Küstenstationen Eutin und Güstrow fliegt die Bell 212.). EC steht dabei für Eurocopter, ein deutsch-französisches Unternehmen, das aus MBB und der Hubschraubersparte der Aérospatiale entstanden und mittlerweile der größte zivile Hubschrauberhersteller der Welt ist. (www.eurocopter.com)

How long has the helicopter type BO 105 been used for air rescue in Germany?

The MBB (Messerschmidt-Bölkow-Blohm) helicopter type BO 105 has been used for air rescue since an air rescue service was set up in Germany in 1970. On November 1 of that year, the rescue helicopter Christoph 1 was put into service in Munich by the German Automobile Club (ADAC). This is the type of helicopter most often used for aerial search and rescue. On 17 February 1967 the first prototype of this helicopter, which was revolutionary back then, made its maiden flight. This helicopter had a rigid titanium rotor head system, plastic rotor blades and two turbine engines.

The most modern (and probably last) version of this helicopter, the EC BO 105 CBS-5, has been flying at 14 of the 16 air rescue bases run by the German Border Police since 1996 (The Bell 212 flies from the coastal bases at Eutin and Güstrow). EC stands for Eurocopter, a German-French consortium resulting from the merger of MBB and the helicopter division of Aérospatiale; it is now the second largest manufacturer of civil aviation helicopters in the world (www.eurocopter.com).

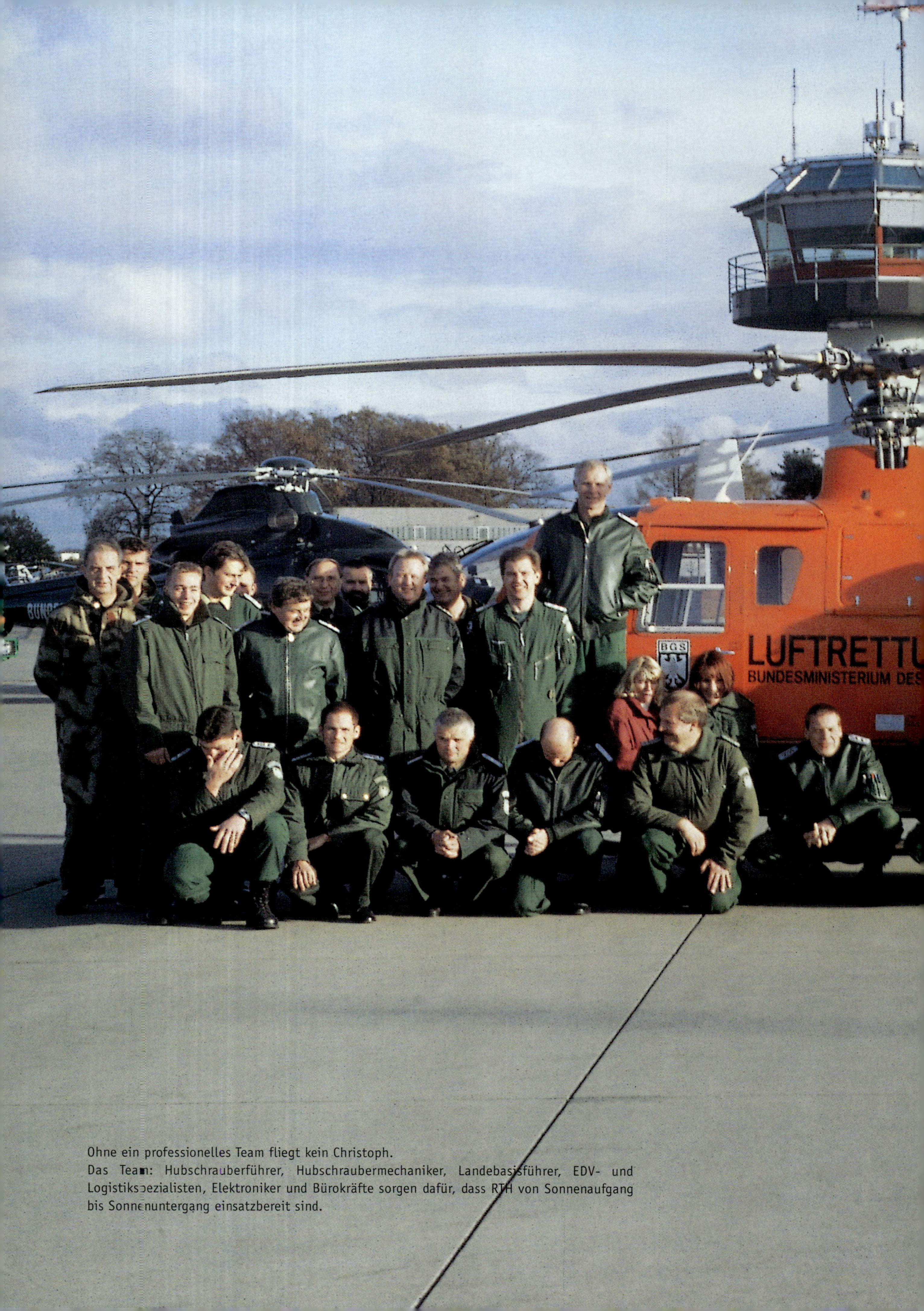

Ohne ein professionelles Team fliegt kein Christoph.
Das Team: Hubschrauberführer, Hubschraubermechaniker, Landebasisführer, EDV- und Logistikspezialisten, Elektroniker und Bürokräfte sorgen dafür, dass RTH von Sonnenaufgang bis Sonnenuntergang einsatzbereit sind.

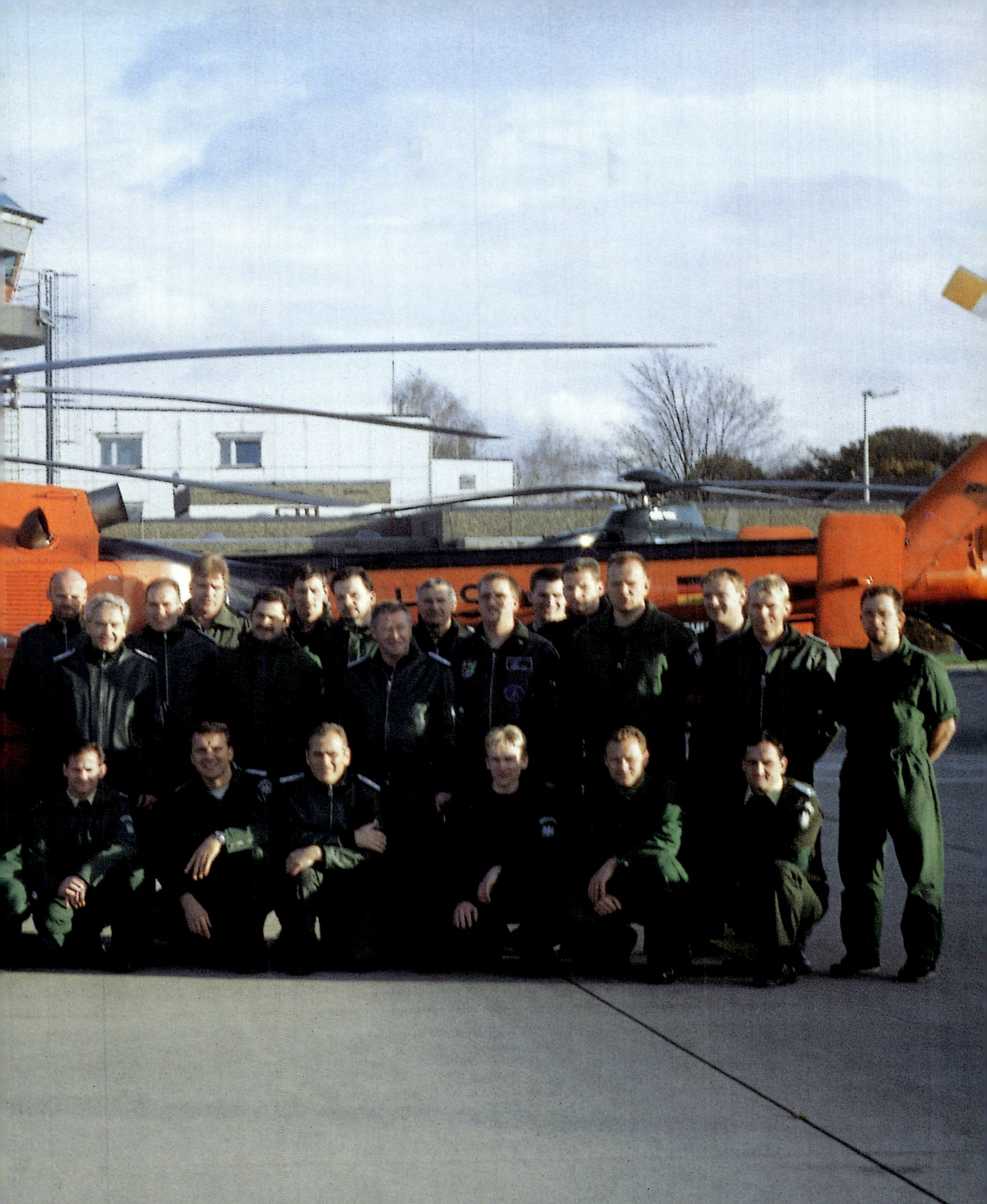

Without a professional team on the ground, the Christoph rescue helicopters would never get into the air. The professional team – consisting of helicopter pilots, helicopter mechanics, the helicopter base manager, computer and logistics specialists, electronic technicians and office staff – sees to it that the rescue helicopter is operational during the hours between sunrise and sunset.

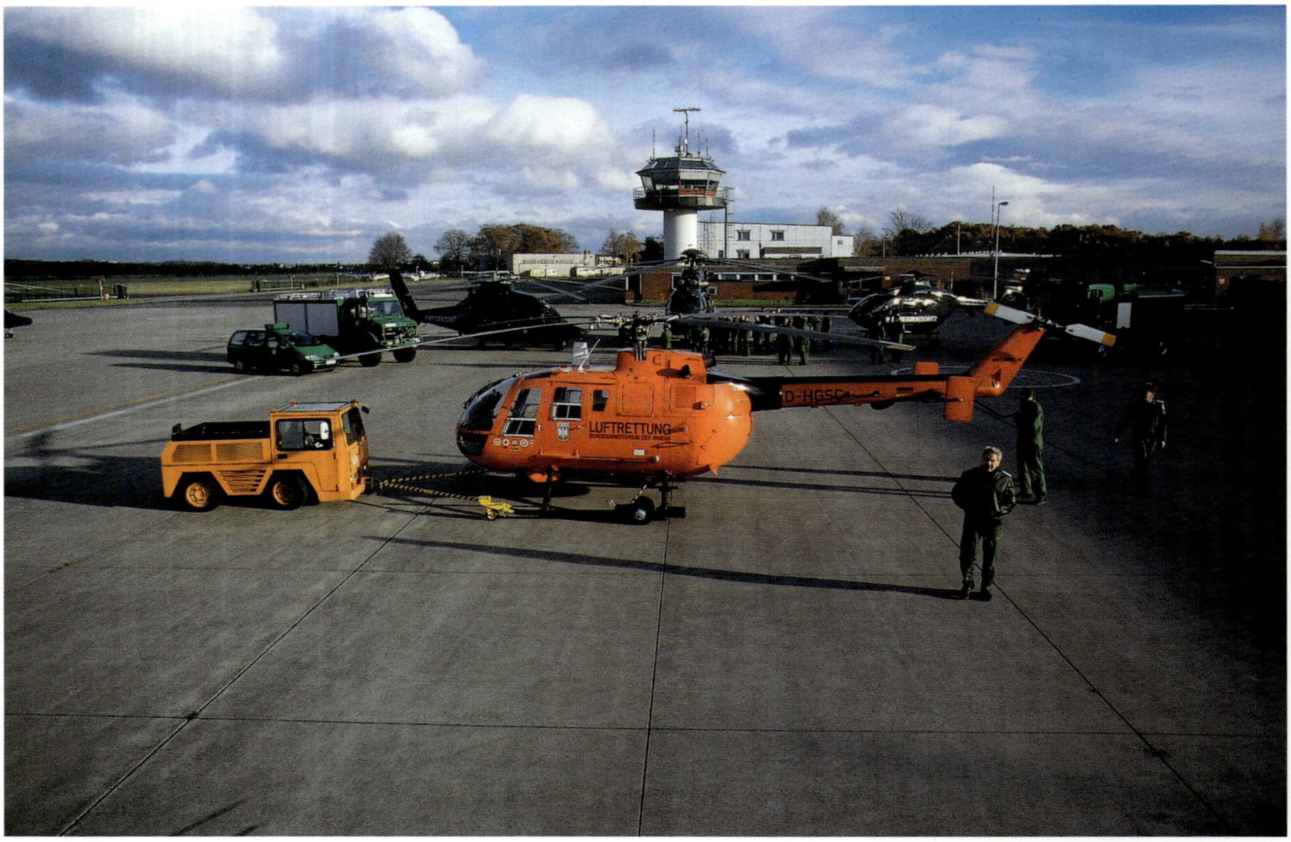

Für seine polizeilichen Aufgaben, den Katastrophenschutz und die Luftrettung betreibt der BGS insgesamt 102 Hubschrauber.

To meet the requirements of its original scope of responsibility, disasterrelief and HEMS, the German Federal Border Police operates 102 helicopters.

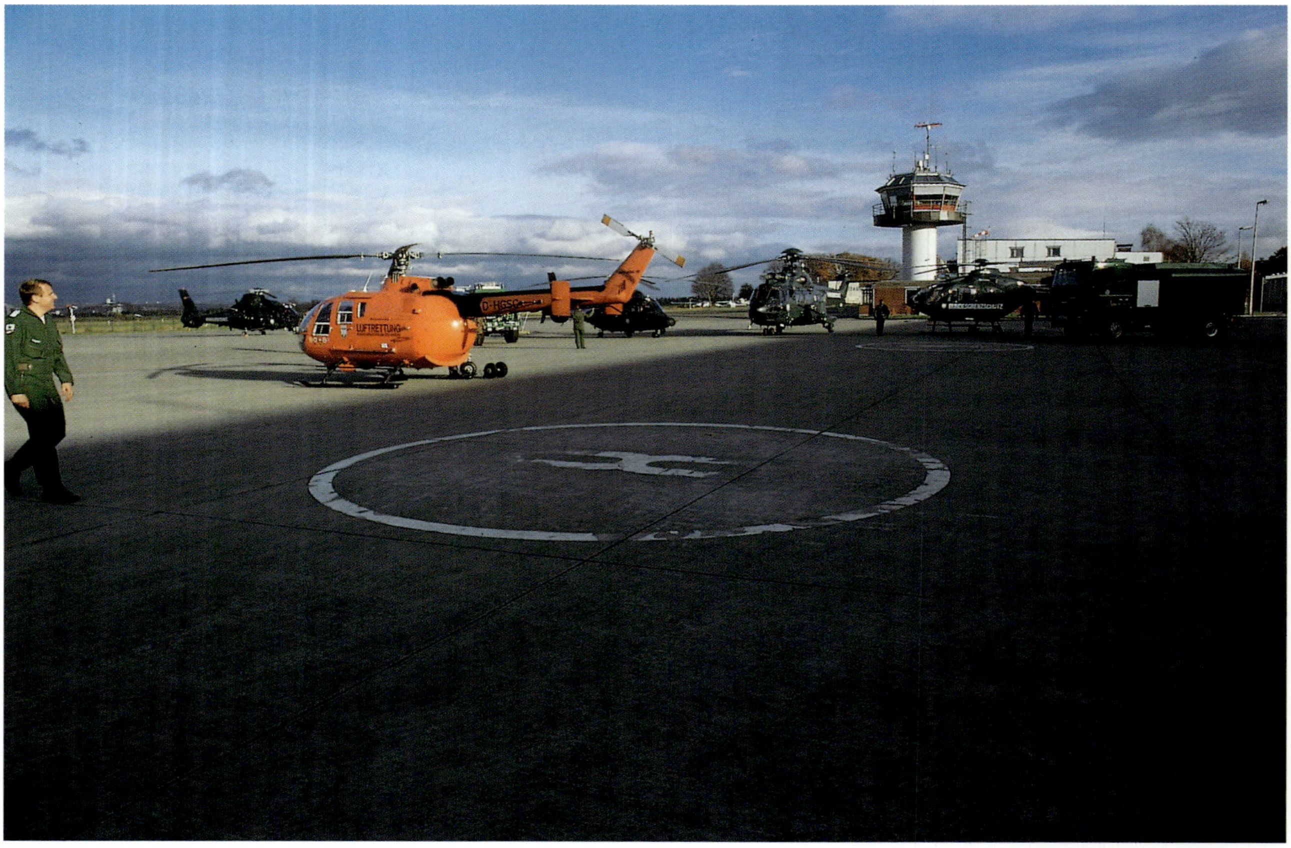

Die Hubschrauberflotte ist nach Indienststellung von EC 135 und EC 155 eine der modernsten.

Following the commissioning of the EC 135 and EC 155, its helicopter fleet is one of the most modern in the world.

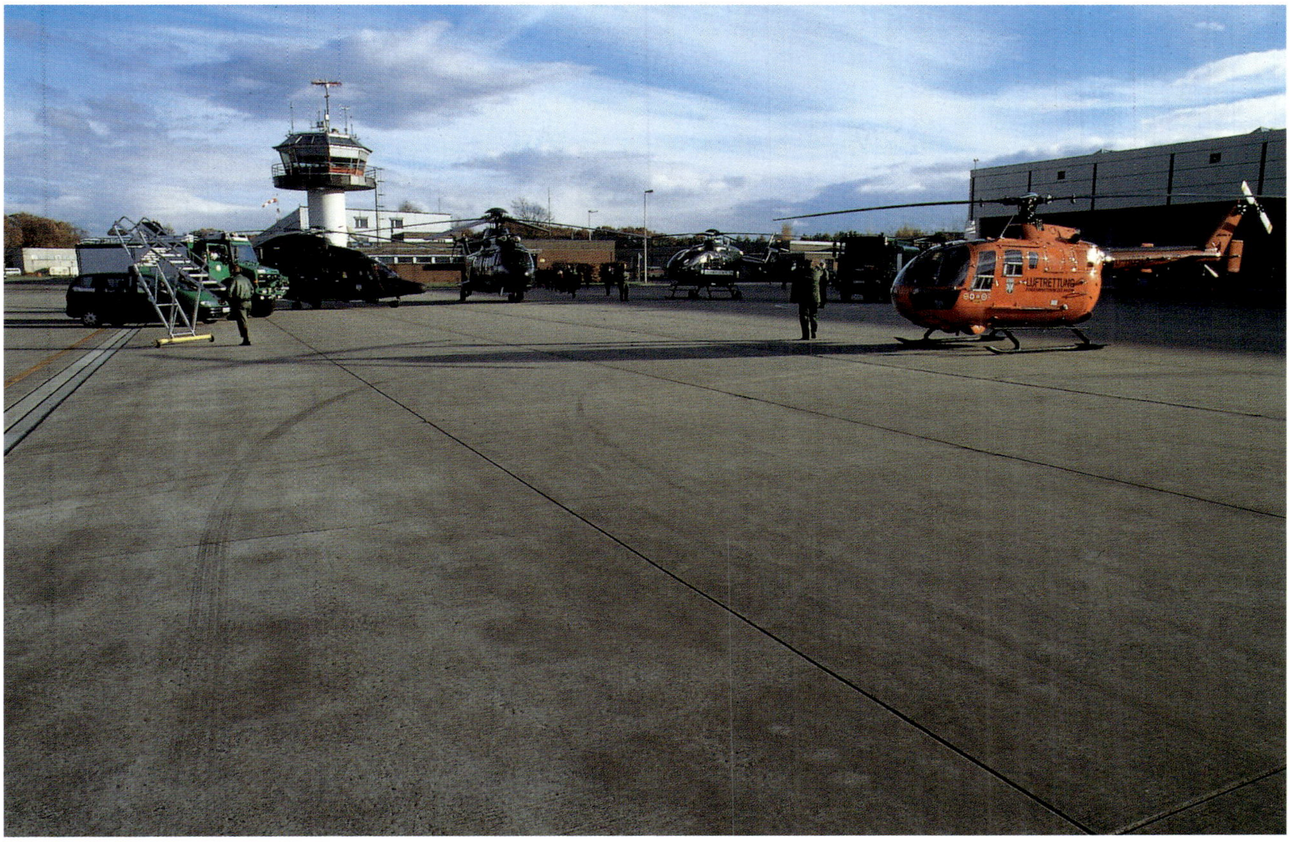

Durch einen modernen Fuhrpark mit einer großen Anzahl von Spezialfahrzeugen, wie Feuerwehrfahrzeuge, Tankfahrzeuge bis zu einem Fassungsvermögen von 40.000 Litern, Sanitätsfahrzeuge, mobile Tower, Werkstattwagen und vielen anderen ist man in der Lage, unabhängig von der Infrastruktur eines Flugplatzes zu operieren.

The German Federal Border Police possesses a state-of-the-art operating fleet containing a large number of special-purpose vehicles, e.g. fire-fighting vehicles, tank trucks with a capacity of 40,000 liters, ambulances, mobile towers, workshop vans, etc. The fleet gives the FBP the capability to operate independently of an airport infrastructure.

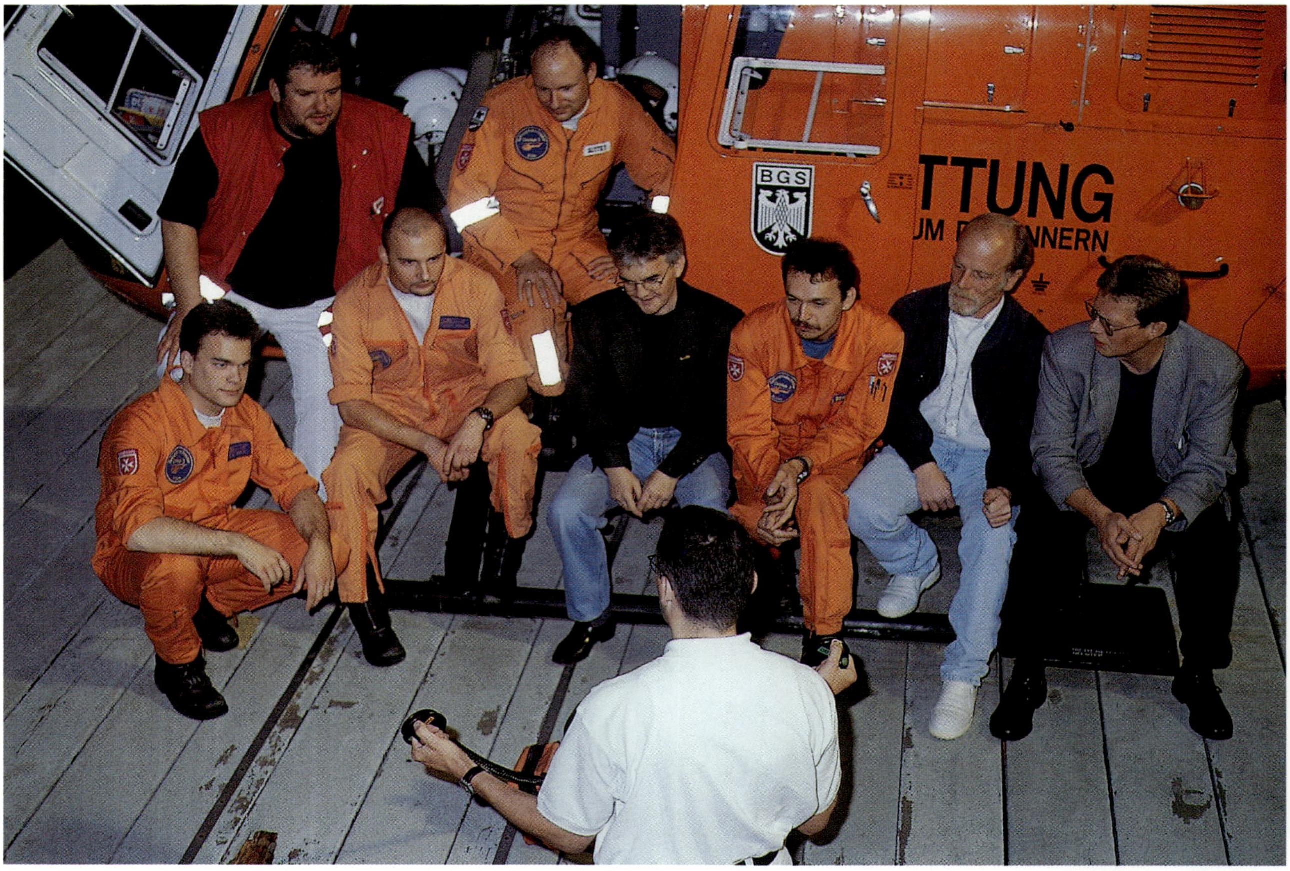

Die Luftrettungsassistenten werden ständig fortgebildet.

The air rescue paramedics constantly improve their knowledge and skills via continued training.

Augenblicke

Nobelviertel. Riesenvilla. Über ein Grundstück, durch das Haus langer Weg zum Patienten. Patient klagt über Luftnot. Ist ansprechbar. Wird versorgt an den RTW übergeben. Wir gehen den langen Weg zurück zum Rettungswagen. Der Patient drückt mir etwas in die Hand. Ist für Sie! Instinktiv öffne ich. Schaue nach. Ein Fünfzigpfennigstück. Darf ich leider nicht annehmen. Gebe es zurück.

Snapshots

A spacious mansion in a rich neighborhood. A long walk over the grounds and through many rooms before we reach the patient. The patient is conscious but is having trouble breathing. We provide emergency medical care and transport him to the rescue ambulance. On the long walk to the ambulance, the patient presses something into my hand with the comment "This is for you". Instinctively, I unclench my fist and have a look. A 50 (less than one single cigarette worth.) pfennig piece. Sorry, I can't accept it. Return the 50 pfennig piece to the patient.

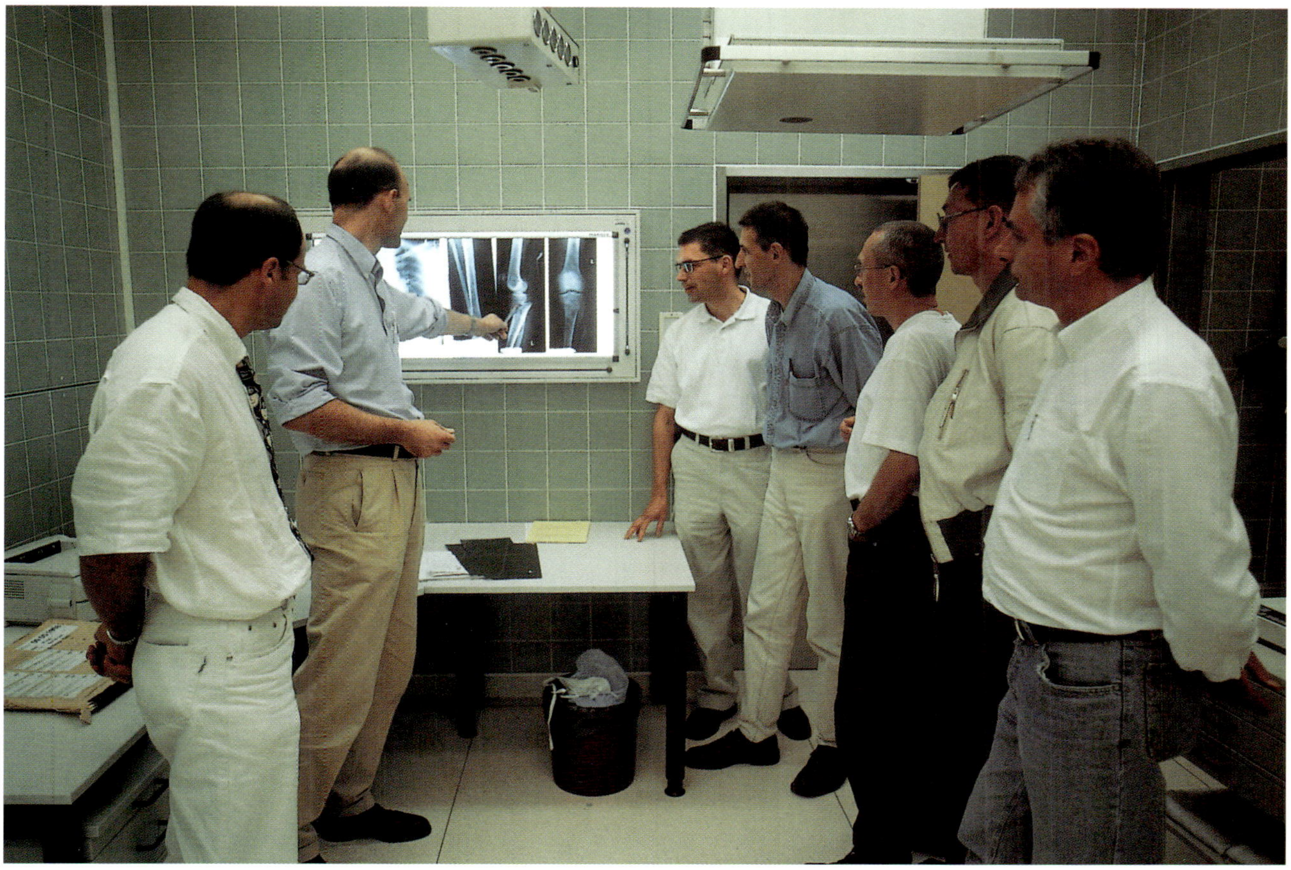

Notärztliche Fortbildung mit dem leitenden Hubschrauberarzt am Fallbeispiel.

Continued education of physicians with emergency & rescue certification: the head emergency physician working on the rescue helicopter presents a case study.

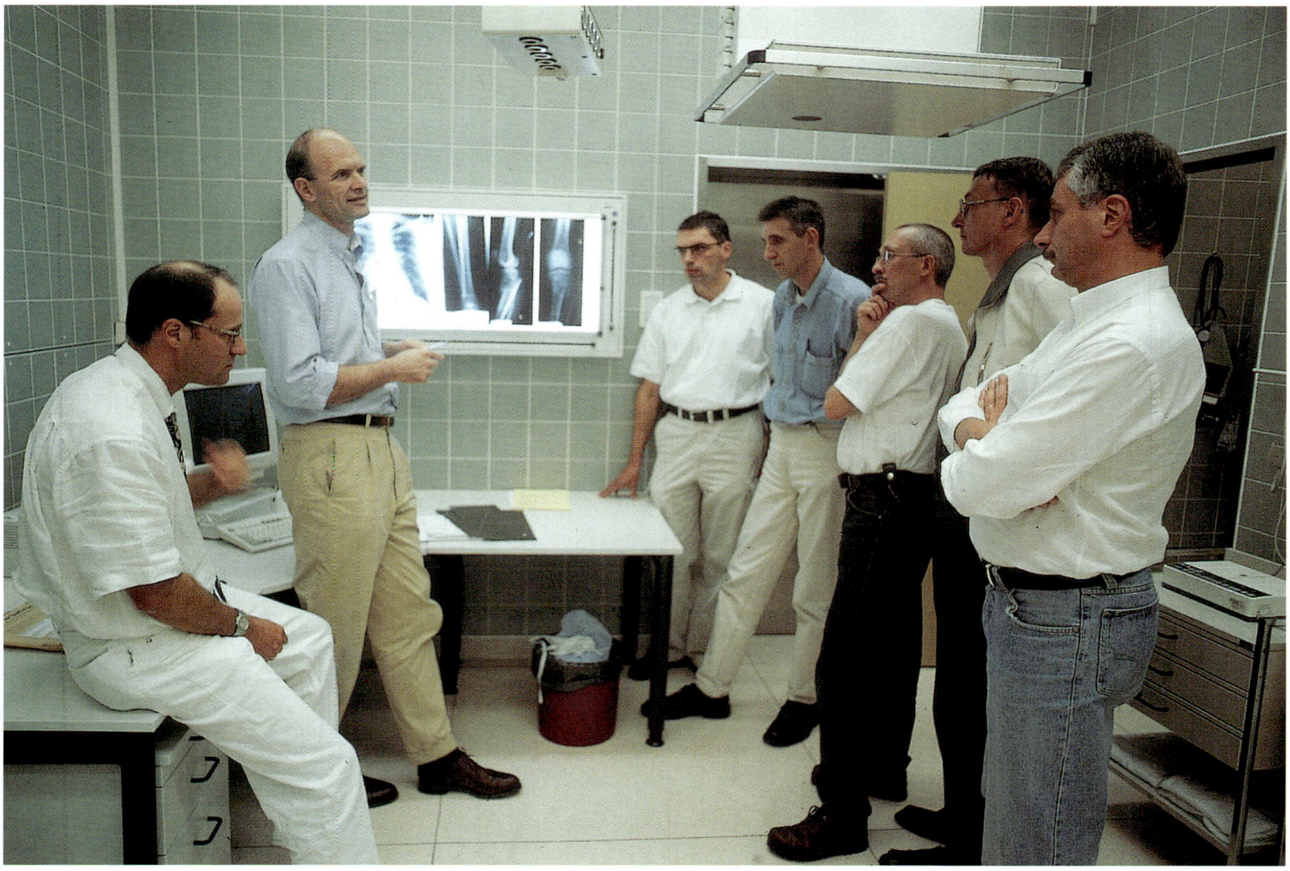

Einsatz für den Rettungshubschrauber
Mission for the Rescue Helicopter

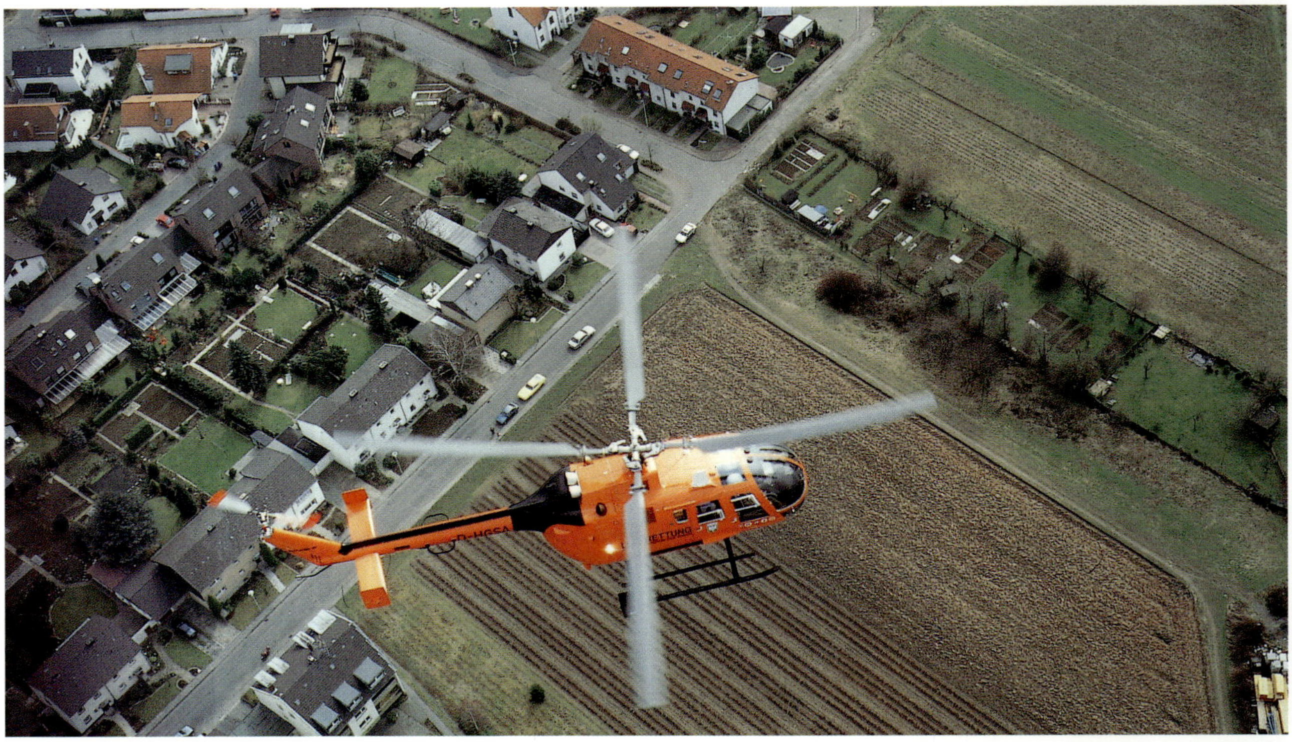

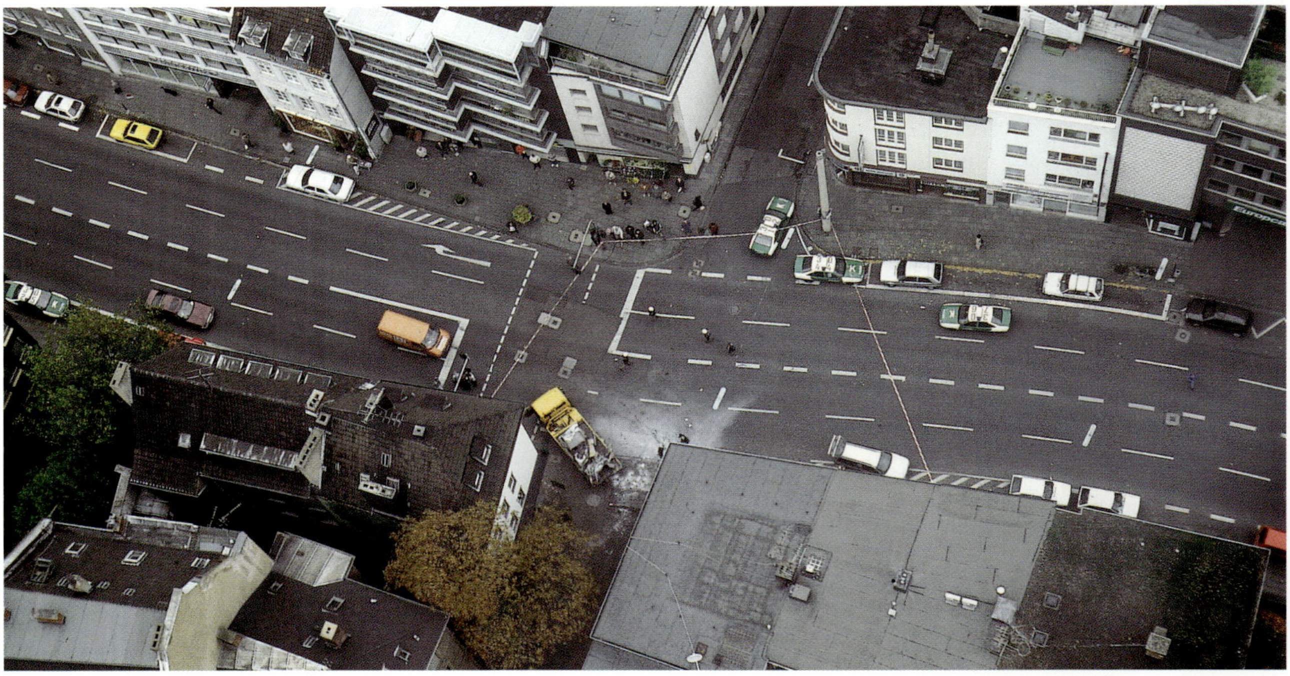

Verkehrsunfall in der Innenstadt.
Wir überfliegen die Einsatzstelle noch einmal, nachdem alle Personen versorgt worden sind. Die Polizei steht noch vor Ort. Die Rettungswagen und Feuerwehrfahrzeuge sind abgezogen. In der Zeitung wird am nächsten Tag stehen: „Ein PKW-Fahrer hat die Gewalt über den Wagen verloren und ist gegen eine Mauer geprallt. Ein auf dem Bürgersteig gehendes gerade verheiratetes Ehepaar wird verletzt, die Frau tödlich."

Traffic accident in the downtown area.
We fly over the accident site once again after all the injured persons have received emergency medical care. The police are still at the scene but the rescue ambulance and fire service vehicles have already left. The story in tomorrow's newspaper will read: "An automobile driver lost control of his car downtown yesterday, running over the sidewalk until the car came to a halt in front of a brick wall. A young couple standing on the sidewalk – married only two weeks ago – were seriously injured; the woman died on the spot."

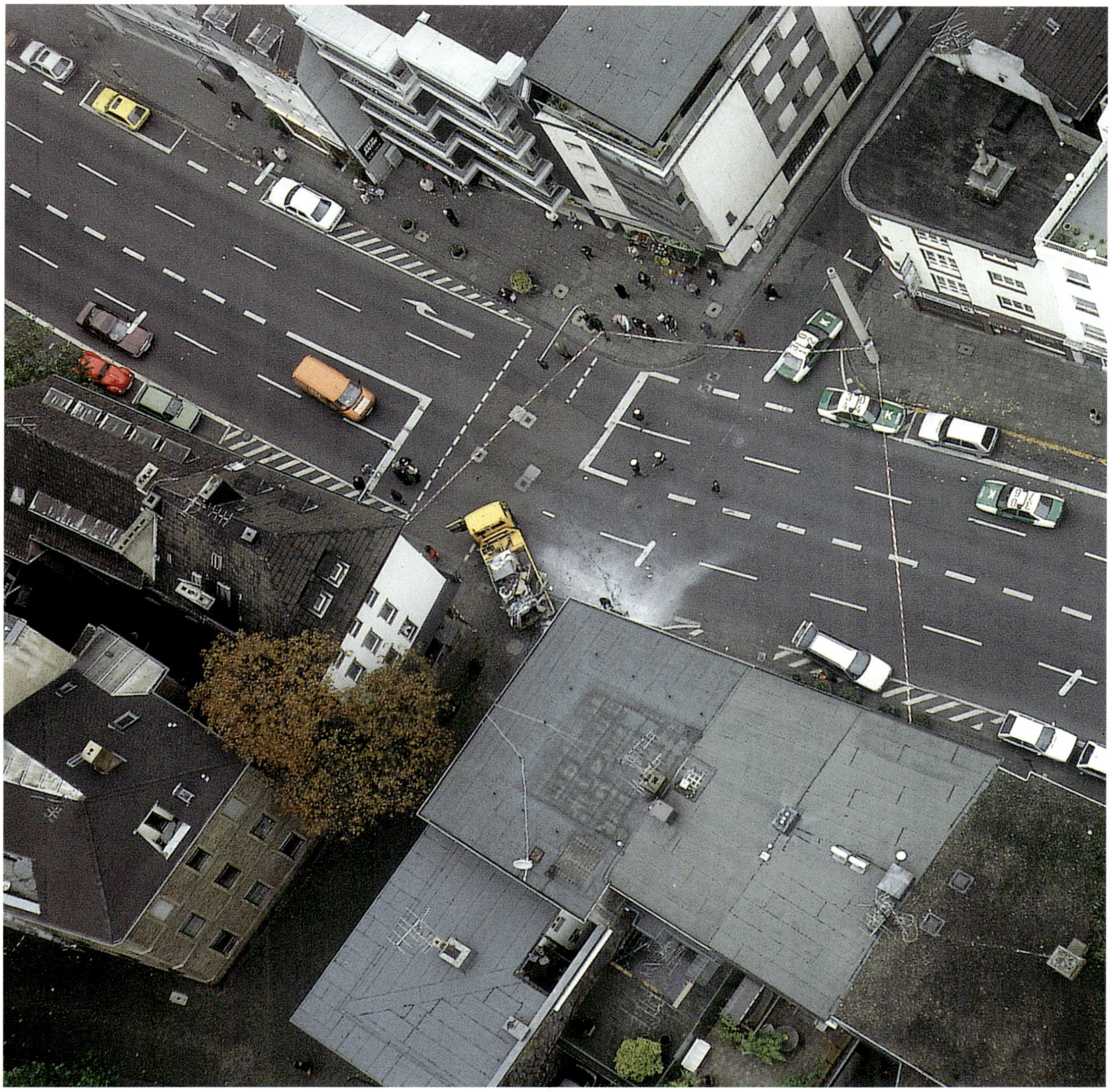

Spektakuläre Ereignisse ziehen naturgemäß viele Beobachter, auch Gaffer, an.

Spectacular events quite naturally attract spectators and even voyeurs.

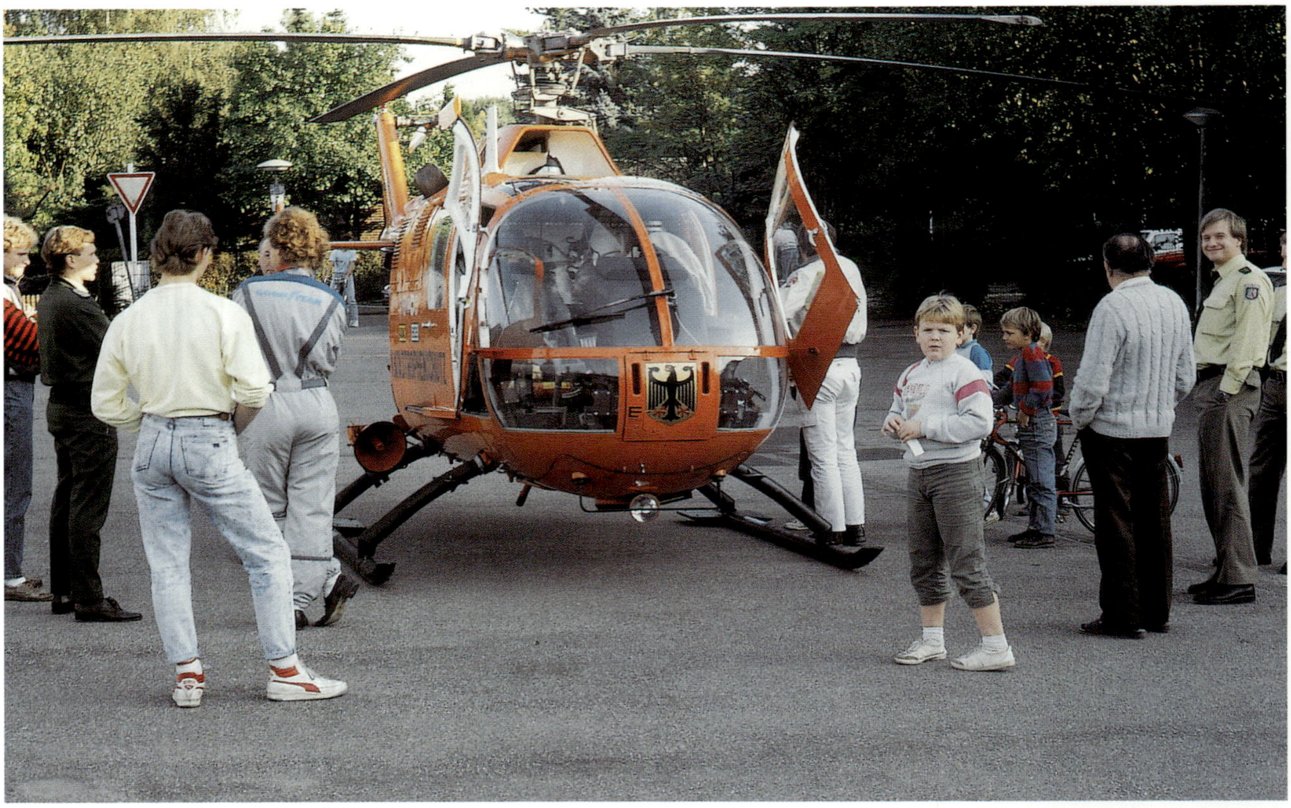

Überall, wo der Hubschrauber landet, findet er sofort Aufmerksamkeit.

Wherever the helicopter lands, it is immediately the center of attention.

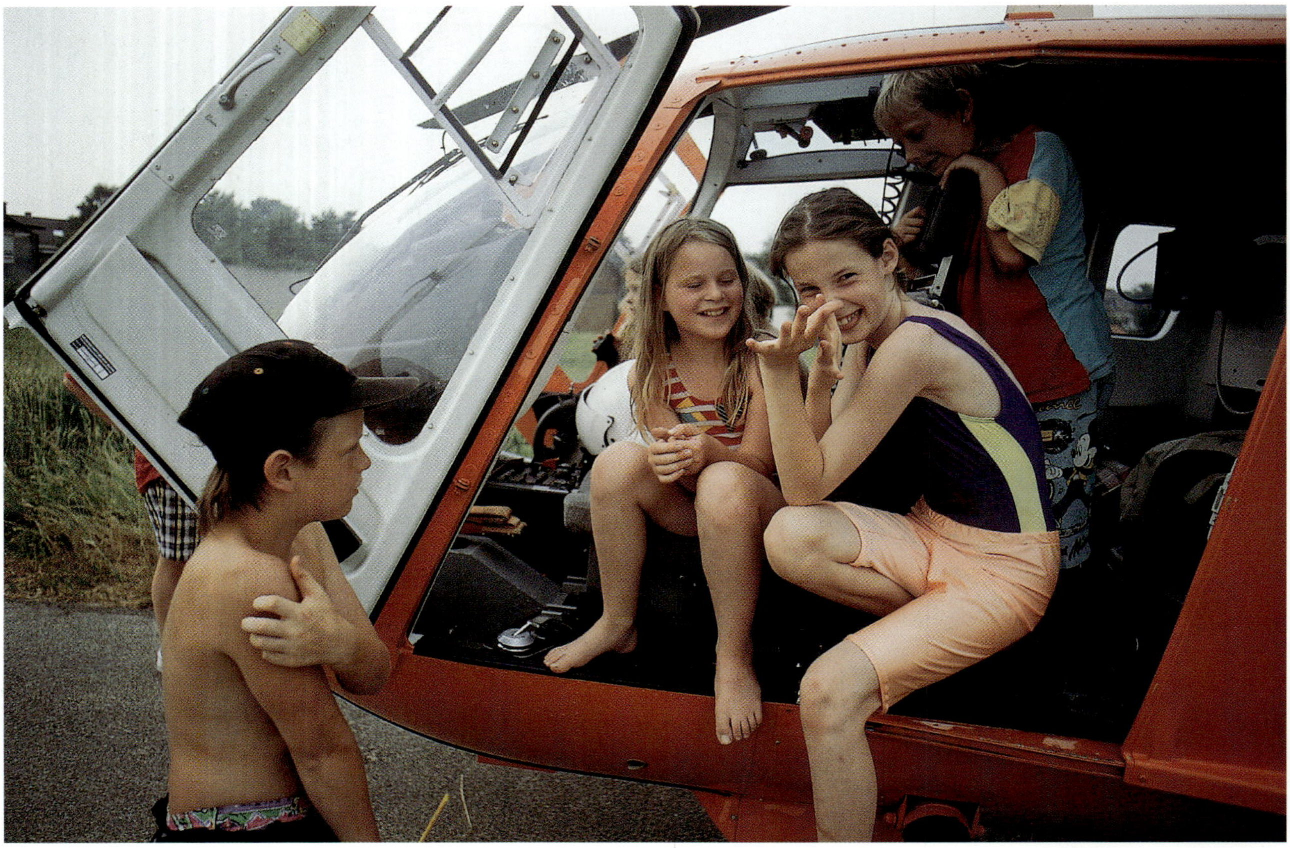

Junge interessierte Öffentlichkeit am Dorfrand.

Young curious spectators just outside the village.

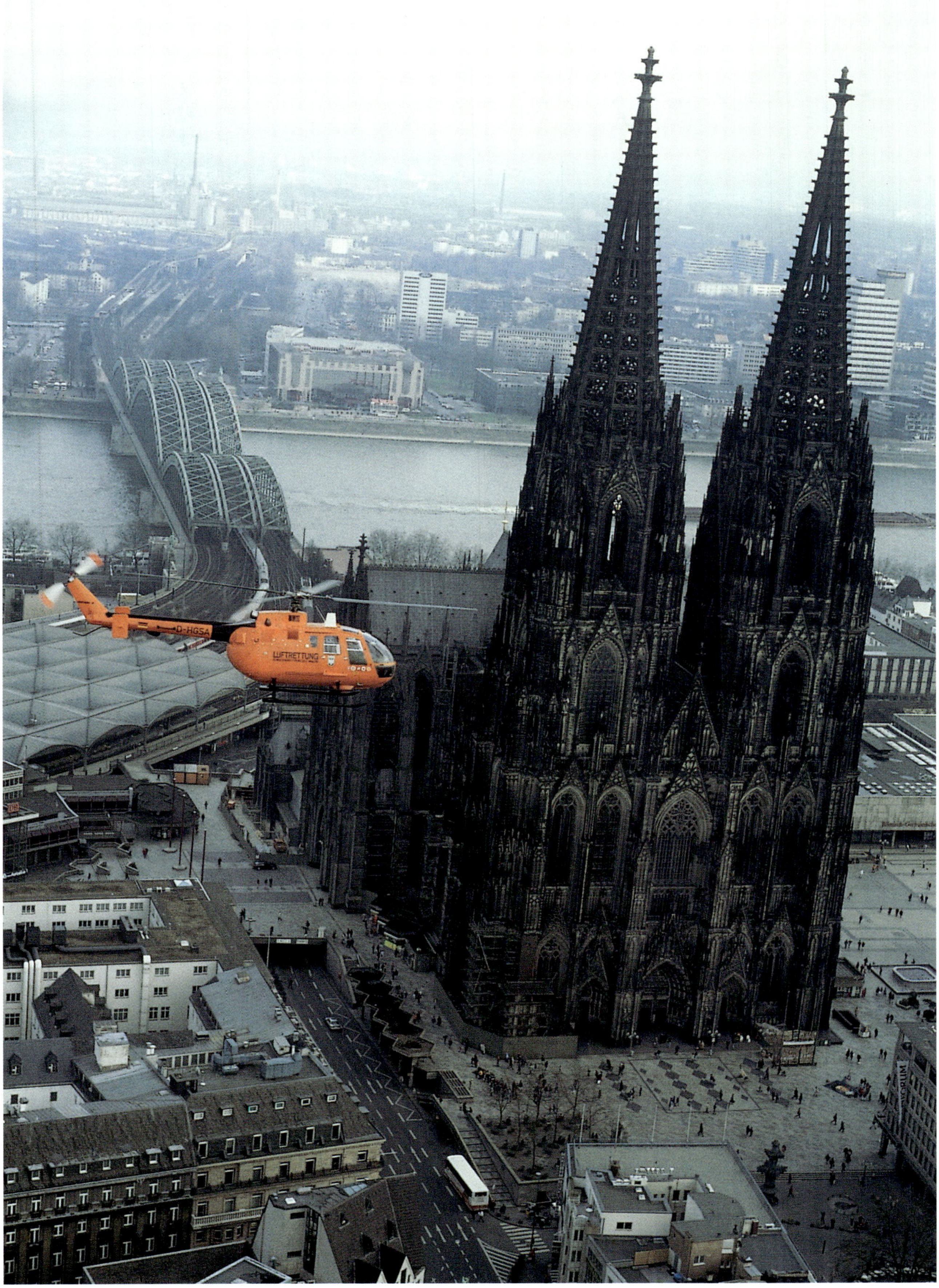

25-Jahresfeier: Der Rettungshubschrauber landet auf der Domplatte.

The 25th anniversary of the helicopter rescue service: the rescue helicopter touches down on the square in front of Cologne Cathedral.

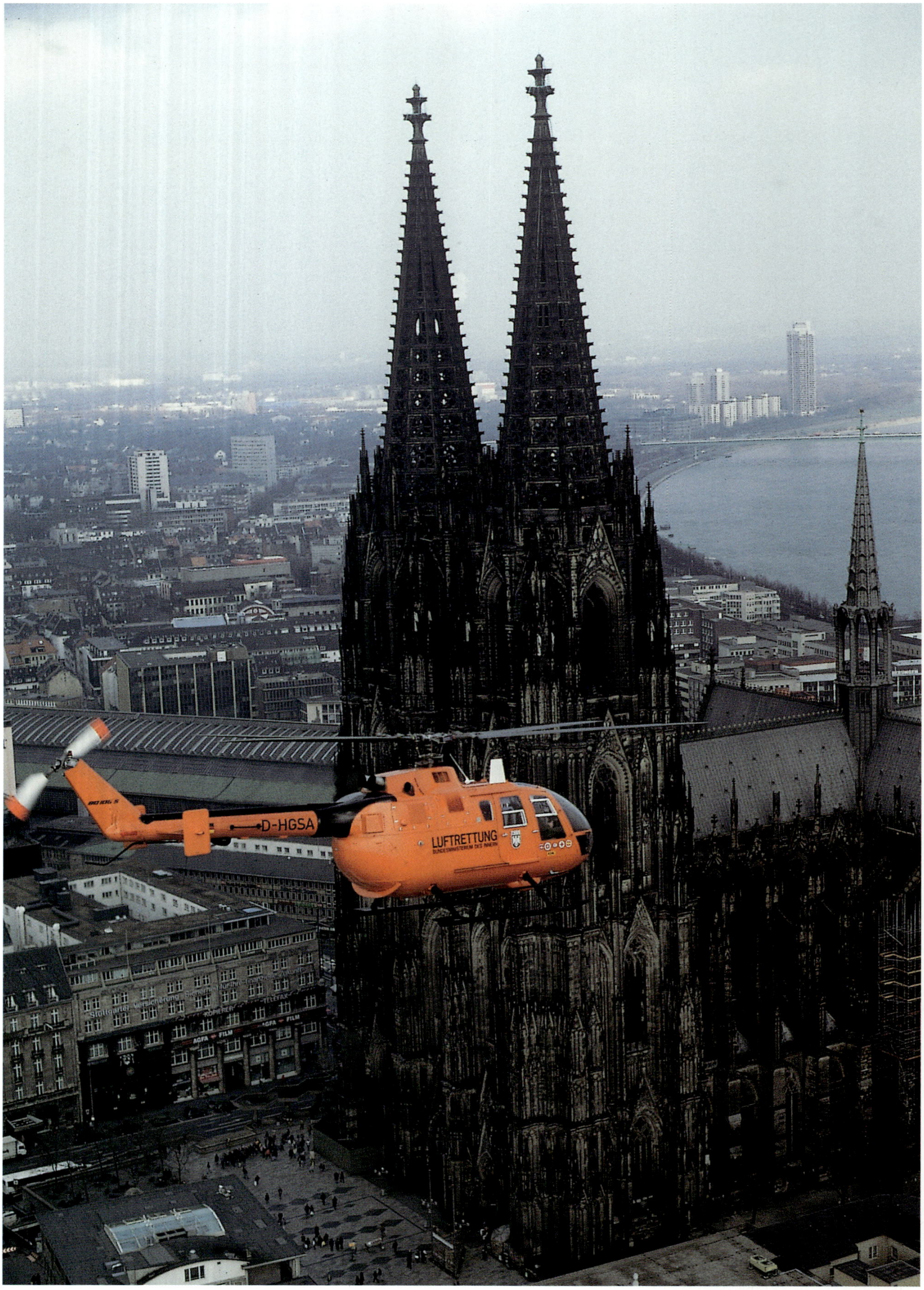

Im Anflug auf den Domvorplatz.

During the approach before landing in front of the cathedral.

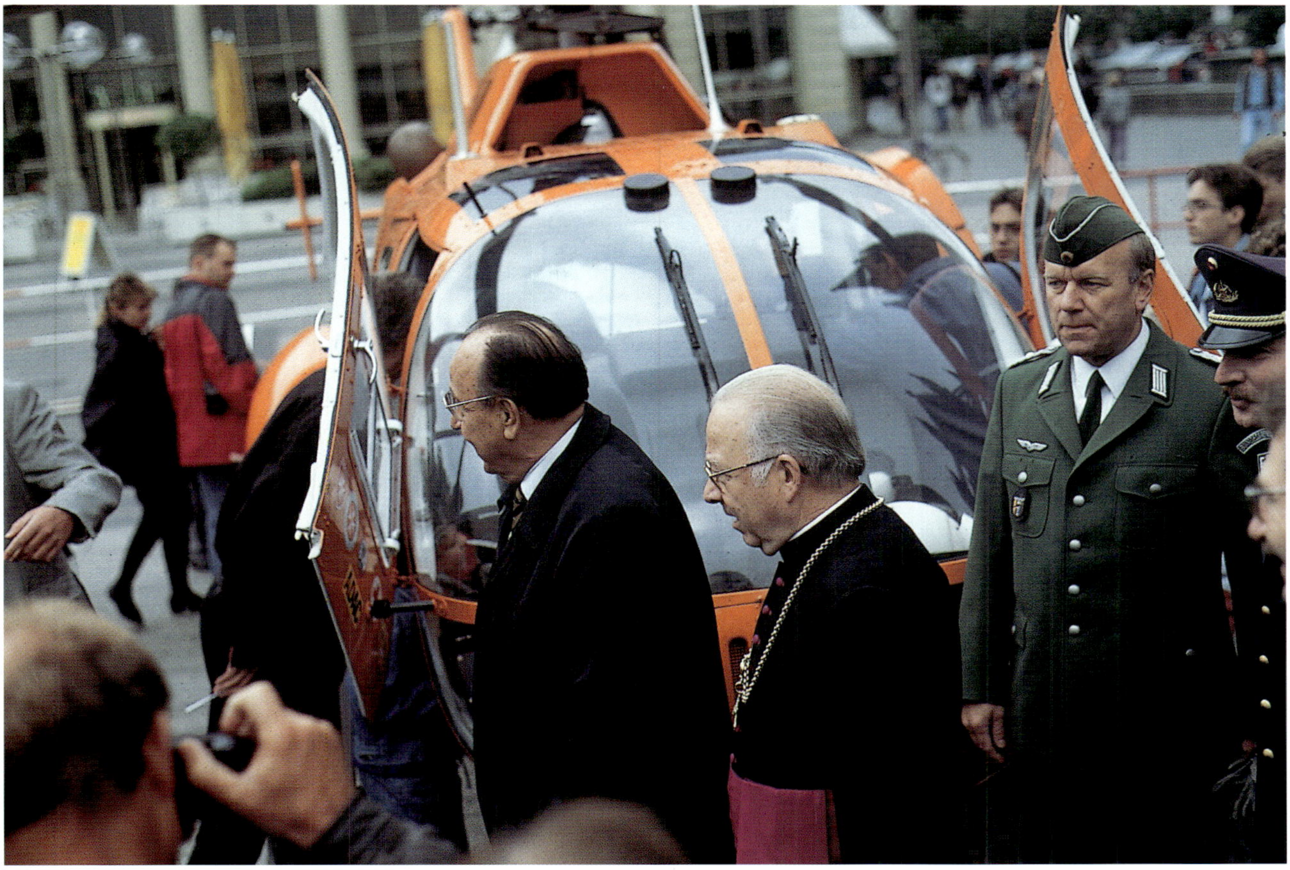

Der Hubschrauber wird auf der Domplatte zum 25jährigen Bestehen gesegnet.

The helicopter receives a blessing on the square in front of the cathedral on the occasion of its 25th anniversary.

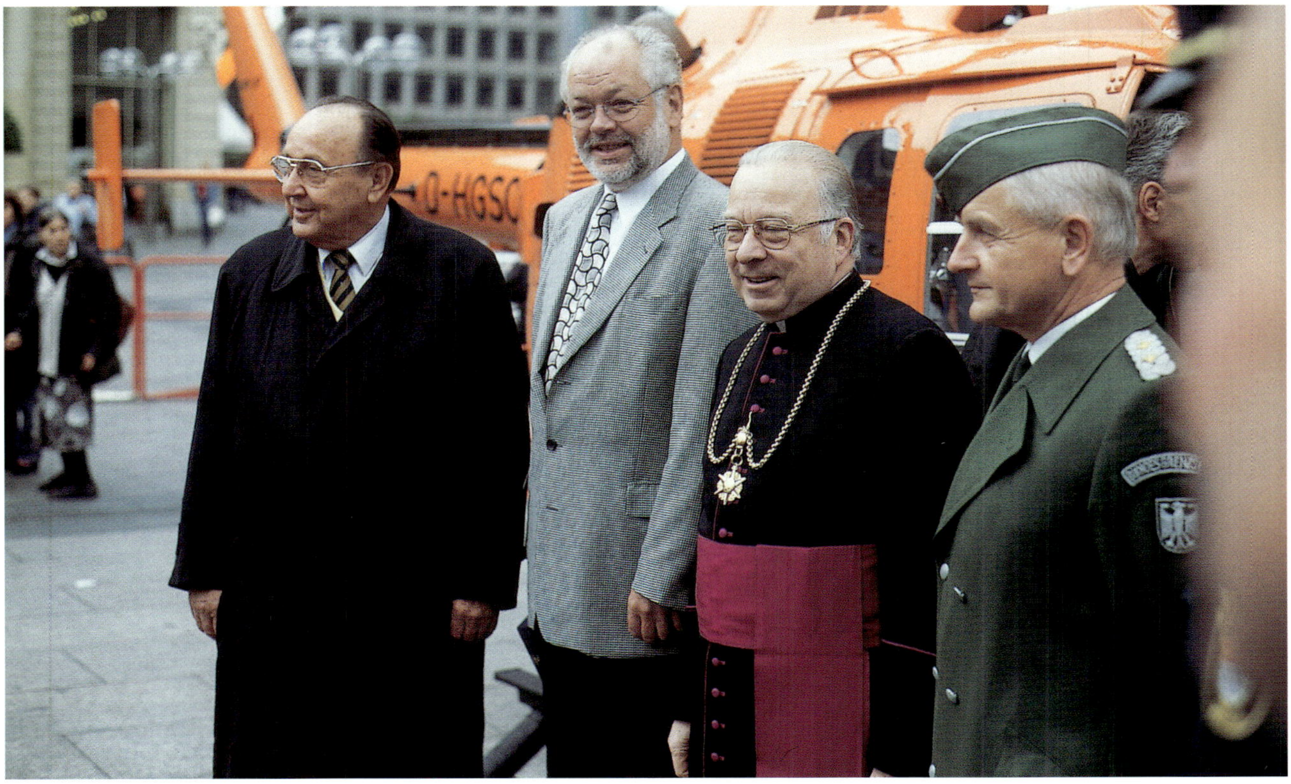

Bundesminister a.D. Genscher, der verstorbene Oberbürgermeister Blum, Domprobst Hendrich und der Kommandeur der Fliegergruppe, Praus, vor dem Rettungshubschrauber.

Group photo taken in front of the rescue helicopter: Hans-Dietrich Genscher, former German Minister; the late Harry Blum, former Senior Mayor of Cologne; Bernhard Hendrich, Dean of the Cathedral; Reinhard Praus, Head of the Aviation Group.

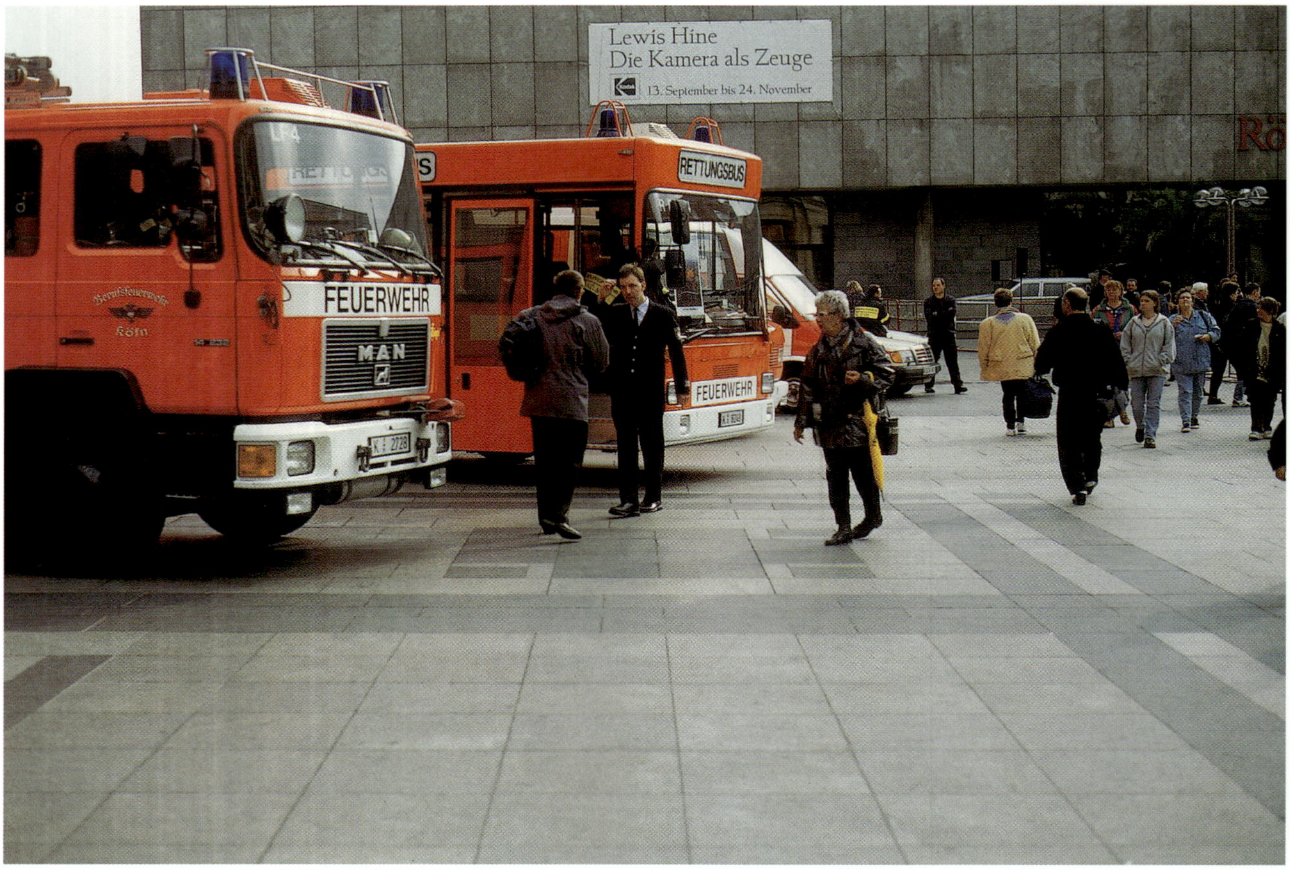

Eine große Aufstellung an Feuerwehrfahrzeugen rundet das Bild ab.

A large exhibition of fire service vehicles completes the picture.

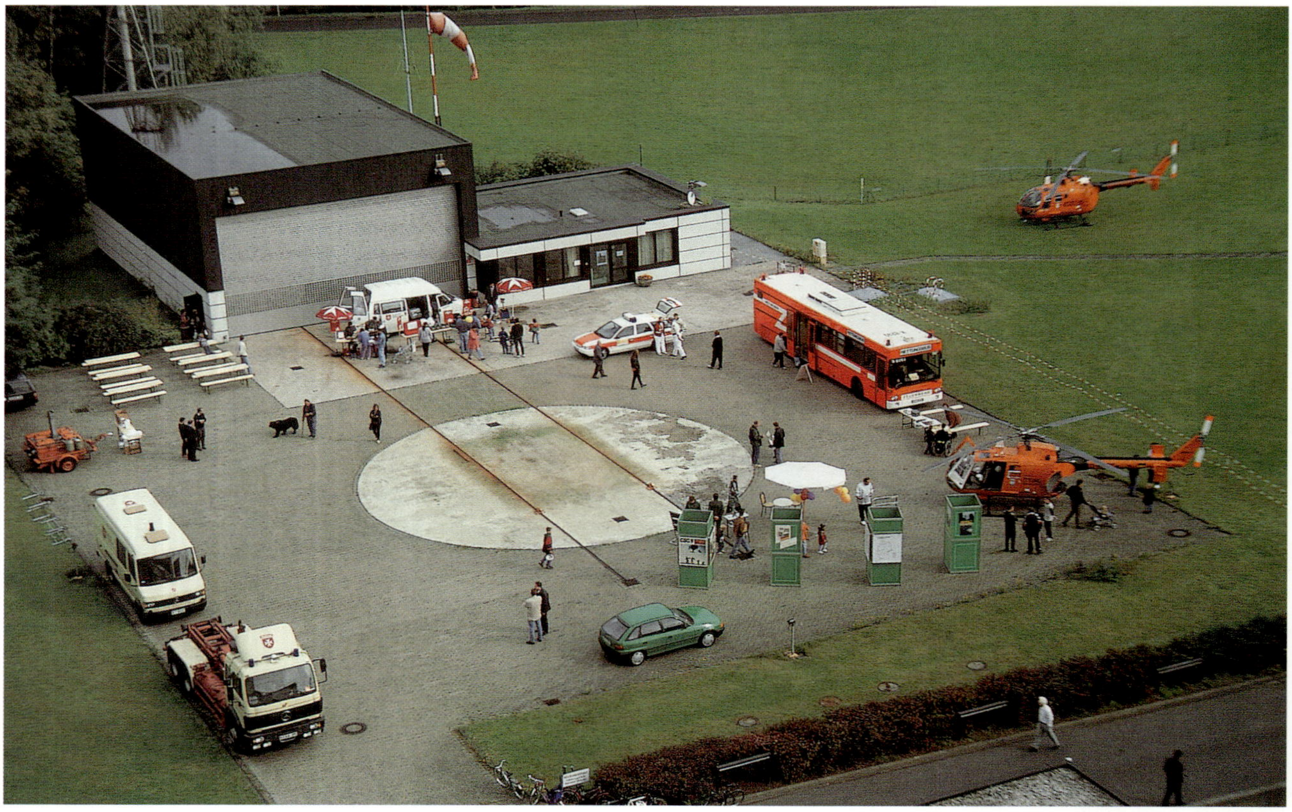

Tag der offenen Tür in der Station Köln. Die Besucher haben die Möglichkeit, sich über Rettungshubschrauber zu informieren.

"Open House" at the Cologne base. The visitors take advantage of this opportunity to find out more about the rescue helicopter.

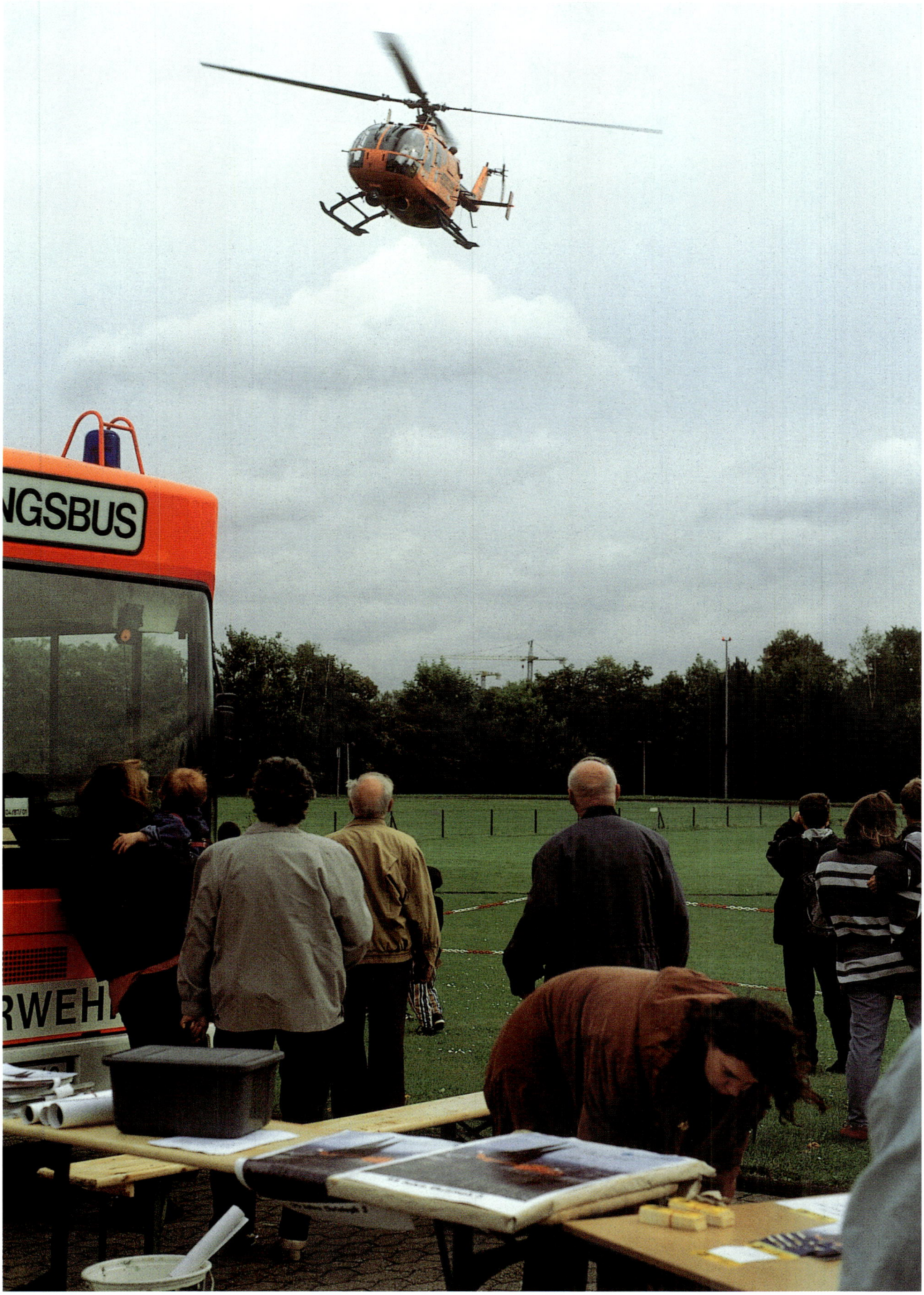

Der Rettungshubschrauberalltag geht natürlich weiter. Einsatz!

The daily work of the rescue helicopter does not grind to a halt because of the "Open House". Emergency call!

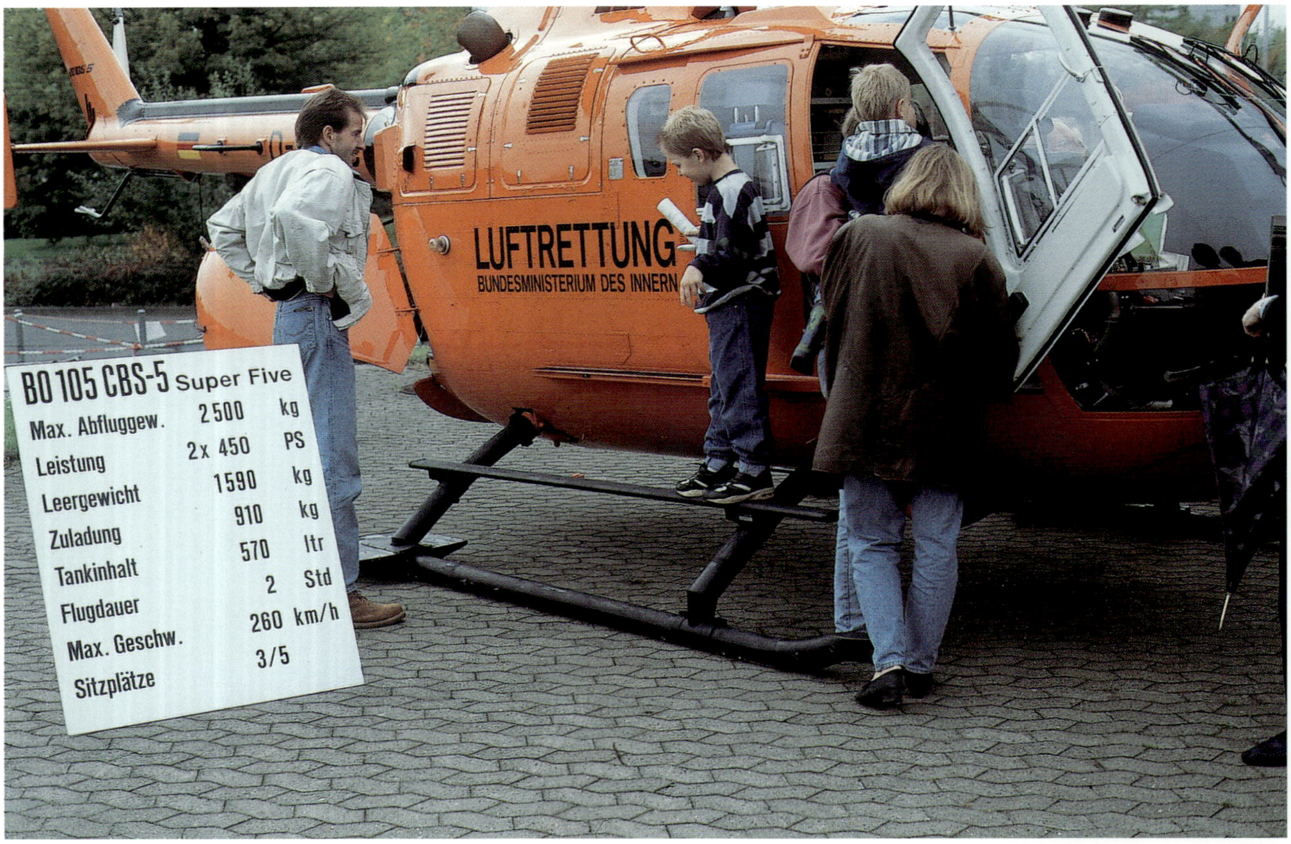
LUFTRETTUNG
BUNDESMINISTERIUM DES INNERN
BO 105 CBS-5 Super Five
Max. Abfluggew. 2 500 kg
Leistung 2x 450 PS
Leergewicht 1590 kg
Zuladung 910 kg
Tankinhalt 570 ltr
Flugdauer 2 Std
Max. Geschw. 260 km/h
Sitzplätze 3/5

Der Hubschrauber im Blickpunkt der Öffentlichkeit.

The helicopter at the center of public attention.

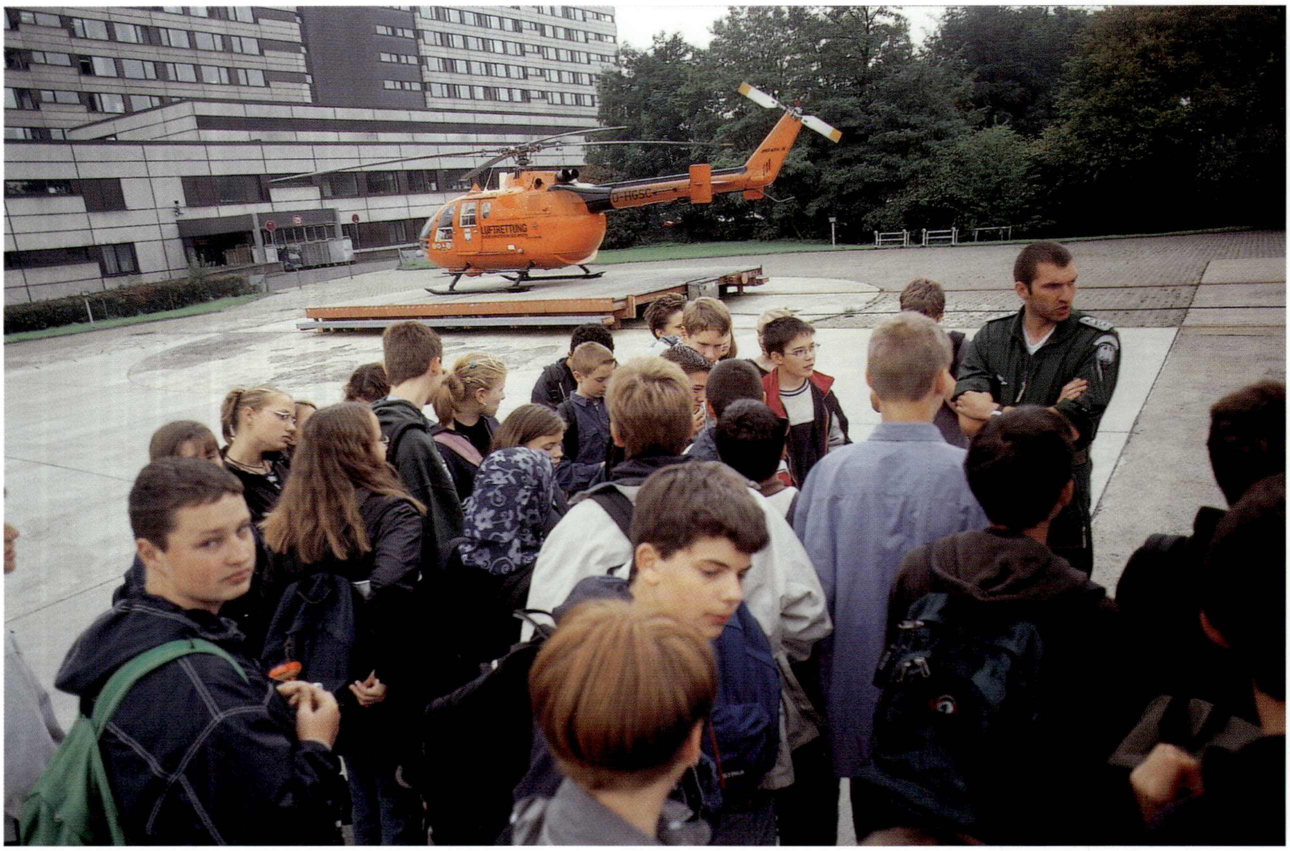

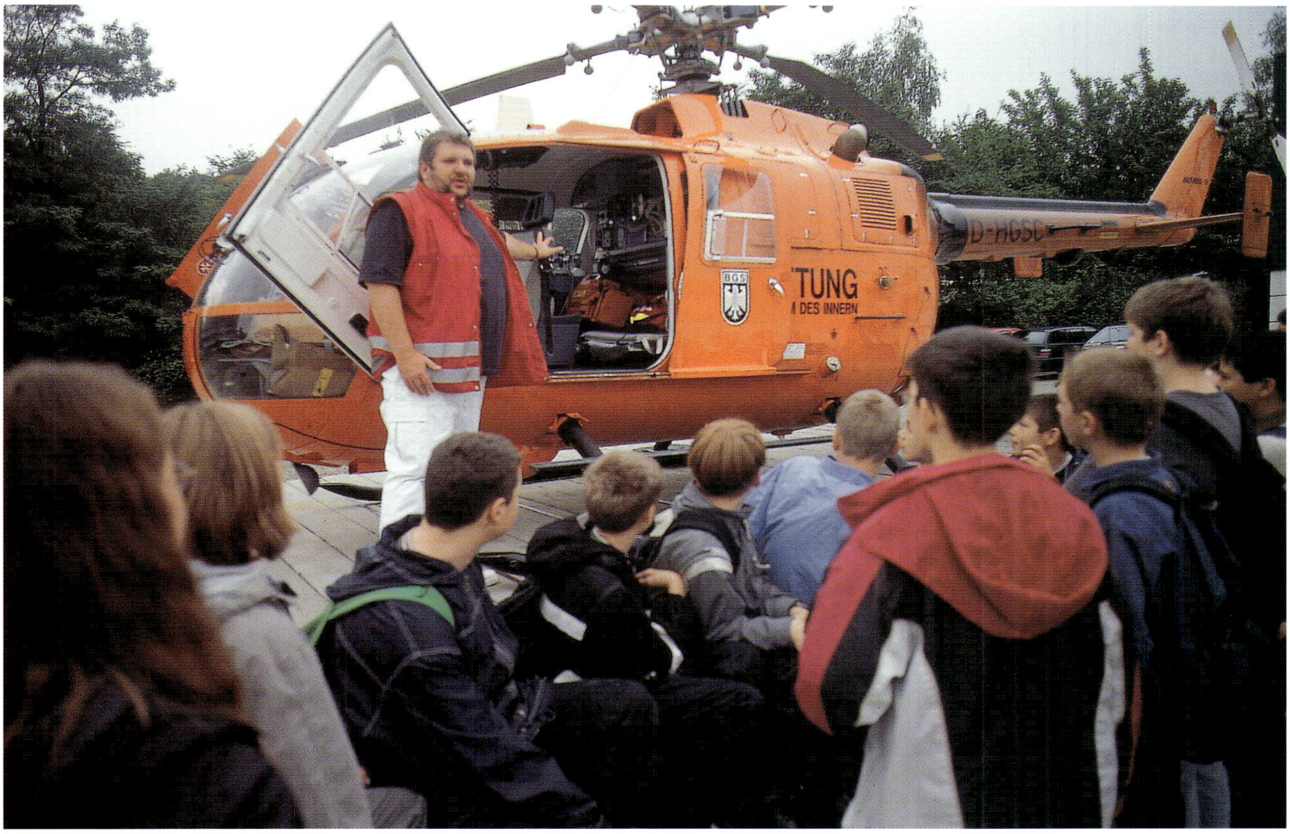

Jede Station informiert auch kleinere Besuchergruppen über Rettungshubschrauber und Rettungsdienst.

Every base is ready to provide information on the rescue helicopter and the rescue service to even small groups of visitors.

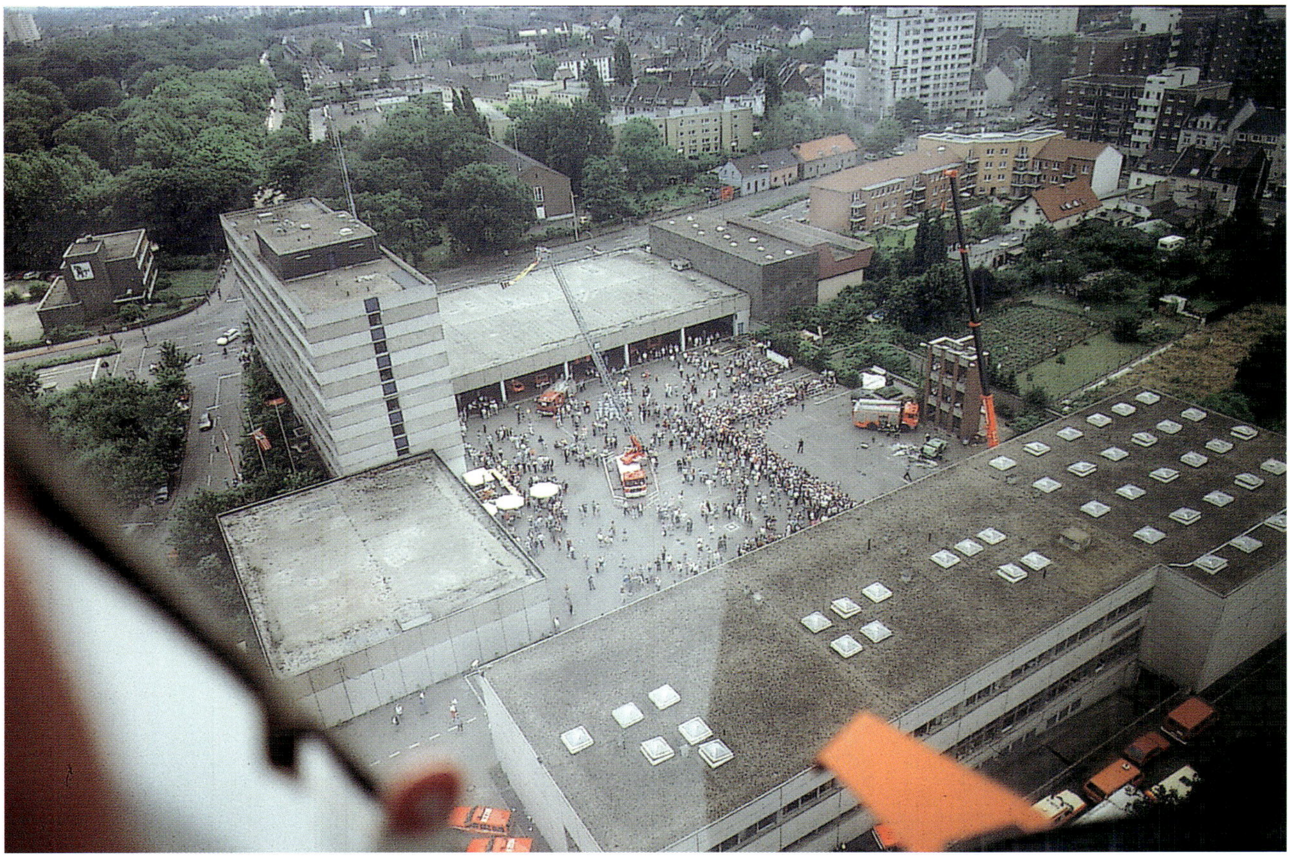

Tag der offenen Tür bei der Berufsfeuerwehr.

Open house at the fire service building.

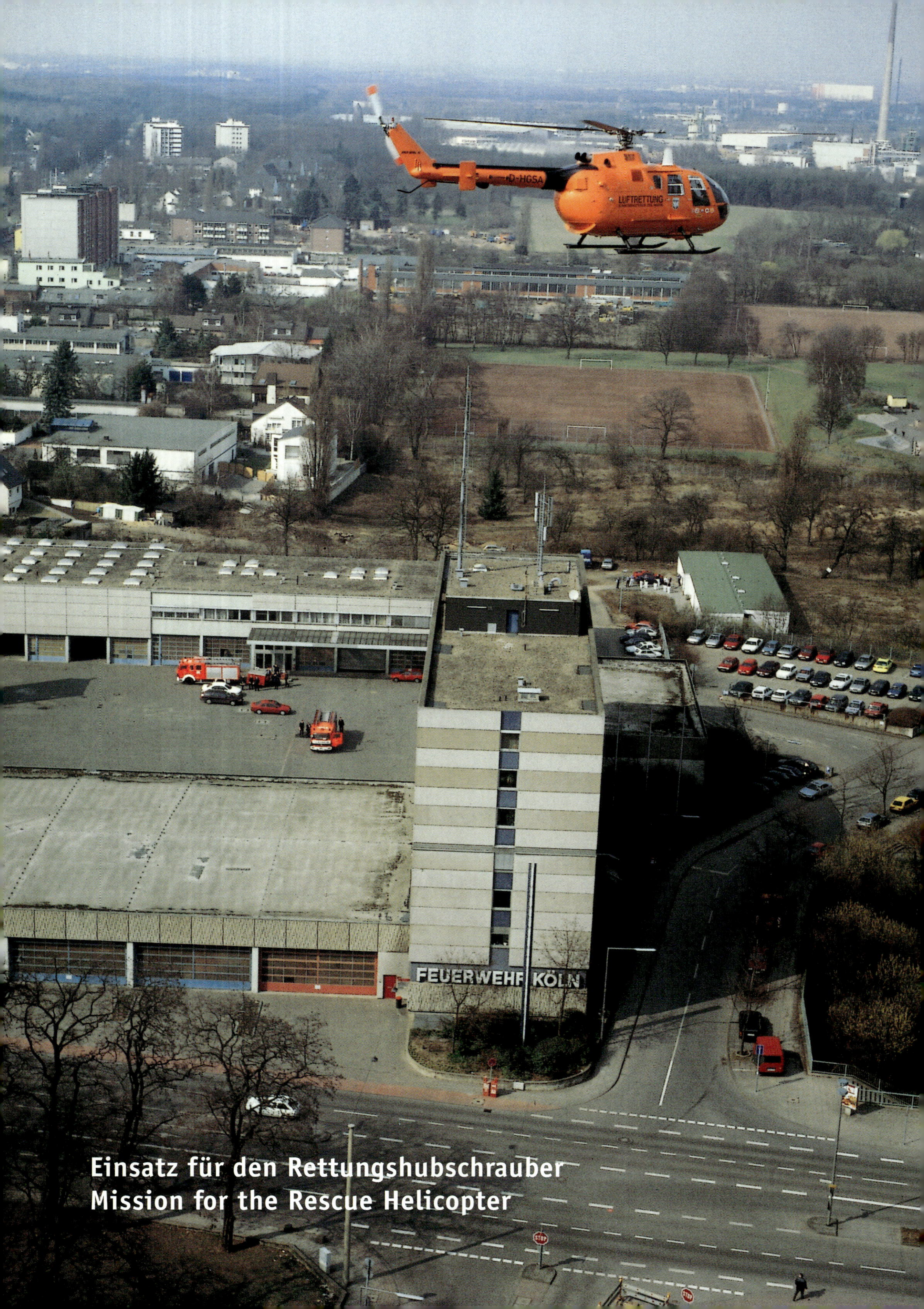

Einsatz für den Rettungshubschrauber
Mission for the Rescue Helicopter

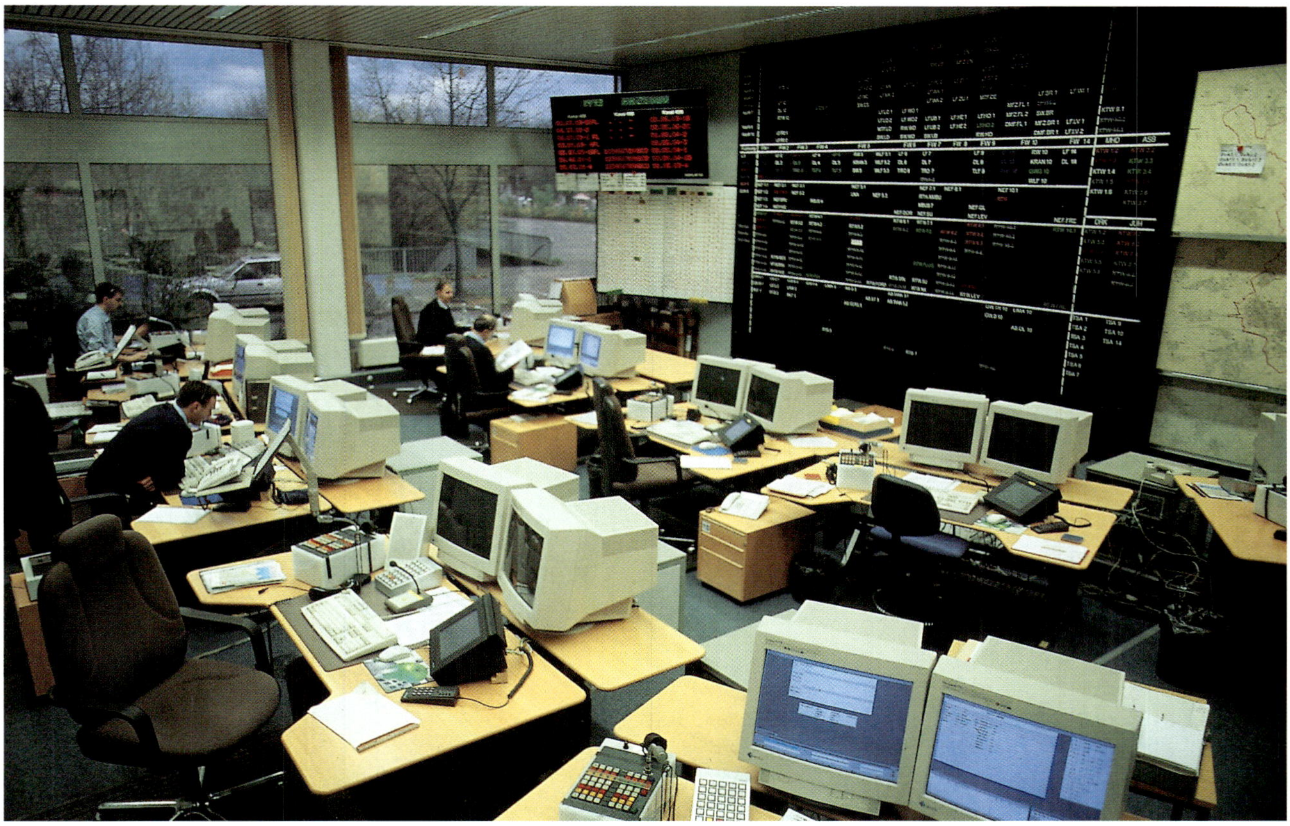

Die Rettungskette wird in Gang gesetzt.
The rescue chain is set into motion.

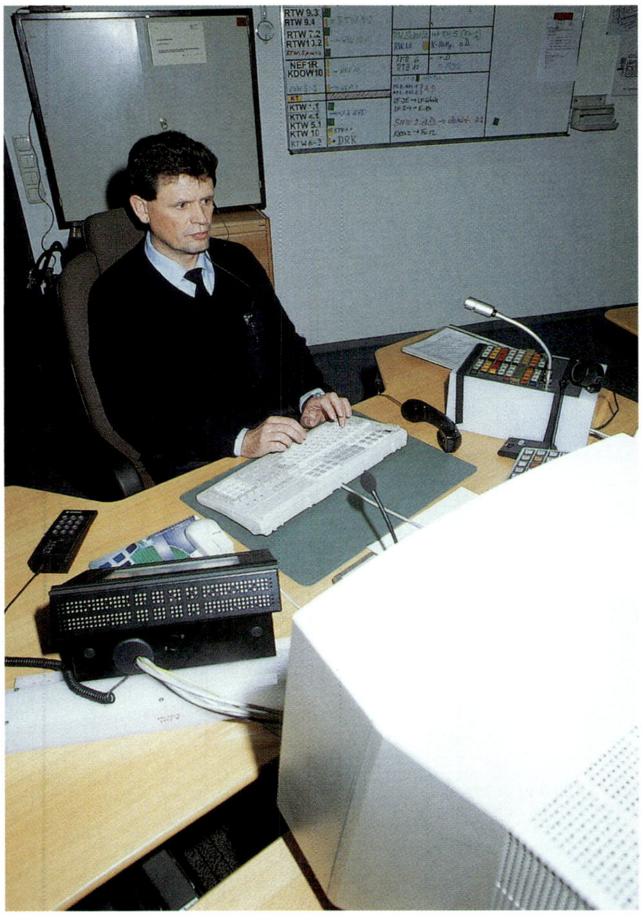

Der Notruf erreicht den Disponenten der (Rettungs-) Leitstelle.

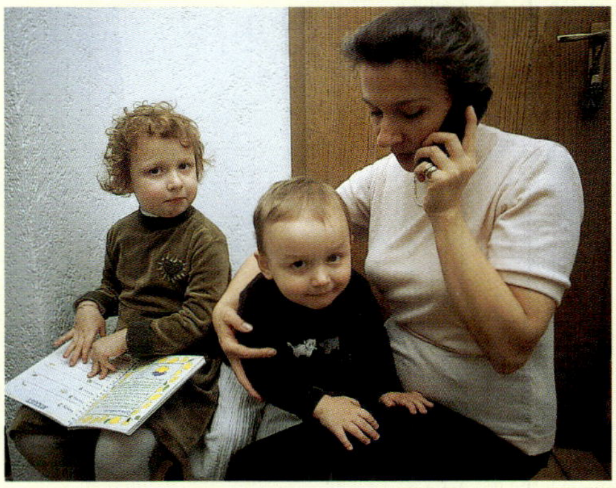

The dispatchers at the Rescue Coordination Center take an emergency call.

Er entscheidet über den Einsatz der Rettungsmittel.

The dispatcher decides which rescue resource is to be employed.

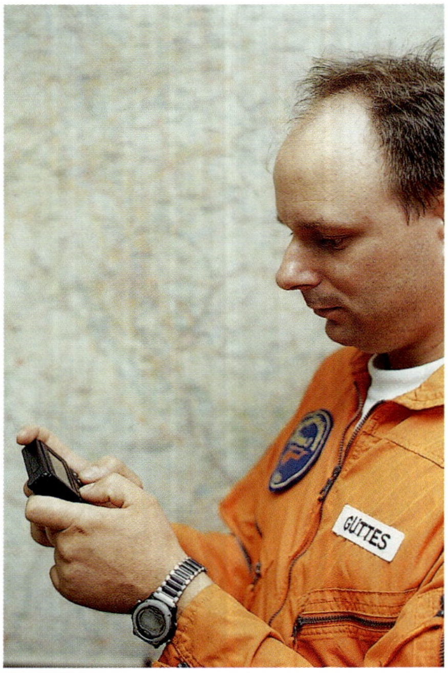

Die Alamierung läuft ein.

The rescue helicopter crews take emergency calls on a pager with a selective call feature.

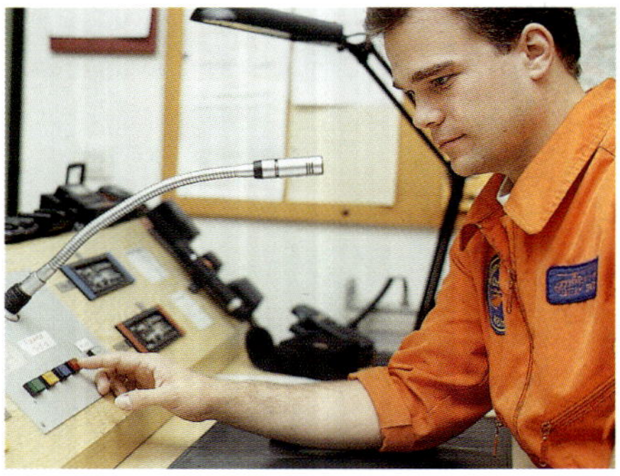

Der Luftrettungsassistent holt genauere Informationen zur Lage der Einsatzstelle ein.

The air rescue paramedic confirms the mission order while the pilot starts the rescue helicopter. The paramedic asks for additional information on the exact location of the emergency site, the radio channel, and the person responsible for liaison on site.

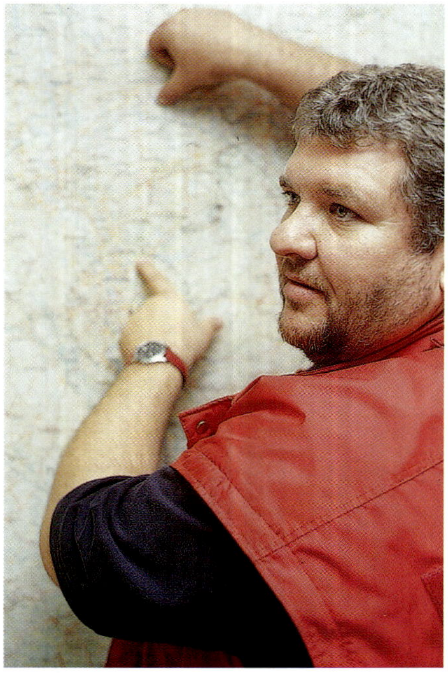

Er misst mit einem Faden, der auf der Generalkarte 1 : 200.000 befestigt ist, den groben Kurs und die Entfernung aus.

A course is plotted with the aid of string on a general map with a scale of 1:200,000.

In Stadtgebieten sucht er die Einsatzstelle im Stadtatlas.

On missions to densely-populated downtown areas, the crew also uses a street atlas for precise navigation.

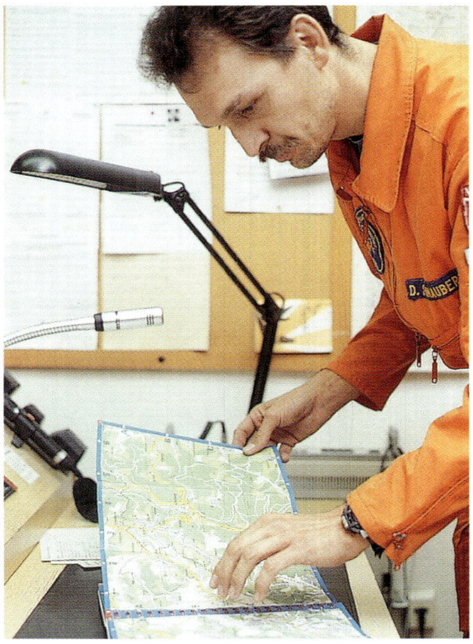

Im RTH gibt er diese Informationen an den Piloten weiter.

Inside the rescue helicopter, he passes on this information.

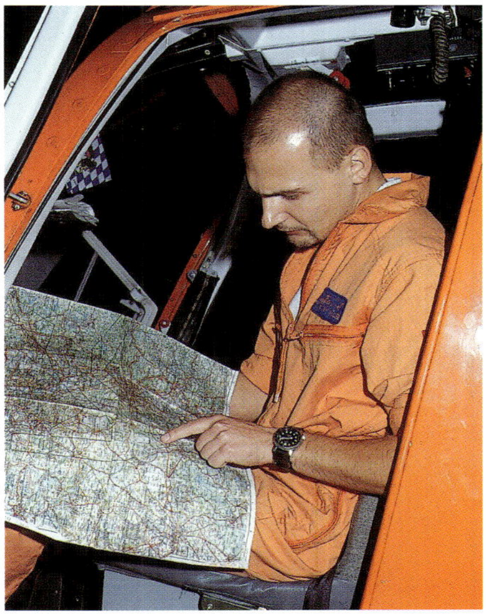

Der Helm ermöglicht Kommunikation innerhalb des Cockpits und zu den Fahrzeugen am Notfallort.

The helmet facilitates communication with the pilot and the physician with emergency & rescue certification in the cockpit as well as with all members of the police and fire service and, of course, all aviation radio partners.

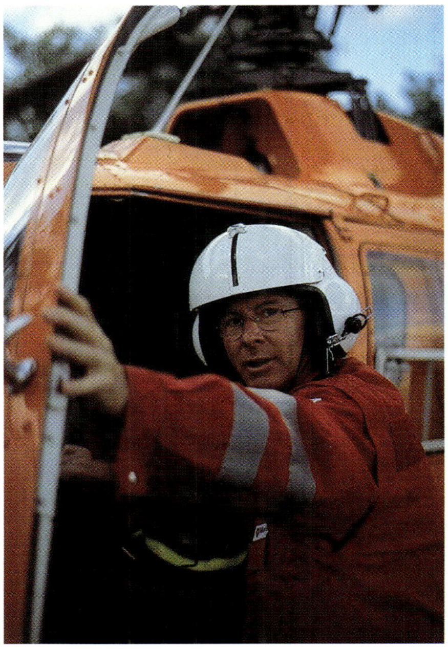

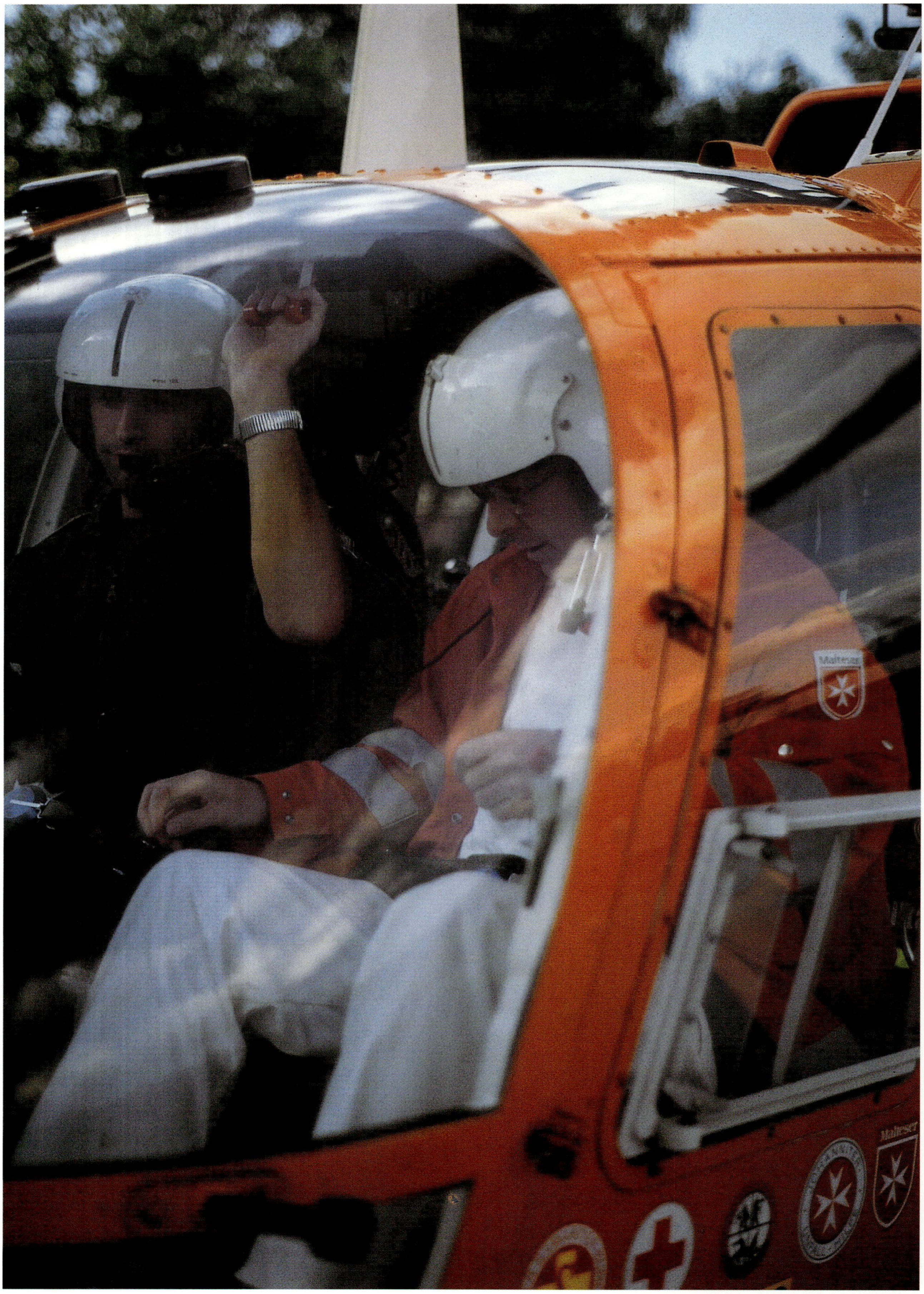

Start, 90 Sekunden nach der Alarmierung.

Only 90 seconds after receiving an emergency call, the helicopter takes off.

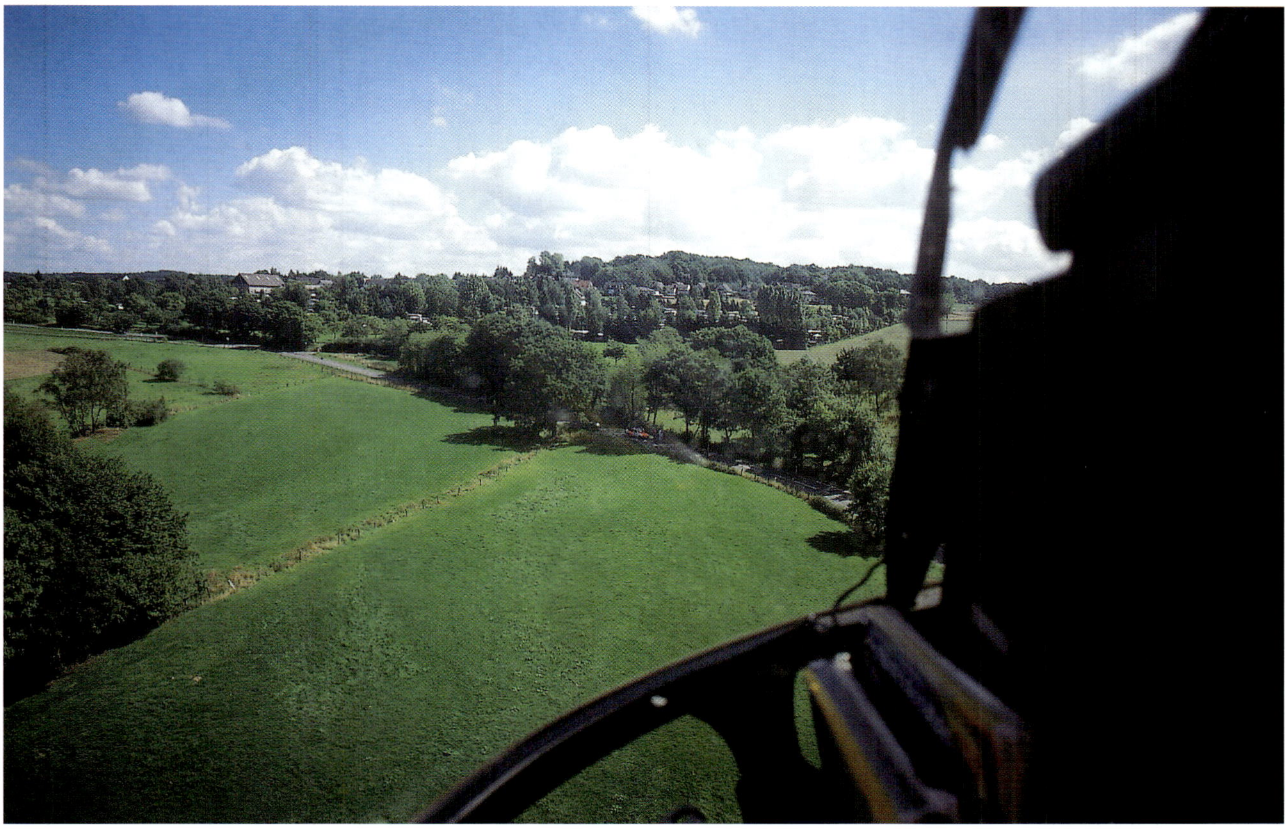

Die häufigsten Fragen an der Einsatzstelle
Frequently Asked Questions

Wieviel Liter fasst eine Tankfüllung und wie lange kann man damit fliegen?

Die Tanks der BO 105 fassen insgesamt 570 Liter. Damit könnte man ca. 2 Stunden und 30 Minuten fliegen. Im Rettungsdienst ist der Tank jedoch nie gänzlich gefüllt, da dies zum einen auf Grund des Einsatzradius von 50 – 70 km nicht erforderlich ist, und zum anderen der Hubschrauber nicht bis zum Gewichtslimit von 2500 kg betrieben werden muss. Dies sichert Leistungsreserven und ermöglicht eine ausreichende Zuladung. Bei einem Leergewicht von 1585 kg, zusätzlich 120 kg an medizinischer Ausstattung sowie drei Besatzungsmitgliedern und einem Patienten wäre bei einem´vollen Tank das zulässige Höchstabfluggewicht überschritten und die Leistungsreserven der Triebwerke (420 PS je Triebwerk) aufgezehrt.

How many liters go into the helicopter's fuel tanks and how far can it fly on this amount of fuel?

The fuel tanks of the BO 105 have a total capacity of 570 liters. With this amount of fuel, the BO 105 can fly for approx. Two hours and 30 minutes. During rescue operations, however, the tanks are never entirely full for two reasons: firstly, this is not necessary for the normal radius of action of 50 – 70 km and secondly, this means that the helicopter does not have to be operated at its weight limit of 2500 kg. This saves the power reserves and allows the helicopter to take on sufficient extra loads. With an unladen weight of 1585 kg in addition to 120 kg of medical equipment, three crew members and one patient, the maximum permissible takeoff weight would be exceeded if the tanks were full and the power reserves of the turbine engines (420 PS per engine) were depleted.

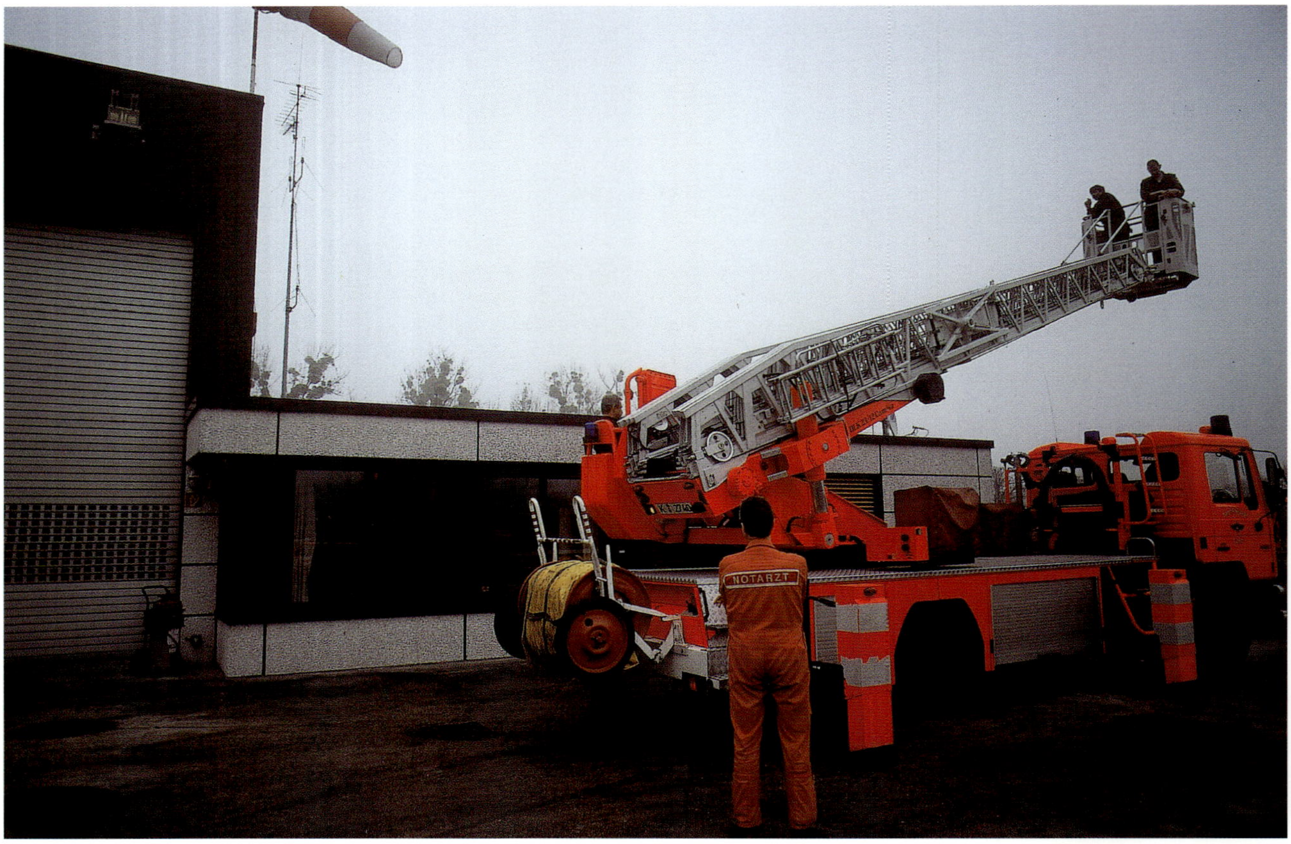

Der Windsack wird erneuert.

The wind sock is repaired.

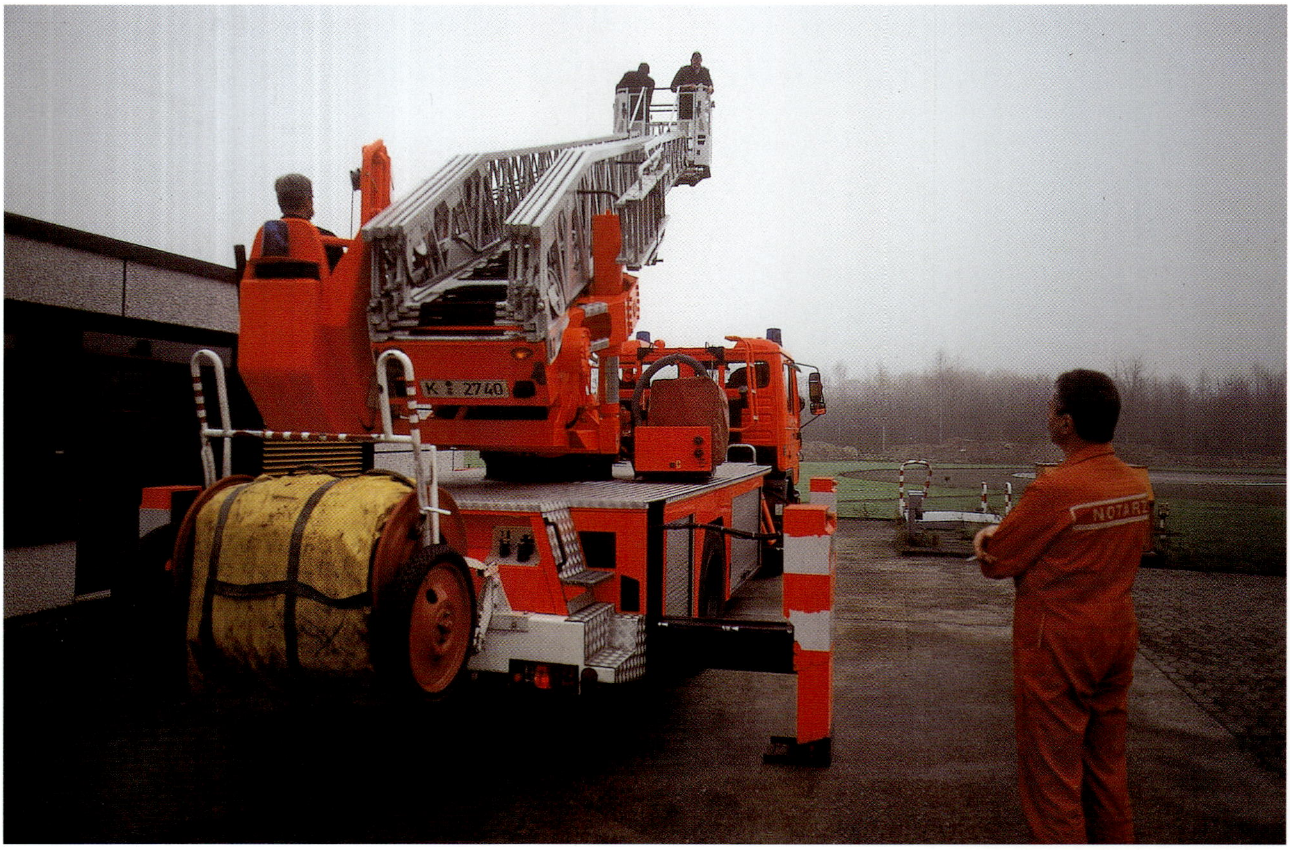

Die Drehleiter der Feuerwehr wird ausgefahren.

The fire service extends their turntable ladder.

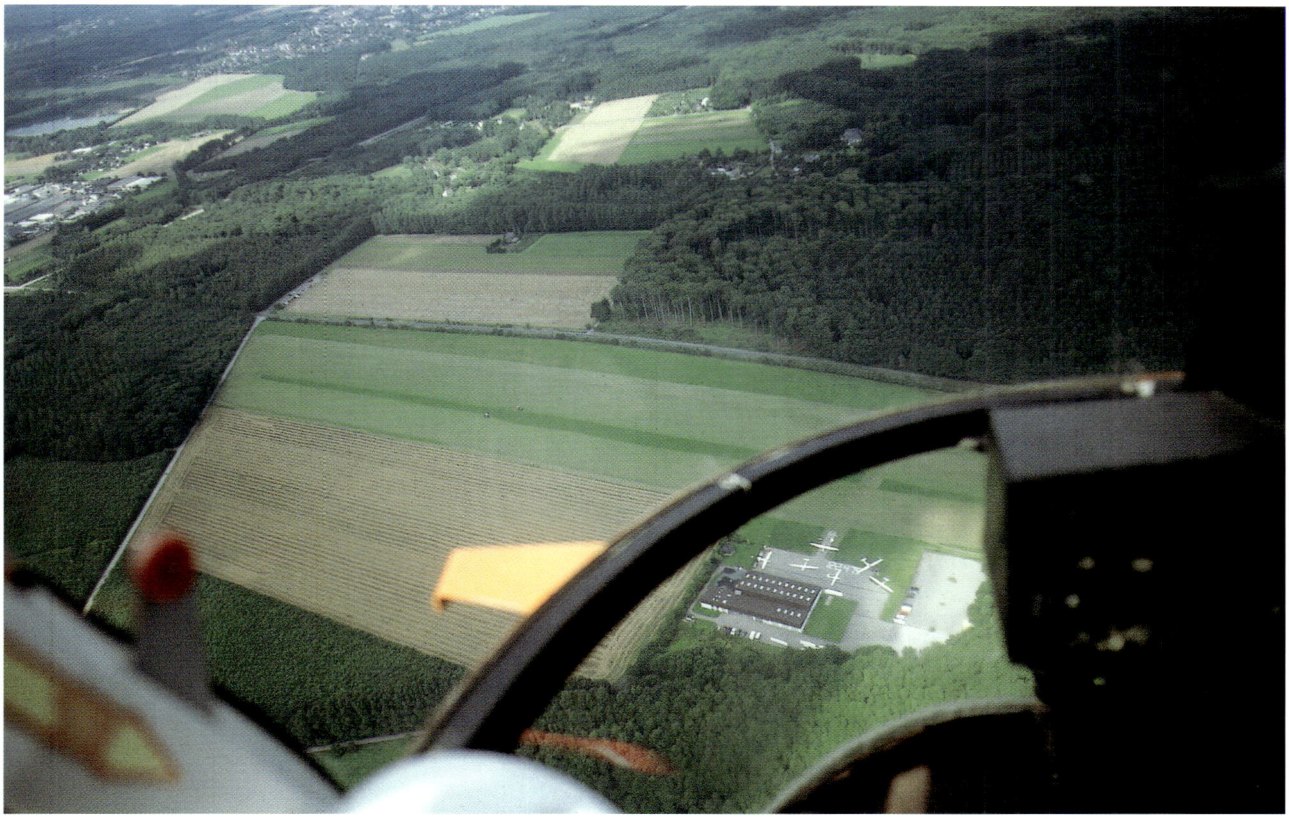

Augenblicke

Alte Frau. Mann verloren. Klagt über Schmerzen. Psychisches Problem. Wir mit Worten versorgt. Menschliche Wärme. Caritas informiert. Seelsorger informiert. Möchte jedem von uns 10,00 DM in die Hand drücken. Das dürfen wir leider nicht annehmen. Frau zutiefst enttäuscht. Wäre wahrscheinlich das Restgeld des Monats gewesen. Rückflug.

Snapshots

An elderly woman. Has lost her husband. Complains of pain. Emotional problem. We administer reassuring words and human warmth. We inform Caritas and her pastor. She wants to give each of us ten Deutschmarks. We explain that we are not allowed to accept money. The woman is very disappointed. It was probably all the money she had left for the month. Return flight.

Einsatz für den Rettungshubschrauber
Mission for the Rescue Helicopter

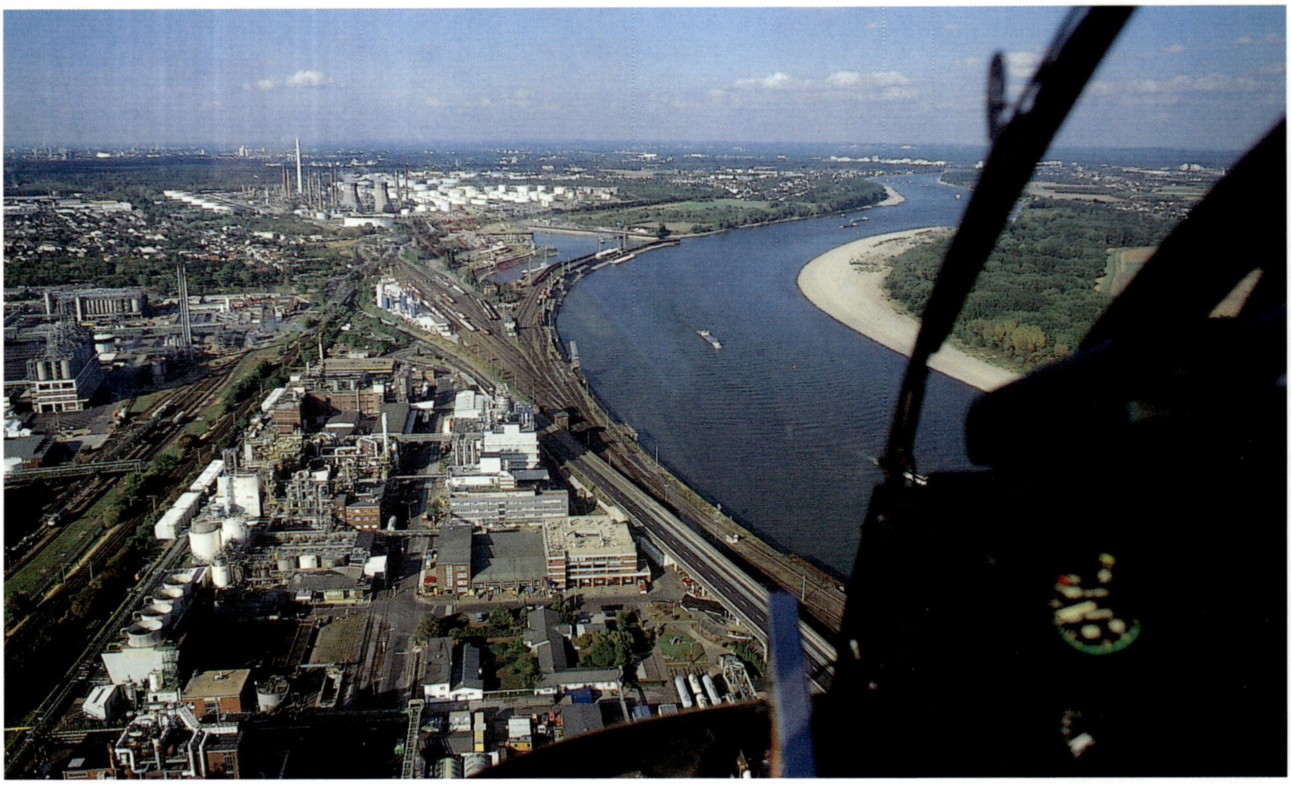

Person im Rhein.

Person in the Rhine.

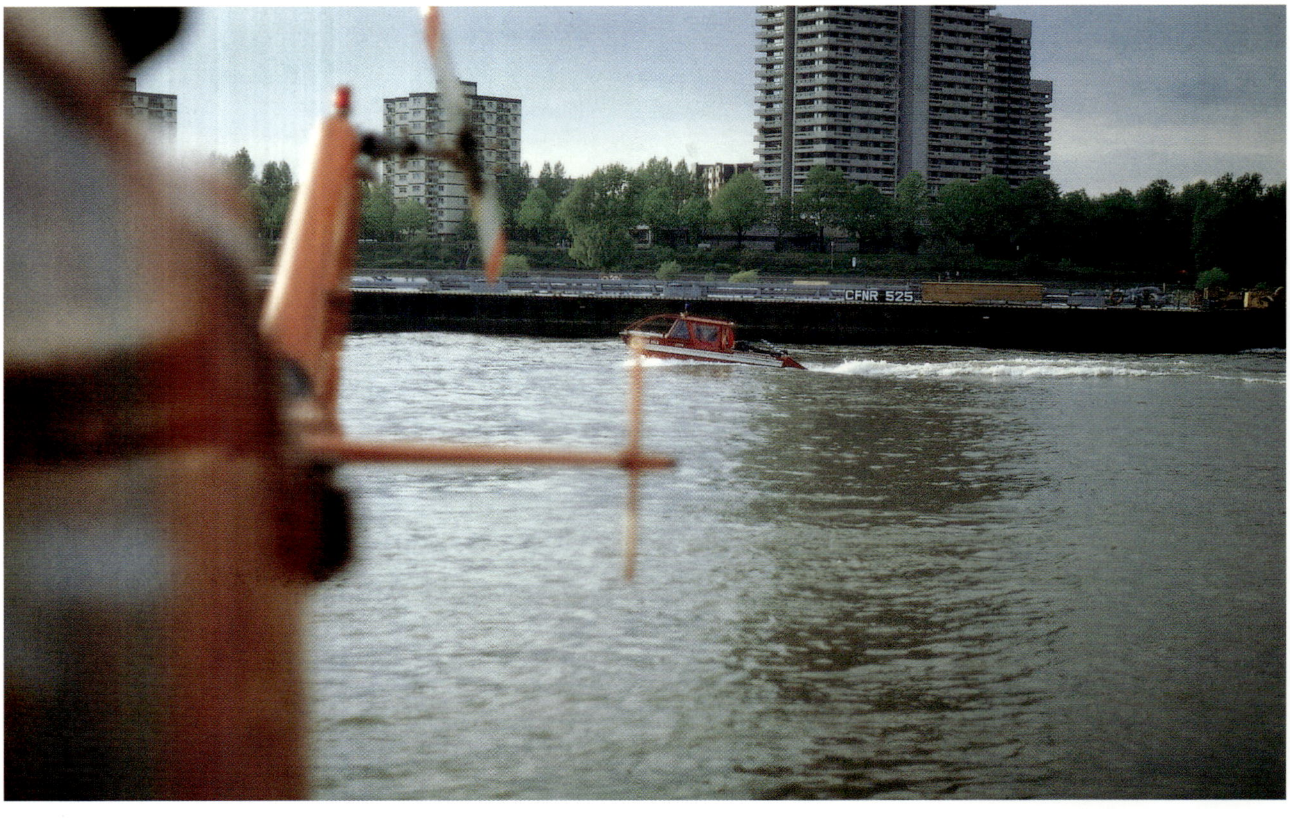

Das Löschboot der Feuerwehr ist auch unterwegs

The fire-fighting boat is already on its way to the scene.

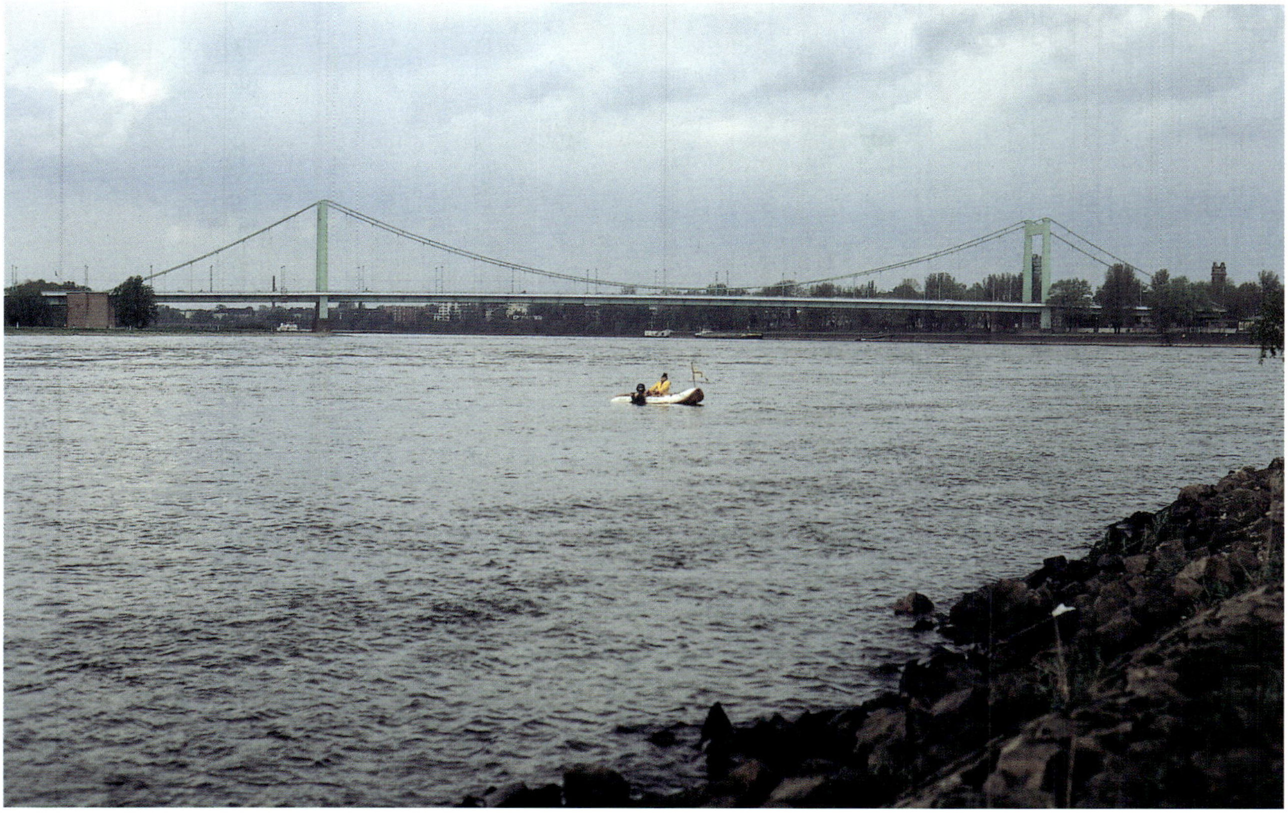

Ein Schlauchbootfahrer hat die Person erkannt.

A man in a rubber dinghy has spotted the person.

Die häufigsten Fragen an der Einsatzstelle
Frequently Asked Questions

Welche Mindestsicht nach vorn und nach unten benötigt der Rettungshubschrauber im Flug?

Der Rettungshubschrauber fliegt nach Sichtflugregeln, im Gegensatz zu Verkehrsflugzeugen, die, von Fluglotsen überwacht, nach Instrumentenflugregeln fliegen. Der Gesetzgeber fordert eine Mindestsicht aus dem Cockpit in Flugrichtung von 800 Metern. Weiterhin muss der Hubschrauberpilot/in, der die alleinige Verantwortung für den sicheren Flugbetrieb des Hubschraubers trägt, Erdsicht haben, es sei denn, er/Sie fliegt über einer geschlossenen Wolkendecke. In diesem Fall muss er/Sie aber mit absoluter Sicherheit wissen, dass er/Sie am Ziel wieder Bodensicht hat. Ähnlich wie für den Notarztwagen auf der Straße gelten jedoch auch für den Rettungshubschrauber Sonderrechte. Der Pilot/in kann deshalb, wenn er/Sie es für erforderlich und verantwortbar hält, die Mindestbedingungen im Rettungseinsatz unterschreiten.

How much minimum visibility does in front and below the rescue helicopter need?

Unlike commercial aircraft, which fly by instrument rules under the surveillance of the air traffic controllers, the rescue helicopters fly according to the visual flight rules. A minimum visibility from the cockpit in the direction of flight of 800 meters is required by law. Furthermore, the helicopter pilot, who carries the sole responsibility for the safe flight operation of the helicopter, must have ground visibility unless he or she is flying above a cloud cover. In this case, the pilot must be absolutely certain, however, that he or she will have ground visibility again at the helicopter's destination. Like the rescue ambulance with a physician with emergency & rescue certification aboard, however, the rescue helicopter enjoys special privileges. For this reason, the pilot is allowed to fall short of the minimum requirements for rescue missions if he or she feels that this is necessary and justifiable.

Einsatz für den Rettungshubschrauber
Mission for the Rescue Helicopter

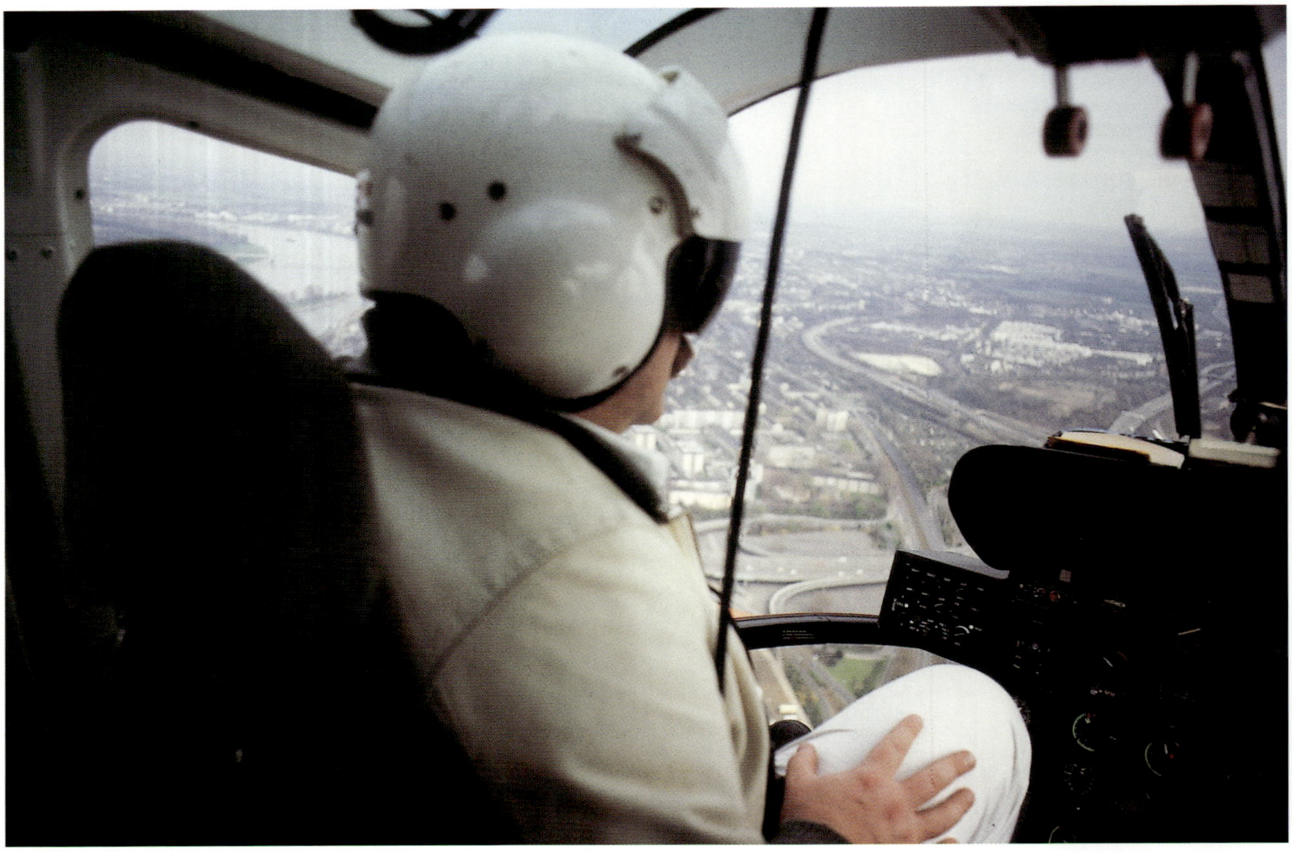

Ein Kind ist vom Wickeltisch gefallen.

An infant has fallen off the diaper-changing table.

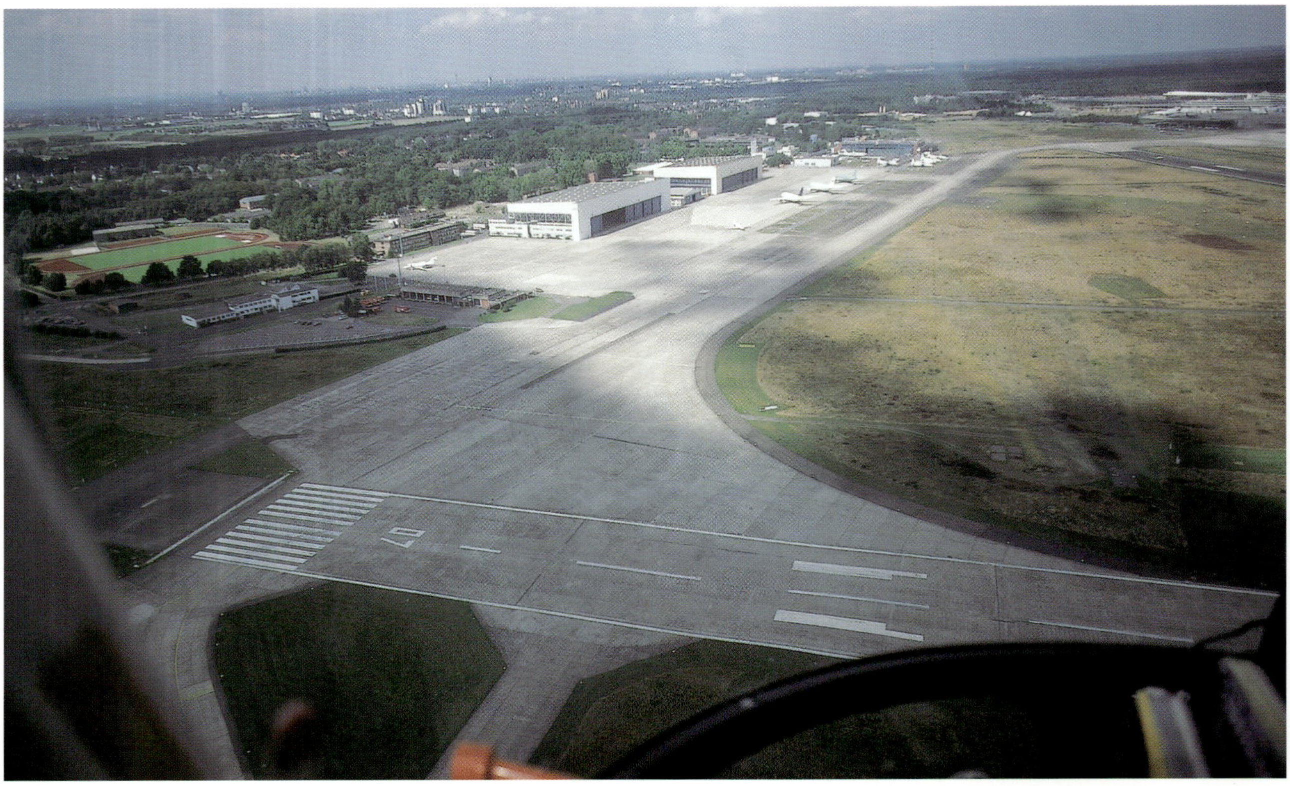

Wir überqueren den Flughafen Köln/Bonn.

We fly over Cologne-Bonn Airport.

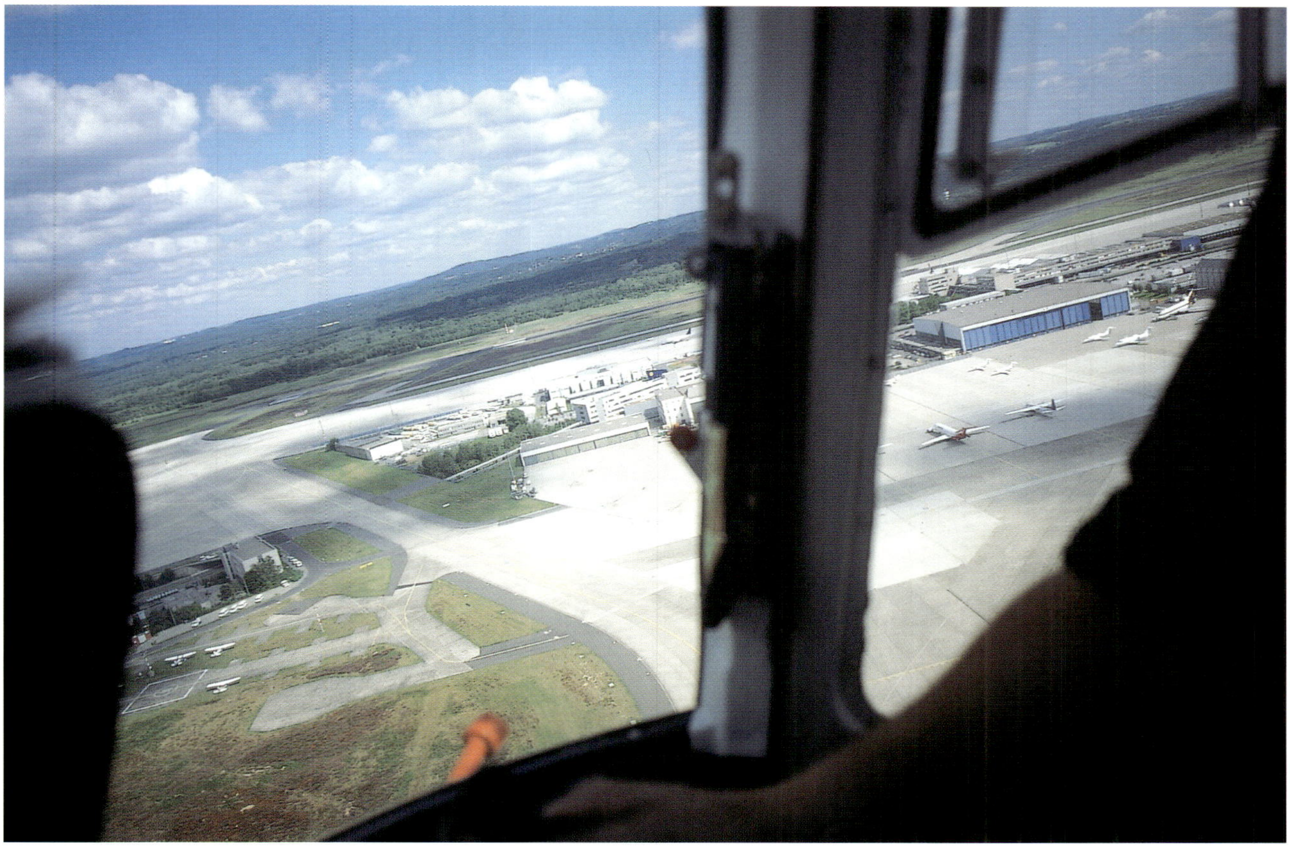

Die häufigsten Fragen an der Einsatzstelle
Frequently Asked Questions

HEMS-Crew-Member? Was heißt das?

Mit der Inkraftsetzung gesamteuropäischer Luftfahrtvorschriften im Jahre 1998 entstand auch eine Vorschrift, die den Betrieb von Rettungshubschraubern regelt. In diesen JAR-OPS 3 (Joint Aviation Requirements - Operations 3) ist die Funktion des Rettungsassistenten als Mitglied der Flugbesatzung geregelt. Vorgeschrieben wird dabei auch, dass er in fliegerische Grundlagen einzuweisen und darin regelmäßig fortzubilden ist, um ihn in die Lage zu versetzen, den Piloten insbesondere als Navigator, Funker und Luftraumbeobachter zu unterstützen. Dies geschieht für die HEMS (Helicopter Emergency Medical Service)- Crewmember von Christoph 3 (Köln), 8 (Lünen) und 9 (Duisburg) durch die Mitarbeiter der BGS-Fliegerstaffel West in Sankt Augustin-Hangelar.

What exactly is an HEMS crew member?

With the enactment of pan European aviation regulations in 1998, a regulation also went into effect governing the operation of rescue helicopters. In the same year, the regulation JAR-OPS 3 (Joint Aviation Requirements - Operations 3) went into force governing the function of the paramedic as a member of the rescue helicopter crew. This regulation also stipulates that the paramedic is to receive instruction in the basic principles of flying to enable him or her to assist the pilot, in particular in the capacity of navigator and radio operator. This instruction is given to the members of the HEMS (Helicopter Emergency Medical Service) crew members of Christoph 3 (Cologne), 8 (Lünen) and 9 (Duisburg) by members of the Flying Squadron West of the German Border Police based in St. Augustin-Hangelar.

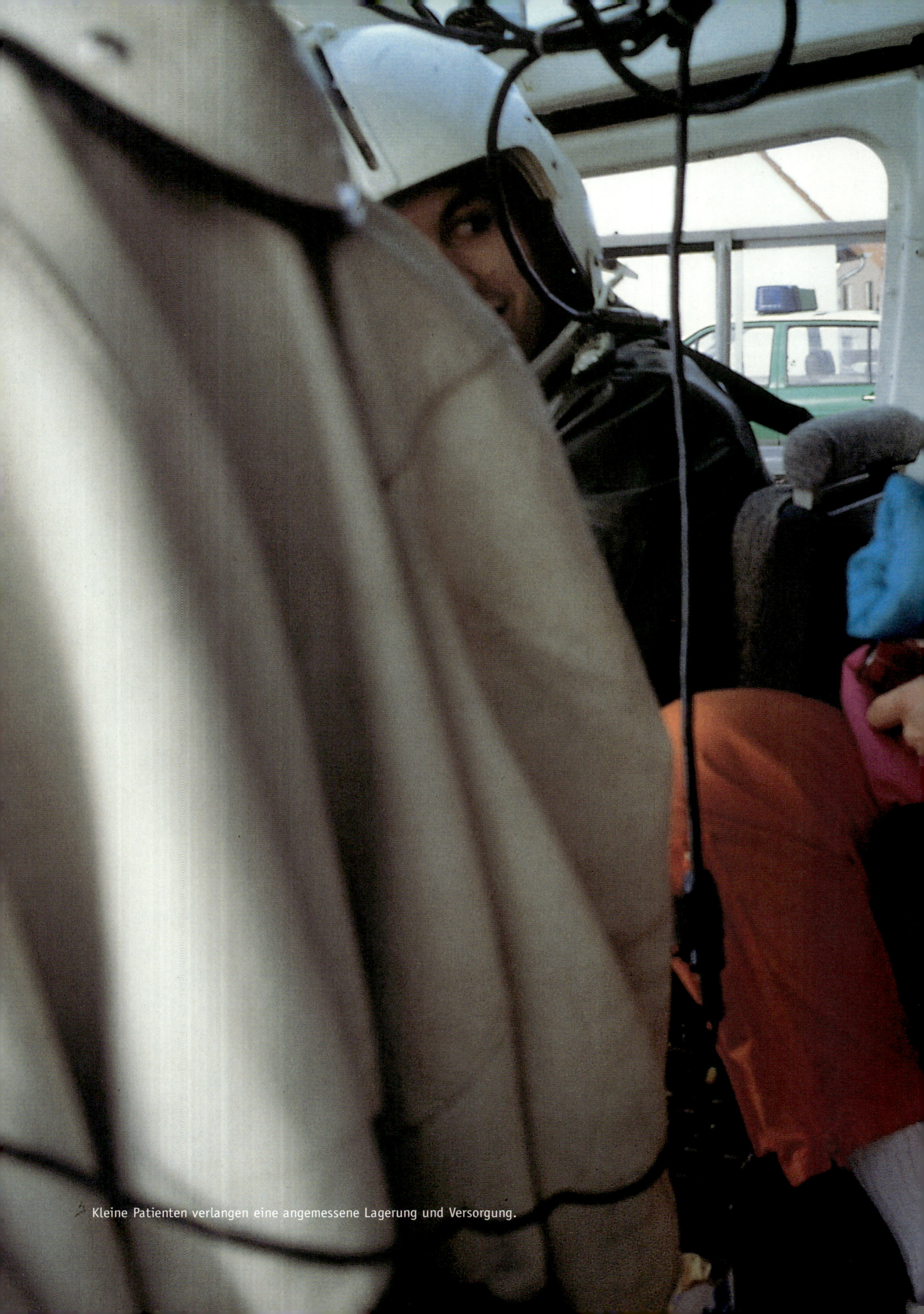

Kleine Patienten verlangen eine angemessene Lagerung und Versorgung.

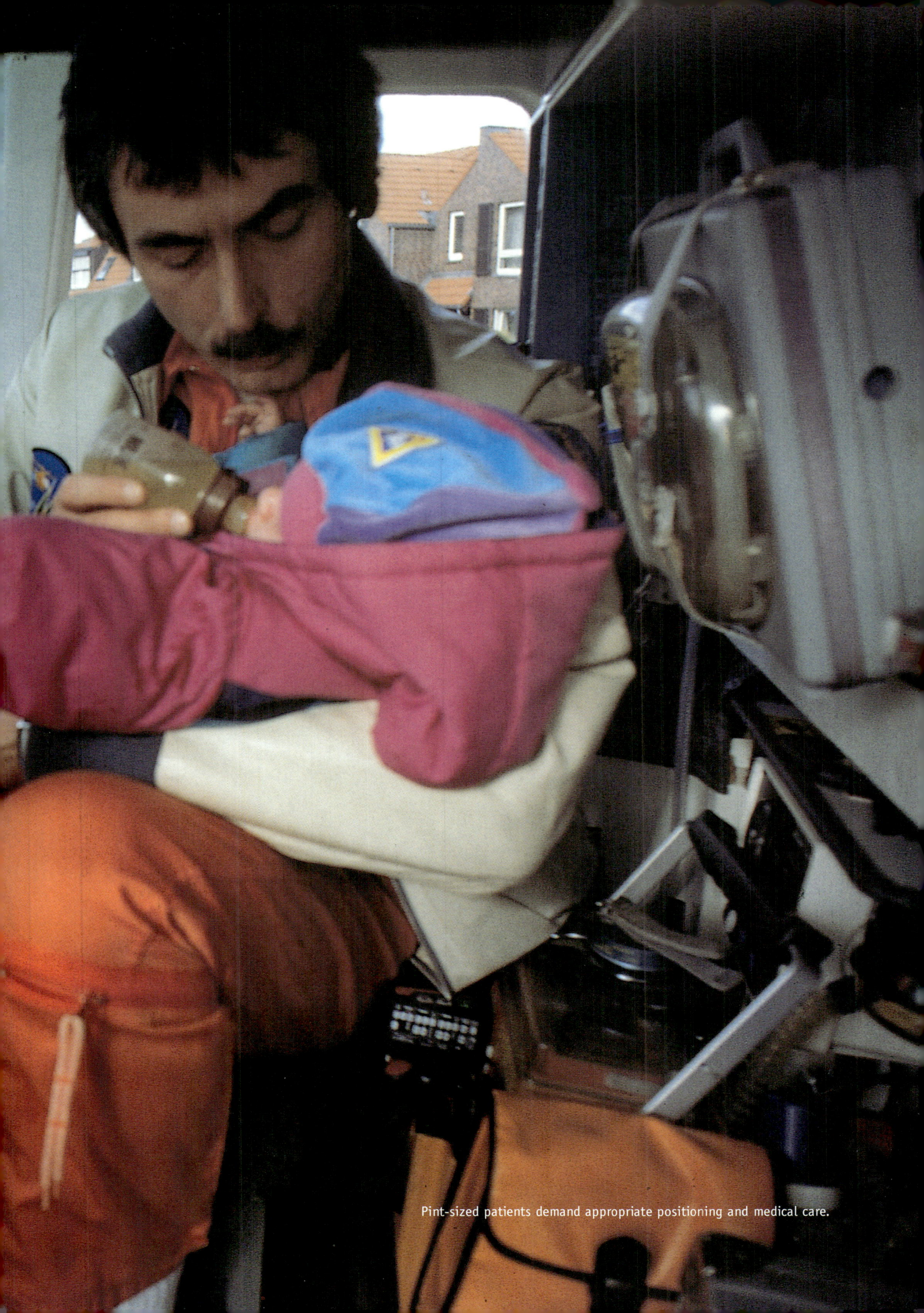

Pint-sized patients demand appropriate positioning and medical care.

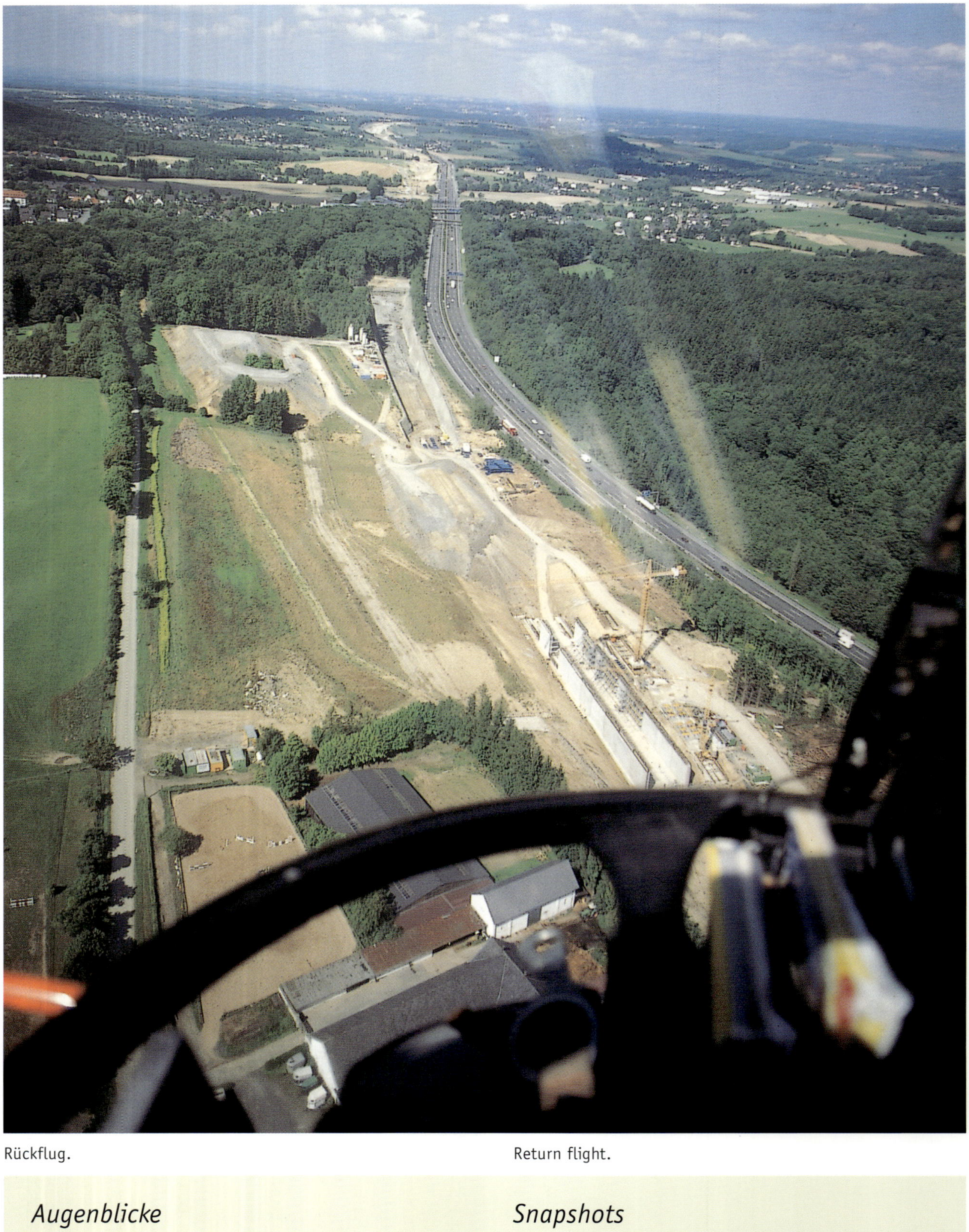

Rückflug.

Return flight.

Augenblicke

Dienstende. Eine ereignisreicher Tag. Viele Einsätze. In einigen Fällen lebensrettend. Morgen Gespräch mit meinem Vorgesetzten. Er wird mir die Welt erklären wollen. Ob das geht?

Snapshots

End of shift. An eventful day with a lot of missions, many of them life-saving. Tomorrow I have a meeting with my boss. He will probably want to explain the universe to me again. Fat chance.

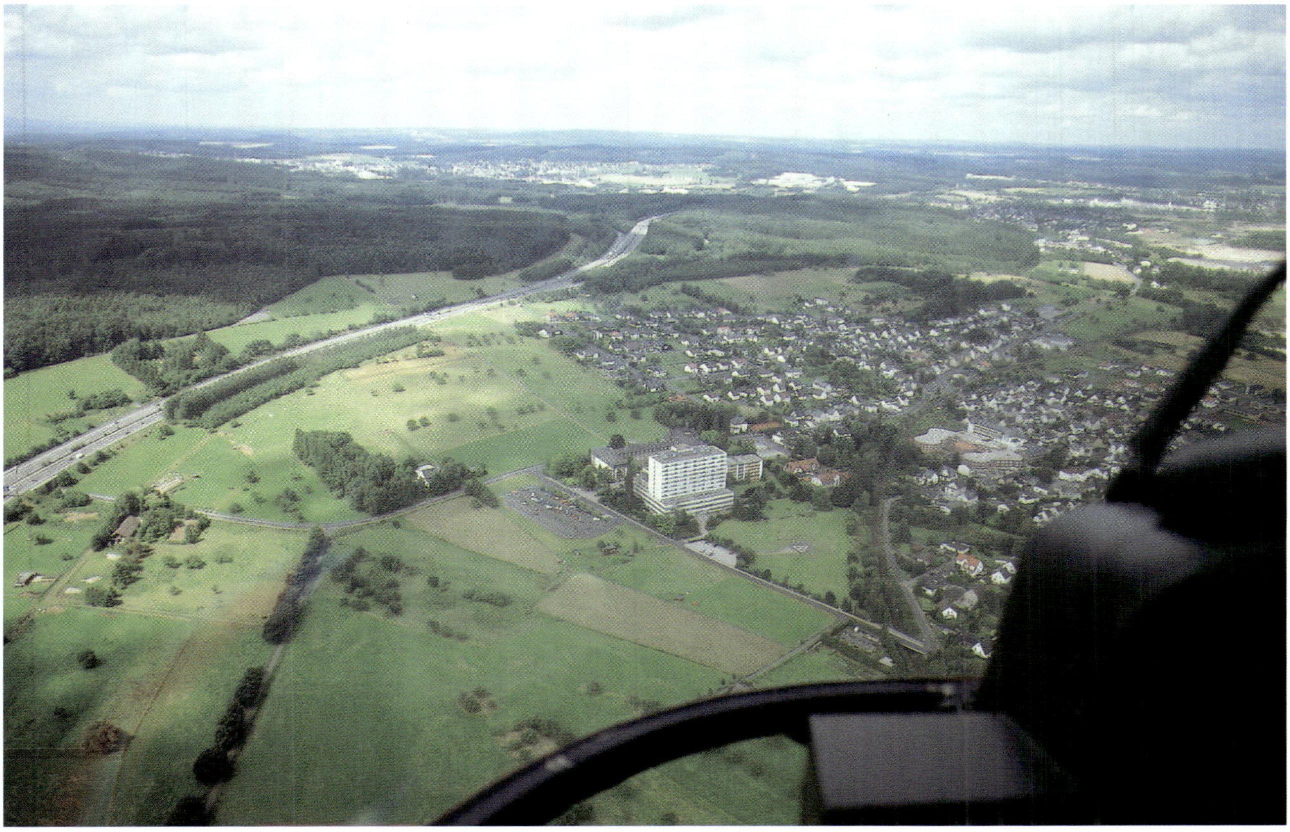

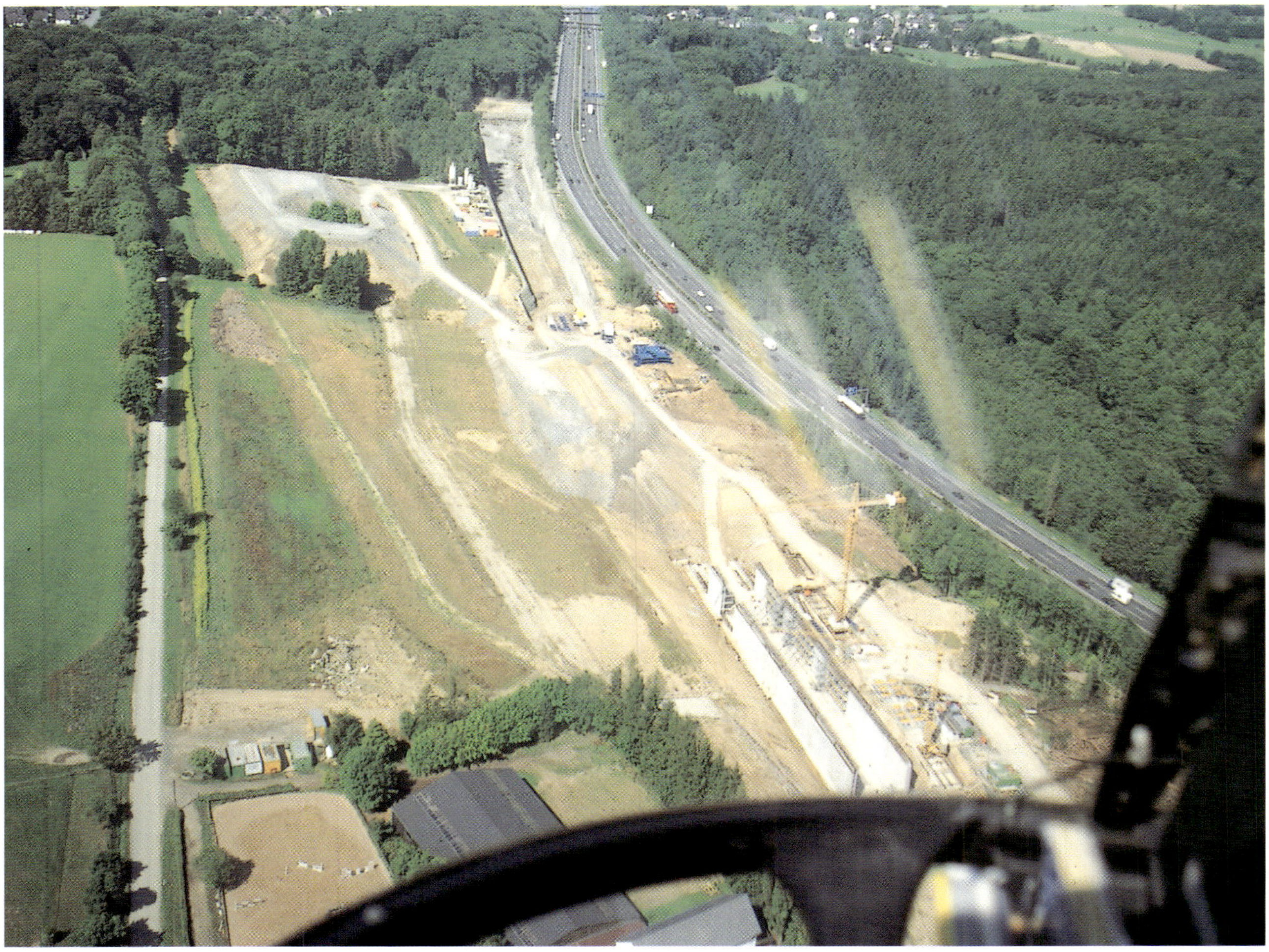

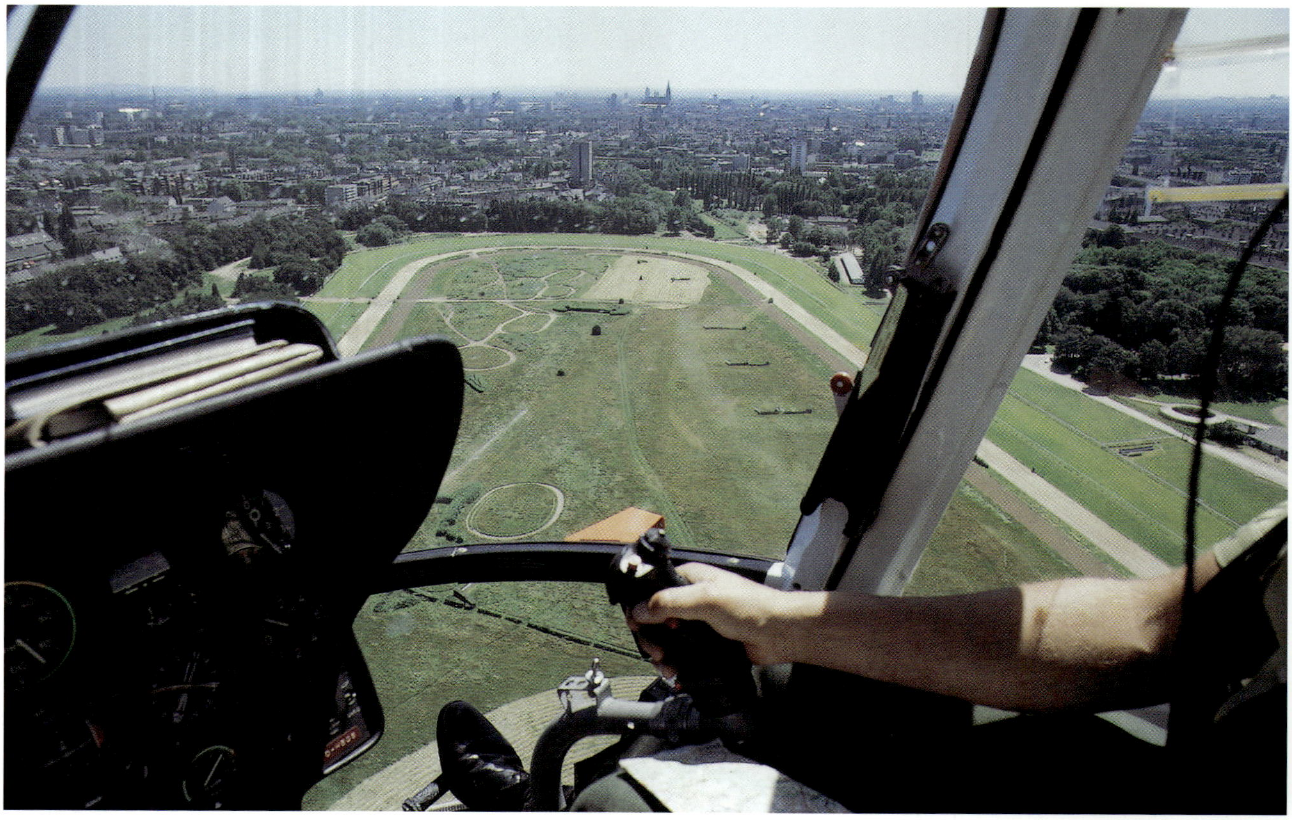

Die häufigsten Fragen an der Einsatzstelle
Frequently Asked Questions

Was bedeutet das Kennzeichen „D-HDOC“ auf dem Heckausleger?

Wie jedes Auto hat auch jedes Luftfahrzeug ein „Nummernschild“. In Deutschland zugelassene zivile Hubschrauber tragen das D für Deutschland und das H für Hubschrauber. Die folgenden drei Buchstaben sind frei wählbar bzw. werden zugeteilt. Die insgesamt 22 Rettungshubschrauber des Zivilschutz/des BGS vom Typ BO 105 tragen die Kennzeichen D-HBGS sowie D-HGSA, D-HGSB, D-HGSC usw.

What is the meaning of the abbreviation “D-HDOC“ on the tailboom?

Like every automobile, every aircraft has its own “license tag“. Helicopters licensed for civil aviation in Germany can be identified by the letter D for Germany (Deutschland) and H for helicopter. The following three letters are issued (they can also be chosen). The total of 22 rescue helicopter of the type BO 105 operated by German Civil Defense authorities and the Federal Border Police (BGS) carry the license tag identification D-HBGS or D-HGSA, D-HGSB, D-HGSC, etc.

Das Institut für Notfallmedizin der Berufsfeuerwehr Köln
The Institute for Emergency Medicine of the Cologne Professional Fire Service

von/by Alex Lechleuthner

Im Dezember 1995 wurde im Amt für Feuerschutz, Bevölkerungsschutz, Rettungsdienst und Katastrophenschutz das „Institut für Notfallmedizin der Berufsfeuerwehr Köln" gegründet und die Leitung dem Ärztlichen Leiter des Rettungsdienstes (ÄLR) übertragen. Zu diesem Zeitpunkt war das Institut noch keine Abteilung, sondern es bestand neben dem Leiter überwiegend aus ehrenamtlichen Kräften. Hauptaufgabe des Instituts war die konzeptionelle Verbesserung des Kölner Rettungsdienstes, die in Form von Konzeptentwicklung und Abstimmung auf verschiedenen Ebenen umgesetzt wurde. So wurden die Aus- und Fortbildung standardisiert und die Behandlungsleitlinien in einer so genannten Standardkommission mit allen am Rettungsdienst beteiligten Organisationen und den weiterbehandelnden Kliniken abgestimmt. Aufgrund der direkten Einbindung in das tägliche Rettungsgeschehen entstanden problemorientierte Projekte aus der täglichen Praxis. Die ersten Projekte waren die Koordination der multizentrischen Untersuchung, wie häufig ein Krankentransport zum Notfall wurde, das Kölner Schlaganfallprojekt (Kölner gegen den Schlaganfall – wir machen mobil), Herzinfarkterkennung und die Prüfung der Möglichkeiten einer verbesserten Leitstellendisposition.

Eine weitere Herausforderung kam im Jahr 1995 auf das IFN zu, als die Sprungrevision des so genannten „Aachener Urteils" Bundesverwaltungsgericht abgewiesen wurde, was dazu führte, dass durch eine Unscharfe Beschreibung im Sozialgesetzbuch V (§ 75 SGB V) die notärztliche Versorgung für gesetzlich Krankenversicherte definitiv dem Sicherstellungsauftrag der Kassenärztlichen Vereinigung zugeordnet wurde. In der Konsequenz hätte das bedeutet, dass – mit Ausnahme von Bayern, das schon immer diese Sonderregelung hatte – alle Rettungsdienstträger fortan die Notärzte nicht mehr selbst hätte organisieren können, sondern diese Aufgabe mit Organisation und Finanzierung den Kassenärztlichen Vereinigungen aufgebürdet worden wäre. Ohne auf die Komplexität der rechtlichen Folgen und Zusammenhänge hier einzugehen, hätte dies in letzter Konsequenz zu einer Zerstörung der

In December 1995 the "Institute for Emergency Medicine of the Cologne Professional Fire Service" was founded at the Office for Fire Protection, Civil Defense, Rescue Service and Disaster Relief; the Medical Director of the Rescue Service was entrusted with the task of heading the new institute. Back then the Institute did not even have departmental status; except for the director, it consisted mainly of volunteers. The main task of the Institute was to improve the basic concept of the Cologne Rescue Service; these efforts were implemented on various levels in the form of concept development and coordination. The programs of basic and continuing education were standardized, for example, and the treatment guidelines coordinated with all the organizations involved in the rescue service and with the hospitals which provided further care by a so-called Standarts Committee. On the basis of its direct involvement in everyday rescue activities, the Institute was able to develop problem-related projects. The first projects entailed coordinating multicentric studies exploring the frequency with which a patient transport developed into an emergency, the Cologne Stroke Project (Citizens of Cologne Mobilize Against Stroke), diagnosis of myocardial infarction, and exploration of possibilities for improved dispatching at the Coordination Centers.

The IEM was presented with an additional challenge in 1995, when the leap-frog appeal of the "Aachener Ruling" was turned down by the Federal Administrative Court. The consequence of this court decision was that, owing to an imprecise description in Volume V of the Code of Social Law (§ 75 SGB V), the emergency care provided by physicians with emergency & rescue certification to patients insured with the statutory health insurance schemes was definitively counted among the services which the Association of Physicians Registered with the Statutory Health Insurance Schemes is obliged to secure. This would have meant that – with the exception of Bavaria, which has always had this special arrangement – all organizations providing rescue services could no longer have organized these services themselves; instead, the onus of organizing and financing these activities would have been transferred to the Association of Physicians Registered with the Statutory Health Insurance Schemes. Without going into the complexity of the legal consequences and interrelationships at this point, we can say, however, that the ultimate consequence would have been the dismantling

flächendeckenden Notarztsysteme geführt. In dünn besiedelten Regionen wäre es zu einer Ausdünnung der Systeme und in dicht besiedelten Gebieten zu einer Vielzahl von teilnahmeinteressierten Ärzten gekommen. Möglicherweise wäre auch – wie in Bayern – der Fahrer des Notarzteinsatzfahrzeugs nicht mehr bezahlt worden etc.. Hier wurde das IFN tätig und hat durch konzeptionelle Vorschläge und Informationen auf verschiedenen politischen Ebenen mit dazu beitragen können, dass letztlich Bundesrecht (im 2. GKV Neuordnungsgesetz) das SGB V geändert wurde und die funktionierenden Strukturen erhalten werden konnten. Die Tätigkeit rechtlicher Analysen und Weiterentwicklung ist bis heute eine Hauptaufgabe des IFN geblieben und führte dazu, dass die rettungsdienstliche Entwicklung in NRW und der Bundesrepublik aufmerksam verfolgt und analysiert wird. Laufende Anfragen von Behörden, Kostenträgern und Fachgruppen zeigen, dass hier ein kontinuierlicher Bedarf besteht.

Bei der Gestaltung des Kölner Rettungsdienstes zeigte sich, dass der Ausbildungsstand des nichtärztlichen Rettungsdienstpersonals in den vergangenen Jahren laufend gewachsen ist. Bedingt durch das Notarzt-Rendez-Vous-System wurde die Standardisierung und hochwertige Ausrüstung der RTW erforderlich. So hatten bereits 1993 alle Rettungswagen EKG-Defibrillatoreinheiten, da routinemäßig der Notarzt vom NEF auf den Rettungswagen steigt und den Patienten dort behandelt und – wenn notwendig – auch begleitet. Es machte taktisch keinen Sinn, EKG-Defibrillatoren nur auf den NEF mitzuführen, da das RTW Personal bei einer Notarzt-Begleitung dann auch mit diesen Geräten arbeiten muß. Insofern war es folgerichtig alle RTWs auch vollständig auszustatten, da damit gewährleistet werden konnte, dass das RTW Personal auch mit den Geräten vertraut ist und darüber hinaus auch Verlegungen zwischen Kliniken mit vollausgestatteten RTWs organisatorisch einfacher zu realisieren ist.

1996 wurde das Kölner Notkompetenzsystem eingeführt, das es ermöglichte, dass die ersteintreffenden Rettungsassistenten noch vor Eintreffen des Notarztes mit den ersten lebensrettenden Maßnahmen beginnen konnten. Dazu gehören die sofortige Defibrillation (Elektroschock-Therapie bei Herzkammerflimmern, das die häufigste Ursache des plötzlichen Herztodes ist), die Intubation (Atemwegssicherung mit einem Beatmungsschlauch bei Wiederbelebun-

of the system guaranteeing emergency care by physicians possessing emergency & rescue certification throughout the entire country. In sparsely populated regions, there would have been a "thinning out" of the system and in densely populated areas, an increase in the number of doctors interested in participating. Quite possibly, the drivers of emergency vehicles would no longer be paid – as is the case in Bavaria, for example. In this situation, the IEM mounted various campaigns; with its recommendations for rescue system concepts and the information it provided on various levels of the political hierarchy, it was partially responsible for the fact that ultimately the federal law contained in Volume 5 of the Code of Social Law was altered (in the 2nd Reform Law on the Statutory Health Insurance Schemes) and that the functioning structures remained intact. Legal analyses and further development have remained the main field of endeavor of IEM and caused the evolution of rescue services in the state of North Rhine-Westphalia and in the Federal Republic of Germany as a whole to be carefully followed and analyzed. The continual inquiries received from authorities, sponsors and professional groups show that there is a continuous demand for such information.

During the design of the Cologne Rescue Service, it was shown that the level of education possessed by non-physician rescue service personnel has risen continuously in recent years. In the wake of the introduction of the rendezvous system for physicians with emergency & rescue certification, the rescue helicopters had to be standardized and furnished with high-quality equipment. In 1993, for example, all rescue ambulances were already equipped with EKG defibrillation units; this was because the physician with emergency & rescue certification riding in the emergency doctor's car routinely entered the rescue ambulance, treated patients in the ambulance and – when necessary – accompanied them to the hospital. It does not make sense from a tactical point of view to only equip the emergency doctor's car with EKG defibrillators since the rescue ambulance personnel would also have to work with this equipment if a physician with emergency & rescue certification came aboard. In this respect, it was a logical and wise decision to fully equip all rescue ambulances. This step was taken to guarantee that rescue ambulance personnel are also familiar with the equipment. Moreover, it is easier to transfer patients from one hospital to another in fully equipped rescue ambulances.

In 1996 the Cologne Emergency Competency System was introduced which allows the first paramedic who is on the scene before the physician with emergency & rescue certification arrives to start the first life-saving measures. These include immediate defibrillation

gen) und die Gabe von bestimmten Medikamenten, die sofort und ohne Zeitverzögerung gegeben werden müssen.

Dies setzt allerdings eine regelmäßige Nachschulung, Leistungskontrolle und Überwachung des laufenden Rettungsdienstbetriebes voraus. Dazu werden alle Rettungsdienstmitarbeiter im Rahmen der gesetzlich vorgeschriebenen 30-Stunden-Fortbildung zentral fortgebildet und zertifiziert.

Im Jahr 1999 wurde eine Umstrukturierung der Berufsfeuerwehr Köln konzipiert, die die Produktverantwortung konzeptionell in den Mittelpunkt der Organisationsstruktur setzte und im Jahr 2000 umgesetzt wurde.

Das Produkt Rettungsdienst wird dabei vom Institut für Notfallmedizin der Berufsfeuerwehr Köln in Form der Trägeraufgaben hergestellt und überwacht.

Zu diesem Produkt gehören die Festlegung des Mindeststandards der rettungsdienstlichen Leistungserbringung und ihre Überwachung. Zusätzlich wurden die Maßnahmen nach dem PsychKG vom Ordnungsamt und die Genehmigungsbehörde für gewerbliche Anbieter nach Abschnitt III des Rettungsgesetzes NW auf das Institut übertragen.

Ebenso fällt seitdem die Zuständigkeit für den Rettungshubschrauber Christoph 3 in den Aufgabenbereich des Instituts für Notfallmedizin, der für 14 Gebietskörperschaften (Trägergemeinschaft) fliegt und von der Stadt Köln als Kernträger nach § 10 RettGes NW verwaltet wird.

In Abbildung 1 ist das Organigramm des Instituts dargestellt.

Nach der Zertifizierungs-Konzeption für das nicht-ärztliche Personal wurde im Jahre 2000 nach Abschluss eines Qualitätssicherungsvertrages mit den notarztstellenden Kliniken die Eingangszertifizierung für die Notärztinnen und Notärzte eingeführt. Dabei werden in Zwei-Tages-seminaren die werdenden Notärztinnen und notärzte auf ihre Aufgaben in Köln vorbereitet, ein Einweisung nach Medizin-Produkte-Gesetz auf alle Geräte und eine theoretische und praktische Zertifizierung durchgeführt.

Als laufende Projekte sind im Jahre 2000 die Erprobung eines mobilen Ultraschallgerätes und die Neukonzeption der Herzinfarkttherapie mit Lysebehandlung zu nennen.

(electroshock therapy for patients with ventricular fibrillation (the most frequent cause of sudden cardiac death), intubation (keeping the respiratory passages open with a tube during resuscitation measures) and the administration of certain medications which have to be given without delay.

However, all of the above presume the existence of regular further training, monitoring of performance and supervision of ongoing rescue operations. For this purpose, all rescue services personnel undergo central further training and certification within the framework of the 30 hours of further training prescribed by law.

In 1999 a concept was drawn up for the restructuring of the Cologne Professional Fire Service. This new concept created an organizational structure focused on product liability; it was put into action in 2000.

In this context, the product "rescue service" is manufactured and monitored by the Institute for Emergency Medicine of the Cologne Professional Fire Service within the scope of sponsoring.

This product includes the establishment of minimum standards for the performance of rescue services and the monitoring of these services. In addition, the responsibility for the rescue measures to be provided pursuant to the Law on the Care & Protection of Patients with Mental Disease has been transferred to IEM by the Office for Public Order and the licensing authorities for commercial rescue services in accordance with Section III of the Law on Rescue Services in North Rhine-Westphalia.

Since then the responsibility for the rescue helicopter Christoph 3 has also fallen within the jurisdiction of the Institute for Emergency Medicine; it flies for 14 regional or local authorities (sponsor collective) and is administered by the City of Cologne as the core sponsor in conformance with § 10 RettGes NW [Law on Rescue Services in North Rhine-Westphalia].

Figure 1 shows the organization chart of IEM

In accordance with the certification concept elaborated for non-physician personnel, certification was introduced as the entrance qualification for physicians with emergency & rescue certification after quality assurance agreements had been concluded with the hospitals providing such physicians. For this purpose, physicians aspiring to attain this certification are prepared for their work in Cologne at two-day seminars. Here they are instructed on the use of all the equipment and undergo certification of their theoretical and practical knowledge in accordance with the Law on Medical Products.

The projects underway in 2000 included the testing of a mobile ultrasonographic unit and the redesign of MI therapy to include lysis methods.

Im Jahre 2001 wird die bereits 1996 projektierte Mobile Datenerfassung (Projekt „Mobidat“) eingeführt, die eine genauere Qualitätssicherung, Abrechnung und Bedarfsplanung für den Kölner Rettungsdienst ermöglichen soll.

Ebenfalls im Jahr 2001 wird in Verbindung mit dem Institut an der Fachhochschule Köln ein neuer Studiengang „Rescue Engineering“ eingeführt, der sich in einen Bachelor- (6 Semester) und einen Masterstudiengang (4 Semester) gliedert. Diese Studiengänge sollen Rettungsdienstmitarbeiterinnen und –mitarbeitern die Möglichkeit geben, sich für Führungsaufgaben in Rettungsdienst, Katastrophenschutz und für internationale Einsatzprojekte zu qualifizieren (näheres auf der Homepage des Instituts http://www.ems-cologne.com und der Fachhochschule Köln http://www.fh-koeln.de, dort im Fachbereich Anlagen- und Verfahrenstechnik.).

The Mobile Data Acquisition Project ("Mobidat Project") already planned in 1996 is getting underway in 2001; this project will permit more precise quality management, invoicing and requirements planning for the Cologne Rescue Service.

In 2001 a new academic program in "Rescue Engineering" is being set up at the Cologne University of Applied Sciences in cooperation with the Institute. Students enrolled in this program will be able to earn a bachelor's degree (B.A.) in six semesters and a master's degree (M.A.) after four additional semesters. These academic programs are intended to give rescue service personnel the possibility to qualify for management positions in rescue services, civil defense and international rescue operations (Additional information can be obtained from the website of the Institute http://www.ems-cologne.com or of Cologne University of Applied Sciences http://www.fh-koeln.de, Department of Plant and Chemical Engineering.)

Institut für Notfallmedizin der Berufsfeuerwehr Köln – Organigramm –
The Institute for Emergency Medicine of the Cologne Professional Fire Service
– Organisation chart –

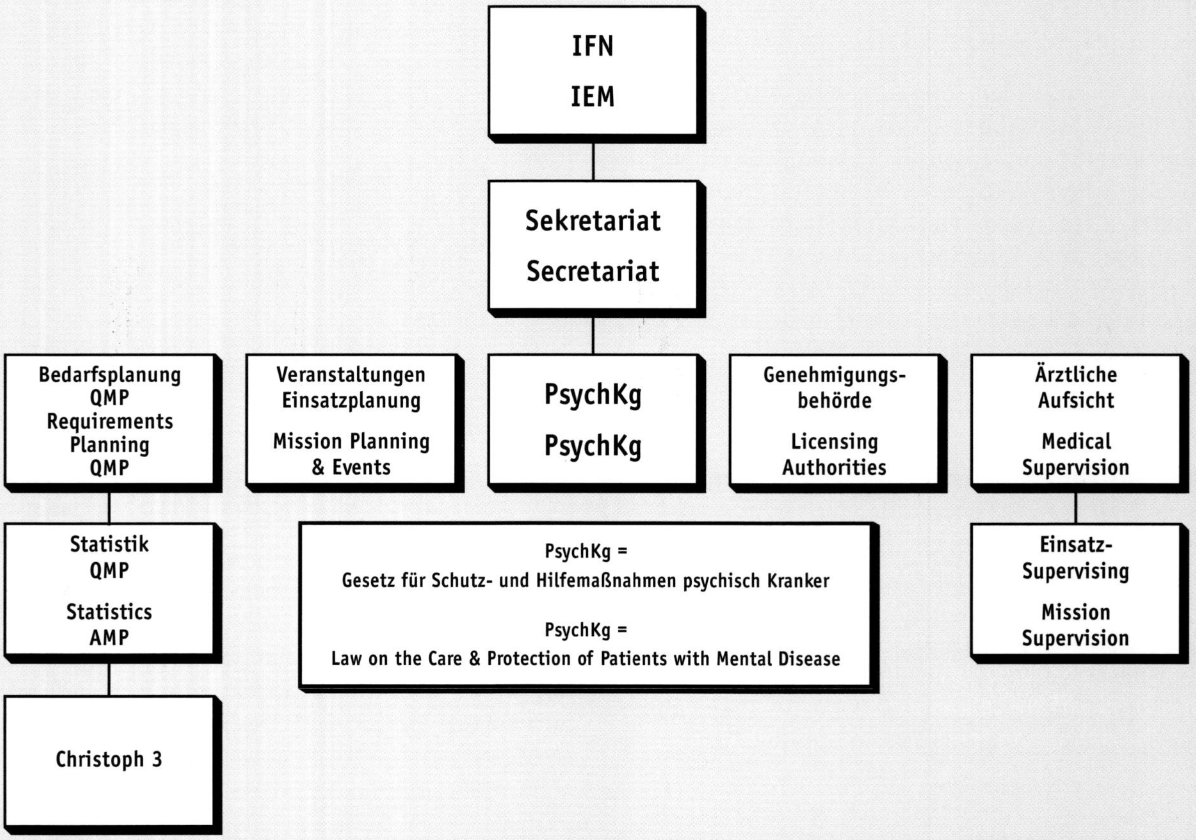

Abbildung 1: Organigramm des Instituts für Notfallmedizin der Berufsfeuerwehr Köln, Scheibenstrasse 13, 50737 Köln

Fig. 1: Organization Chart of the Institute of Emergency Medicine of the Cologne Professional Fire Service, Scheibenstrasse 13, 50737 Cologne, Germany

Die ersten Einsätze

von Wolfgang Nowak

21. Dezember 1971 – Ein ganz besonderes Geschenk macht kurz vor Weihnachten der damalige Bundesinnenminister Hans-Dietrich Genscher, als er in Köln den ersten Rettungshubschrauber des Katastrophenschutzes in Dienst stellt. Im wahrsten Sinne des Wortes als „Feldversuch“ startet Christoph 3 (damals noch „Johannes- Köln 1“ gerufen) im ersten Jahr vom Feld-/ Segelflugplatz Leverkusen-Kurtekotten aus. „Feldmäßig“ ist auch die Verpflegung. Vom Malteser-Krankenhaus Köln-Mülheim, das auch die Notärzte stellt, wird das Mittagessen in einem alten VW-Käfer zur RTH-Besatzung gebracht. Soll es noch warm ankommen, werden bei der rasenden Fahrt spätestens auf den letzten 300m holprigen Feldwegs die Portionen stark dezimiert.

Von den Piloten des Bundesgrenzschutzes sind erst wenige auf den neuen Hubschraubertyp BO 105 umgeschult. Herbert Klein kommt von der Fliegerstaffel Küste, um 2 Wochen lang „Christoph 3“ zu fliegen. Schon am dritten Tag beherrscht dichter Nebel das Wetter im Raum Köln/Bonn. Arzt und Sani warten vergebens auf den dritten Mann zum Skat, bei dem der Küchendienst „ausgespielt“ wird. Doch dann ein vertrautes Geräusch, und plötzlich taucht aus dem Nebel die Silhouette der BO vor dem Fenster der Luftaufsichtsbaracke auf. Seitdem hält sich hartnäckig das Gerücht: Herbert Klein fliegt noch, selbst wenn die Vögel schon zu Fuß gehen.

The First Rescue Missions

by Wolfgang Nowak

On December 21, 1971 – a few days before Christmas – Hans-Dietrich Genscher, then German Minister of the Interior, made the inhabitants of Germany a very special Christmas present by inaugurating the country's first rescue helicopter within the framework of disaster relief services. The first missions of the rescue helicopter "Christoph 3" (still called "Johannes Cologne 1" at that time) represented "field trials" in the truest sense of the world. The helicopter took off literally from an open field at the Leverkusen-Kurtekotten gliding field. The food service was also reminiscent of the military. A warm lunch was delivered to the rescue helicopter crew every noon from the kitchen of the Malteser Hospital in Cologne-Mülheim, the same hospital that supplied the physicians with emergency & rescue certification for the helicopter missions. The food was transported in an ancient VW beetle. Even on the rare occasions when the food was still warm by the time it reached the flying field, the portions were decimated by the rough ride at breakneck speed down the last 300 m of bumpy dirt road.

The rescue helicopter "pioneers" went on missions with the handful of German Border Police pilots who had undergone further training qualifying them to fly the new helicopter type BO 105.

Herbert Klein was sent to Cologne by the Coastal Flying Squadron to fly "Christoph 3" for two weeks. On the third day after his arrival, the Cologne-Bonn area was covered by fog as thick as pea soup. The doctor and emergency medical technician were waiting without much hope for the third man they needed to play a hand of "skat" – it had been agreed that the loser had to do the washing up. Suddenly, they heard a familiar noise; they looked out of the window of the air controller's barracks and saw the silhouette of the BO emerging from the fog. That was the day Hubert Klein gained his reputation as a pilot who would fly on days when even the birds decided to go on foot.

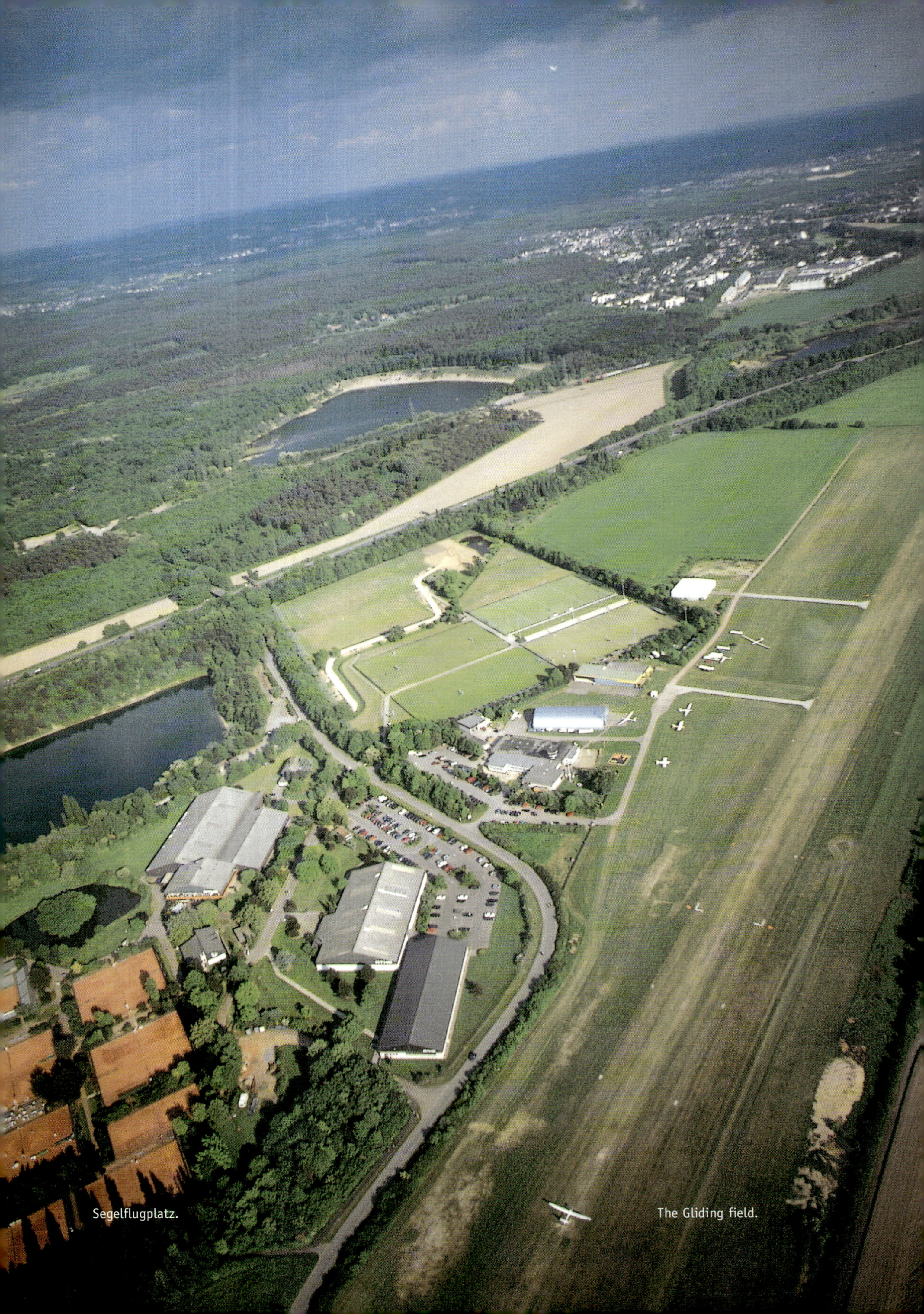

Segelflugplatz.

The Gliding field.

Der Modellversuch Rettungshubschrauber
The Rescue Helicopter Model Program

von/by Ernst Brück

Nach 30 Jahren Luftrettungsdienst spricht niemand mehr über die Anfangsschwierigkeiten. An den Pioniergeist der damaligen Zeit erinnert auch heute noch vieles. Gestartet als zunächst ungeliebtes Kind der Landesregierung, der Stadt und der Anrainer am Standort hat sich der Rettungshubschrauber heute als fester Bestandteil des Rettungsdienstes bewährt. Es war auch der feste Glaube an dieses Rettungsmittel,der alle Beteiligten der Aufbaujahre zusammenschweißte und Skeptiker und Gegner von der Einsatzeffektivität dieses Rettungsmittels letztendlich überzeugte.

Am 21.12.1971 wurde der Rettungshubschrauber Christoph 3 mit dem Funkrufnamen Johannes-Köln-1 und mit dem legendären Hubschrauberkennzeichen D-HDOC durch den damaligen Bundesinnenminister Hans-Dietrich Genscher im Rahmen eines Modellversuchs im Beisein zahlreicher Persönlichkeiten auf dem Segelflugplatz Leverkusen nahe der Kölner Stadtgrenze dem damaligen Leiter des Malteser Hilfsdienstes (MHD), Graf Landsberg-Velen, übergeben und in Dienst gestellt. Zeitgleich ereignete sich auf der nahen Autobahn ein schwerer Verkehrsunfall mit tödlichen Folgen, ohne dass der RTH gerufen wurde. Das neue Rettungsmittel Hubschrauber war den eingesetzten Polizeibeamten zu diesem Zeitpunkt noch suspekt und fremd. Man hatte Angst, zu den Kosten herangezogen zu werden.

Nach Indienststellung wurde der leitende Beamte der Autobahnpolizei tätig und informierte seine Kollegen über den Einsatz des Rettungshubschraubers. So geschah es nicht wieder, dass bei solch schweren Verkehrsunfällen auf der Autobahn der Rettungshubschrauber nicht gerufen wurde. Die Polizei war bis zum Inkrafttreten des Landesrettungsgesetzes geradezu Anwalt für den Einsatz des RTH und es ist besonders ihr mitzuverdanken, dass der RTH schnell einen Platz in der Bevölkerung erhielt.

Die Akzeptanz in der Region war geteilt. In einigen Landkreisen war man dankbar auf dieses Rettungsmittel zurückgreifen zu können, da die Dichte der bodengebundenen Notärzte nicht so hoch wie heute war. Man bedauerte es, dass der RTH nicht auch noch nachts kommen konnte. Andere Kreise, Krankenhäuser und Rettungs-

After 30 years of air rescue service in Germany, no one talks any more about the teething problems of the "rescue helicopter model". The pioneer days of helicopter rescue are still vivid in the memories of the rescue helicopter pioneers, however. From its origins as a project viewed with skepticism by the state government, the Cologne city government, and the owners of property abutting the helicopter base, the rescue helicopter service has grown to become an accepted part of the rescue system. It was, in fact, the firm belief in this type of rescue which welded together all the participants in those early years and ultimately convinced both skeptics and opponents of the effectiveness of helicopters for rescue missions.

On 21 December 1971 the rescue helicopter Christoph 3 with the radio call "Johannes-Cologne-1" and the legendary helicopter ID "D-HDOC" was inaugurated by the former Minister of the Interior Hans-Dietrich Genscher within the scope of a model program. A large audience and numerous VIPs attended the inauguration ceremony held at the Leverkusen Gliding Field near the Cologne city limits. At this ceremony, Genscher officially commissioned Christoph 3 and handed it over to Count Landsberg-Velen, then Director of the Malteser Hilfsdienst (MDH). Almost simultaneously, a serious automobile accident took place on the nearby autobahn in which several persons were killed. The rescue helicopter was not called in; the police officers who rushed to the scene still viewed the rescue helicopter with suspicion and mistrust. There was also a certain fear that any organization which called in a rescue helicopter would have to pay part of the resulting costs.

Once the rescue helicopter was officially in service, however, the highest ranking police officer on the autobahn police force mounted his own information campaign. This police officer explained the role of the rescue helicopter to all of his colleagues; after that, the police never failed to summon the rescue helicopter to the scene of a serious accident on the autobahn. The police were, in fact, the main advocates of the employment of the rescue helicopter prior to the enactment of the State Rescue Law and they deserve a large part of the credit for the acceptance the rescue helicopter soon enjoyed among the general population.

The initial reaction to the rescue helicopter was mixed. In several rural districts, the population was grateful for this new rescue possibility – especially since the network of physicians with emergency & rescue certification on the ground was not as tightly meshed as it is today. The members of this group were sad that the rescue helicopter

wachen hatten Angst, der RTH würde ihnen Patienten wegnehmen.

Die Aufbauarbeit der ersten Jahre wurde getragen von einem beispiellosen Pioniergeist aller am Luftrettungsdienst Beteiligten.Der Glaube an dieses Rettungsmittel und seinen Nutzen für die Bevölkerung war und ist bis heute geblieben. Neben der großen Akzeptanz des RTH bei der Polizei war es auch der Bezirksregierung zu verdanken, dass der RTH eingesetzt wurde. Immer wieder ließen sich leitende Beamte bei Einsätzen mit offensichtlich Schwerstverletzten darüber berichten, warum der RTH nicht gerufen worden ist.So wichtig dieses Nachhaken für die Arbeit des RTH war, so problematisch war es für die Zusammenarbeit mit den bodengebundenen Rettungskräften. Hier bedurfte es eines langen Atems in der Aufklärungsarbeit für die Luftrettung bei Krankenhäusern und Rettungsdiensten.

Ganz andere Schwierigkeiten warteten auf die Beteiligten auf der Suche nach einem festen Standort. Vom Segelfluggelände der ersten Tage suchte man Kontakt zu dem Heilig-Geist Krankenhaus, dass dem Malteser Hilfsdienst sehr nahe stand. Ordensschwestern und Chefärzte sagten nach einer gewissen Bedenkzeit ihre Unterstützung zu. Aus leidvoller Erfahrung mit Anrainern waren sie bezüglich einer Zustimmung sehr zurückhaltend. Hervorzuheben ist hier eine Ordensschwester, die dem Ansinnen sehr skeptisch gegenüberstand. Erst als der Grenzschutzpilot sie zu einem Rundflug über Köln und zu den Türmen des Kölner Doms einlud, wich die Skepsis und sie unterstützte nachhaltig das Stationierungsersuchen.

Anrainer und ein Ortsverein beschwerten sich recht schnell über Geräusch- und Geruchsbelästigung. Es wurde der gerichtliche Klageweg beschritten, der vor dem Oberverwaltungsgericht letztinstanzlich endete. Das Oberverwaltungsgericht wies daraufhin, dass das Interesse der Öffentlichkeit an der Aufrechterhaltung des Hubschrauber-Rettungsdienstes vorrangige Berücksichtigung gegenüber dem privaten Interesse der Antragsteller verdiene, von Lärmbelästigung freizubleiben, da es sich beim Luftrettungsdienst um eine humanitäre Einrichtung von weit tragender Bedeutung handle. Die Anbindung des Rettungshubschraubers an ein Krankenhaus erhöhe die Effektivität und sei sinnvoll.

could not fly at night. However, there were other districts, hospitals and rescue stations which viewed the rescue helicopter as a competitor who might take patients away from them.

The work of building up the rescue helicopter system in those early days was propelled by the unprecedented pioneering spirit displayed by everyone involved in air rescue. The belief in this rescue modality and in its value for the population has remained unchanged. In addition to the police, among whose ranks the rescue helicopter enjoyed a high degree of acceptance from the start, the district government was instrumental in promoting the use of the rescue helicopter. Repeatedly, high-ranking officials in the district government asked why the helicopter had not been called in to serious accidents with severely injured persons. As valuable as this insistence was to the rescue helicopter crews on the one hand, it did not make the collaboration with the land-based rescue crews any easier. During this difficult transition period, the rescue helicopter crews learned to take the long view and await the results of information campaigns mounted among hospital and rescue service personnel to explain the role played by air rescue on the overall rescue scene.

Another major problem confronting the air rescue pioneers was the search for a fixed base. From their first temporary quarters at the gliding field, the rescue helicopter team took up contact to Heilig-Geist [Holy Spirit] Hospital, an institution with which the Malteser Hilfsdienst maintained excellent relations. After asking for time to consider, the medical directors and the Catholic nuns running the hospital pledged their support. The hospital administrators were skeptical on the basis of their previous negative experience with the hospital's neighbors. One nun, in particular, viewed the project with intense mistrust. Her skepticism turned to ardent support, however, after the helicopter pilot from the Federal Border Police invited her to a helicopter flight over Cologne topped off by a spin around the towers of Cologne Cathedral. After this flight the nun staunchly backed the rescue helicopter's efforts to obtain approval for the establishment of a rescue helicopter base at the hospital.

Owners of abutting properties and a local citizen's group were quick to complain about the air and noise pollution caused by the helicopter. The resulting litigation went all the way to the Higher Administrative Court (OVG). This court ruled that the public interest in the maintenance of the helicopter rescue service took priority over the right of the parties initiating the action not to suffer from noise pollution. In its explanation of this ruling, the court pointed out that the air rescue service is a humanitarian institution of far-reaching importance. The stationing of

Ein weiterer Umzug wurde dennoch erforderlich und es gelang unbürokratisch, auf dem Gelände der belgischen Streitkräfte etwa einen Kilometer Luftlinie vom alten Standort aus ein neues Refugium zu finden. In einem angekauften Bauwagen wurde die Crew untergebracht und musste unter schwierigen Umständen vorerst von dort aus den Rettungsdienst versehen. Täglich wurden zwei Transferflüge bei Dienstbeginn von Hangelar nach Köln und nach Dienstende zurück erforderlich. Bei allen Unzulänglichkeiten waren die Beteiligten jedoch froh,dass der Luftrettungsdienst ohne Einschränkungen fortgesetzt werden konnte.

Seit nahezu zwanzig Jahren fliegt der Rettungshubschrauber nun von dem bisher letzten Standort am Krankenhaus Köln-Merheim aus und wieder scheint sich eine Veränderung abzuzeichnen: In der Diskussion um Landeplatzvorschriften und dem Neubau einer großen Siedlung um den Standort herum wird die Einrichtung eines Dachlandeplatzes nicht ausgeschlossen. Es bleibt den nachfolgenden Chronisten vorbehalten, die Entwicklung seit den ersten Tagen hier fortzuführen.

a rescue helicopter at a hospital increased the effectiveness of this service and was a justifiable measure.

Nevertheless, the rescue helicopter crew had to move again. They succeeded in finding a new home – with a minimum of bureaucracy – on the grounds of a Belgian military base located about one kilometer as the crow flies from their former base. The crew's new quarters consisted of a second-hand construction-site trailer. The helicopter made the transfer flight from Hangelar to Cologne every morning and from Cologne to Hangelar every evening. Despite these difficult circumstances, all participants was glad that the air rescue service could be continued without any restrictions.

For almost 20 years now, the rescue helicopter has been stationed at its (up to now) last base, Cologne-Merheim Hospital. Now there is talk of a major change. In the wake of the discussion of landing site regulations and the construction of a large housing estate near the site, consideration is being given to the erection of a rooftop heliport. It will be up to future chronicle-writers to carry on the story of the rescue helicopter which began in those early days.

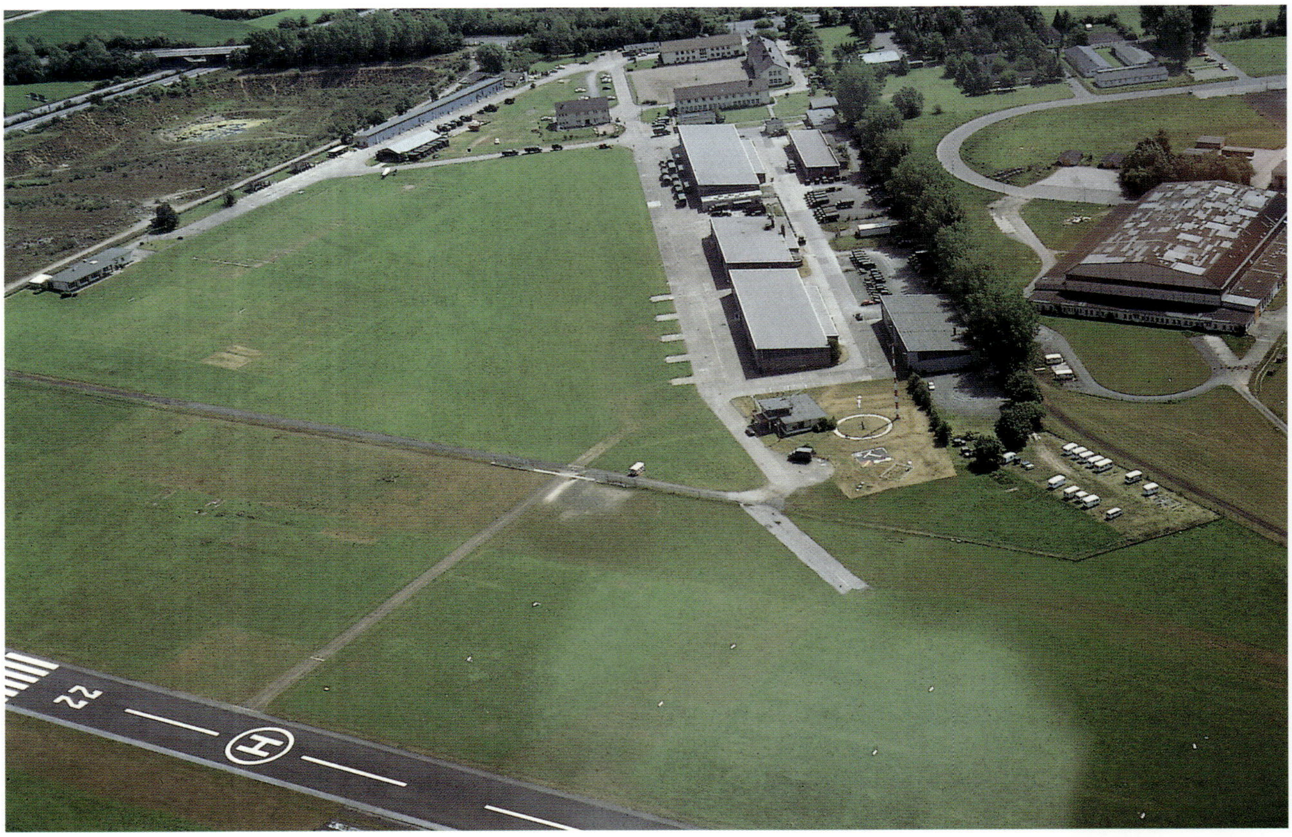

Der Flugplatz Butzweilerhof, unser Refugium von 1979 bis 1983.

Butzweilerhof Flying Field. Our home from 1979 to 1983.

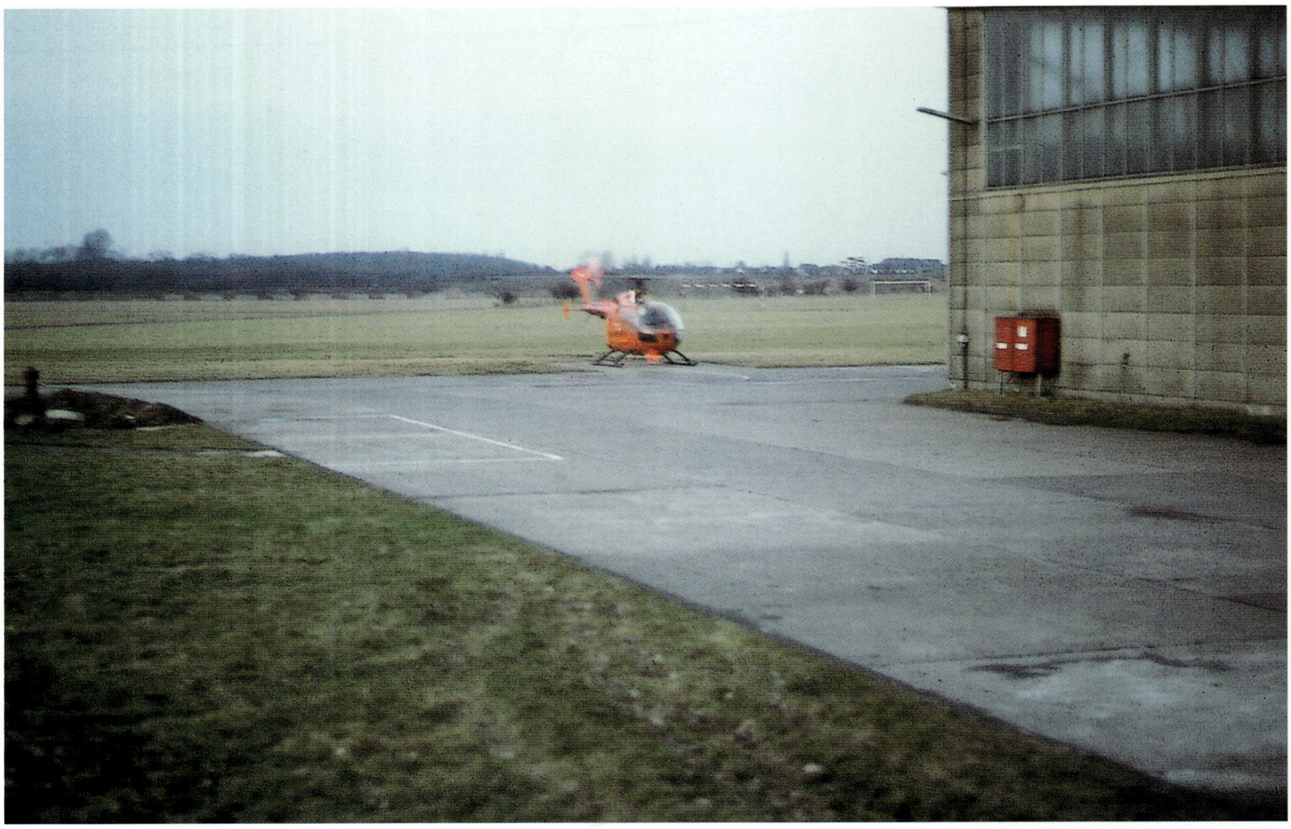

Der Blick aus dem Bauwagen auf den Hubschrauber.

View of the helicopter from inside the construction-site trailer.

Die Bauwagenzeit des RTH
The Early Days of Air Rescue

von/by Peter Simon

In dem oben erwähnten Zeitraum startete der Rettungshubschrauber Christoph 3 nicht von einem Standortkrankenhaus, sondern von dem Gelände Butzweilerhof der belgischen Streitkräfte. Dieser Flugplatz war seinerzeit in einen militärischen und in einen zivilen Bereich unterteilt, wobei Christoph 3 auf dem militärischen Teil stationiert war. Dieser unterstand den belgischen Streitkräften, die dort ebenfalls Hubschrauber und Flugzeuge stationiert hatten. Es handelte sich um ein umzäuntes und vom Militär bewachtes Gelände, das nur nach vorheriger Anmeldung beim diensthabenden Wachposten betreten werden durfte. Alle Besatzungsmitglieder hatten spezielle Ausweise, die jedesmal beim Betreten und Verlassen des Geländes registriert wurden.

Der Hubschrauber überflog ohne Notarzt und Sani an jedem Morgen um 6.30 Uhr, nur mit dem Piloten besetzt, das Wachgebäude, um danach auf einer vom militärischen Tower vorgegebenen Position zu landen. Nach Sonnenuntergang geschah dieses Verfahren in umgekehrter Reihenfolge, wobei die Maschine dann zum Standort der Bundesgrenzschutzfliegergruppe in Hangelar zurückflog. Dies hatte zur Folge, dass „Christoph 3" in der Regel nicht bei seiner kleinen Luftrettungsstation Butzweiler übernachtete, sondern jeden Morgen und jeden Abend diesen Transferflug durchführen mußte. Gründe hierfür waren u.a. ein fehlender Hangar, die dann von den Technikern des Bundesgrenzschutzes in St. Augustin-Hangelar durchgeführt werden konnten.

Die eben erwähnte kleine Luftrettungsstation bestand anfangs aus einem alten Funkwagen mit Hanomag-Fahrgestell der 5,5 Tonnenklasse. Dieses ältere, geländegängige Fahrzeug war seitens der Malteser vom Bundesgrenzschutz erworben und in Eigenleistung zu einem sog. Funkwagen umgebaut worden. Im hinteren bzw. Kofferaufbau des Funkwagens waren Tische, Stühle und Beleuchtung eingebaut. Da das Fahrzeug im weiteren über mehrere Sprechfunkgeräte verfügte, wurde somit eine kleine Verbindungsstation zur eigentlichen Einsatzleitstelle auf Funkkanal „Johannes Köln" des Malteser-Hilfsdienstes betrieben. Damit die Besatzung nicht den ganzen Tag in diesem Wagen sitzen mußte,

During the period between 1978 and 1983 the rescue helicopter Christoph 3 was not stationed at a hospital; instead, it took off for missions from the Belgian military base Butzweilerhof. At that time this military airport was divided into a military and a civil aviation sector; Christoph 3 was stationed in the military part. This part of the base fell under the jurisdiction of the Belgian armed forces, who had also stationed helicopters and other aircraft there. The military base is surrounded by a barbed-wire fence and guarded by military personnel; no one is allowed to enter the grounds without reporting to the guard on duty. All of the helicopter crew members had special identity cards; their ID numbers were recorded every time they entered or left the base.

Every morning at around 6.30 a.m. the helicopter – with only the pilot aboard – flew over the guardhouse and landed at the position assigned to it by the military control tower. The physician with emergency & rescue certification and the rescue paramedic were not yet on board. After the sun went down, this sequence of events was repeated in the opposite order. In this case the aircraft flew back to the base of the Aviation Group of the German Border Police in Hangelar. As a consequence, Christoph 3 usually did not spend the night at its small air rescue base in Butzweiler, since it has to carry out this transfer flight every morning and evening. One important reason for this situation, among others, was the extensive maintenance which had to be carried out by flight mechanics of the German Border Police at St. Augustin-Hangelar.

The small air rescue base mentioned above initially consisted of an old radio truck with a Hanomag chassis of the 5.5 ton class. The Malteser Hilfsdienst had bought this older 4WD vehicle from the German Border Police and had converted it themselves into a radio truck. Lights, chairs and a table had been built into the rear part of the truck, which is normally used to carry loads. Since the truck contained several walkie-talkies, it served as a small relay station linking the crew to the Coordination Center over the "Johannes Cologne" radio channel operated by the Malteser-Hilfsdienst. Our Belgian friends

durften wir mit freundlicher Genehmigung der belgischen Freunde deren Gesellschaftsräume (eine kleine Fliegerkneipe) mitbenutzen. Dies war im Winter 1979 von großem Vorteil, da es sich um schneereiche und kalte Wochen handelte. Es passierte in dieser Zeit durchaus des öfteren, daß wir nicht die orangefarbene BO 105, sondern eine grenzschutzgrünlackierte Bell UH-1D zur Verfügung hatten. Dies war immer dann der Fall, wenn eine BO 105 in Reparatur oder Wartung war. Die komplette Ausrüstung nebst den zwei Krankentragen wurden in die Bell geräumt und nach der Landung um 6.30 Uhr auf dem Butzweilerhof durch den Rettungssanitäter (Sani) dann möglichst optimal eingebaut. Da zu der Bell stets ein Bordwart des BGS gehörte, bestand die Besatzung des Christoph 3 an diesen Tagen aus vier Personen. Der Sani saß hinten beim Arzt quer auf einer Bank und das Platzangebot zur Versorgung und Betreuung des Patienten während des Fluges war auf einmal riesig. Die Verwandtschaft dieses Fluggerätes zu den SAR-Maschinen der Bundeswehr (diese flogen ebenfalls Bell UH-1 D) war unverkennbar. Bereits auf dem Hinflug zur Einsatzstelle erkannten Insider des Rettungsdienstes im laufenden Funkverkehr das vibrierende Geräusch in der Stimme des funkenden Sanis oder Bordwartes. Ein typisches Zeichen für die Bell UH-1 D. Auch der Anflug auf die Einsatzstelle war von dem typischen „Flapp-Flapp" begleitet. Die Landeplätze mußten etwas größer als üblich sein und der Rotorabstrahl einer Bell UH-1 D ist auch nicht zu unterschätzen. Da wir in Köln seit Anfang der 80iger Jahre vermehrt Einsätze im Stadtgebiet fliegen, waren wir jedoch nicht unglücklich, wenn wir unsere alte organgefarbene BO 105 wieder zur Verfügung hatten. Der sehr wendige und etwas kleinere Hubschrauber bietet hier doch große Vorteile.

Nach einigen Wochen Behelfsunterkunft im Funkwagen und in der Kneipe der Belgier wurde uns als eigene Behelfsunterkunft ein Bauwagen mit Strom- und Wasseranschluß sowie Gasversorgung mit einem LKW auf den Butzweilerhof gezogen. Dieser Bauwagen, der ansonsten für Großbaustellen zur behelfsmäßigen Unterbringung von Architekten, Büros etc. dient, wurde links neben dem Tower der belgischen Streitkräfte abgestellt. Er sollte dort vier Jahre lang als Unterkunft dienen. Im Inneren war er mit einem eingebauten Schreibtisch, zwei Funkgeräten, einem Telefonanschluß in der einen Ecke ausgestattet. In der anderen Hälfte dieser

generously allows us to use their social facilities (consisting at that time of a small pilot's pub) so that the helicopter crew did not have to sit in the radio truck all day. This invitation was greatly appreciated during the long, cold and snowy winter of 1979. During this period, we frequently flew with a Bell UH-1 D painted green, the color of the German Border Police, instead of our orange BO 105. This was always the case when a BO 105 was being repaired or serviced. Our complete equipment, including two stretchers, was loaded into the Bell; after the aircraft landed at Butzweilerhof around 6.30 a.m., the emergency medical technician had the job of fitting all of the equipment in the helicopter in an optimal manner. Since the Bell always had a flight technician from the German Border Police on board, the crew of Christoph 3 consisted of four persons on those days. After the emergency medical technician has taken his or her seat on a bench directly behind the pilot, there was suddenly a huge amount of space available for taking care of patients during the flight. The similarity between this aircraft and the SAR helicopters of the German Army (who also flew Bell UH-1 D helicopters) was undeniable. On the helicopter's flight to the scene of an emergency, rescue service insiders already recognized the telltale vibrato in the radio voice of the EMT or flight technician. This was an unmistakable sign of the Bell UH-1 D. Another typical characteristic of this aircraft was the "flap-flap" noise heard during the approach. The landing site had to be a bit larger than usual and the rotor wash of a Bell UH-1 D should not be underestimated. Since we had to fly an increased number of missions in urban areas in Cologne starting in the early 1980s, however, we were not sad when we had to use our old orange BO again. This very maneuverable and somewhat smaller helicopter has great advantages for rescue work in cities.

After spending several weeks in provisional quarters consisting of the radio truck and the Belgian pilots' pub, a construction-site trailer was towed onto the Butzweiler Hof for our own use; this new accommodation, although also provisional, boasted its own electricity, water and gas supply. The trailer – which normally housed architects and office personnel on large construction sites – was parked next to the Belgian military control tower. The trailer was to be our home for four years. Inside the trailer, there was a built-in desk, two radio units and a

Unterkunft befanden sich ein kleines Materiallager, ein WC und im Rahmen des Aufenthaltsbereiches war noch eine kleine Junggesellenküche vorhanden, die sogar über einen Elektroboiler zur Warmwasseraufbereitung verfügte. Im Winter fror uns regelmäßig die Gasleitung ein und im Sommer war es in dieser nur mäßig isolierten Unterkunft sehr warm. Wir verlagerten dann unsere Aktivitäten sehr oft auf die Wiese, wo wir mit Campingstühlen und einem Campingtisch unsere Tage verbrachten. Trotz all dieser Widrigkeiten war es meistens eine schöne Zeit, die den Zusammenhalt des kontinuierlich anwesenden Arztes mit Sani und Pilot in ein sehr kameradschaftliche Bahnen lenkte.

telephone connection in one corner. The other half of the trailer was occupied by a small materials storage area and a W.C. The crew area contained a small efficiency kitchen which even had a hot water boiler. In the winter the gas lines routinely froze up; in the summer it was often unbearably warm inside the poorly insulated trailer. On warm summer days, we often moved outdoors and did our paperwork seated on camping chairs around a foldup table. Despite all these hardships, the crew members who experienced these pioneer days look back with nostalgia to the extraordinary camaraderie between the pilots, physicians and paramedics.

Abfragebogen Sekundärtransporte

Abgebende Klinik:	Adresse, Telefonnummer, Arzt
Patient:	Name, Geburtsdatum, Anamnese, Diagnose
Arzt-Arzt-Gespräch	**(Hubschrauberarzt – Klinikarzt)**
Fragen:	◆ Zweck der Verlegung? ◆ Vitalfunktionen: Atmung, Bewußtsein, Kreislauf? ◆ Venöser Zugang? ◆ Intubation, Beatmung? ◆ Medikation? ◆ Papiere für Verlegung fertig? ◆ Aufnehmende Klinik, Arzt? ◆ Hubschrauberlandeplatz vorhanden?

Questionnaire for Secondary Transport

Hospital of origin:	Address, Phone, Contact physician
Patient:	Name, DOB, History, Diagnosis
Dr.-Dr. discussion:	**(Helicopter physician – hospital physician)**
Questions:	◆ Reason for transfer? ◆ Vital functions: respiration, alertness, cardiovascular system? ◆ Venous access? ◆ Intubation, ventilation? ◆ Medication? ◆ Papers ready for the transfer? ◆ Accepting hospital, physician? ◆ Heliport available?

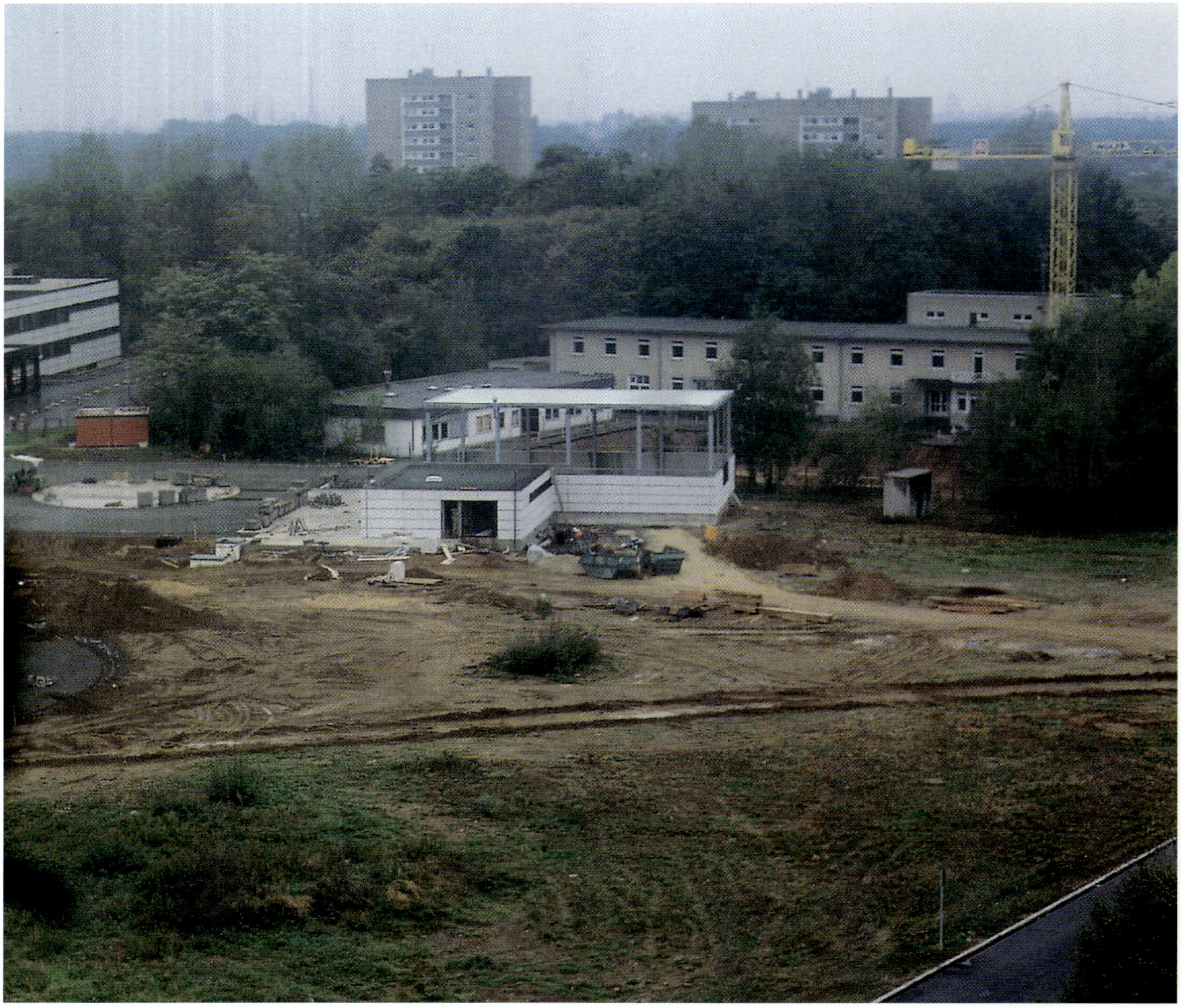

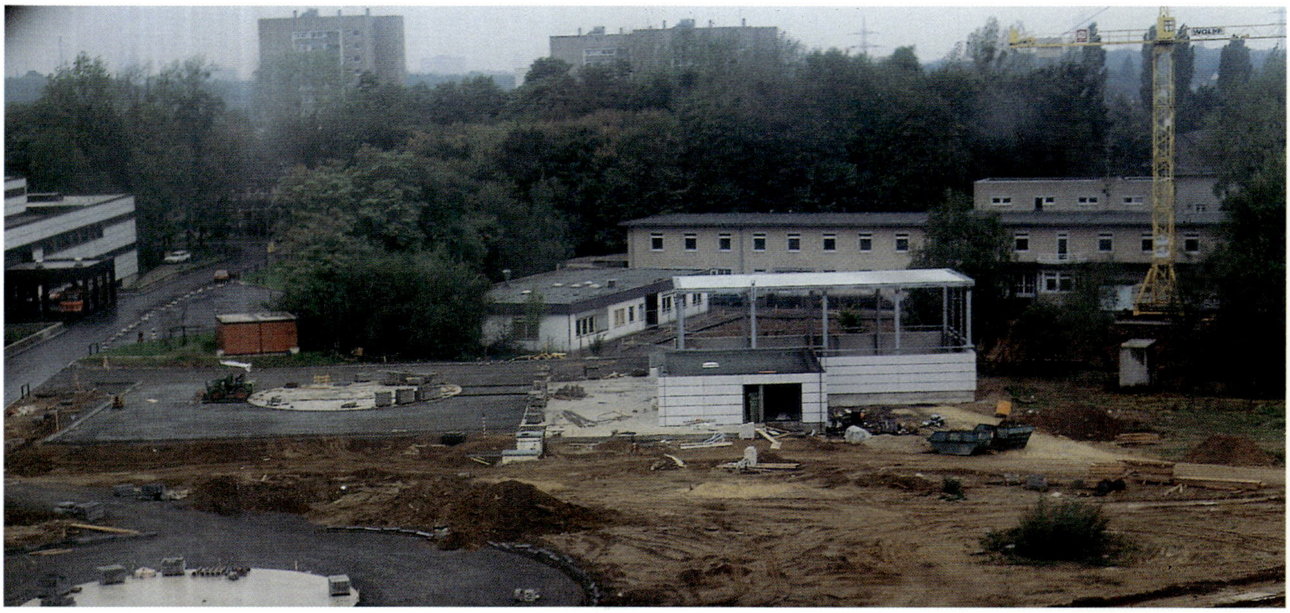

Die Station in Köln-Merheim wird gebaut. Construction of the base in Cologne-Merheim.

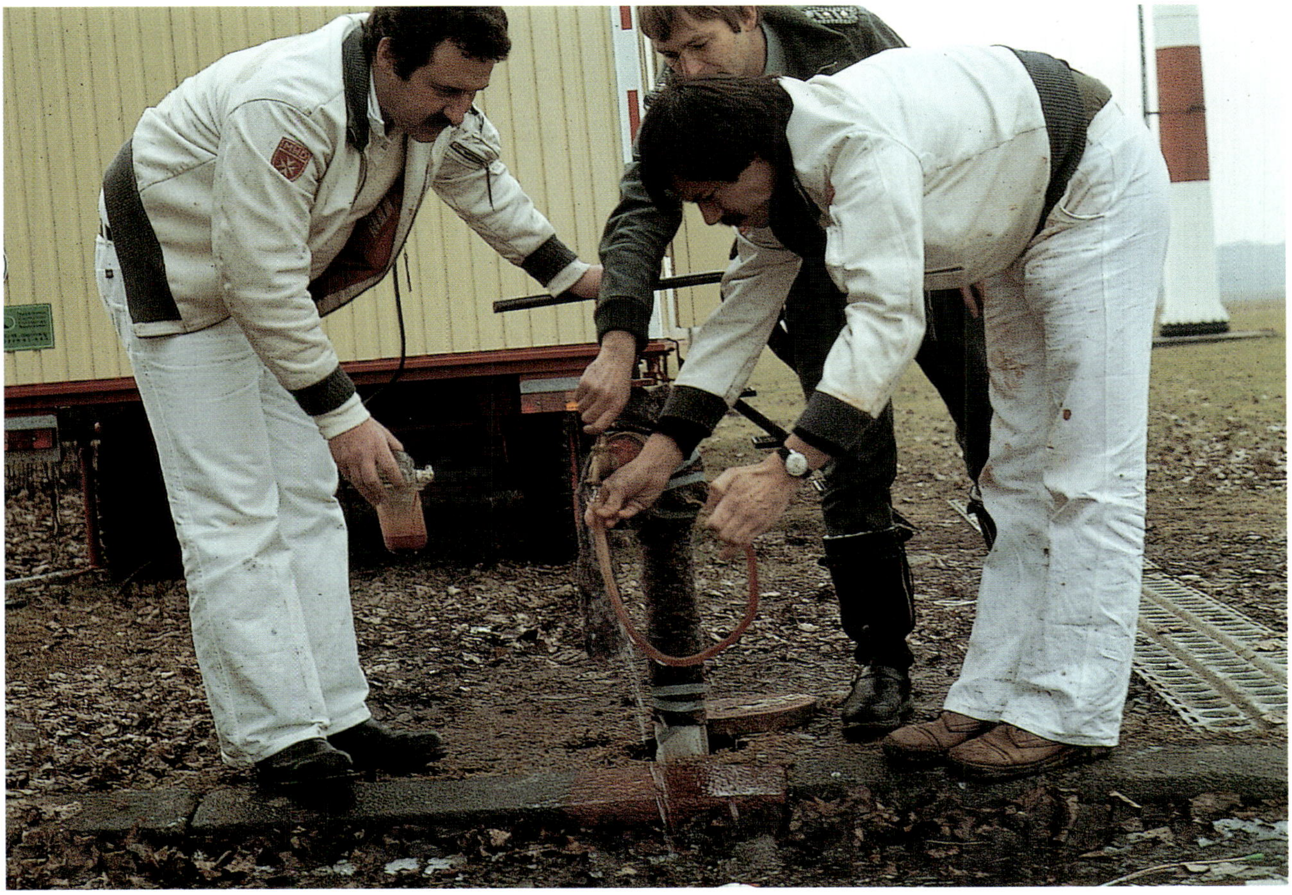

Der Bauwagen. Schwierige Verhältnisse.

The construction-site trailer. Difficult conditions.

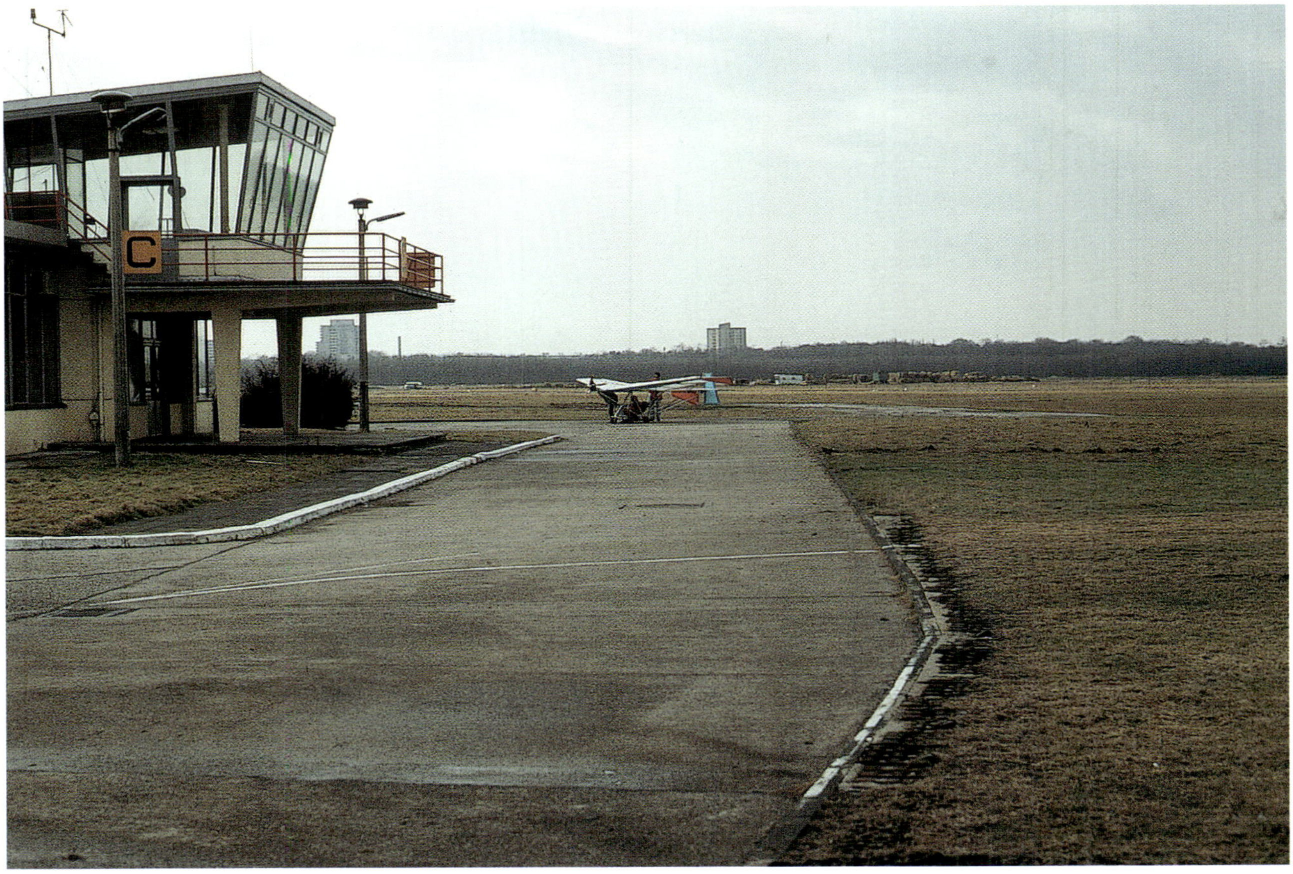

Butz Tower.

Butz Tower.

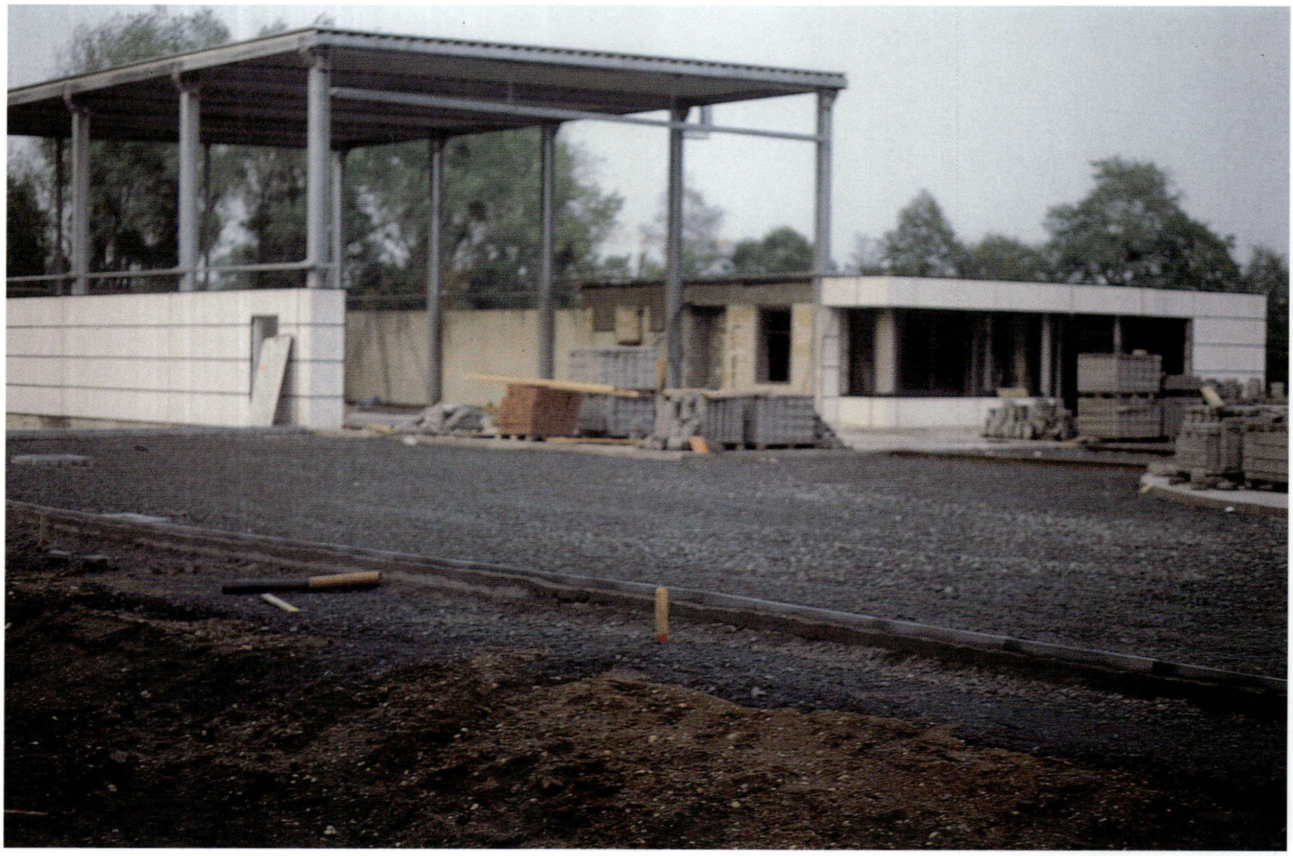

Wann wird die Station wohl fertiggestellt?

When will it ever be finished?

Die häufigsten Fragen an der Einsatzstelle
Frequently Asked Questions

Wieviel Abstrahl entsteht bei Start und Landung des Rettungshubschraubers?

Messen kann man die Stärke des Abstrahls weniger. Man müsste die Windgeschwindigkeit in Stundenkilometern oder in den üblichen Maßen für die Windstärke ausdrücken, dies gibt aber den Eindruck der Verwirbelungen in der Nähe eines startenden und landenden Hubschraubers nicht wieder. Der Abstrahl entsteht durch den Auftrieb, den der Hauptrotor erzeugen muss, um das Abheben zu ermöglichen. Startet der Hubschrauber mit einem tatsächlichen Gewicht von 2200kg, so müssen eben diese 2,2 Tonnen Auftrieb erzeugt werden. Von einem Orkan kann man deshalb in unmittelbarer Nähe wohl sprechen. Und dieser Orkan ist um so größer, je schwerer der Hubschrauber ist.

How much downwash is produced during the takeoff and landing of a rescue helicopter?

It is very difficult to measure the amount of downwash. For this purpose you would have to express the wind velocity in kilometers per hour or in other commonly used measures of wind velocity; however, this would not reproduce the impression of turbulence created in the vicinity of a helicopter that is taking off or landing. The downwash is produced by the lift which has to be generated by the main rotor to enable the helicopter to take off. If the helicopter takes off with an actual weight of 2200 kg, 2.2 tons of lift have to be generated. It is accurate to say that "hurricane-like winds" are generated in the immediate vicinity of a helicopter. The heavier the helicopter, the stronger the hurricane-like winds.

Landeplätze im Einsatz.
Landing sites During Rescue Missions.

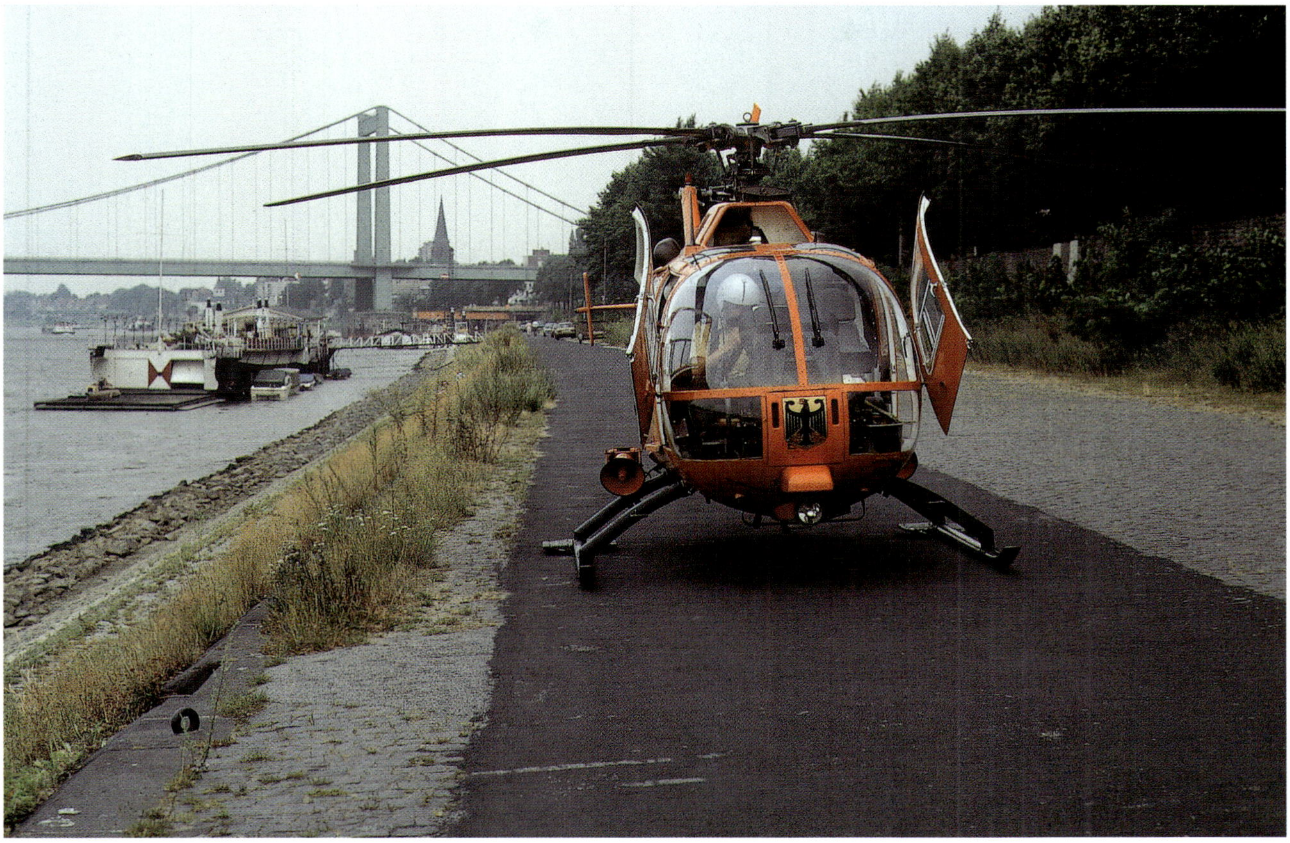

Landeplatz Rheinufer. Ein internistischer Notfall im angrenzenden Dorf.

Landing site on the banks of Rhine. A medical emergency in a nearby village.

Die häufigsten Fragen an der Einsatzstelle
Frequently Asked Questions

Mit welchem Kartenmaterial navigiert die Besatzung des Rettungshubschraubers?

Benutzt werden die vorgeschriebene Luftfahrtkarte im Maßstab 1:500.000, die auch den Autofahrern bekannte Generalkarte 1:200.000 sowie Stadtatlanten. Unterstützt wird die Navigation durch ein Satellitennavigationsgerät, das der Besatzung u.a. den Kurs, die Entfernung und auch die Flugzeit zu einem eingegebenen Ziel sowie eventuelle Abweichungen anzeigt. Diese Technik unterliegt einer ständigen Weiterentwicklung und wird in absehbarer Zeit die üblichen Karten ersetzen.

What kind of maps do the crews of the rescue helicopters use for navigation?

They use the stipulated aerial navigation maps on a scale of 1:500,000, the general maps on a scale of 1:200,000 which are also used by motorists, and city atlases. Today helicopter navigation is supported by a satellite navigation system providing the crew, by means of a display, with important information such as the aircraft's course, the distance and flying time to the stated destination, and possible deviations. This technology is undergoing rapid development and will replace normal maps within the near future.

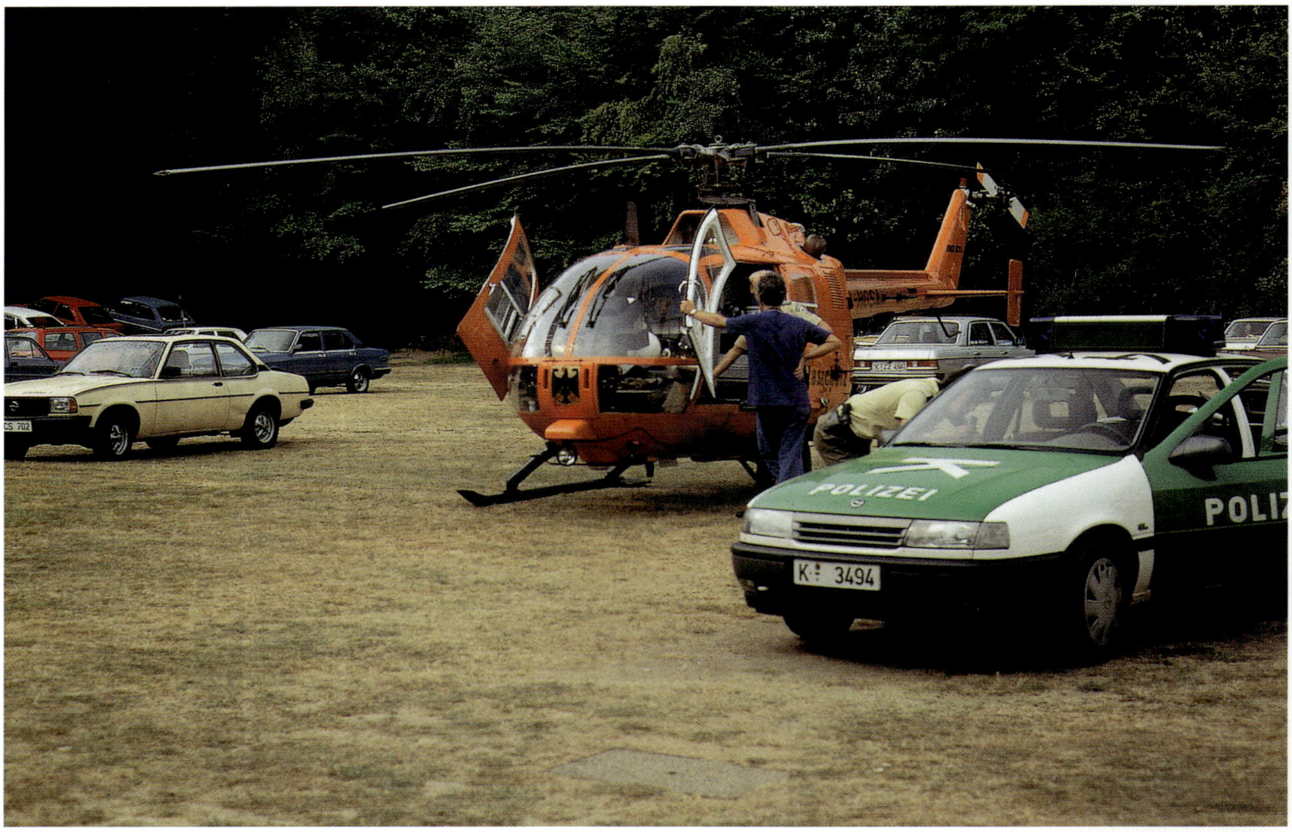

Landeplatz Schwimmbad.
Eine Person schwimmt nahe dem Beckenrand. Kopfsprung einer anderer Person. Querschnittslähmung.

Landing site at a swimming pool.
A person was swimming close to the edge of the pool. Another person dove in head first. Paraplegia resulting from a high-level spinal cord injury.

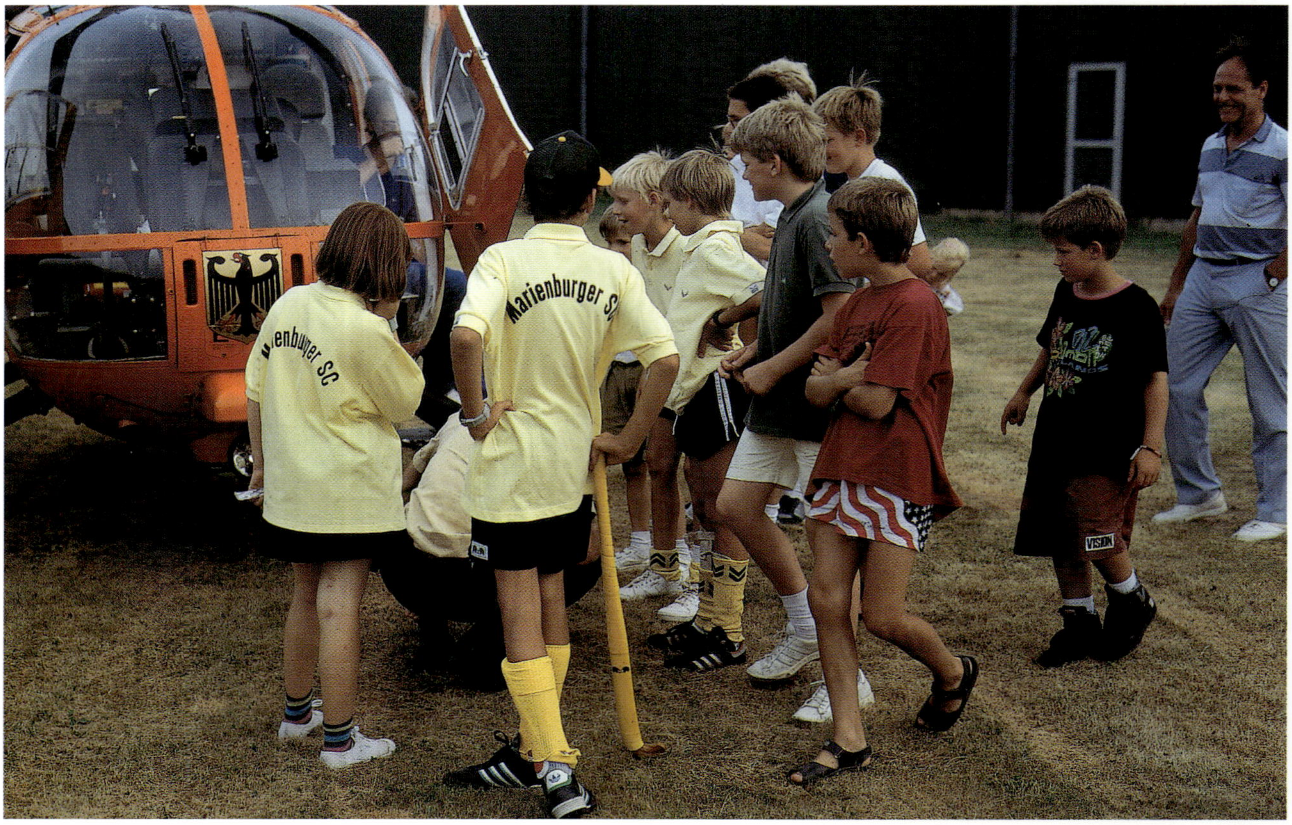

Landeplatz Sportplatz.

Landing site on an athletic field.

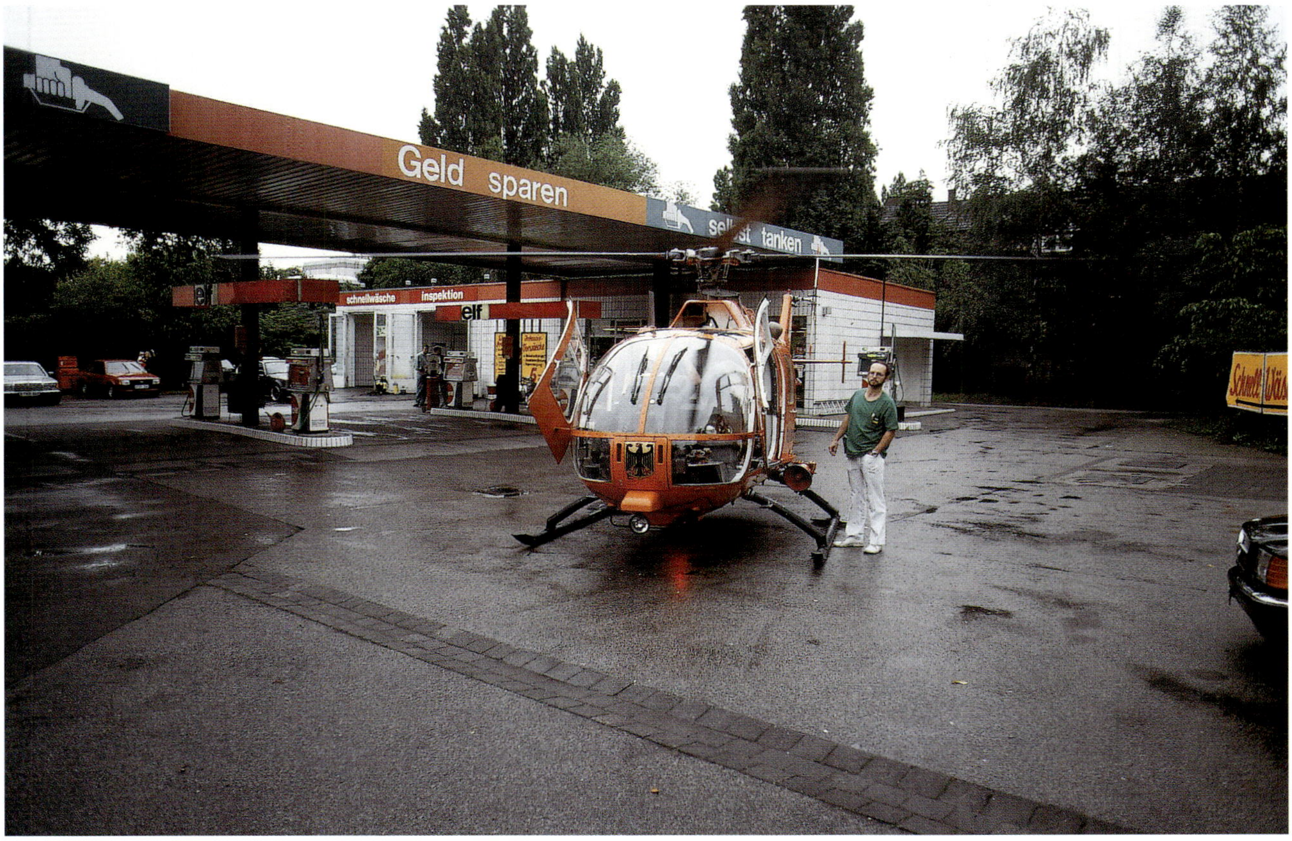

Landeplatz Tankstelle

Landing site at a filling station.

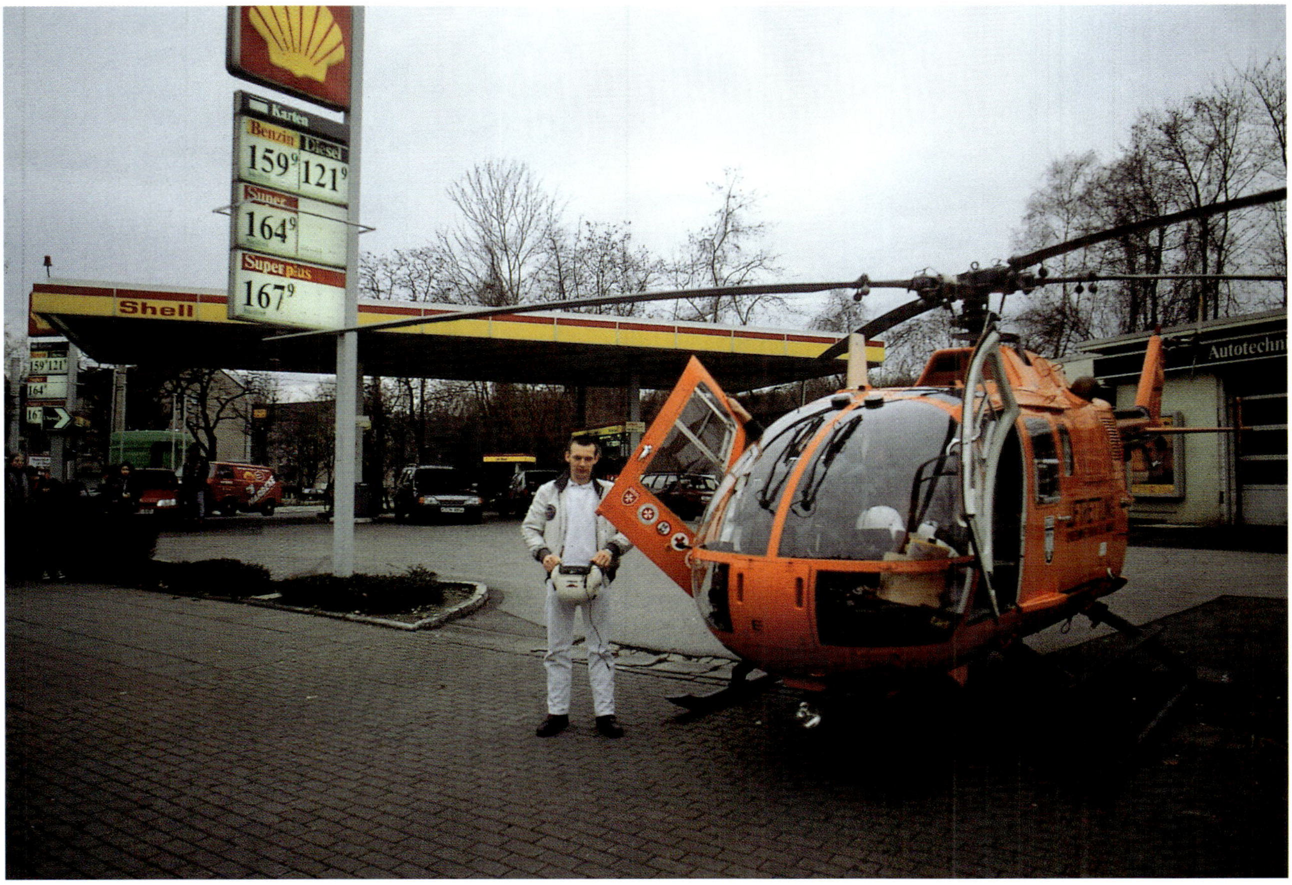

Jahre später. Landeplatz Tankstelle – einzige Änderung: der Preis.

Landing site at a filling station years later – the only thing that has changed is the prices.

Die häufigsten Fragen an der Einsatzstelle
Frequently Asked Questions

Warum tragen alle Rettungshubschrauber den Rufnamen Christoph?

Der Heilige Christopherus (wörtl.: „der Christus trägt") ist in der katholischen Kirche der Schutzpatron der Reisenden und fand sich in Form einer Plakette bis vor nicht allzu langer Zeit in fast jedem Auto. Da eines der ursprünglichen Ziele der Luftrettung die Reduzierung der großen Zahl von Unfalltoten zu Beginn der Siebzigerjahre war, ist dies wohl der Hintergrund der Entstehung dieses Rufnamens.

Why do all the rescue helicopters have the name Christoph?

According to Catholic theology, St. Christopher (literally: "he who carries Christ") is the patron saint of travelers. Until very recently medals or small statues of St. Christopher were found on the dashboards of most automobiles. One of the original reasons for establishing an air rescue service was to reduce the large number of traffic accident fatalities in the early 1970s. Against this background, the name was an apt choice.

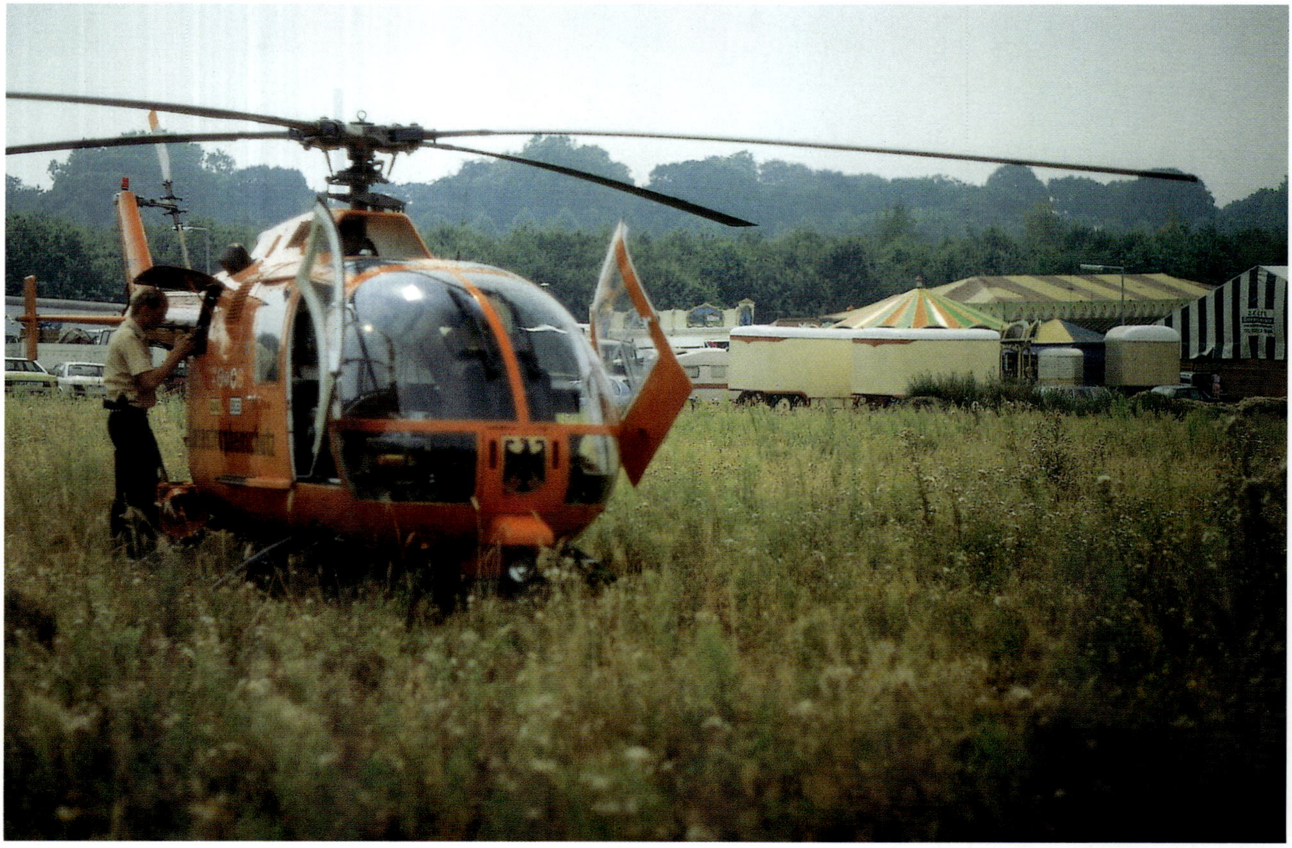

Landeplatz vor der Kirmes

Landing site in front of a carnival.

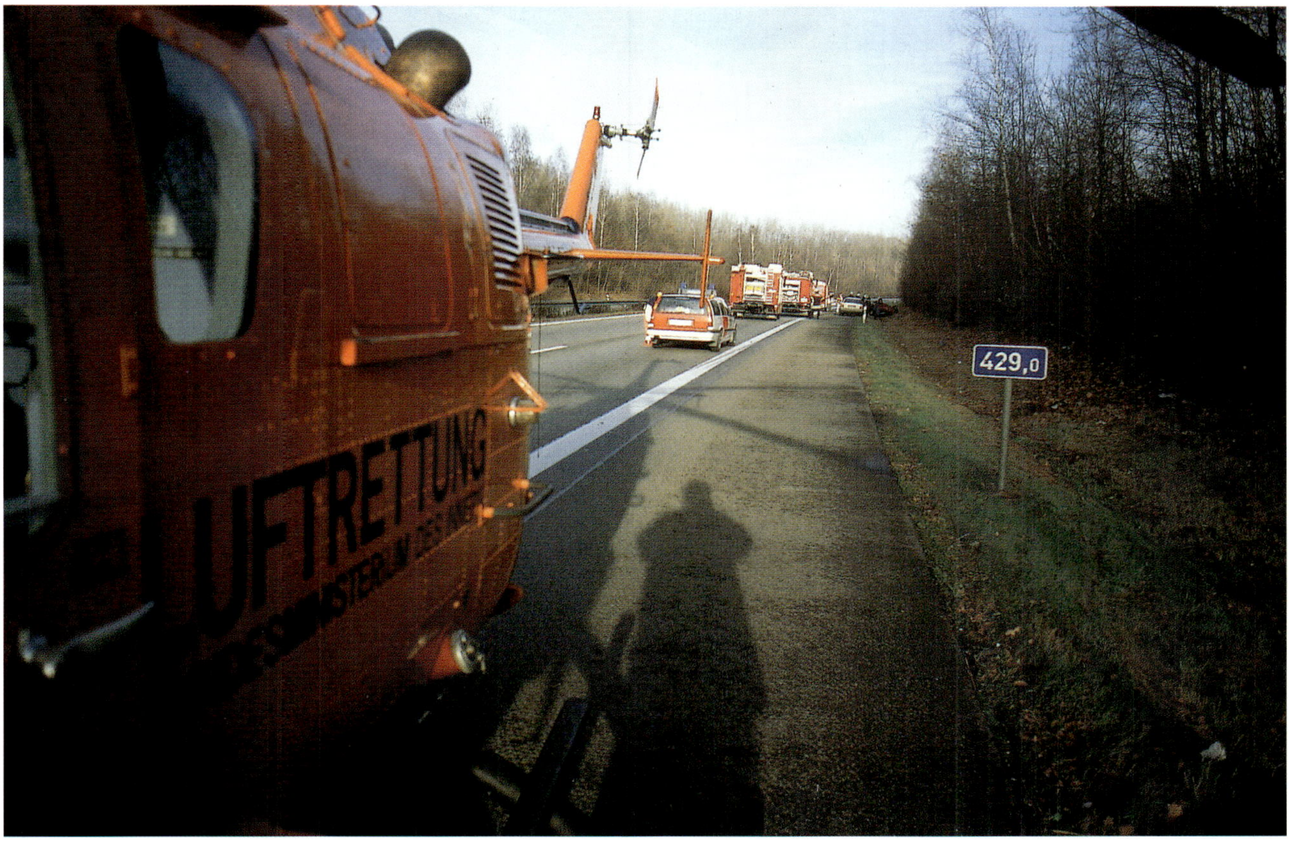

Landeplatz Standstreifen.

Landing site in the emergency lane of a highway.

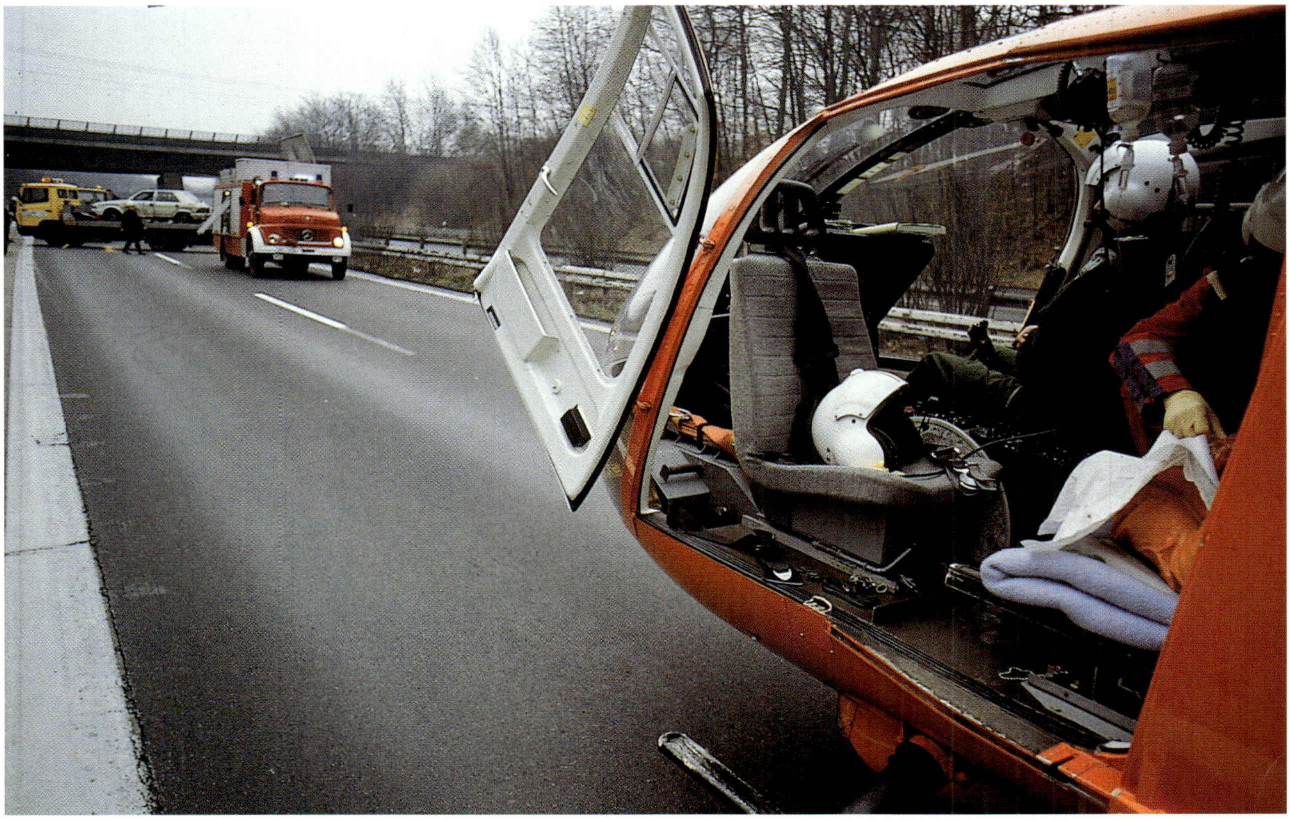

Landeplatz Fahrspur. Der Sitz links vorne ist gedreht, damit beim Patiententransport Notarzt und Luftrettungsassistenten am Kopf des Patienten sind.

Landing site in the traffic lane of a highway. The left front seat is turned so that the physician with emergency & rescue certification and the air rescue paramedic are at the patient's head during the transport flight.

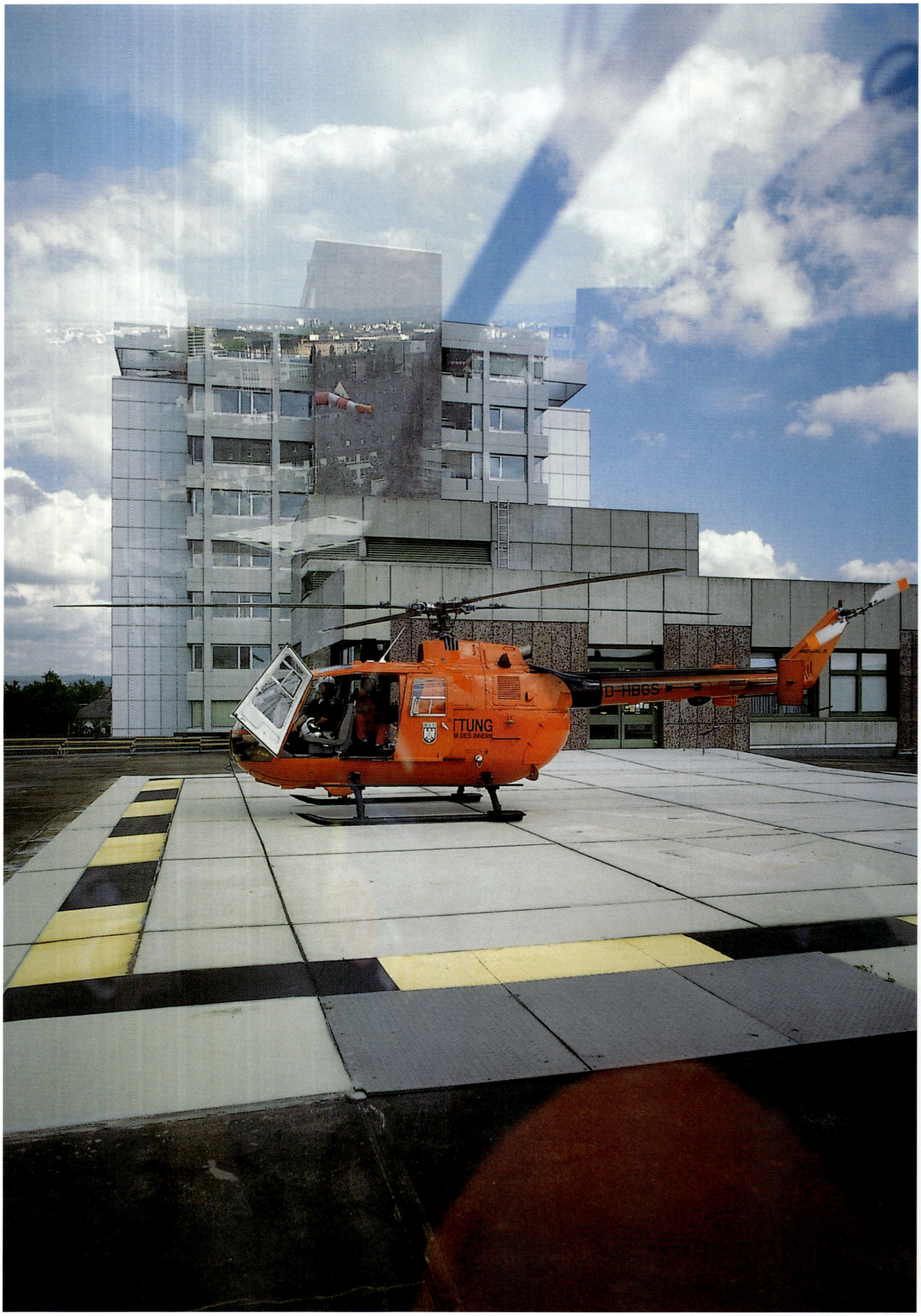

Landeplatz auf dem Dach der Klinik.

Landing site on a hospital roof.

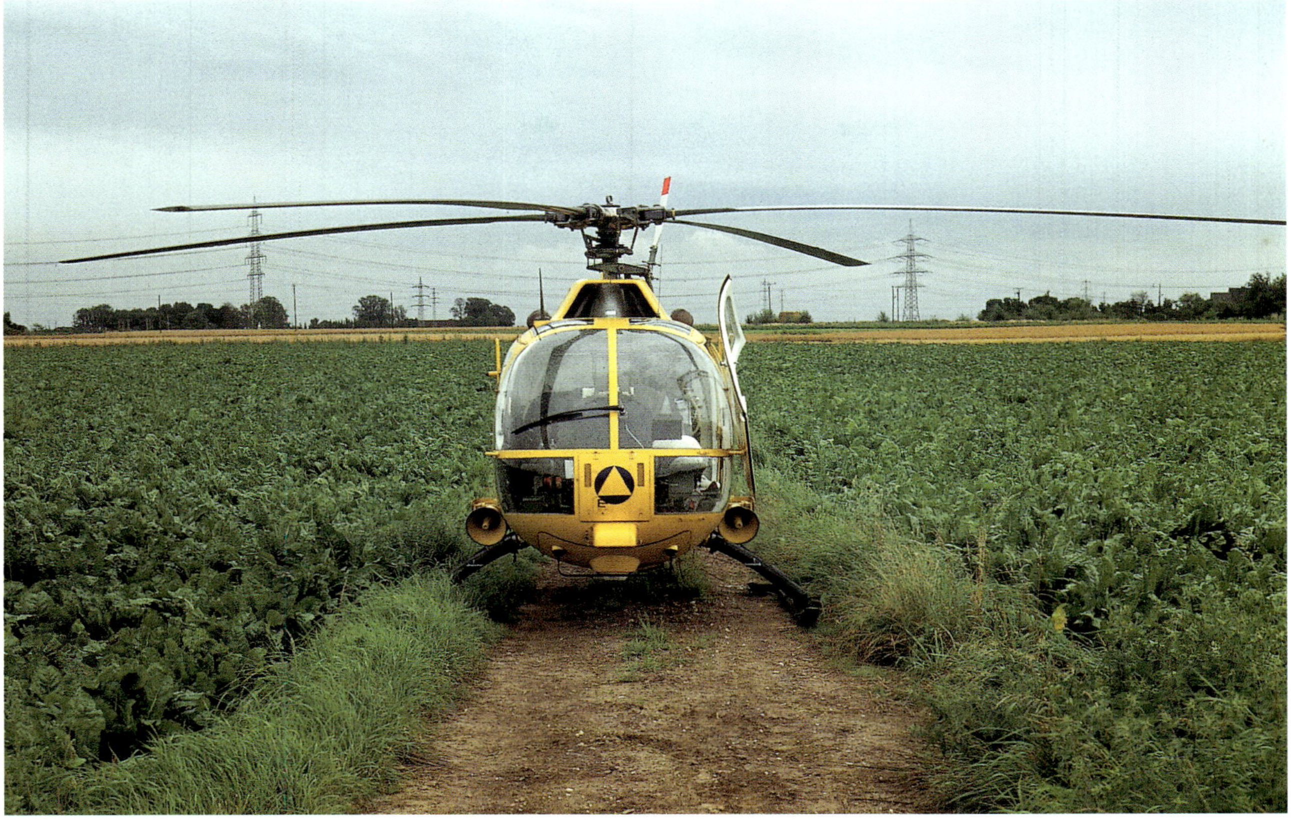

Landeplatz Feldweg.

Landing site on a dirt-road.

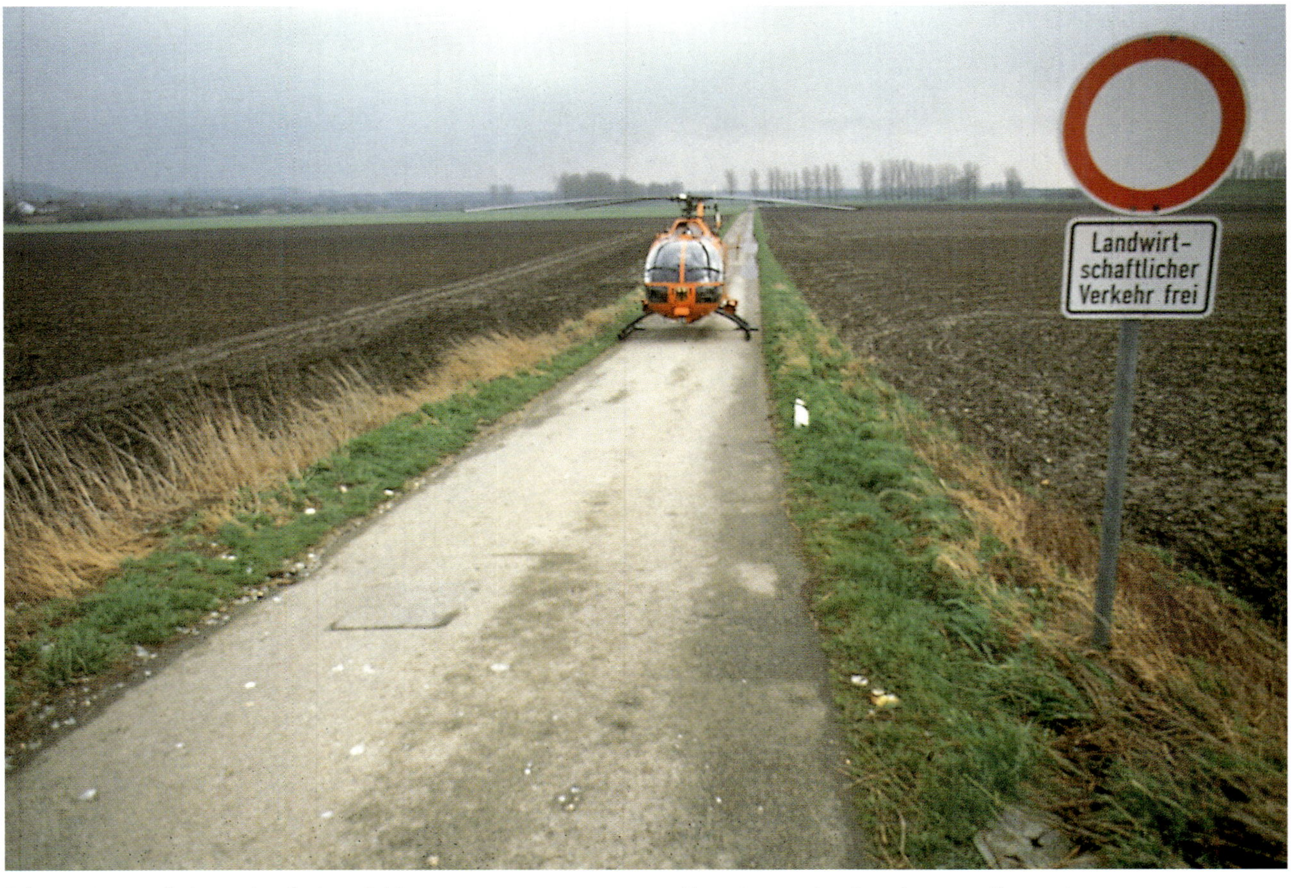

Jahre später – wiederum Landeplatz Feldweg.

Years later – landing site on a dirt-road.

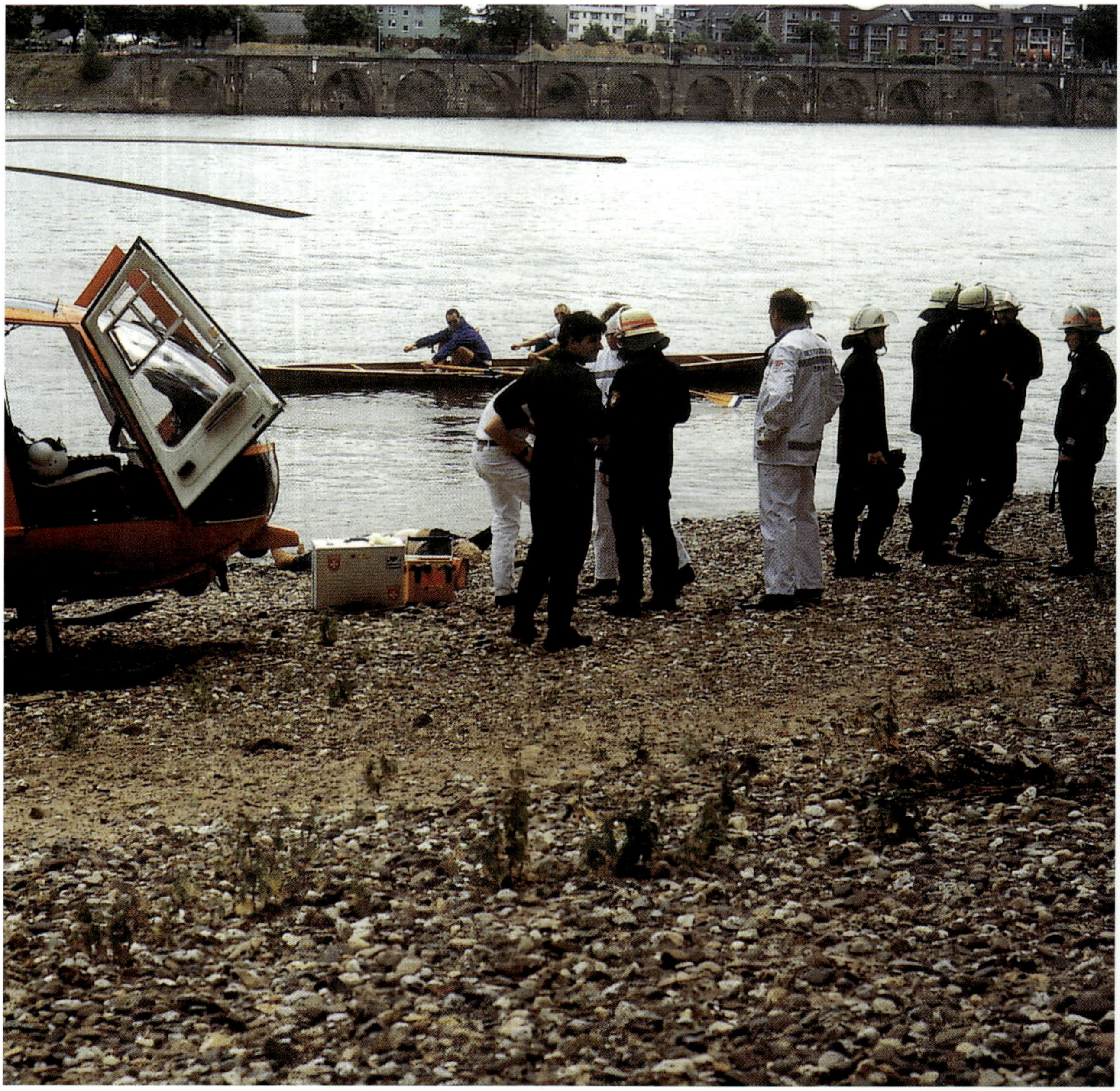

Landeplatz Rheinufer.

Landing site on the banks of the Rhine.

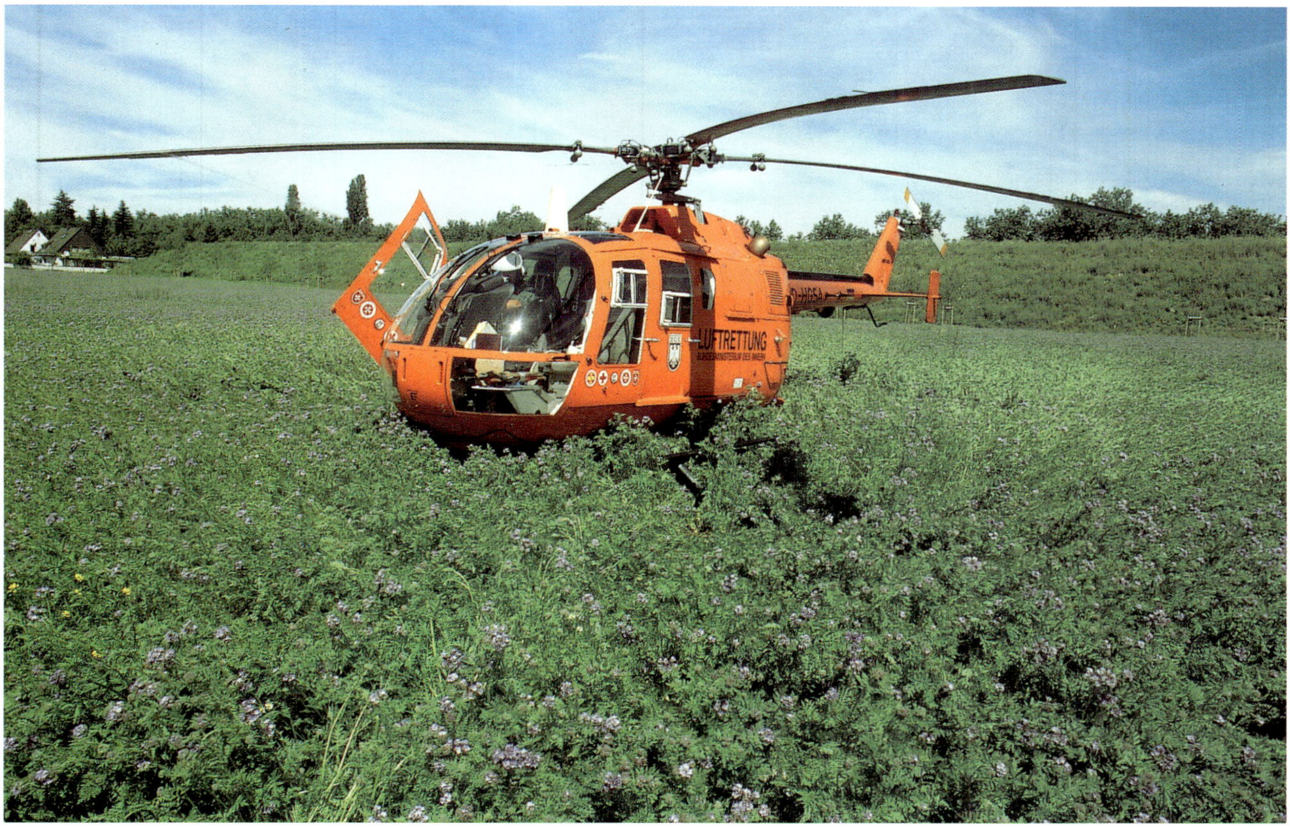

Landeplatz Acker.

Landing site on a field.

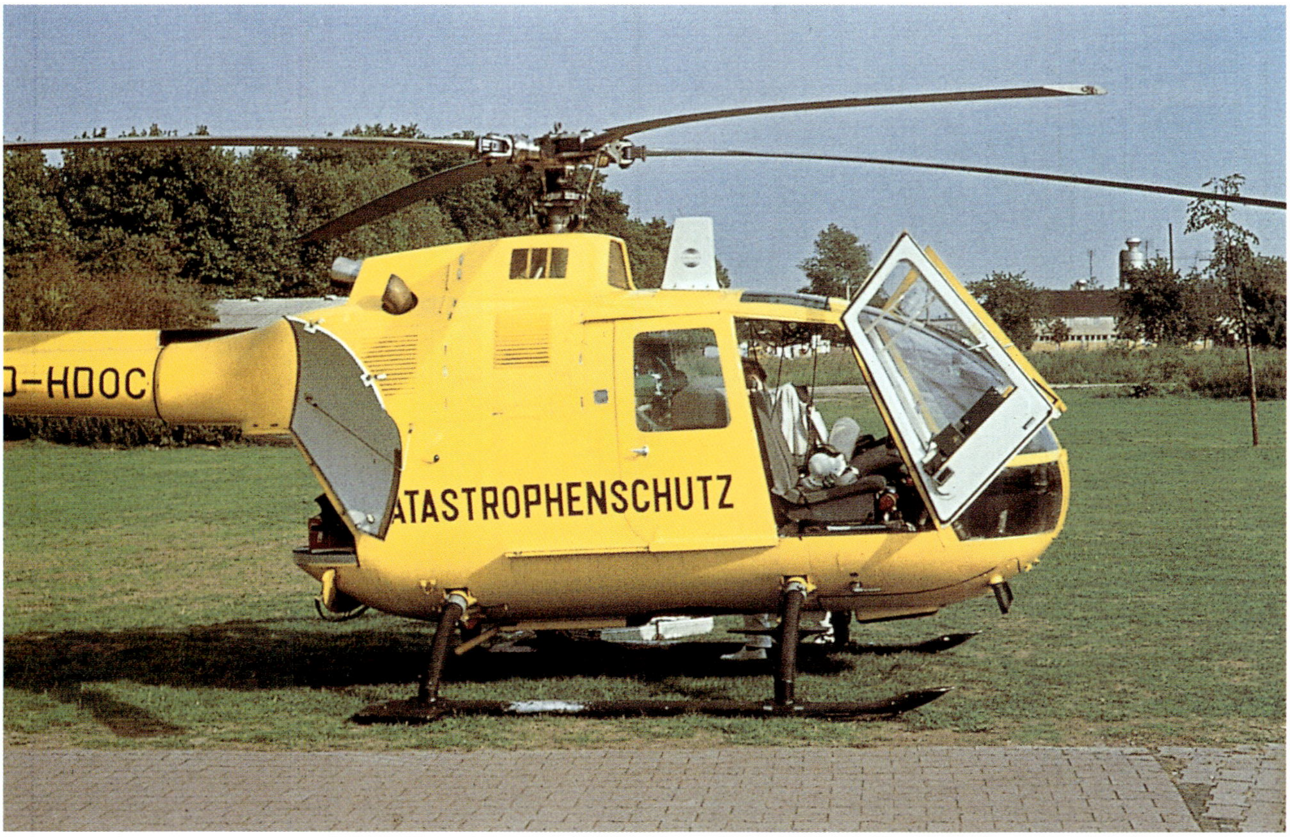

Landeplatz Uniwiese.

Landing site on a university campus.

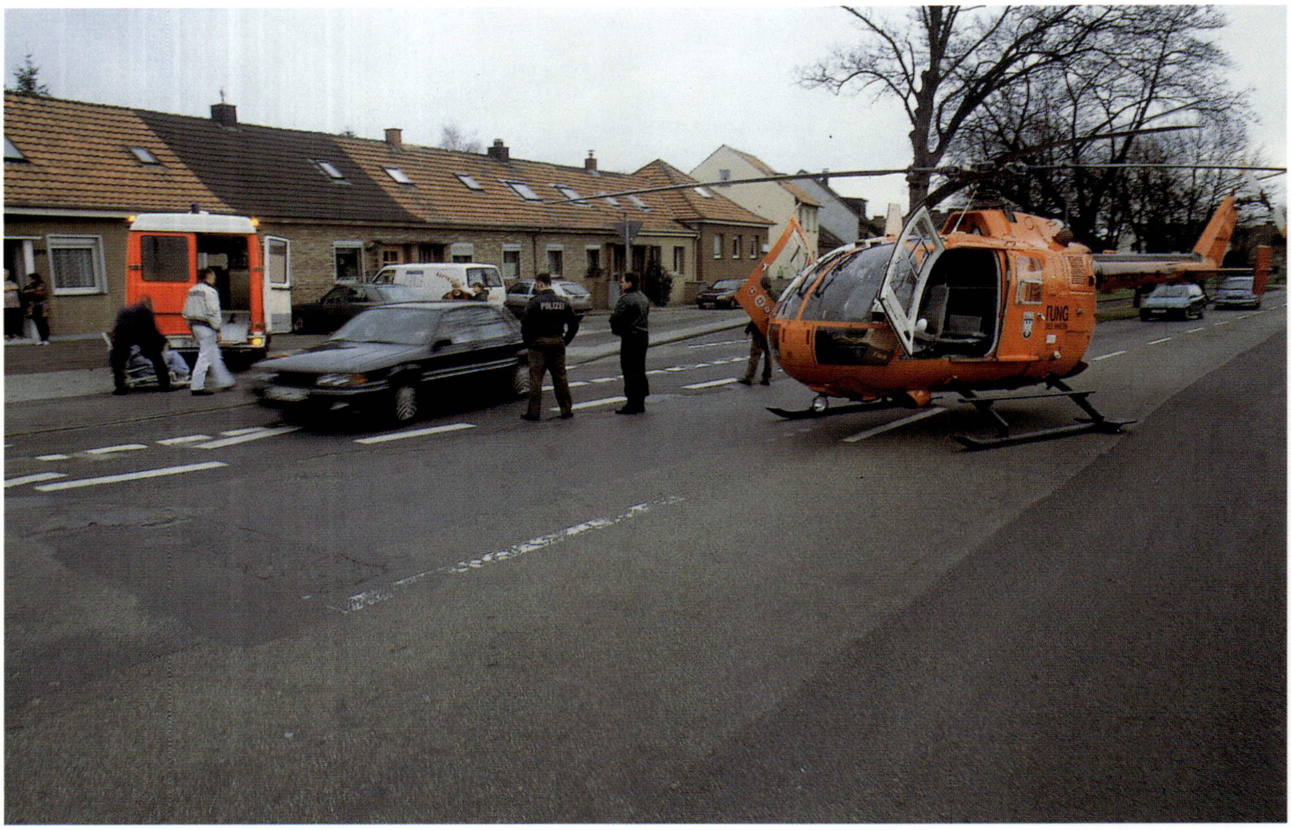

Landeplatz Innenstadt. Landing site in a downtown area.

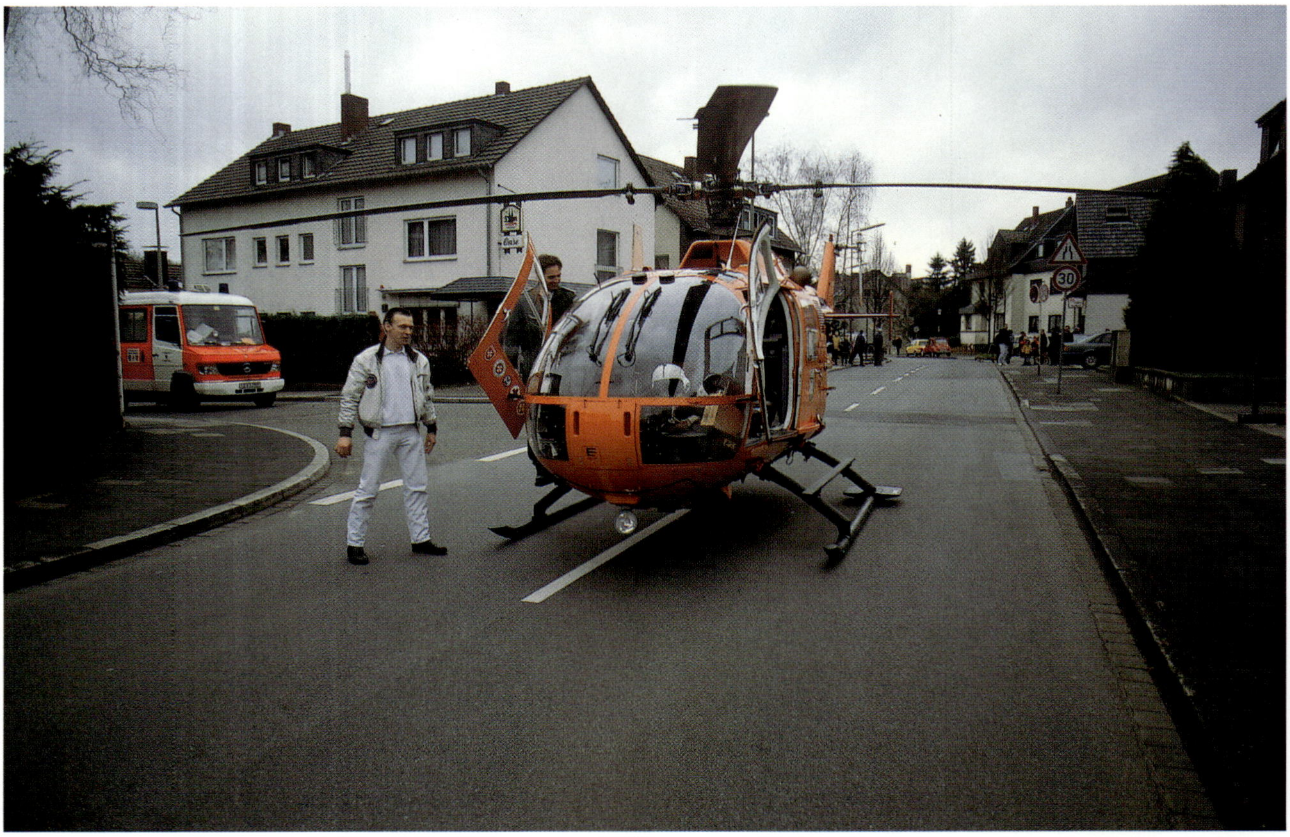

Landeplatz im Dorf. Landing site in a village.

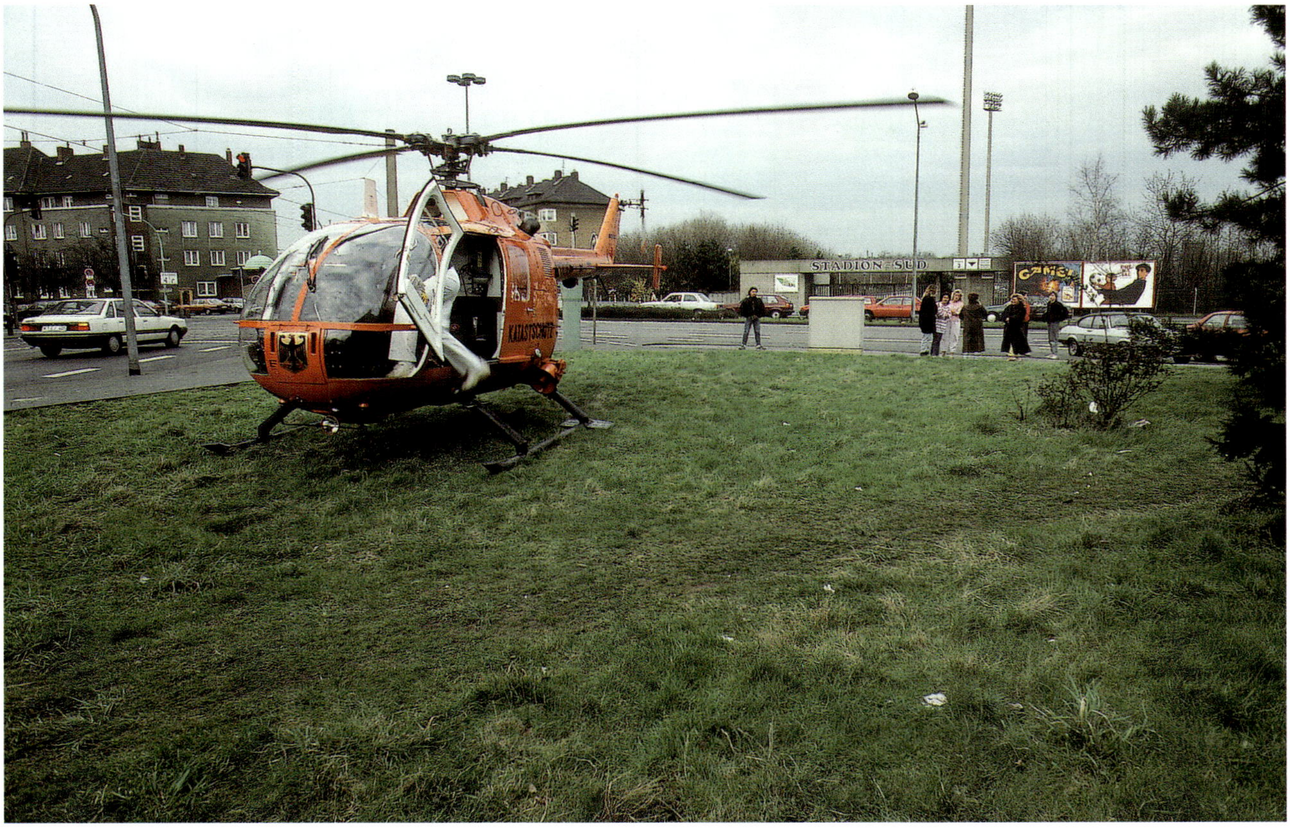

Landeplatz auf einer kleinen Wiese.

Landing site on a small grassy area.

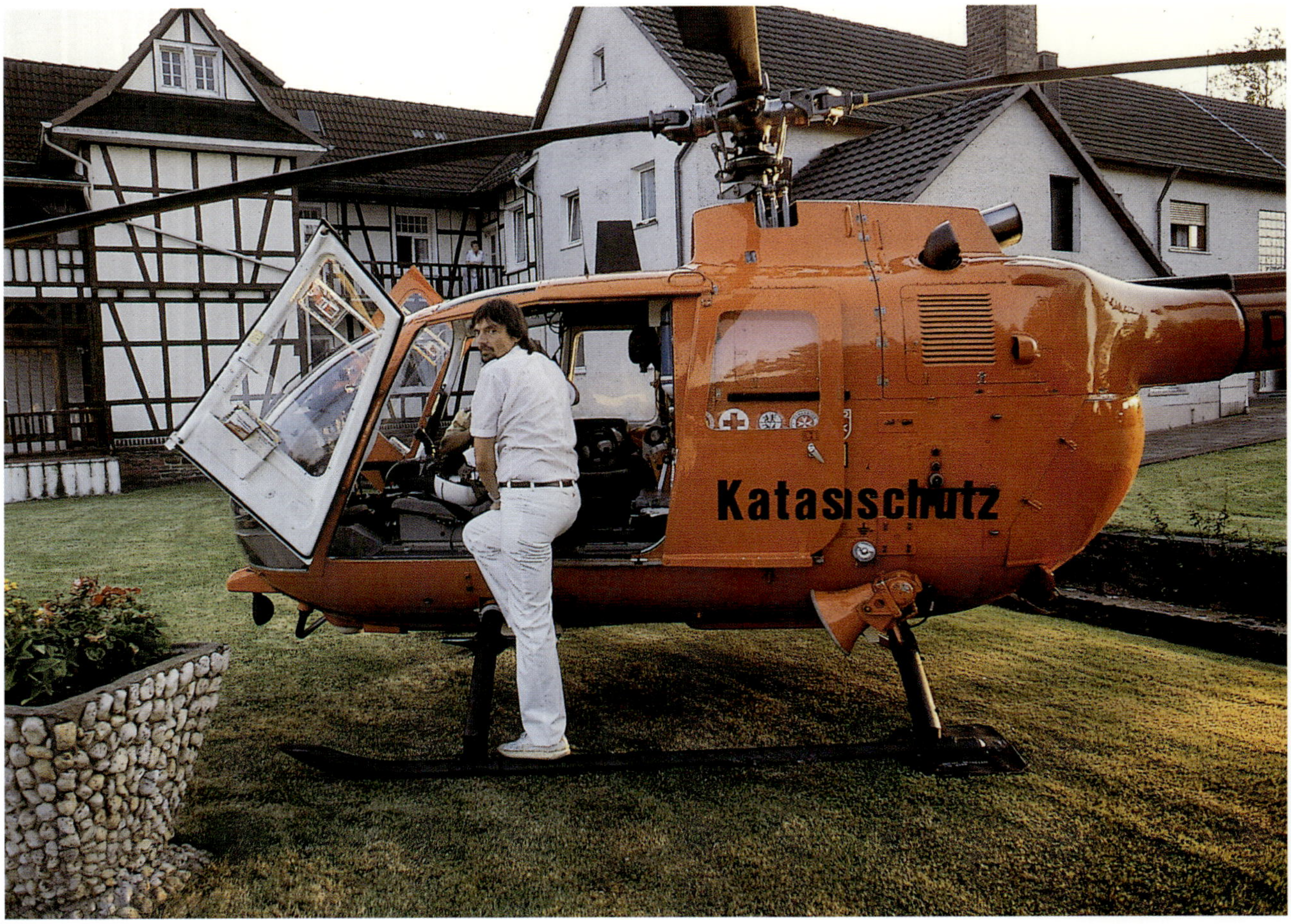

Landeplatz im Dorf.

Landing site in a village.

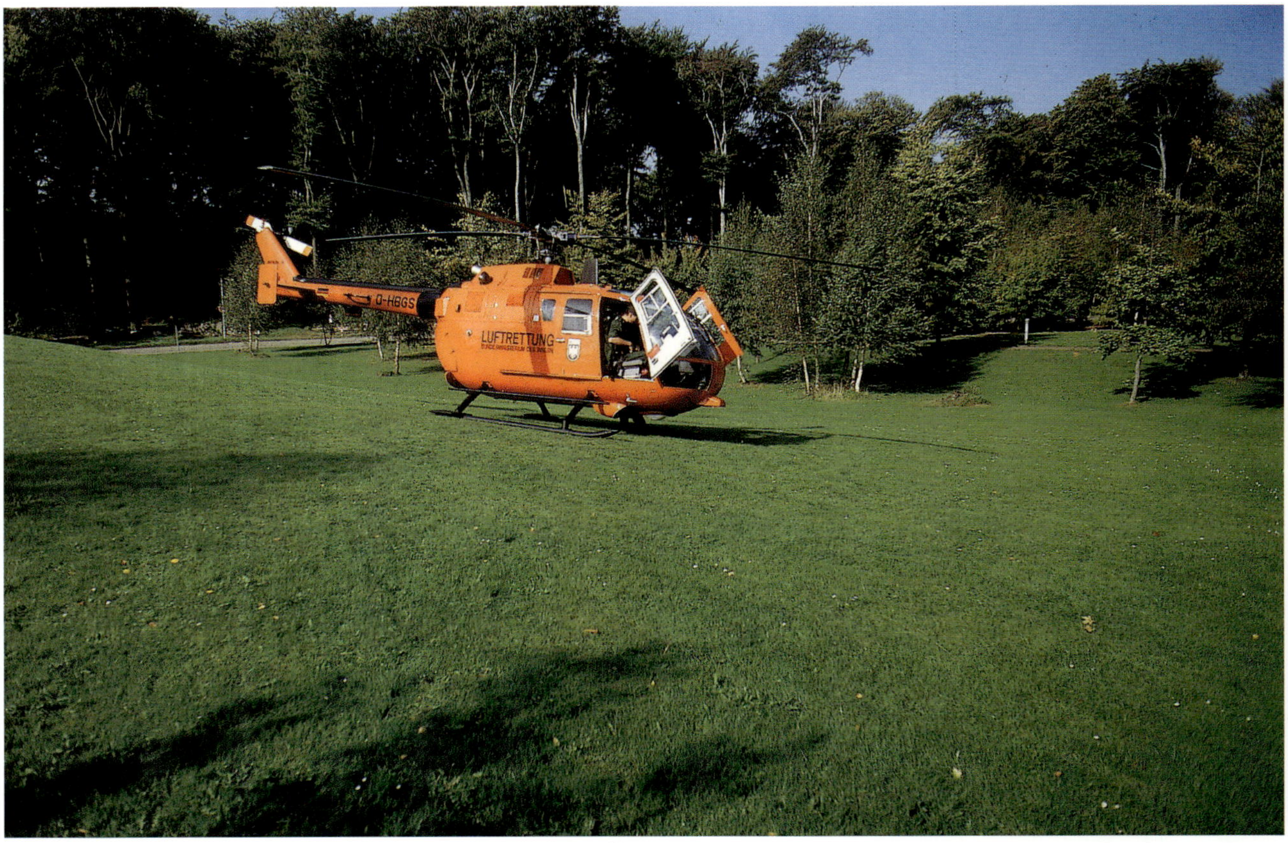

Landeplatz Waldrand.

Landing site on the edge of a forest.

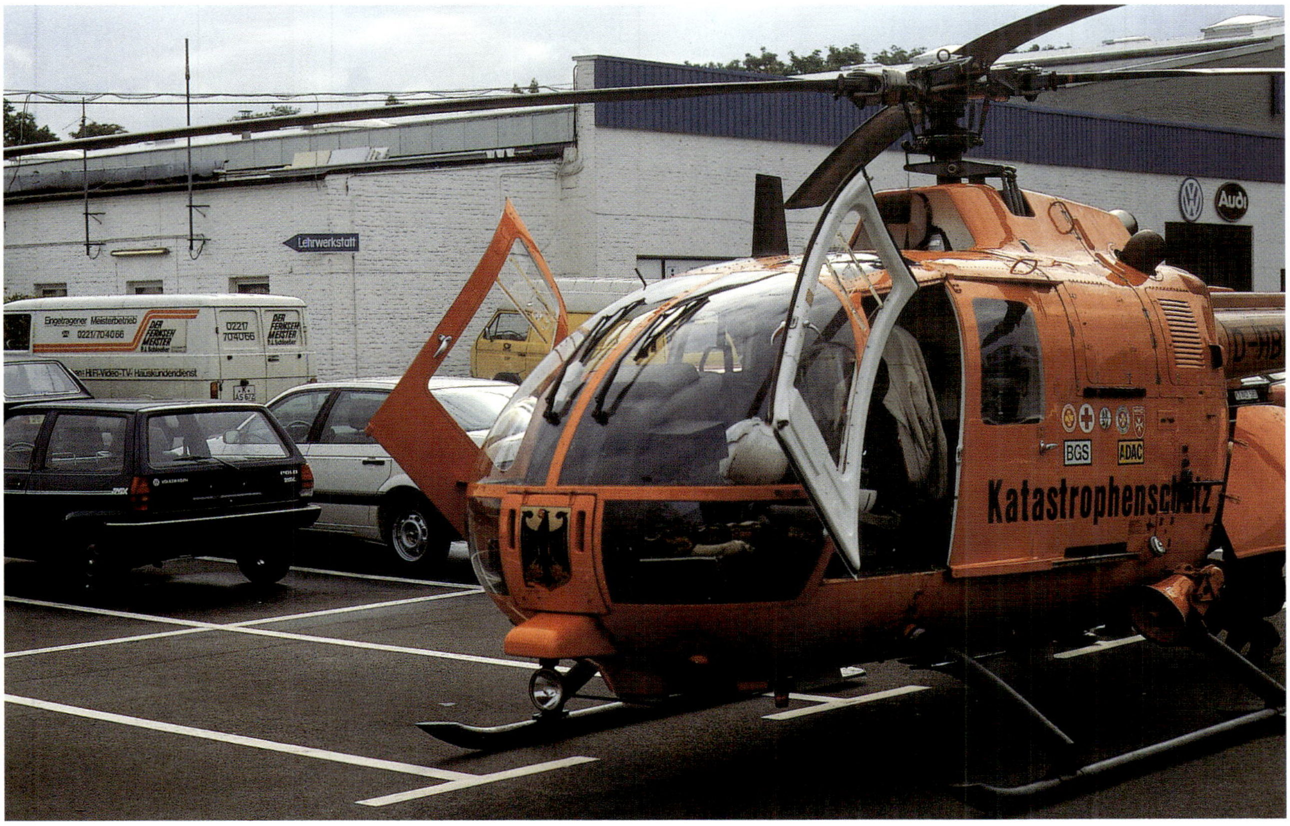

Landeplatz Autowerkstatt.

Landing site at an automobile garage.

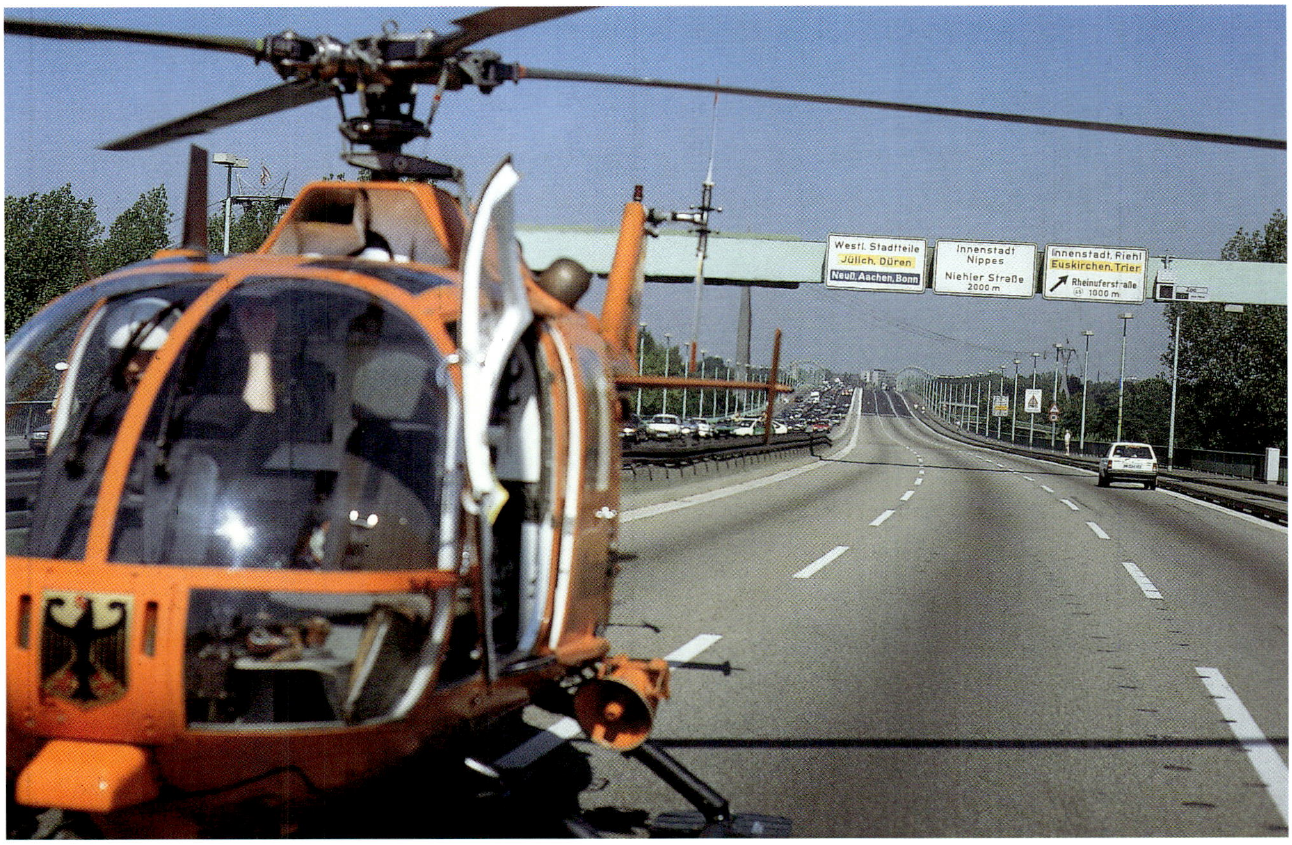

Landeplatz Brücke.

Landing site on a bridge.

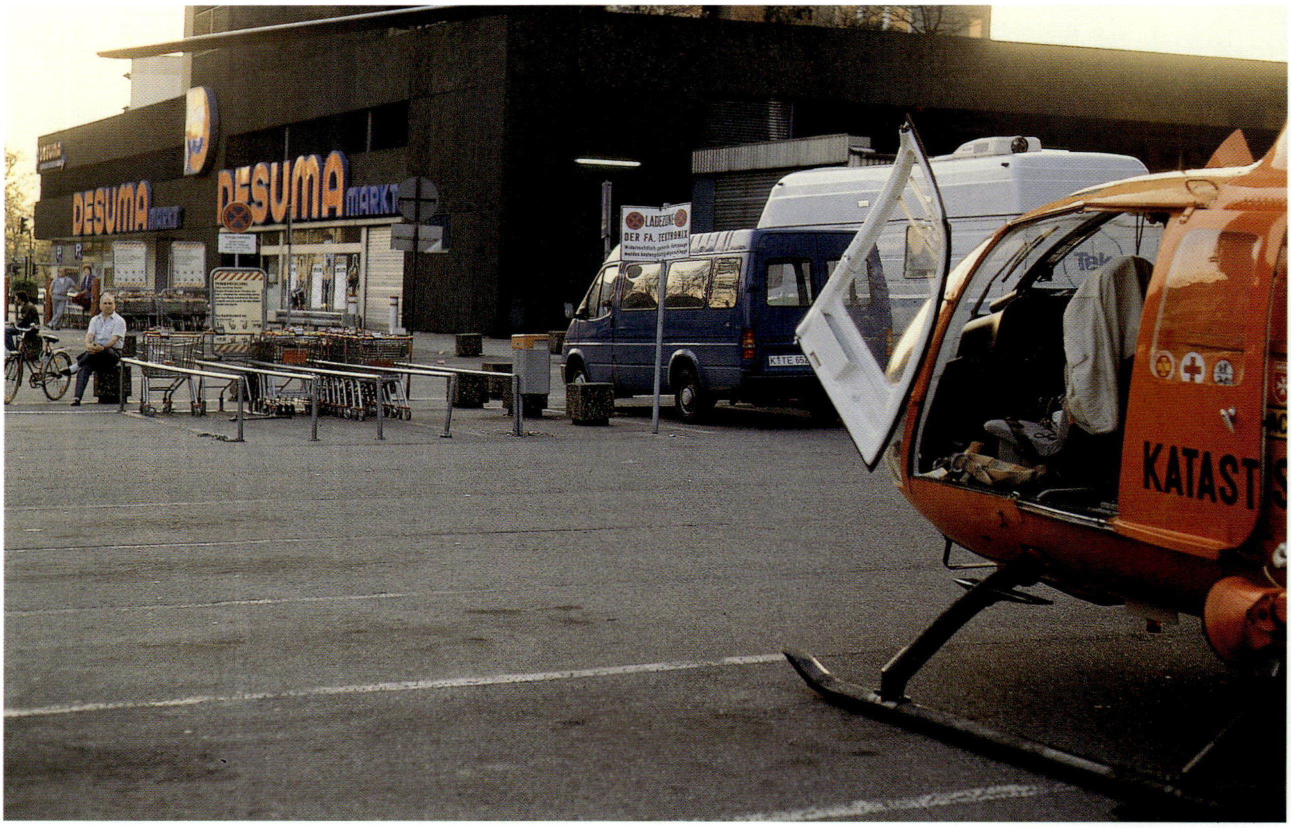

Landeplatz Supermarkt.

Landing site in front of a supermarket.

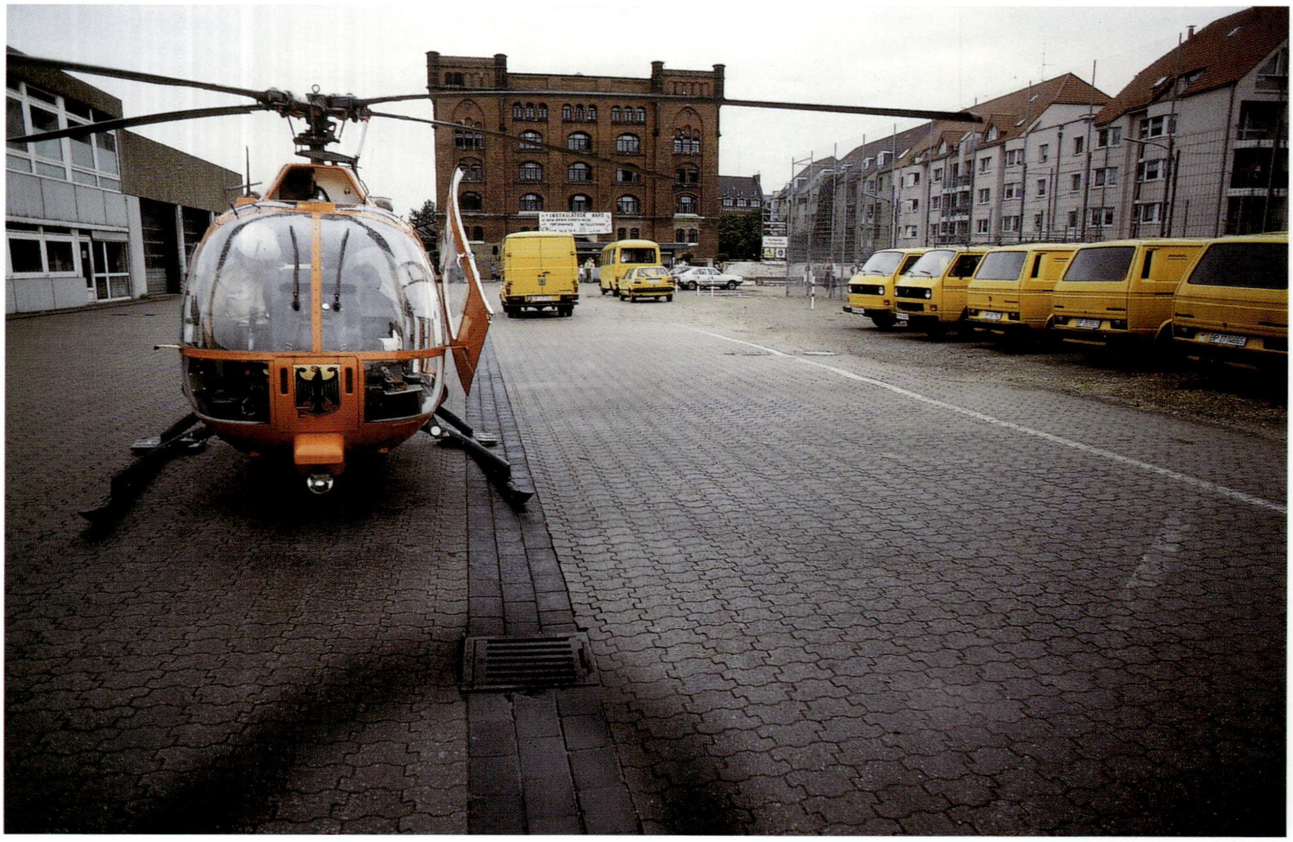

Landeplatz Postamt.

Landing site at a post office.

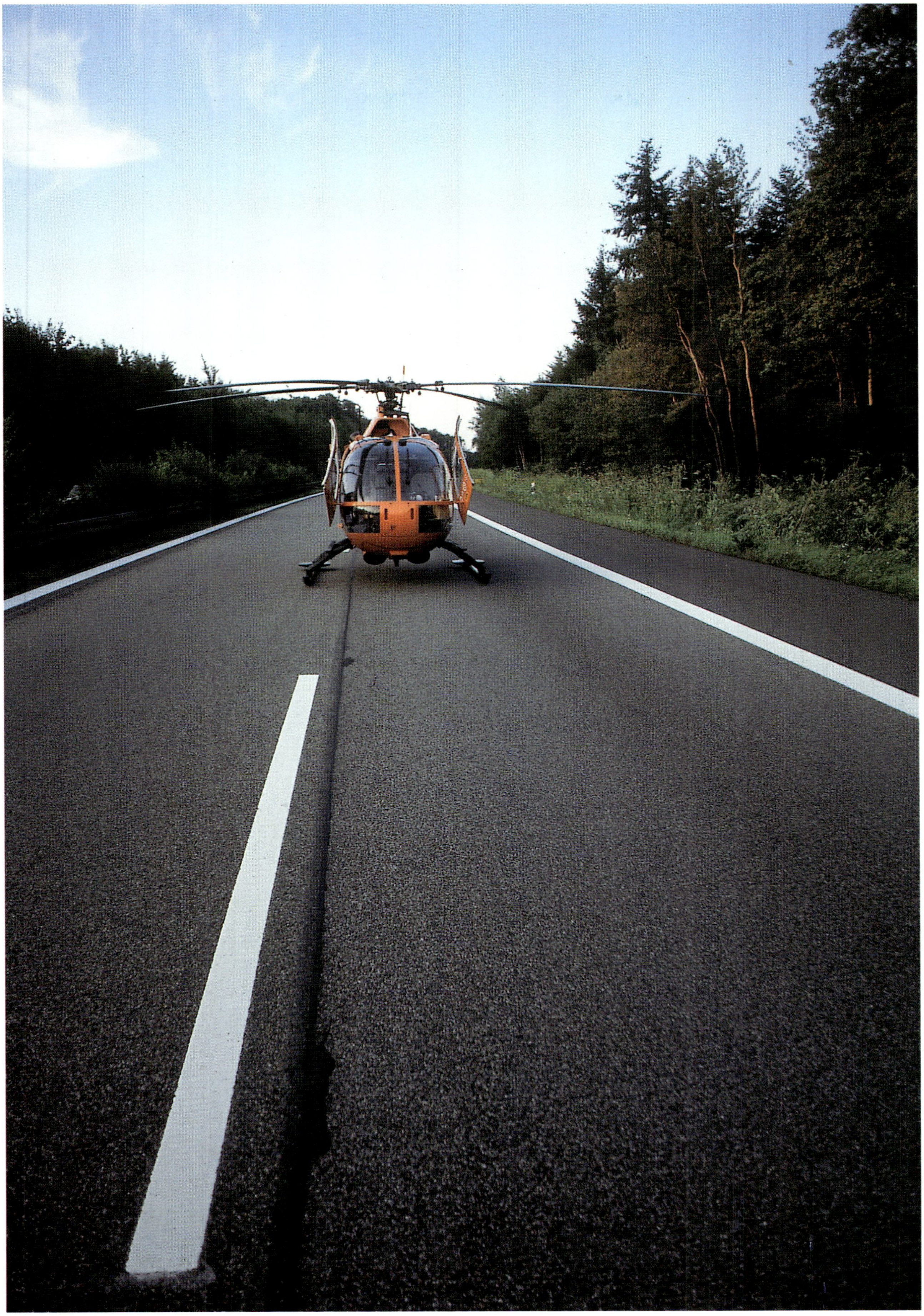

Landeplatz Autobahn.

Landing site on the autobahn.

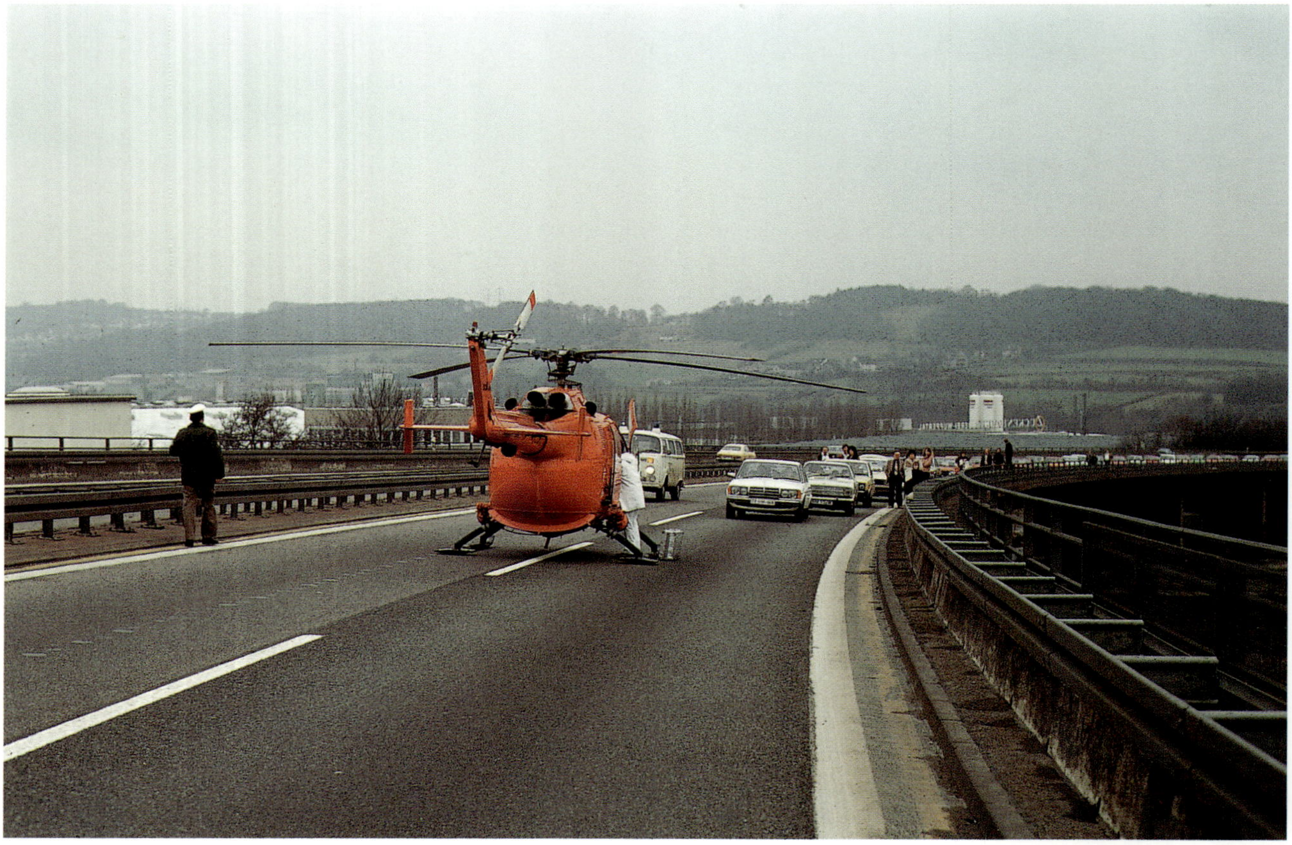

Landeplatz Brücke.

Landing site on a bridge.

Die häufigsten Fragen an der Einsatzstelle
Frequently Asked Questions

Wie oft wird der Hubschrauber gewartet?

Nach jeder Landung macht der Pilot einen Rundgang um die Maschine, um die Flüssigkeitsstände (Triebwerköl, Getriebeöl, Hydrauliköl) zu überprüfen und um eine Sichtkontrolle durchzuführen.

Am Ende eines jeden Einsatztages kontrolliert der Pilot den Hubschrauber anhand einer umfangreichen Checkliste. Dies dauert mit notwendigen Reinigungsmaßnahmen eine halbe bis dreiviertel Stunde. Dabei kann er nach Rücksprache mit der zuständigen Fliegerstaffel des BGS und dem verantwortlichen Techniker auch kleinere Beanstandungen beheben.

Alle 50, 300 und 600 Flugstunden wird der Hubschrauber teilweise sehr umfangreichen Wartungsmaßnahmen unterzogen, die periodisch wiederkehren. Bei erreichten 6000 Flugstunden wird der Hubschrauber grundüberholt.

How often is a helicopter serviced?

After each landing the pilot walks around the aircraft to check the fluid levels (e.g. engine oil, transmission oil, hydraulic oil) and to conduct a visual inspection.

At the end of every operational day, the pilot inspects the helicopter with the aid of a comprehensive checklist. Together with the necessary cleaning procedures, this checklist takes between 30 and 45 minutes. After checking back with the flying squadron of the German Border Police, the pilot can correct small problems.

After every 50, 300 and 600 hours of flying time, the helicopter is subjected to periodic maintenance procedures, some of which are very extensive. After 6,000 hours of flying time, the helicopter undergoes a total overhauling.

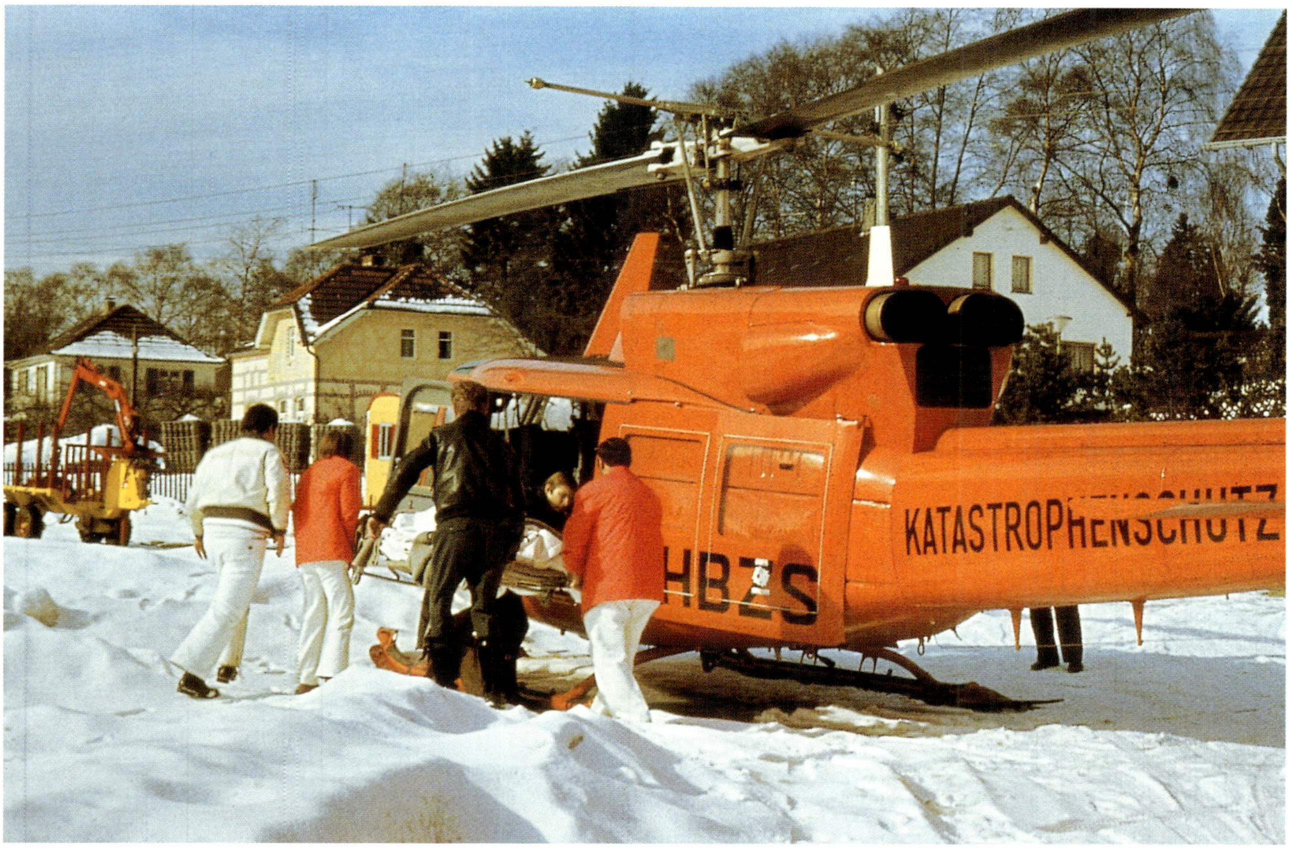

Die Christoph 3 Crew im Einsatz mit der Bell 212. Es sollte 1981 erprobt werden, ob die Bell alternativ zur BO 105 im Gebiet bei Innenstadteinsätzen eingesetzt werden könnte. Die Christoph 3 Station fliegt aber seither weiter mit der BO 105.

The crew of Christoph 3 on a mission with the Bell 212. In 1981 trials were conducted to determine whether the Bell could be employed as an alternative to the BO 105 in urban areas. Following these trials, the rescue helicopter crews based in Cologne continued flying with the BO 105.

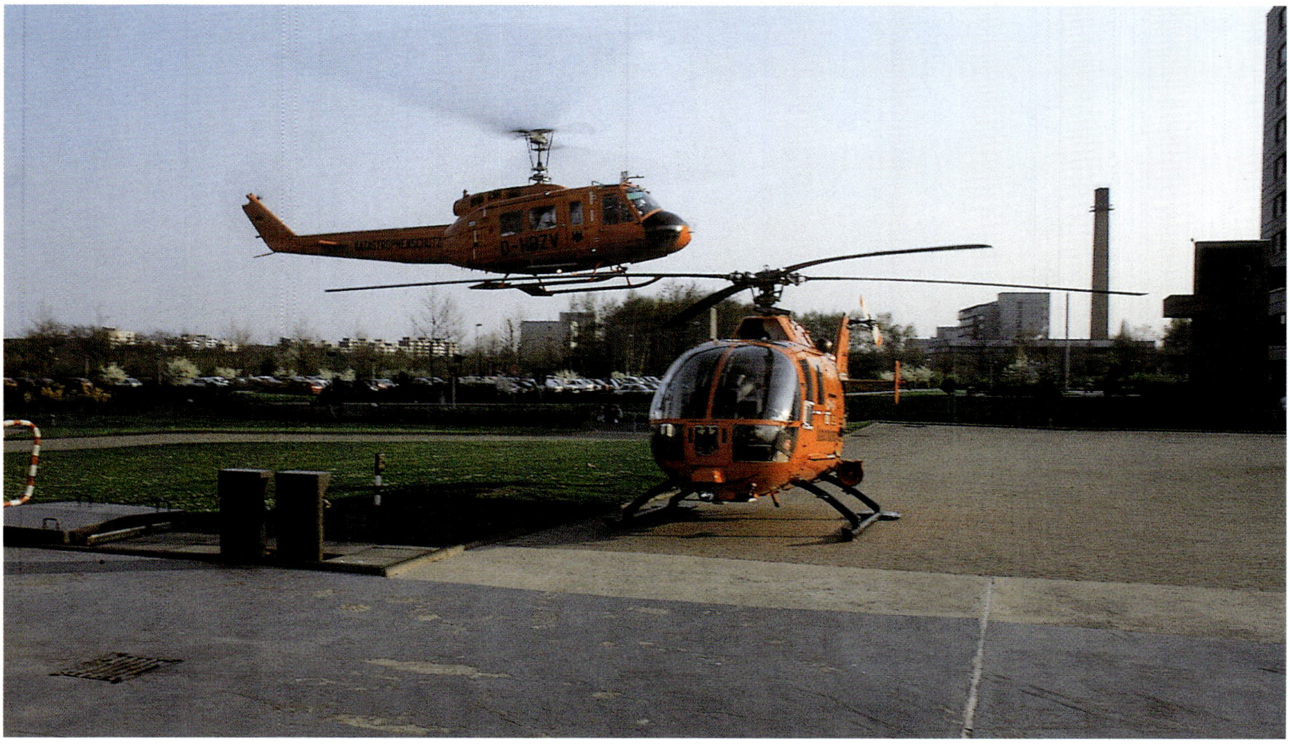

Die Bell UH-1D von einer anderen Rettungshubschrauberstation bringt einen Patienten in das Schwerverbranntenzentrum am Standortkrankenhaus von Christoph 3.

A Bell UH-1D from another rescue helicopter base transports a patient to the Burns Center at the hospital where Christoph 3 is based.

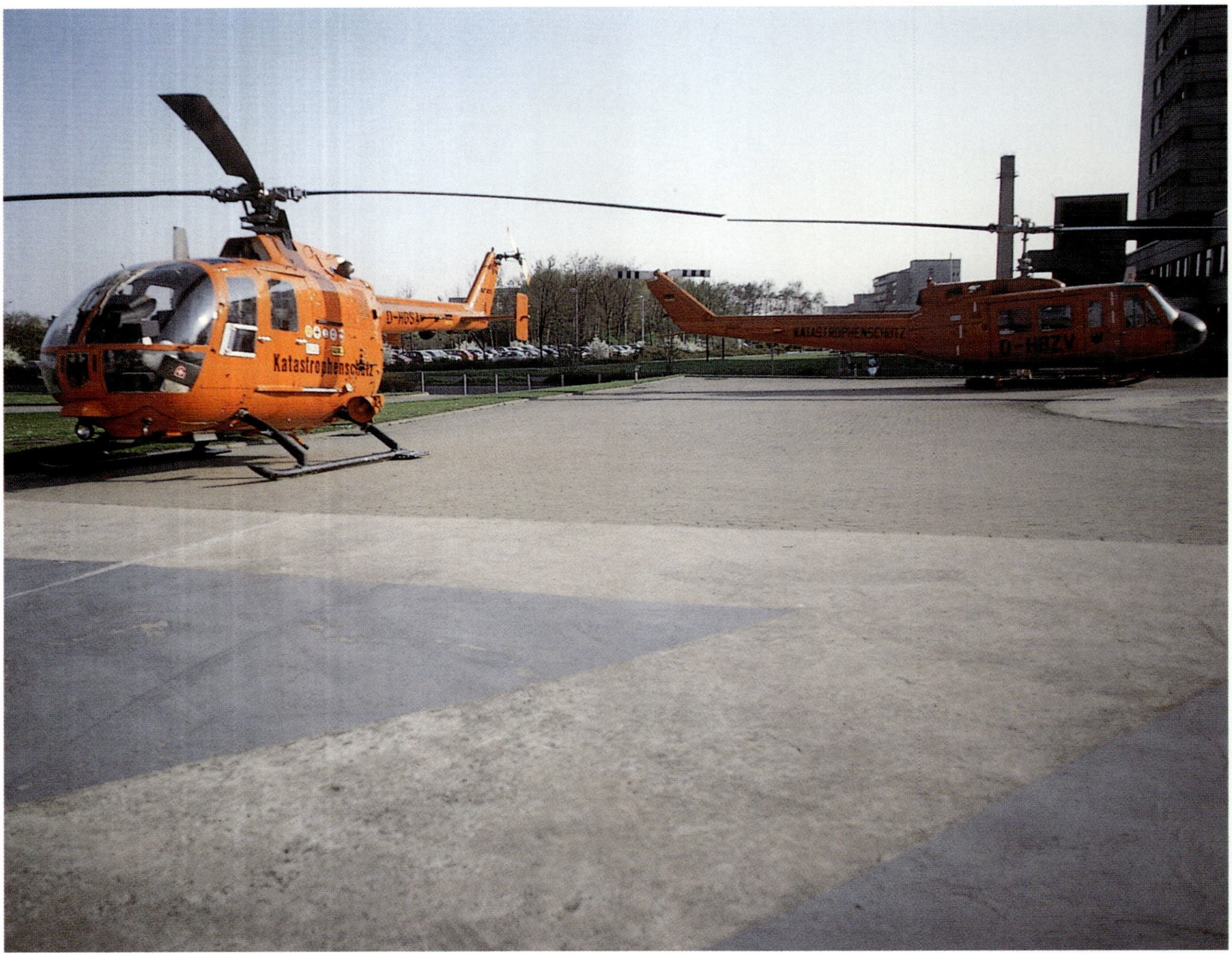

Die häufigsten Fragen an der Einsatzstelle
Frequently Asked Questions

Kann der Hubschrauber auch bei Gewitter fliegen?

Der Pilot wird immer versuchen, einem Gewitter auszuweichen, weil es unkalkulierbare Risiken wie schwere Turbulenzen, so genannte Scherwinde, Wind in Orkanstärke, Hagel und Blitzschlag birgt.

Zwar ist ein Hubschrauber, wie auch jedes Auto, ein so genannter Faradayscher Käfig, ein Blitzschlag würde jedoch mit großer Wahrscheinlichkeit die Instrumente, die Elektronik und auch die Rotorblätter beschädigen.

Große Gewitterfronten, schwere bodennahe Turbulenzen, Nebel, vereisender Regen und dichter Schneefall sind die Wettererscheinungen, die den Flug des Rettungshubschraubers verhindern.

Can the helicopter fly during a thunderstorm?

The pilot will always try to stay out of a thunderstorm since such storms pose incalculable risks such as strong air turbulence, shear winds, hurricane-force winds, hail and lightning. It is true that a helicopter, like all motor vehicles, serves as a Faraday cage; nevertheless, if the helicopter were struck by a bolt of lightning, the instruments, the electronic system and the rotor blades would most certainly be damaged.

Major weather fronts, fog, sleet and heavy snowfall are weather conditions which ground the helicopter.

Einsatz für den Rettungshubschrauber
Mission for the Rescue Helicopter

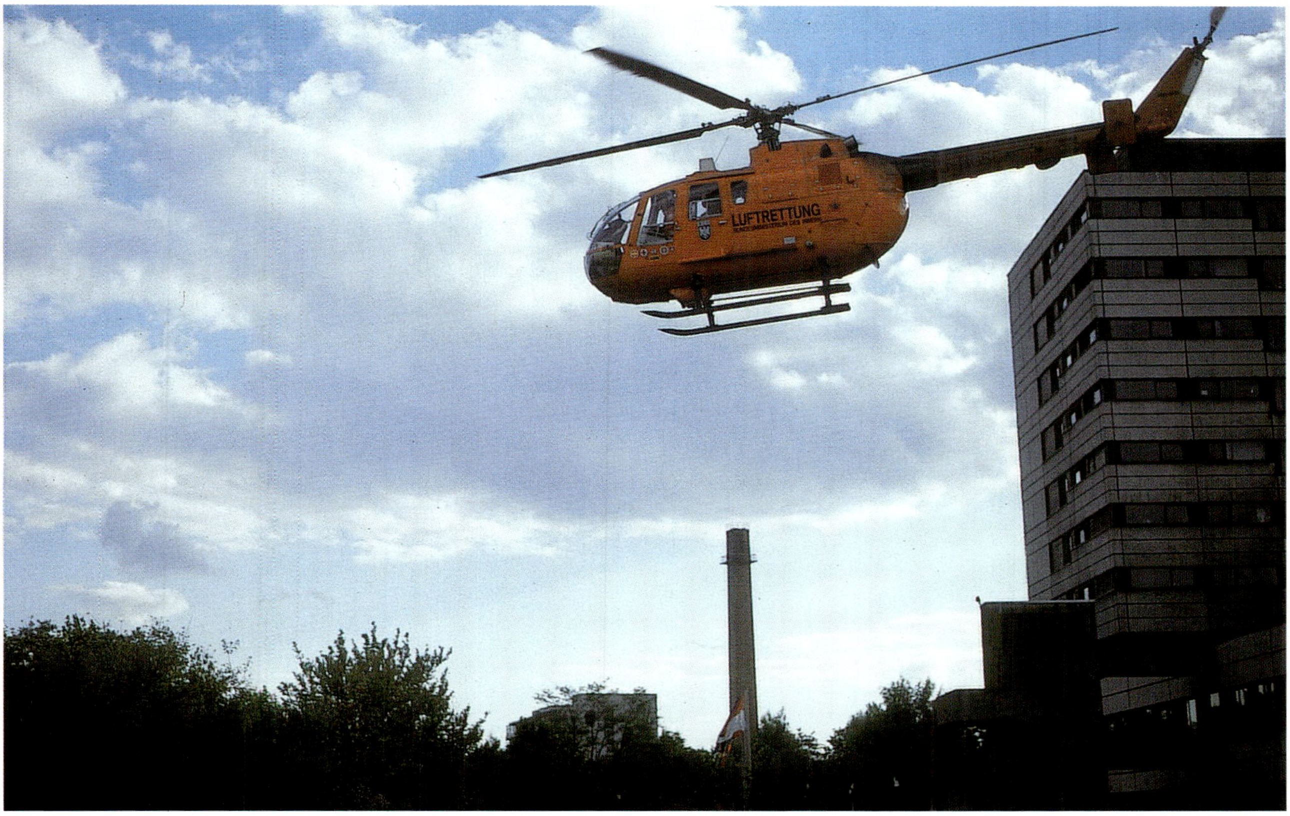

Suchflug: Ein Ruderboot ist gekentert.

Search-and-rescue flight: a rowing boat has capsized during a flood.

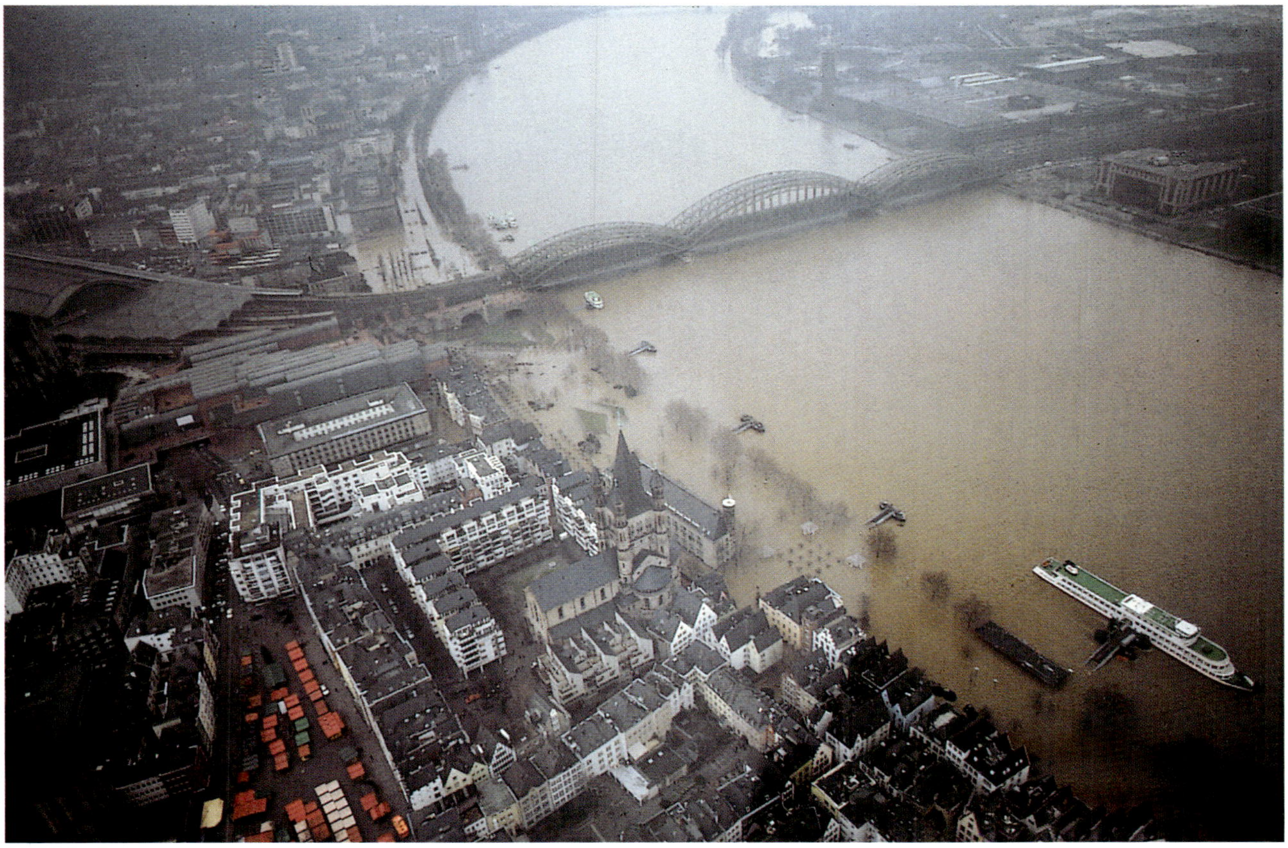

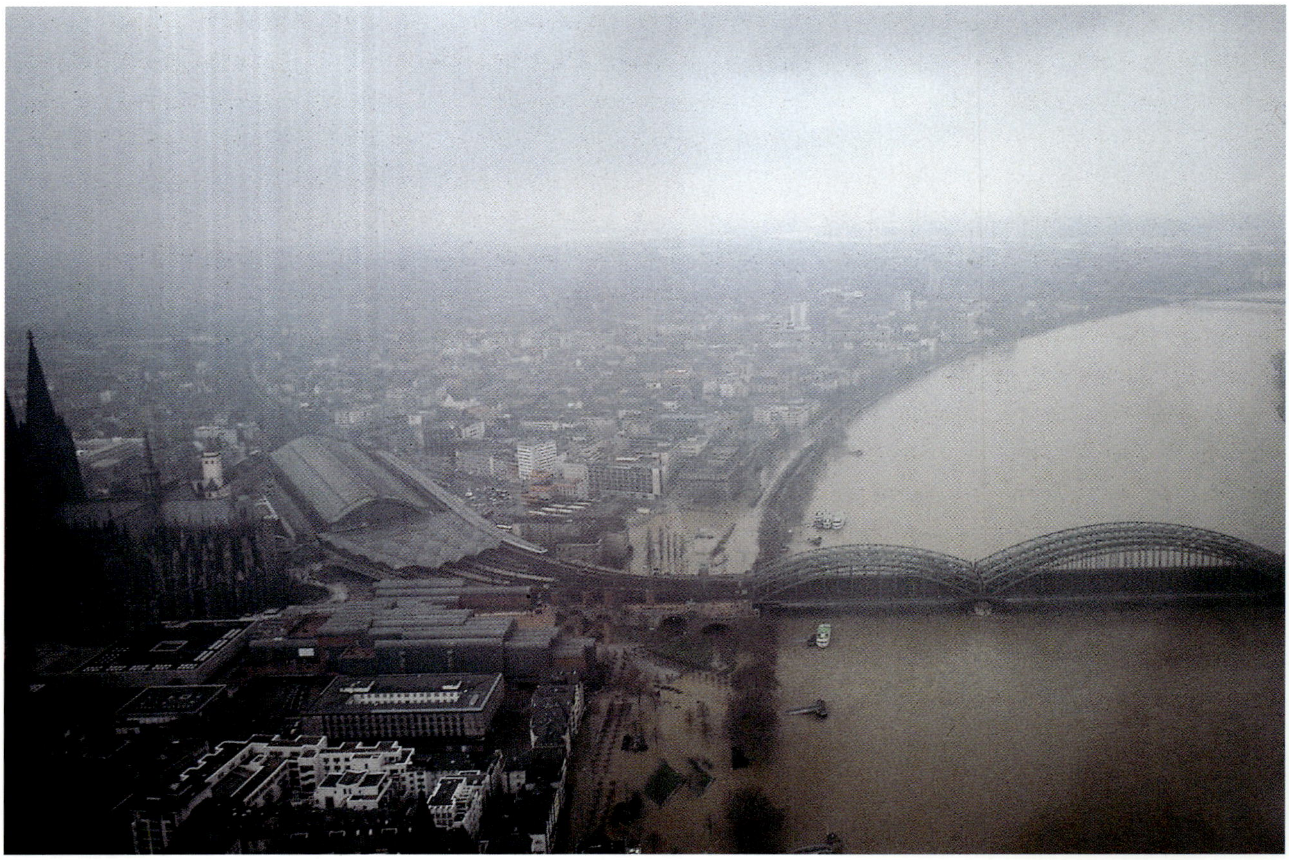

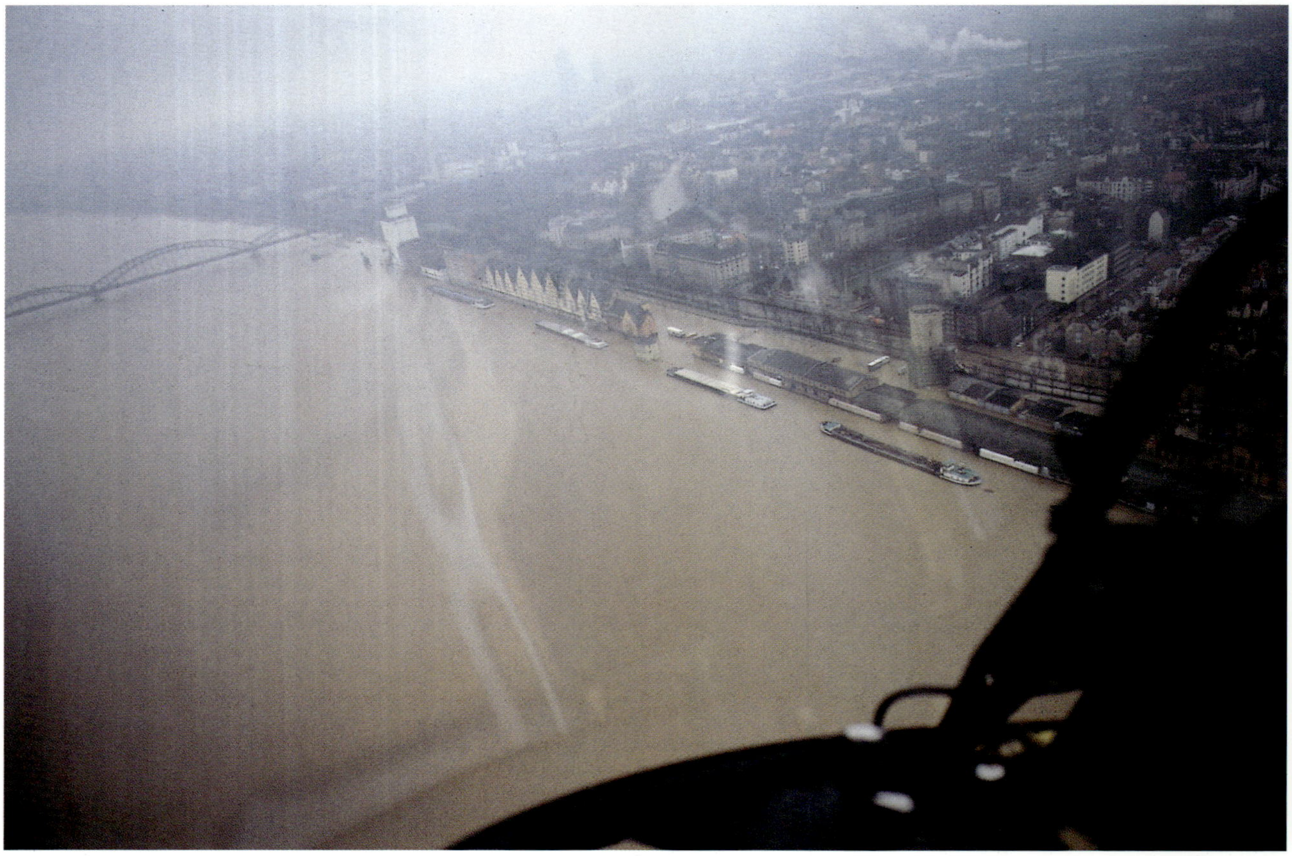

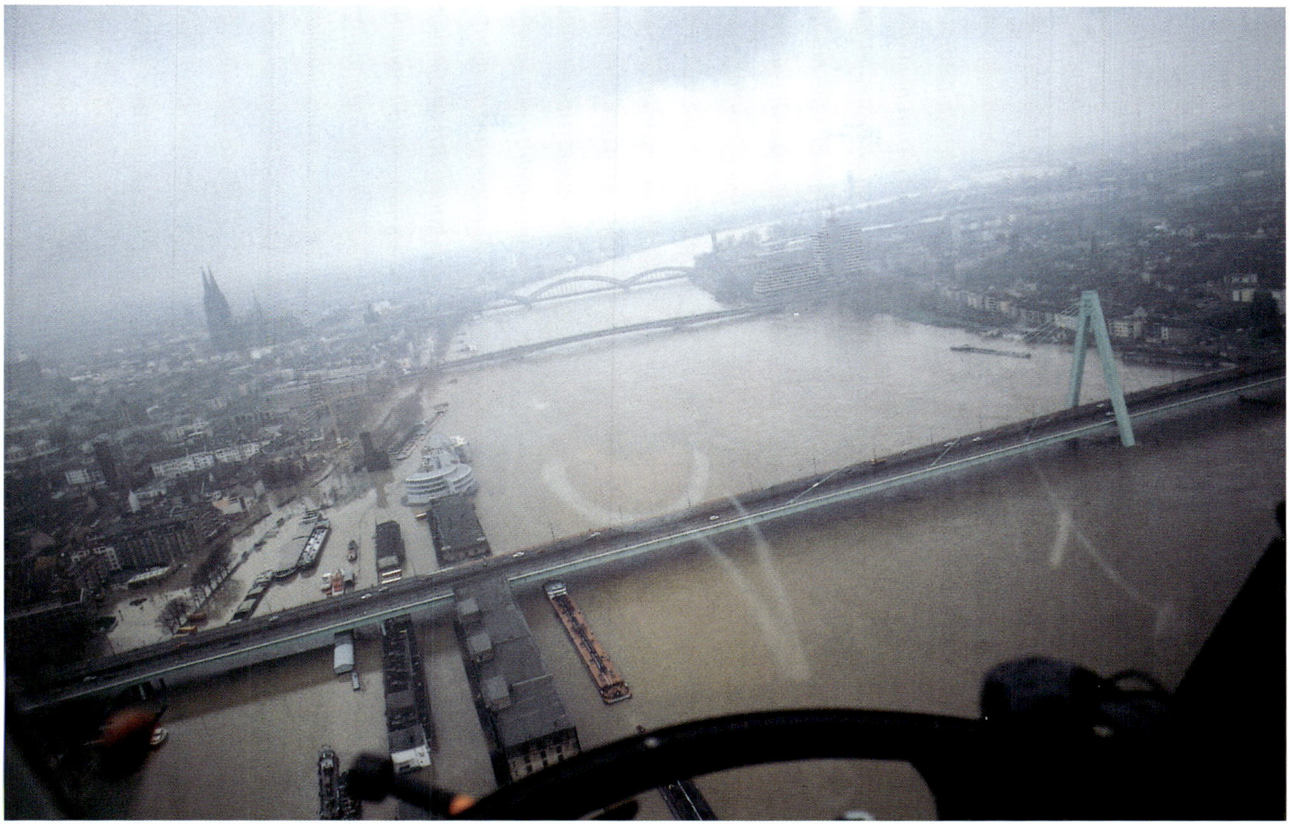

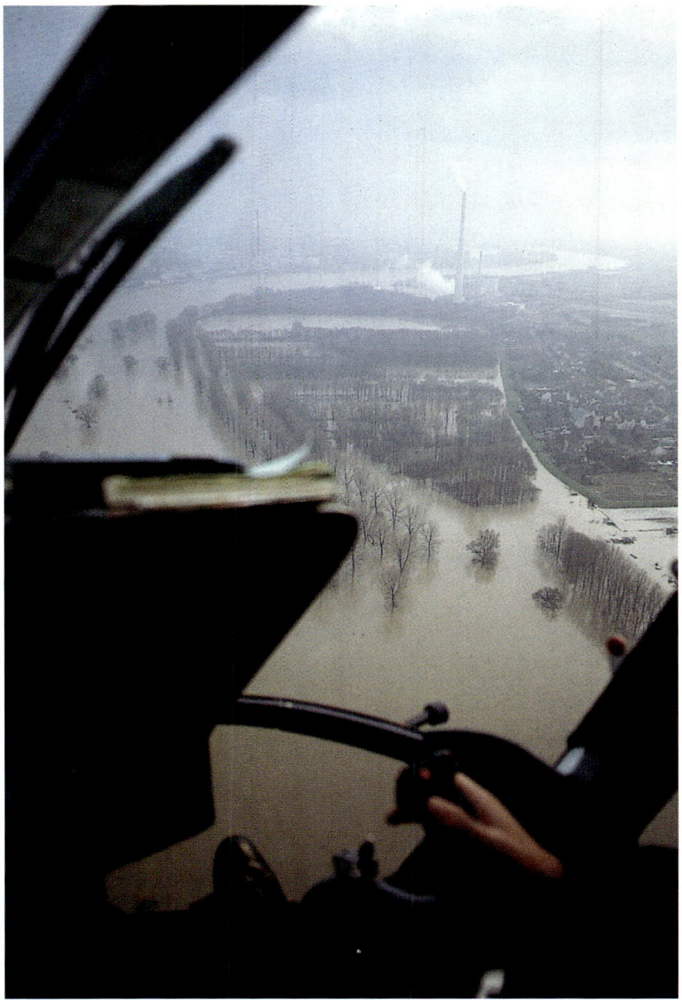

Die häufigsten Fragen an der Einsatzstelle

Frequently Asked Questions

Wie schnell fliegt eine BO 105?

Die Reisegeschwindigkeit im Horizontalflug beträgt etwa 125 Knoten, d.h. 125 Nautische Meilen in der Stunde(1 Nautische Meile = 1,85 km) oder 230 km/h. Im Bahnneigungsflug ist die BO 105 bis zu einer Geschwindigkeit von 145 Knoten oder 270 km/h zugelassen.

How fast does the BO 105 fly?

This helicopter has a cruising speed during horizontal flight of about 125 knots, i.e. 125 nautical miles per hour (1 nautical mile = 1.85 km) or 230 km/h. The BO 105 is licensed for a speed of 145 knots or 270 km/h in the dive.

Einsatz für den Rettungshubschrauber
Mission for the Rescue Helicopter

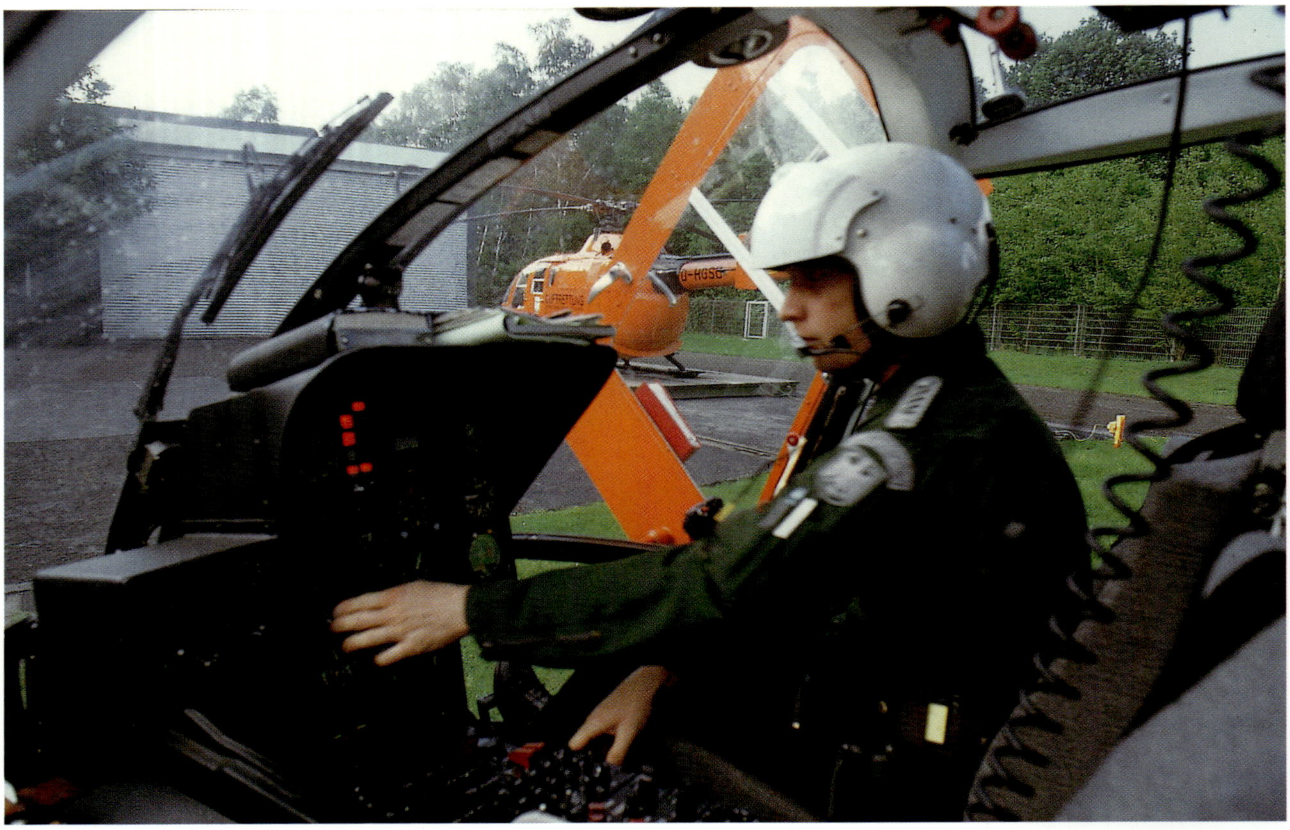

Der Rettungshubschrauber hat einen Patienten in ein anderes Krankenhaus mit einem anderen Rettungshubschrauber gebracht. Der Pilot führt seine Vorflugchecks durch.

The rescue helicopter has transported a patient to a hospital where another rescue helicopter is based. The pilot goes through the pre-flight checklist.

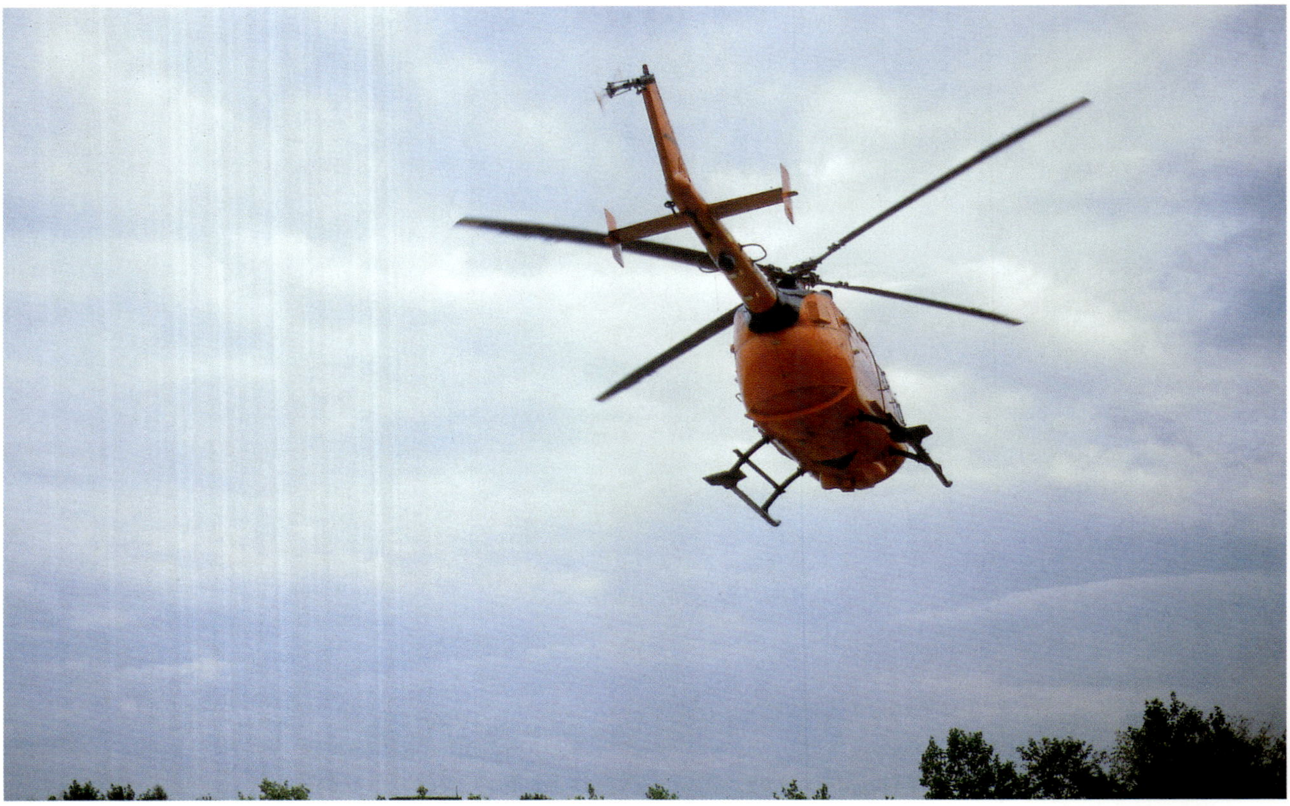

Die häufigsten Fragen an der Einsatzstelle
Frequently Asked Questions

Welche Absprachen müssen beim Start mit einem sehr nahe gelegenen internationalen Verkehrsflughafen getroffen werden?

Die Luftrettungsstation Köln liegt innerhalb der so genannten Kontrollzone des Flughafens. Dies bedeutet u.a., dass jedes Luftfahrzeug, das sich innerhalb dieses Luftraums bewegt oder in diesen ein- oder ausfliegen will, Funkverbindung zum Kontrollturm des Flughafens aufnehmen muss, um Weisungen für die Flugführung einzuholen. Dies gilt grundsätzlich auch für Christoph 3. Um aber den Rettungseinsatz nicht zu behindern, wurde ein erleichtertes Verfahren festgelegt.

Beim Hochfahren der Systeme schaltet der Pilot einen „Transponder“ ein, der einen bestimmten vierstelligen Code abstrahlt. So erkennt der Fluglotse im Kontrollturm den Hubschrauber schon, bevor er überhaupt gestartet ist. Noch am Boden, spätestens jedoch im Start, nimmt der Pilot Funkverbindung mit dem Tower auf und teilt dem Lotsen die Abflugrichtung und das Ziel mit. Er erhält dann postwendend die „Clearance“, d.h. Genehmigung für seinen Flug.

Grundsätzlich kann der Rettungshubschrauber für Flüge in Kontrollzonen Vorrechte reklamieren.

What issues have to be cleared with the tower when the helicopter takes off in the proximity of an international airport?

The Cologne Air Rescue Base is located within the control zone of Cologne-Bonn International Airport. Every aircraft flying within this control zone – or aspiring to enter or leave it – has to take up radio contact to the control tower to get flight control instructions from the air traffic controllers. This important rule applies to Christoph 3 as well. To avoid obstructing rescue operations, however, the aviation authorities have established a simplified procedure for rescue helicopters.

When running up all helicopter systems, the pilot switches on a „transponder“ emitting a certain four-digit code. On the basis of this code, the air flight controller in the control tower identifies the helicopter before it has even taken off. While the helicopter is still on the ground – or at the very latest when it is starting its engines – the pilot takes up radio contact to the tower, informing the air traffic controllers of the aircraft's direction of takeoff and destination. He or she is then usually given clearance immediately for the intended flight. As a matter of principle, the rescue helicopter can claim priority over other flights in control zones.

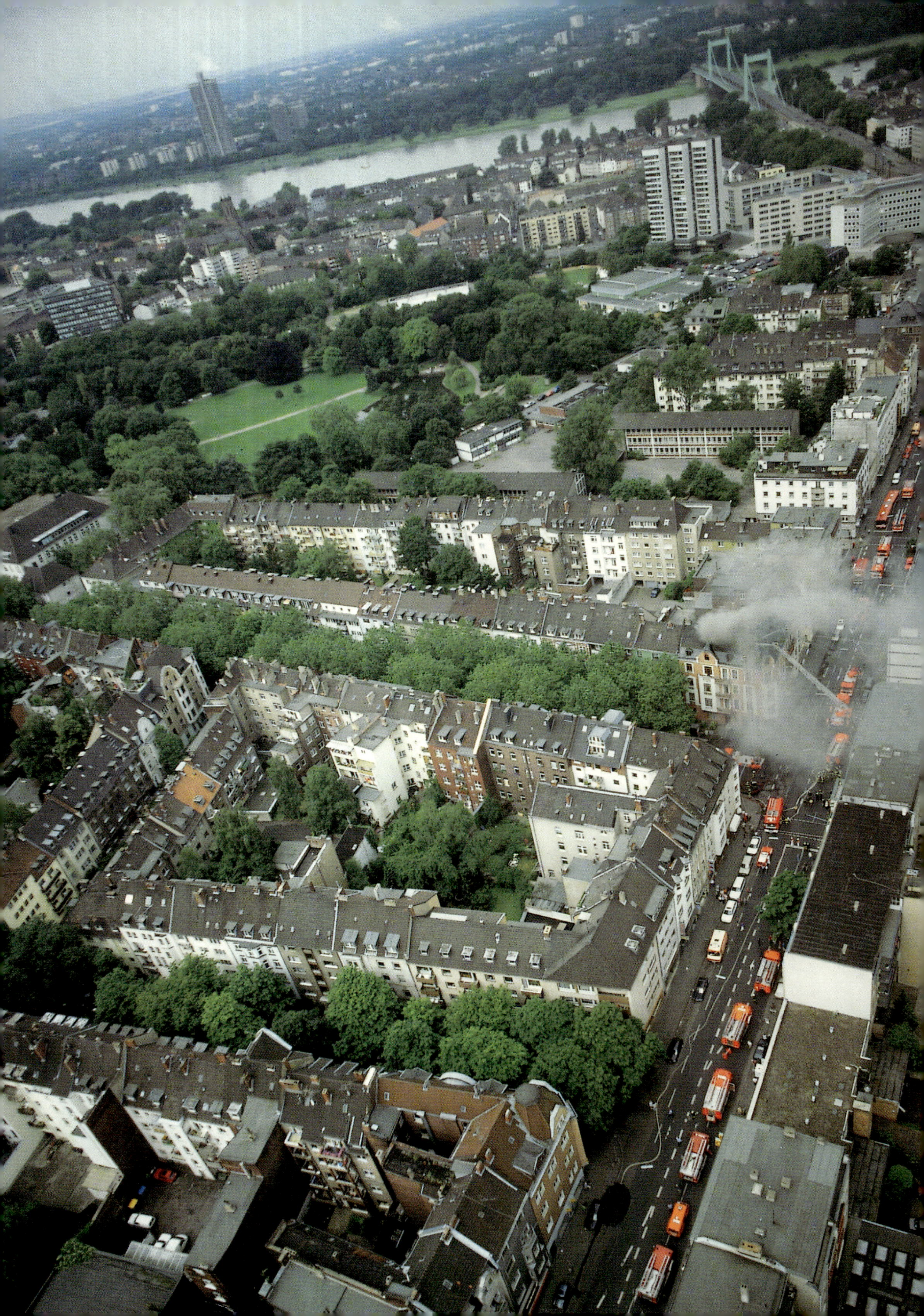

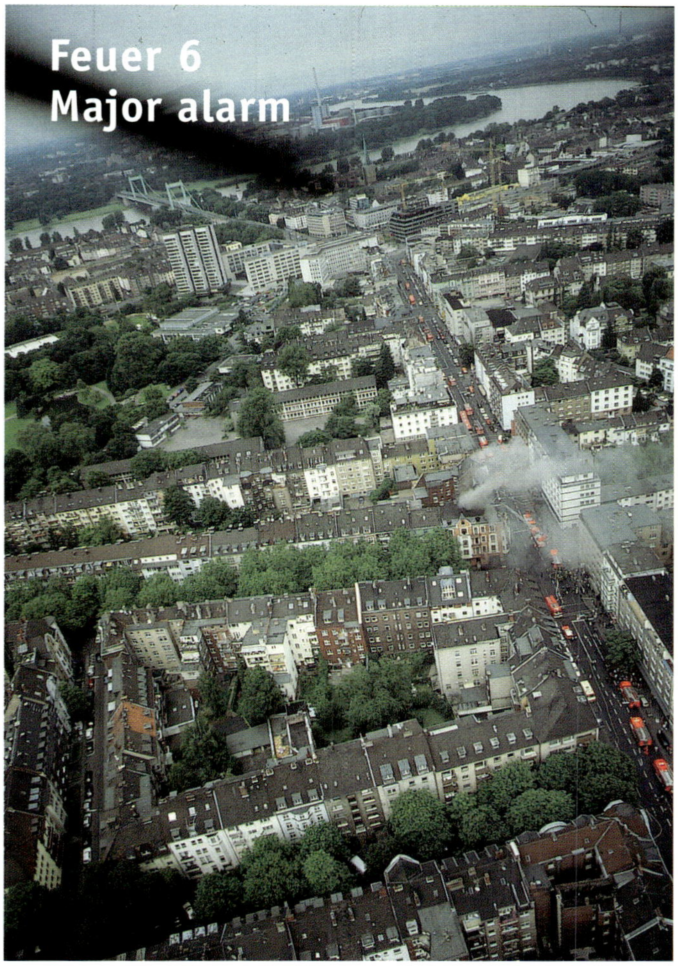

Die häufigsten Fragen an der Einsatzstelle

Frequently Asked Questions

Wie hoch fliegt eine BO 105?

Im Rettungseinsatz fliegen wir, soweit es das Wetter zulässt, in Höhen von 500 bis 2000 Fuß (1 Fuß = ca. 30 cm) über Grund. Dies sind ca. 150 bis 600 m. Die maximal mögliche Flughöhe beträgt 17.000 Fuß oder 5.600 m über dem Meeresspiegel.

How high can the BO 105 fly?

During rescue operations we fly, weather permitting, at altitudes of 500 to 2000 feet (1 foot = approx. 30 cm) above ground. That is about 150 to 600 m. The maximal possible flight altitude is 17,000 feet or 5.600 m above sea level.

6 Feuerwachen sind im Einsatz bei einem Feuer in einem Wohnhaus mitten in der Innenstadt. Das Gebäude droht einzustürzen. Rettungswagen und weitere Notärzte sind in unmittelbarer Nähe der Einsatzstelle.

Major alarm: 6 fire-fighting units have been called in to fight a fire in an apartment building in the downtown area. The building is in danger of collapsing. Rescue ambulances and additional physicians with emergency & rescue certification are in the immediate vicinity of the emergency site.

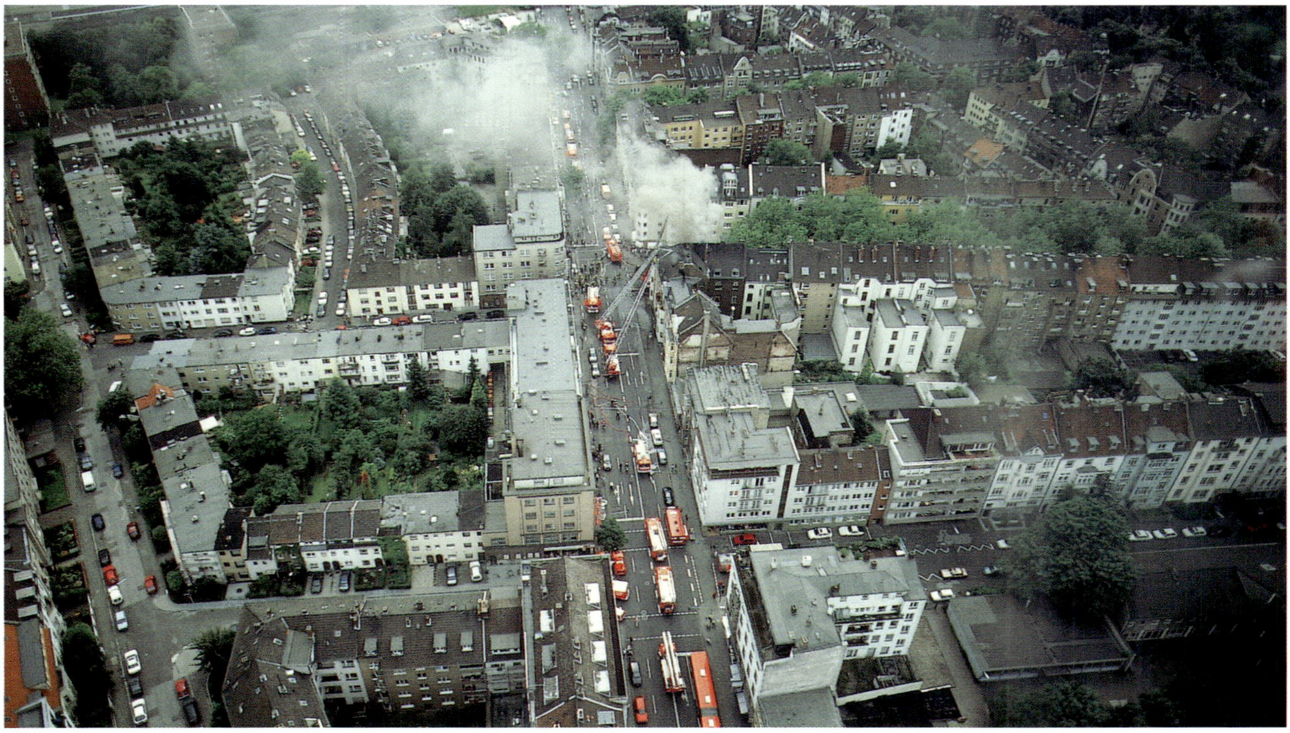

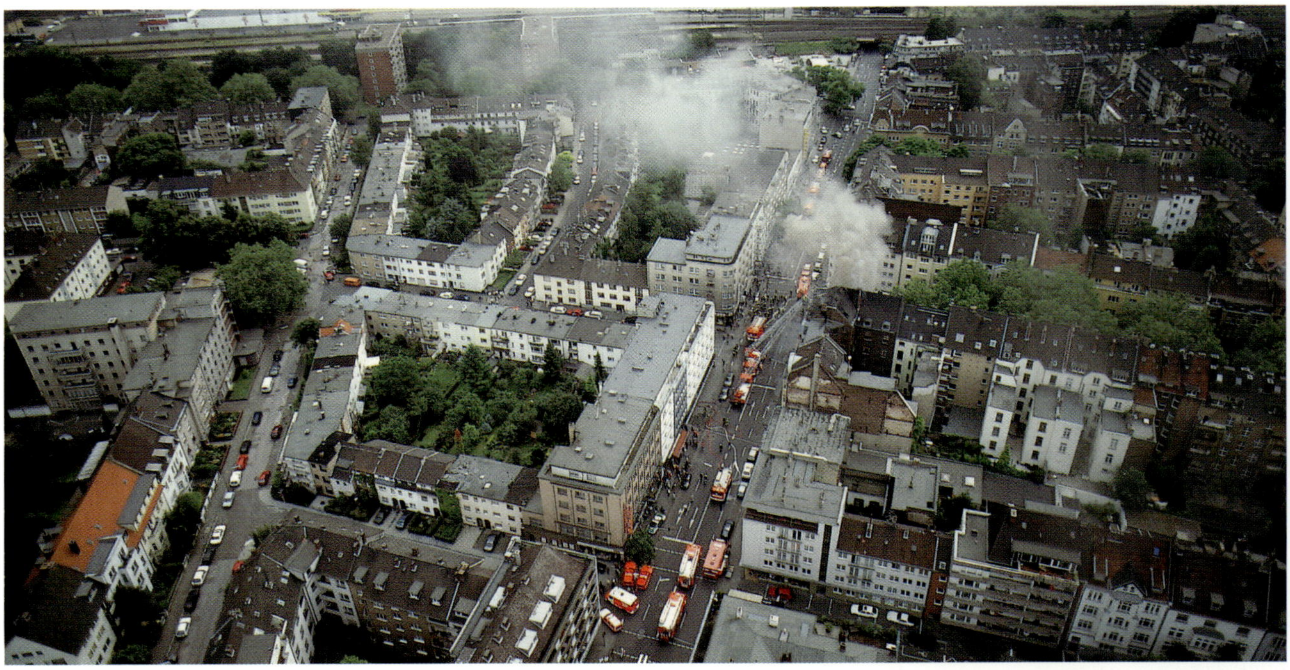

Drohender Gebäudeeinsturz: Feuer 6. Die Feuerwehr ist zu diesem Brand mit 6 Löschzügen, Rettungswagen und Notarztwagen ausgerückt. Wegen der extremen Hitze droht das Gebäude einzustürzen.

Building in danger of collapsing: Fire Alarm 6. The fire service has moved 6 fire-fighting trucks, a rescue ambulance and an emergency physician car (NEF) to the site.

Die häufigsten Fragen an der Einsatzstelle
Frequently Asked Questions

Seit wann trägt Christoph 3 die Aufschrift „Luftrettung – Bundesministerium des Innern"?

Mit dem Aufbau der Luftrettungsstationen in den neuen Bundesländern zu Beginn der Neunzigerjahre trugen die ersten Rettungshubschrauber des Bundes diese Aufschrift. In Köln löste er das Logo „Katastrophenschutz", das Christoph 3 von Anbeginn trug, mit dem Wechsel zur neuesten Version der BO 105 im Jahre 1996 ab. Das Bundesamt für Zivilschutz, ebenso zum Geschäftsbereich des Bundesministeriums des Innern gehörend wie der Bundesgrenzschutz (www.bundesgrenzschutz.de), hat die im Rahmen der Notfallvorsorge beschafften Hubschrauber den Bundesländern für den Luftrettungsdienst zur Verfügung gestellt. Bekanntermaßen werden die Hubschrauber von Mitarbeitern des Bundesgrenzschutzes geflogen und gewartet.

Von der ursprünglichen Zweckbestimmung rührt auch die orange Farbe (RAL 2004) her, es ist die internationale Farbe für den Zivilschutz. Diese Farbe tragen die Rettungshubschrauber des Bundes seit Mitte der Siebzigerjahre. Vorher waren sie gelb.

How long has Christoph 3 carried the lettering "Air Rescue – Federal Minister of the Interior"?

With the establishment of air rescue bases in the new German states at the beginning of the 1990s, the first federal rescue helicopters carried this lettering. In Cologne the "Disaster Services" logo which Christoph 3 had carried from the very beginning was replaced by the present logo when the switch was made to the latest type of BO 105 in 1996.

The Federal Office of Civil Defense – which, like the Federal Border Police (www.bundesgrenzschutz.de), is under the aegis of the Federal Minister of the Interior – contributed helicopters which were purchased within the framework of the emergency and disaster planning of the individual German states. As everyone knows, the helicopters are flown and serviced by members of the German Border Police.

The orange color (RAL 2004) of the helicopter is also a relic of these early days: orange is the international color for civil defense. The rescue helicopters operated by the German federal government have been painted orange since the mid-1970s; before that they were yellow.

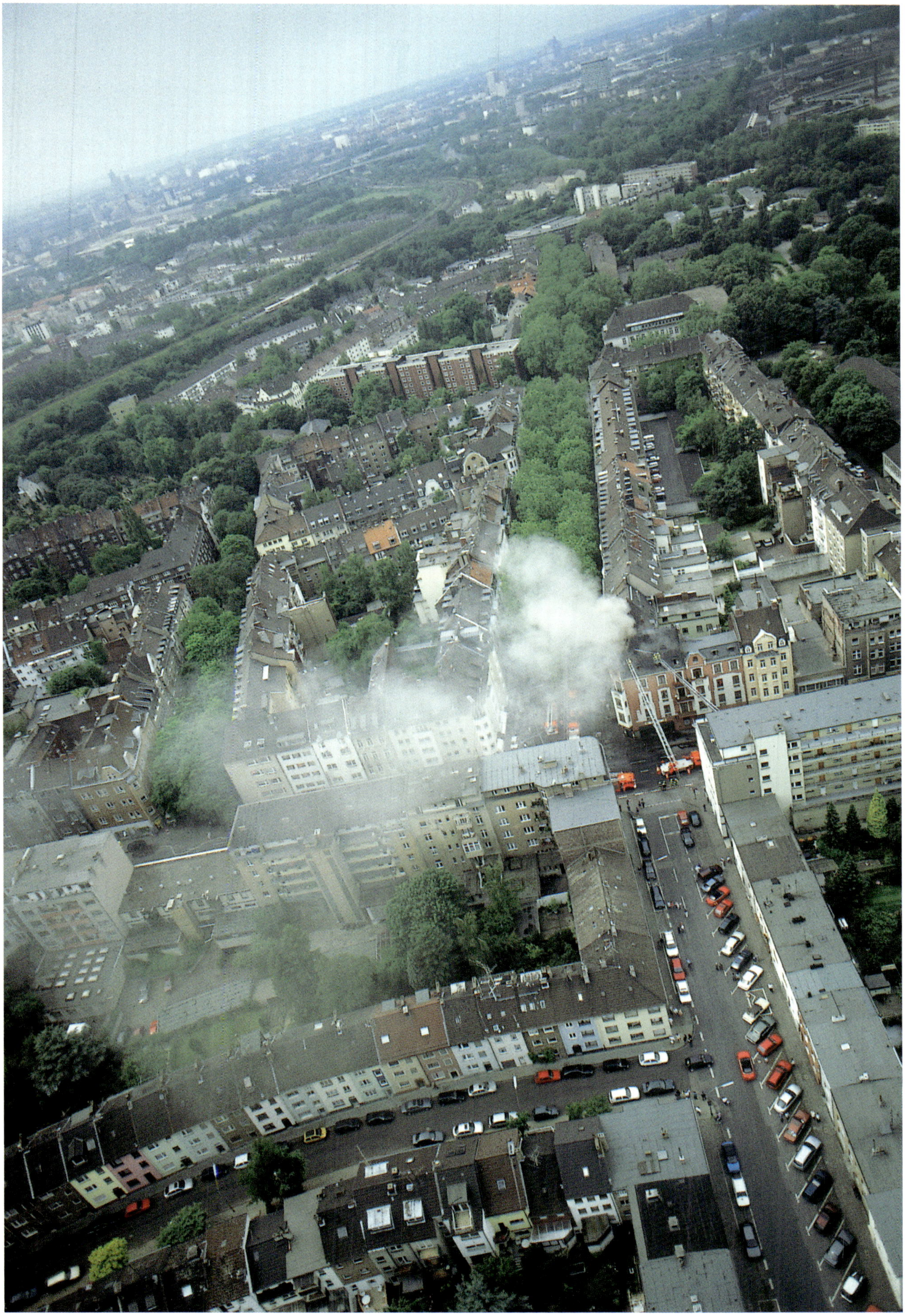

Einsatz für den Rettungshubschrauber
Mission for the Rescue Helicopter

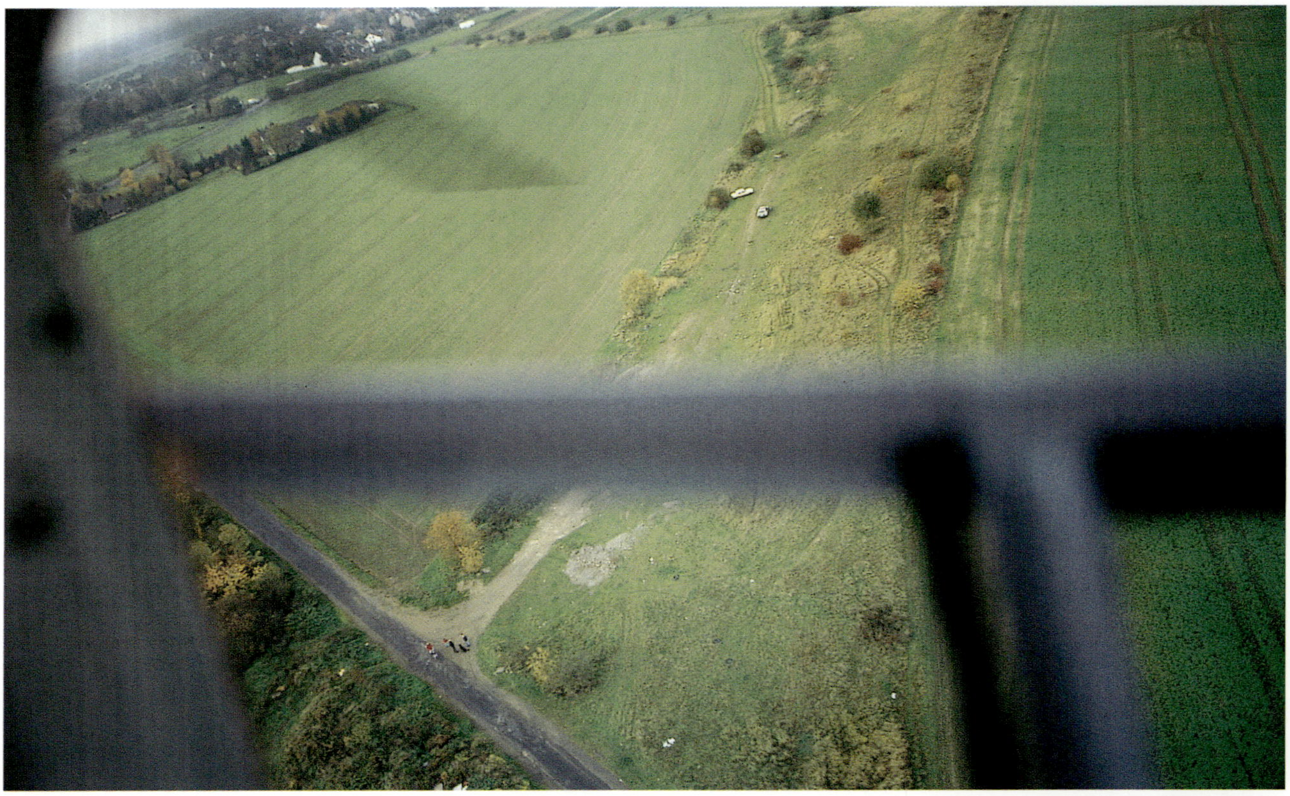

Suchflug – In einem Pkw soll ein lebloser Patient liegen. Spaziergänger haben die Scheiben des Pkw eingeschlagen. Neben dem Patienten liegt ein Abschiedbrief an seine Ehefrau, die sich von ihm getrennt hat.

Search-and-rescue flight: a lifeless man has been sighted inside a locked automobile. Several people out for a walk had smashed the car window in an attempt to rescue the man. On the seat next to him they found a suicide note to his estranged wife.

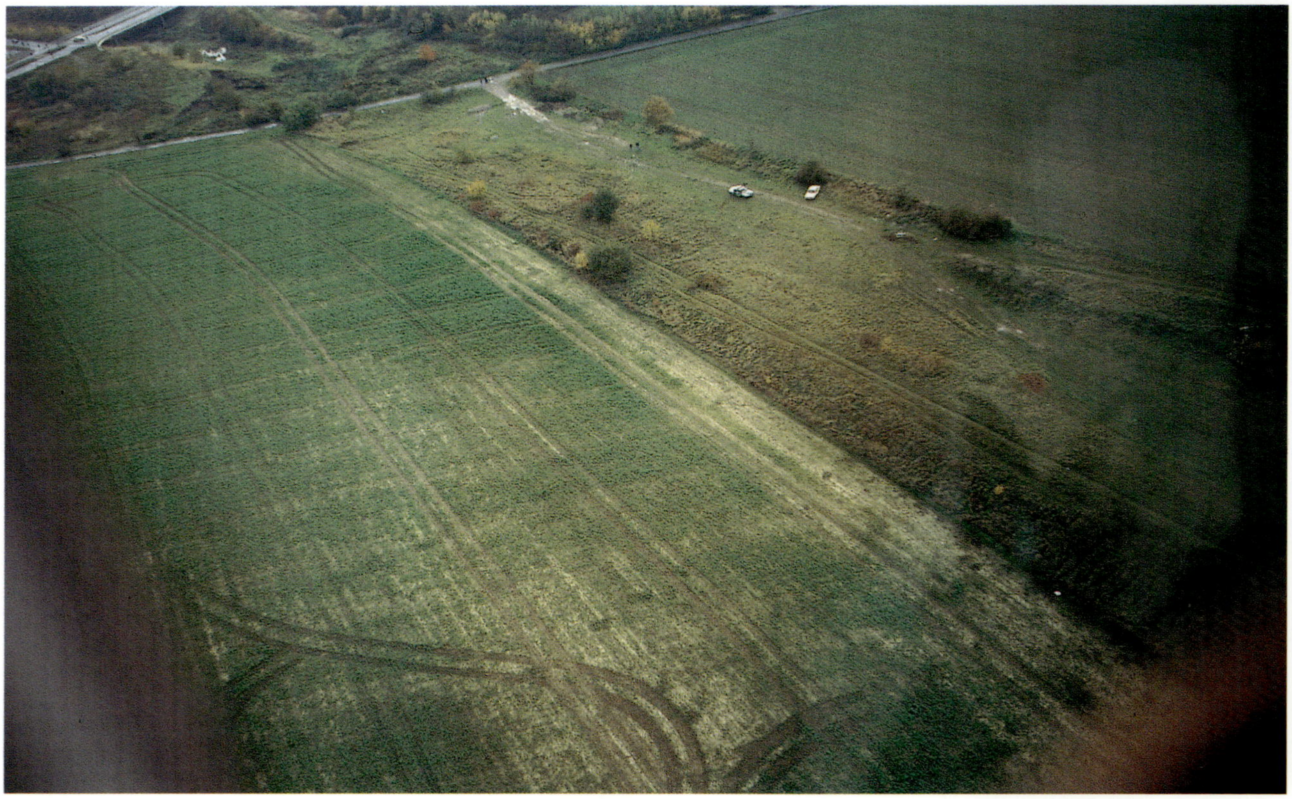

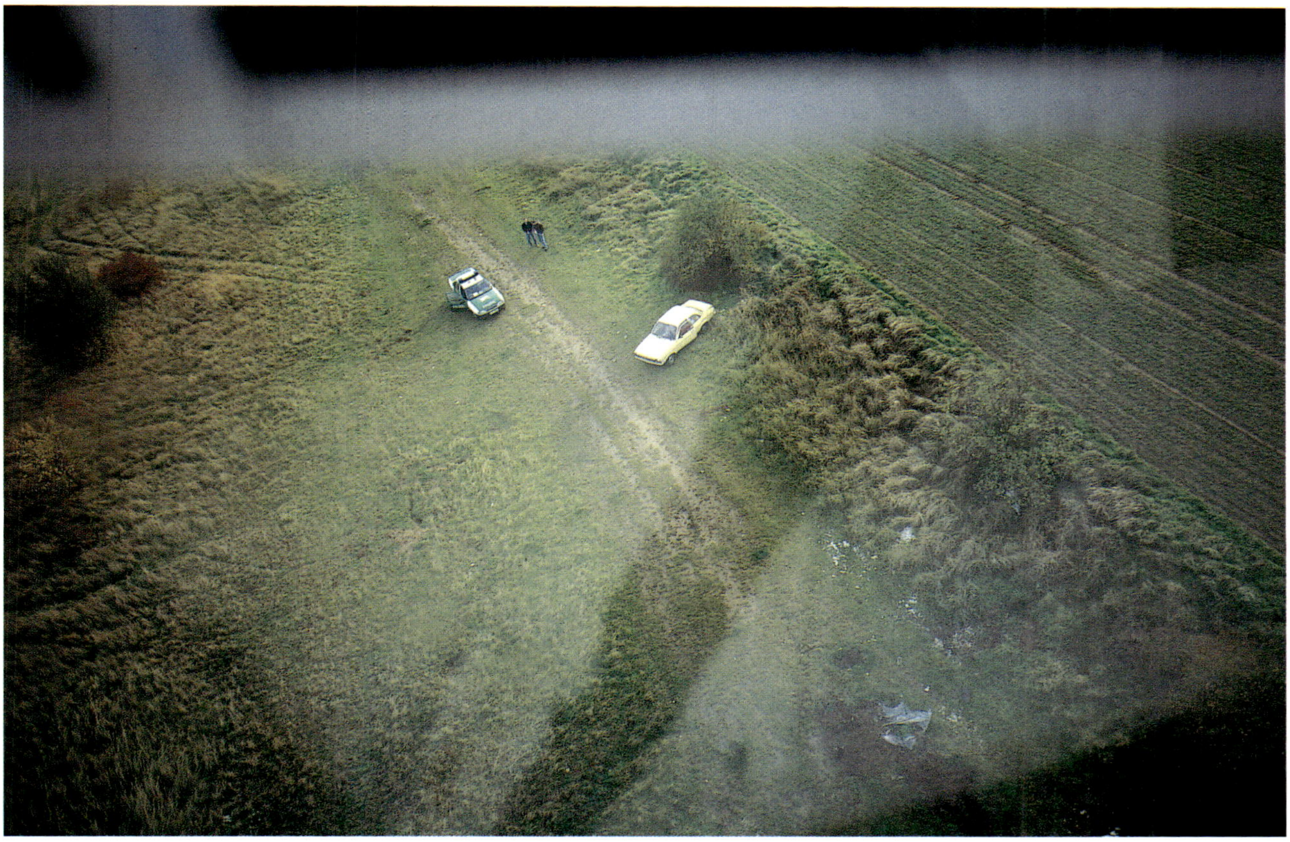

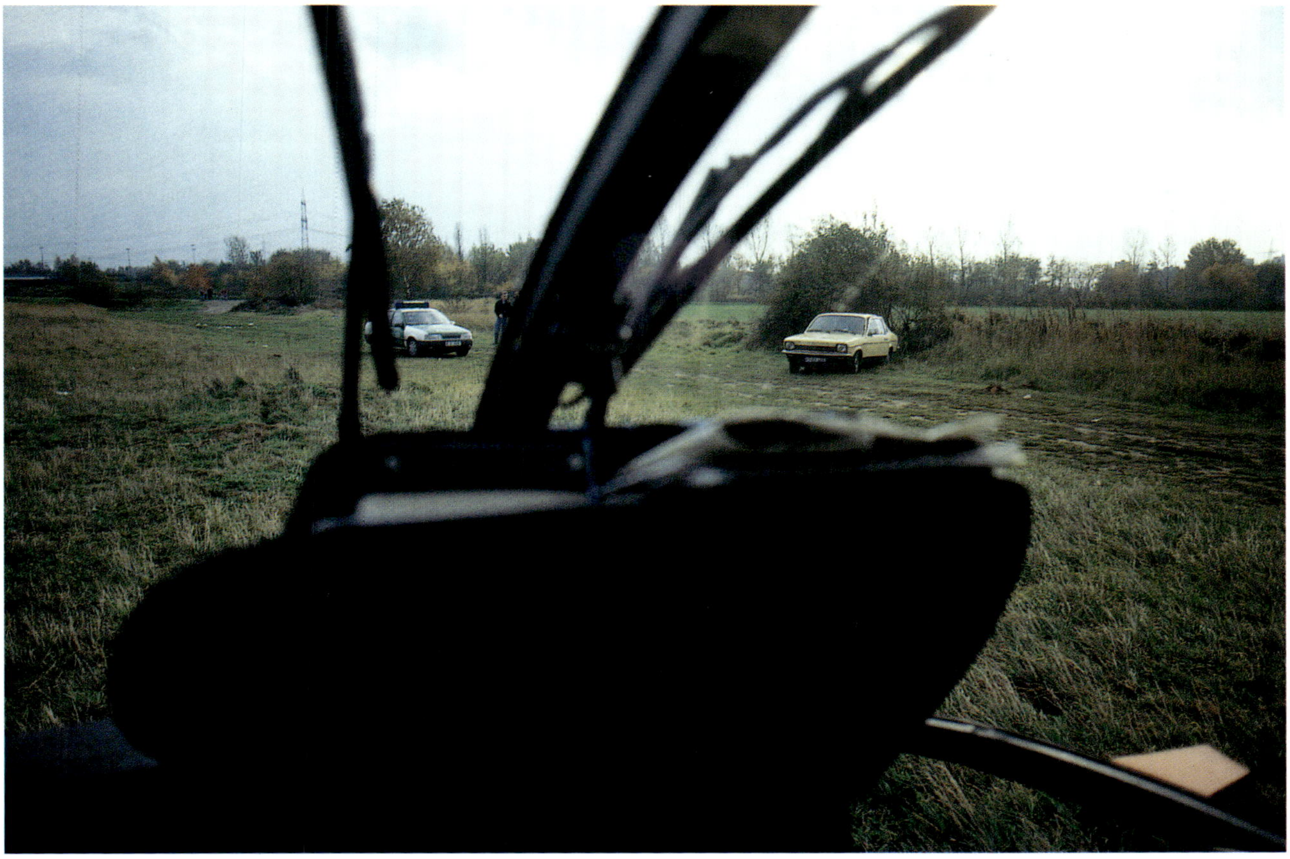

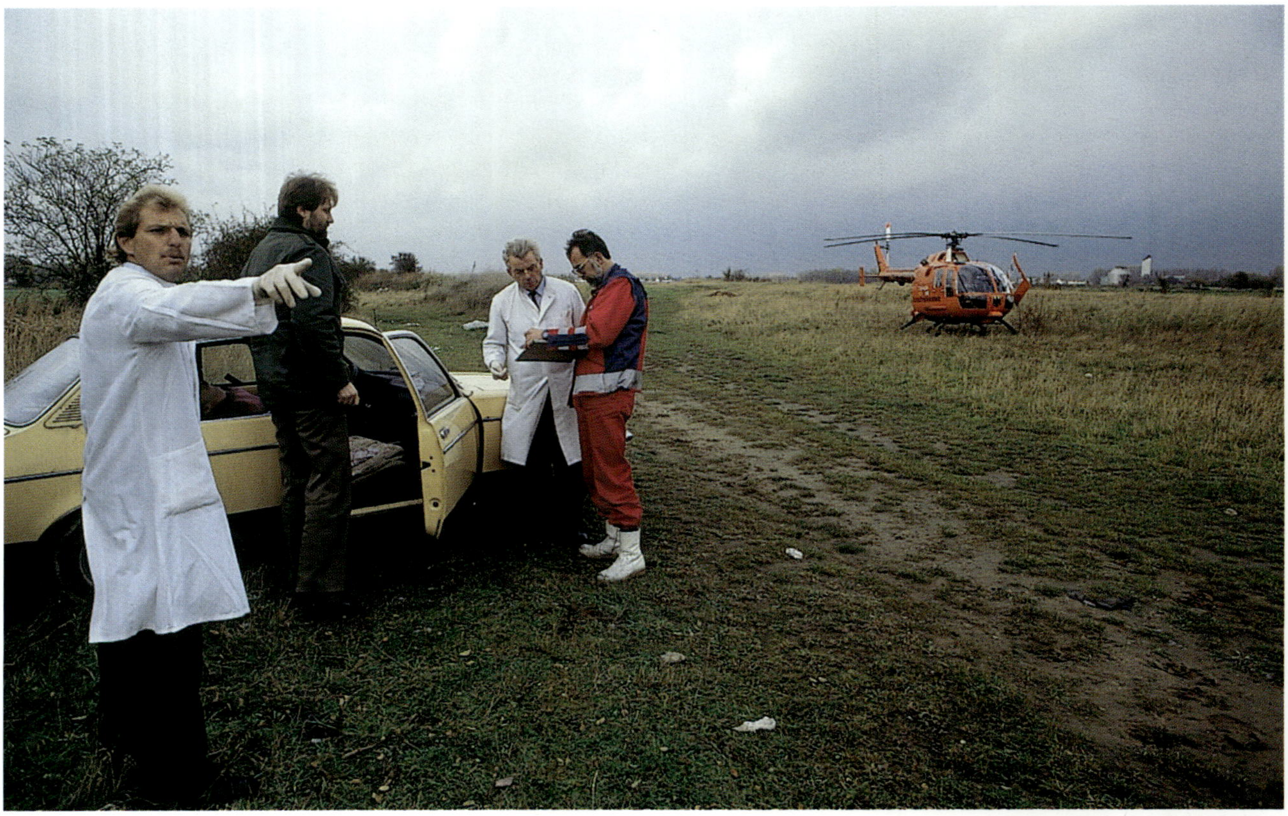

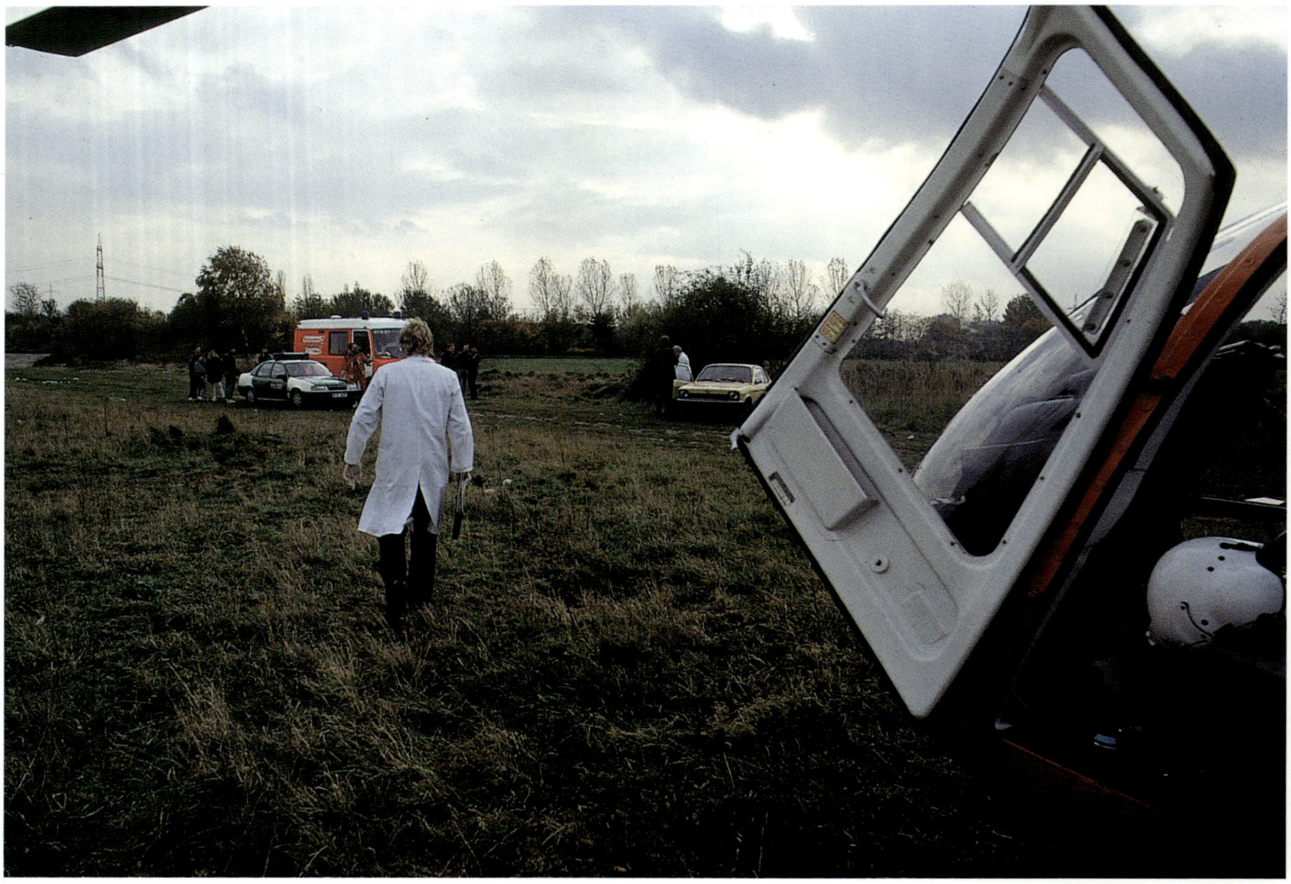

Augenblicke

Dienstbeginn. Sonntagmorgen 5.30 Uhr. Fahrt zur Station. Die Luft ist wunderbar. Die Autobahn ist frei. Ruhe.

Snapshots

Beginning of the Sunday morning shift at 5:30 a.m. Drive to the base on the empty autobahn. The early morning air is wonderful. A peaceful moment.

Einsatz für den Rettungshubschrauber
Mission for the Rescue Helicopter

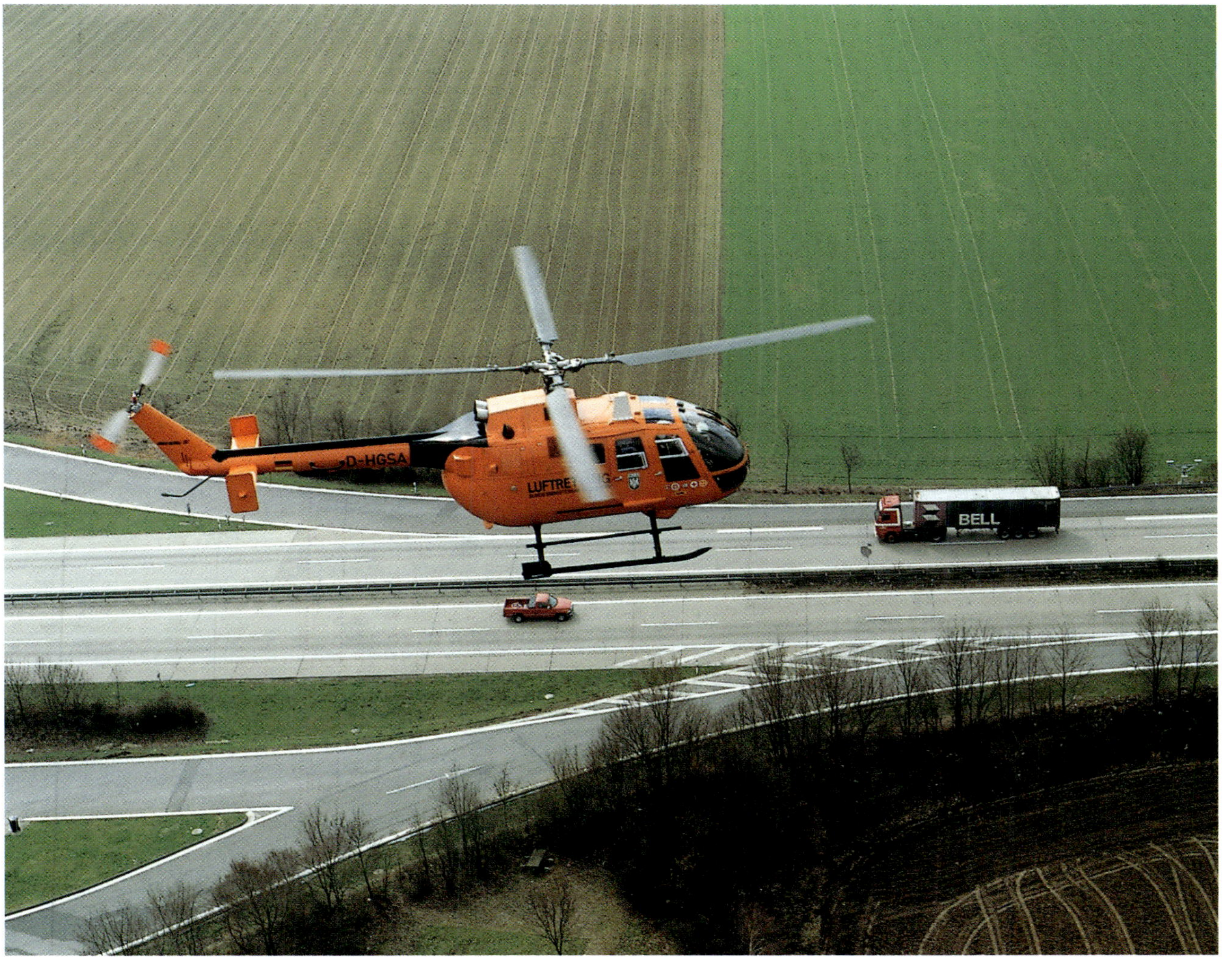

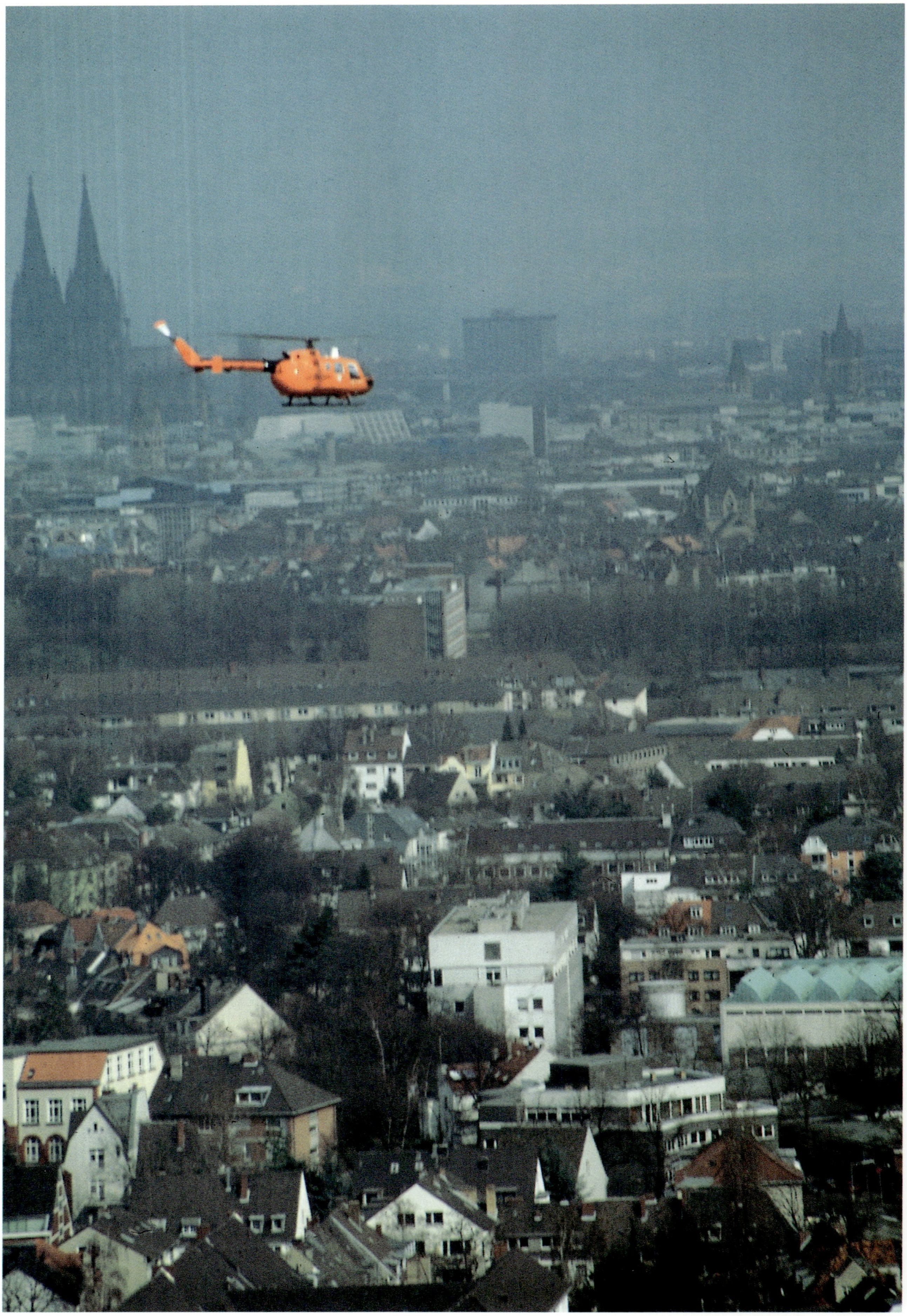

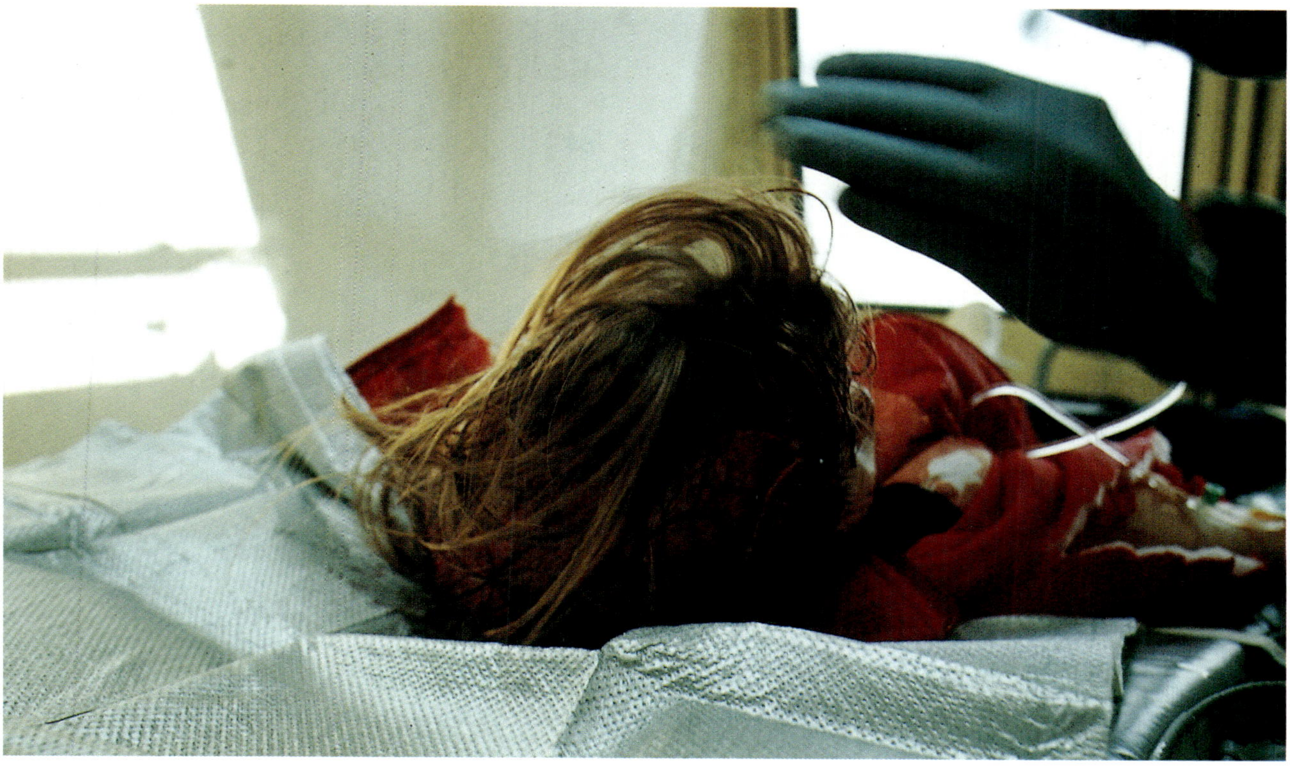

Der eigene Schäferhund hat ein kleines Mädchen skalpiert, das beim Fressen in den Hundezwinger gestiegen ist. Glück im Unglück: Die Kopfhaut kann komplikationslos wieder angenäht werden.

A little girl was literally "scalped" by the family's German shepherd when she climbed into the dog pen while the dog was feeding. This story had a happy ending: surgeons succeeded in reattaching the girl's scalp.

Die häufigsten Fragen an der Einsatzstelle
Frequently Asked Questions

Kann man bei Ausfall eines der beiden Triebwerke noch landen oder starten?

Eine Landung mit einem Triebwerk ist grundsätzlich immer möglich. Abhängig vom Gewicht des Hubschraubers muss aber ggf. eine Ausgleitstrecke in Kauf genommen werden, weil ein Schwebeflug aus Gewichtsgründen nicht möglich ist. Ein Start mit nur einem Triebwerk ist bei zweimotorigen Hubschraubern durch den Hersteller, bei Vorliegen gewisser Umstände, auf absolute Ausnahmen beschränkt.

Selbst beim Ausfall beider Triebwerke ist der Hubschrauber voll steuerbar. Durch Drücken des „pitch" werden die Hauptrotorblätter so angestellt, dass der Luftstrom im Sinkflug den freilaufenden Rotor antreibt. Dies nennt man Autorotation und es ermöglicht die Notlandung auf einem dann hoffentlich vorhandenen hindernisfreien Gelände.

Can the helicopter still take off and land if one of the engines fails?

It is basically always possible to land a helicopter with only one engine. Depending on the weight of the helicopter, however, the helicopter may have to glide for a certain distance since it cannot hover with only one engine, owing to its weight. In two-engine helicopters, takeoff with one engine is permitted by the manufacturers only in very exceptional situations.

Even in the event of a failure of both engines, the helicopter is completely controllable. By pressing the pitch lever, the pilot can adjust the pitch of the main rotor blades in such a way that the air current drives the freely moving rotor during descending flight. This state of affairs is called autorotation and allows the helicopter to make an emergency landing on an available site which is (hopefully) free of obstacles.

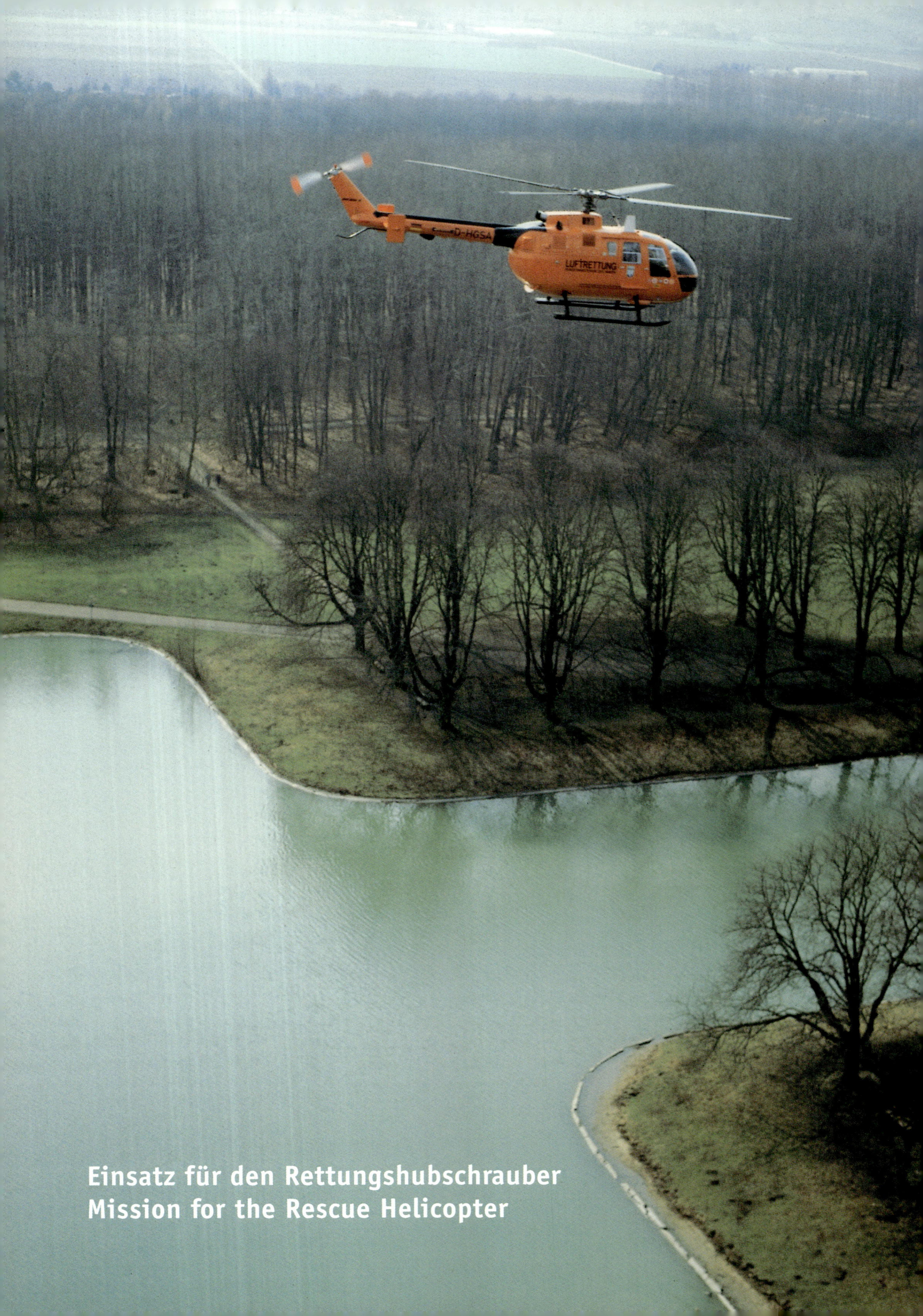

Einsatz für den Rettungshubschrauber
Mission for the Rescue Helicopter

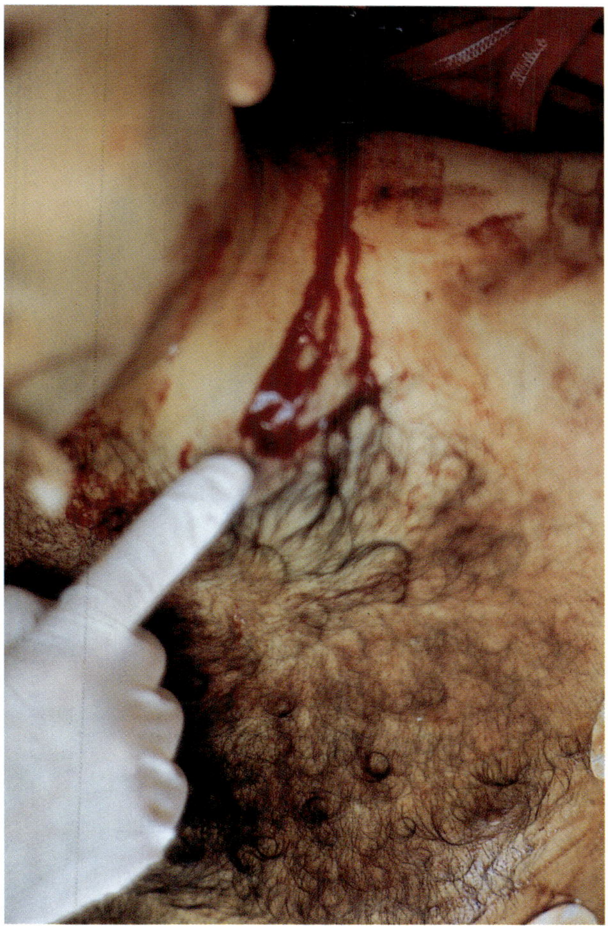

Für den Rettungsdienst ist es eine Schußverletzung. Für Polizei und Staatsanwalt ist es ein Tötungsdelikt zum Nachteil von Herrn A. Für den Richter ist es Mord. Für die Yellow Press ist es Mafiamord.

Gunshot wounds: for the rescue service the emergency call is a gunshot injury with unsuccessful resuscitation efforts, for the police it is homicide committed by XY, for the public prosecutor it is premeditated murder, for the yellow press it is a murder in the drug scene.

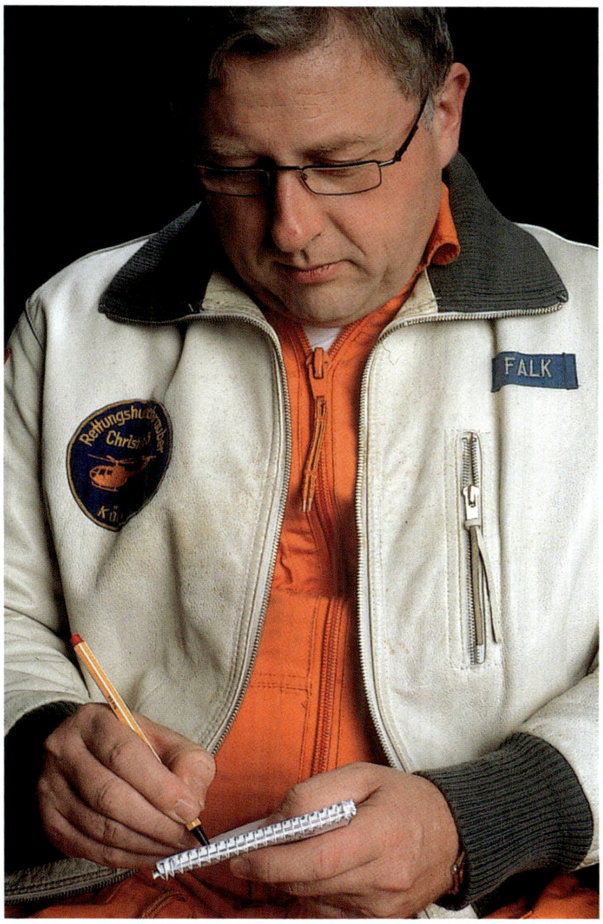

Ermittlung der Patientendaten.

Recording of patient data.

Augenblicke

Sommermittag. Hitze. Im Biergarten Reanimation. Ehepaar hat schon das Auto in den Autoreisezug verladen und will nach Spanien. Ehemann nicht reanimierbar. Ehefrau muß in dieser Situation viele Dinge lösen. Rückkehr.

Snapshots

A hot summer afternoon. Resuscitation efforts in a beer garden. A married couple had already loaded their car onto a train to Spain, where they planned to take a vacation. The resuscitation efforts are unsuccessful. Think of all the things the wife has to take care of. Return flight.

Wartungsarbeiten / Maintenance Work.

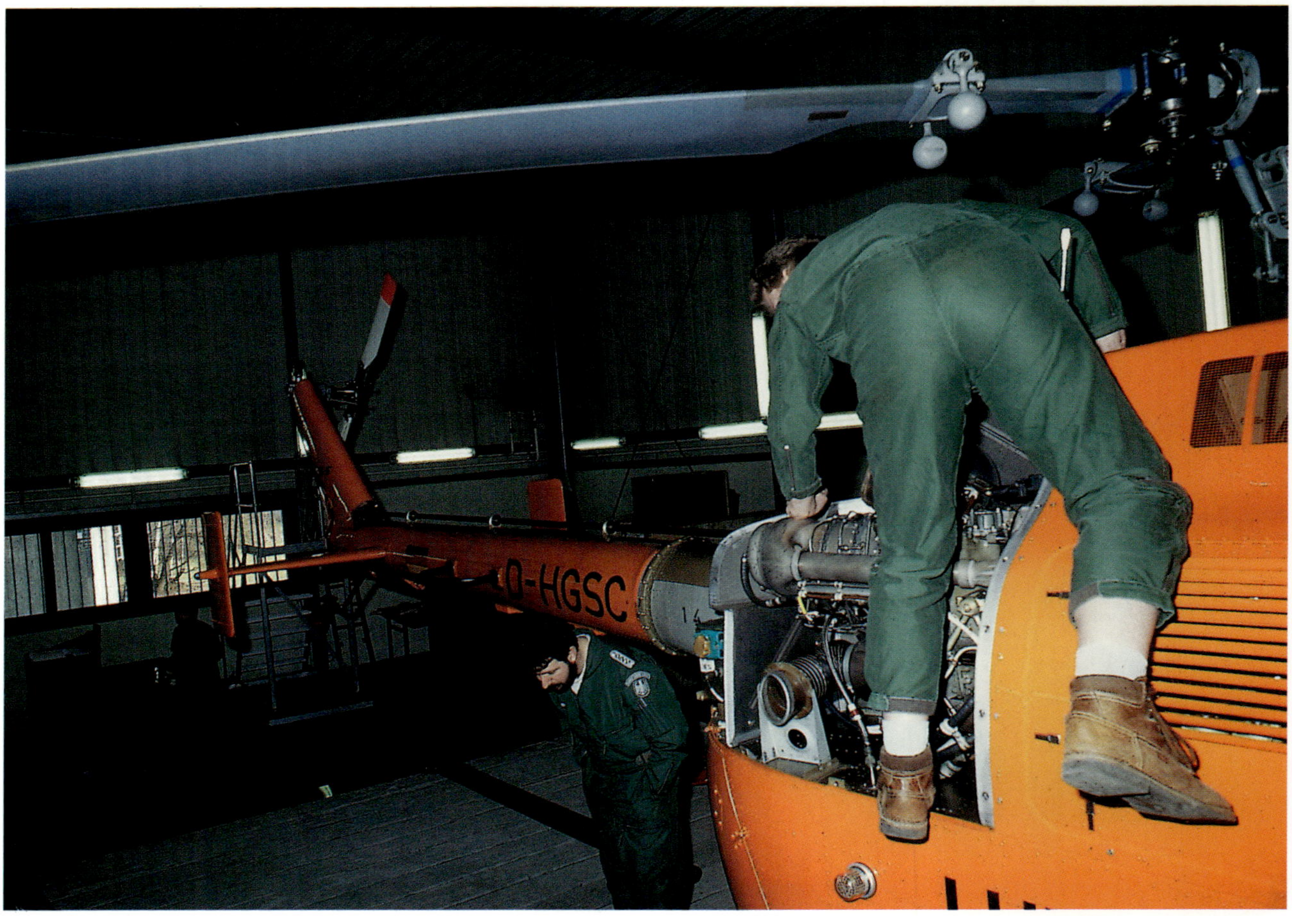

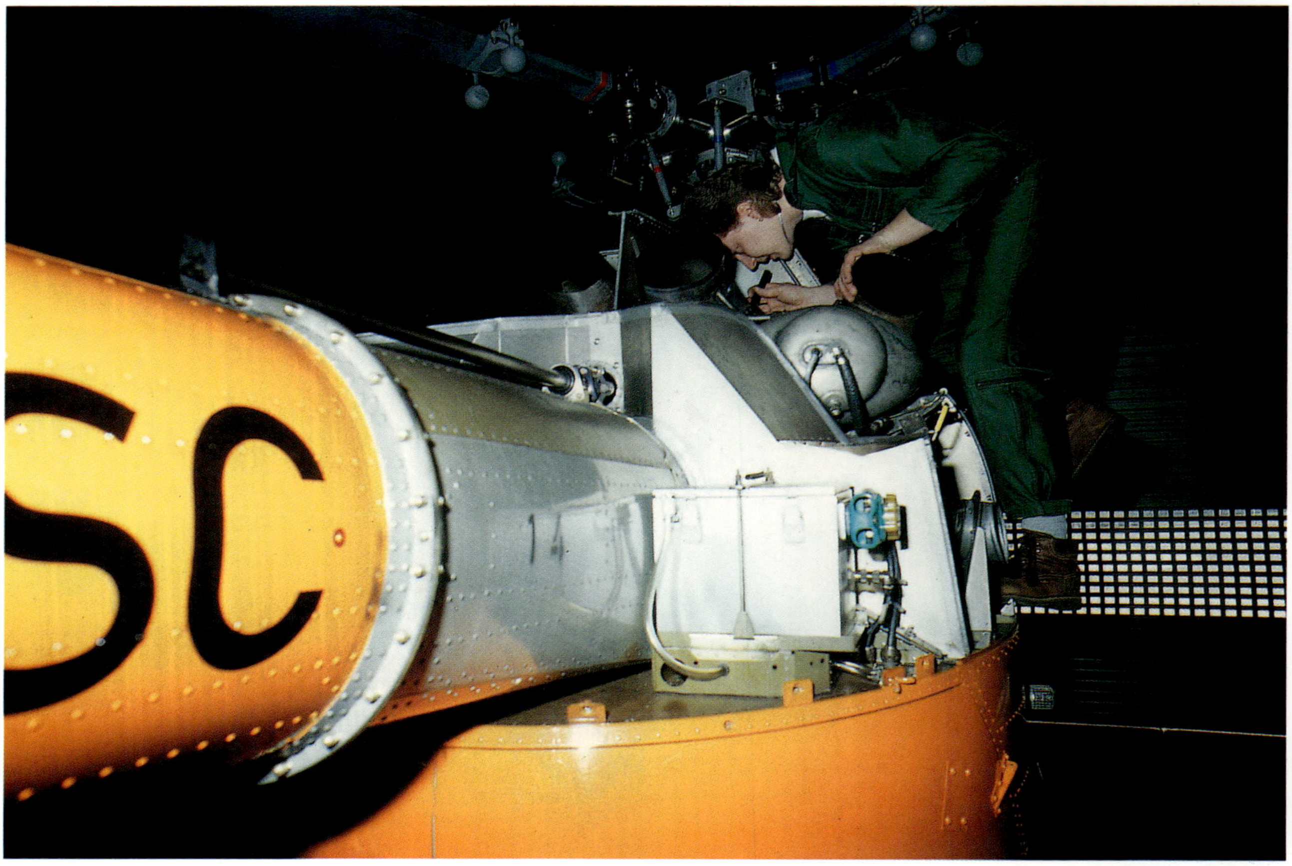

Die häufigsten Fragen an der Einsatzstelle
Frequently Asked Questions

Warum fliegt der Rettungshubschrauber nachts keine Primäreinsätze?

Die Einsatzzeit aller Christoph-Rettungshubschrauber in Deutschland beginnt täglich um 07.00 Uhr, im Winter mit Sonnenaufgang und endet mit Sonnenuntergang.

Ein Primäreinsatz, also der Flug zu einem akuten Notfall, führt in der Regel immer zu einer Landestelle, die für die Besatzung unbekannt und in den allerseltensten Fällen ein Flugplatzgelände ist. Deutschland ist mit unzähligen Hindernissen, insbesondere mit Masten und Leitungen übersät, die in der Nacht aus der Luft nicht erkannt werden können und deshalb ein unkalkulierbares Risiko für den Hubschrauber seine Insassen und für die Menschen am Boden bilden.

Die Technik ist inzwischen weit fortgeschritten. So genannte Bildverstärker (BiV)-Brillen sind in der Lage auch minimalstes Restlicht so zu verstärken, dass die Besatzung auch in der Nacht unbekanntes Gelände anfliegen könnte.

Es stellt sich jedoch die politisch zu beantwortende Frage, ob perspektivisch von einer Einsatzfähigkeit von Hubschraubern zu allen Tages- und Nachtzeiten auszugehen ist. Es wäre dann zu klären, wer die hohen Investitionskosten für die erforderliche Technik und die erhöhten Personalkosten (der Bundesgrenzschutz fliegt in der Nacht mit BiV-Brillen mit einer professionellen Flugbesatzung von mindestens zwei Mann, ein Schichtdienstsystem wäre einzuführen etc.) trägt.

Bisher führen die Rettungshubschrauber in der Nacht nur Verlegungsflüge zwischen bekannten und beleuchteten Landeplätzen durch.

Why doesn't the rescue helicopter fly any primary missions at night?

The operational period of all the Christoph rescue helicopters in Germany starts at 7.00 a.m., in winter with sunrise, daily and ends at sunset. A primary mission, i.e. a flight to an acute emergency, generally leads to a landing site with which the crew is unfamiliar and only in rare cases to an airport. The territory of Germany is strewn with countless obstacles, in particular masts and power lines, which cannot be recognized at night and thus pose an incalculable risk to the helicopter, its passengers, and people on the ground.

Helicopter technology is now very advanced. For example, night vision goggles are able to intensify even minimal residual light to such an extent that the crew is able to fly into unknown territory even at night.

A question that has to be answered in a political context, however, is whether the basic assumption is that rescue helicopters should be operational and ready to take off at all hours of the day and night. It needs to be clarified, moreover, who will cover the higher investment costs for the required technology and for the higher personnel costs (the Federal Border Police fly at night with night vision goggles and a professional crew of at least two persons, a shift system would have to be introduced, etc.). So far rescue helicopters have only carried out night transport flights between familiar well-lighted landing sites.

An dieser Stelle ein kleiner Ausflug in die Physik und die Aerodynamik. Wieso fliegt eigentlich ein Hubschrauber? Weshalb kann er in der Luft auf der Stelle stehen, sich um die eigene Achse drehen und vorwärts, rückwärts und seitwärts schweben?

Die BO 105 verkörpert die Standardbauweise von Hubschraubern, die der russisch-amerikanische Konstrukteur Igor Sikorsky geprägt hat. Wie auch der größte in Serie hergestellte Hubschrauber der Welt, die Mil Mi 26 „Halo", die das 20-fache (!) Höchstabfluggewicht der BO 105 hat, hat Christoph 3 einen Haupt- und einen Heckrotor.

Die beiden Turbinentriebwerke der BO, die sich mit ca. 53.000 U/Min. drehen, übertragen ihre Energie über Wellen an das Hauptgetriebe, dessen wesentlicher Bestandteil der Hauptrotormast ist. Durch ein Planetengetriebe reduziert, dreht sich der Hauptrotor der BO 105 mit 420 U/Min. Aus dem Hauptgetriebe wird über eine Welle auch der Heckrotor angetrieben. Haupt- und Heckrotor drehen sich immer im gleichen Verhältnis von etwa 1 : 5, d.h. der Heckrotor dreht sich fünfmal schneller als der Hauptrotor.

A small excursion into physics and aerodynamics is appropriate at this point. How exactly does a helicopter fly? How can it hover in the air, turn on its own axis, and fly forward, backward and sideward?

The BO 105 embodies the standard helicopter design developed by the Russian-American designer Igor Sikorsky. Like the largest helicopter manufactured in series in the world – the Mil Mi 26 Halo, which has 20 times (!) the maximum takeoff weight of the BO 105 – Christoph 3 has a main rotor and a tail rotor.

The two turbine engines of the BO have a speed of approx. 53,000 RPM. They transfer their energy via shafts to the main gear system, the most important component of which is the main rotor mast. The rotational speed is stepped down by planetary gears; the main rotor of the BO 105 turns at a speed of 420 RPM. This main gear box also drives the tail rotor via a shaft. The speeds of the main rotor and tail rotor are always in a ratio of about 1 : 5, i.e. the tail rotor turns five times as fast as the main rotor.

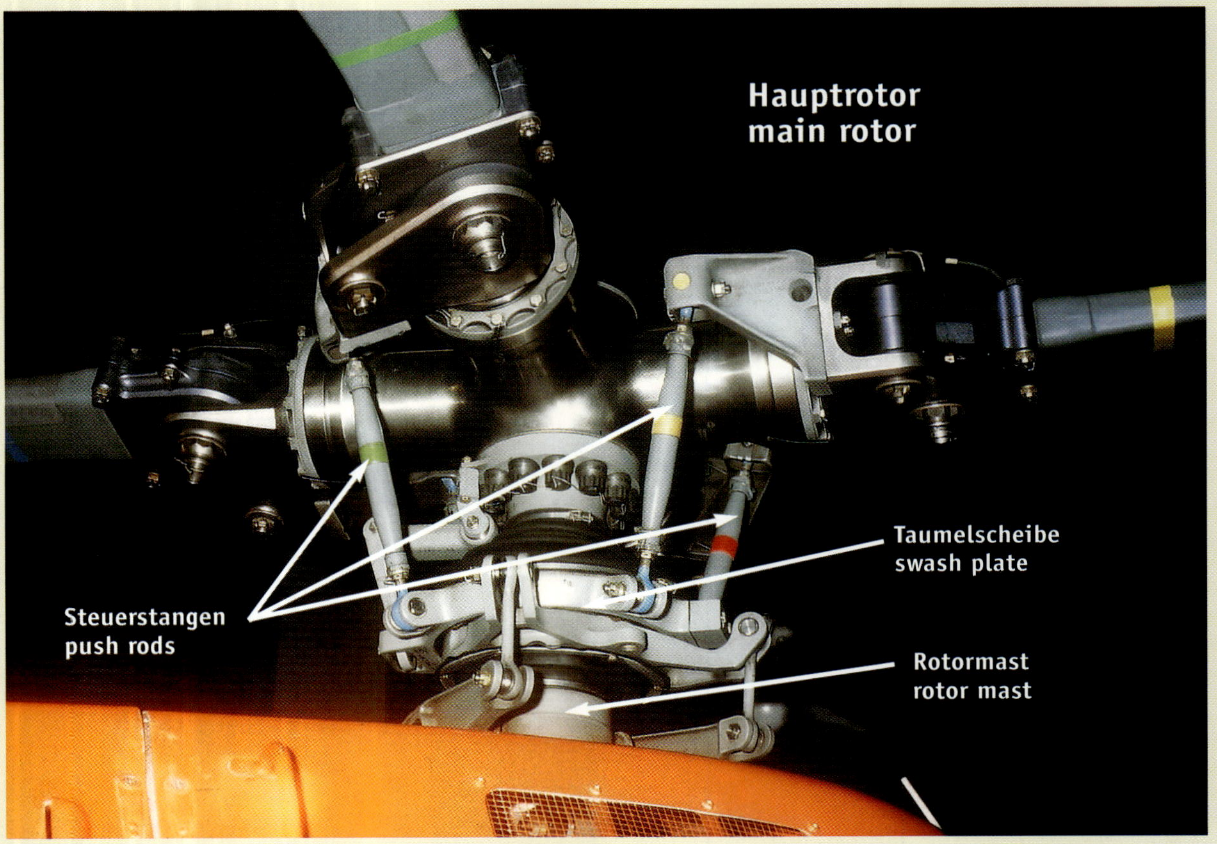

Der Hauptrotor als zentraler Bestandteil des Hubschraubers sorgt nicht nur für den Auftrieb, sondern ist auch das entscheidende Steuerelement. Anders als Flugzeuge, die grundsätzlich stabil fliegen, erkauft sich der Hubschrauber seine einzigartigen Fähigkeiten mit einer aerodynamisch nicht zu lösenden Instabilität, d.h. er muss zum Fliegen „gezwungen" werden. Um also seinen Flugweg beizubehalten, muss der Pilot, der im Hubschrauber übrigens rechts sitzt, ständig korrigierend eingreifen.

Dies tut er, anders als beim Flugzeug, über insgesamt drei Steuerorgane. Über den Steuerknüppel (engl.: stick) und die Steuerstangen kann die Taumelscheibe in alle Richtungen geneigt und somit die Bewegungsrichtung des Hubschraubers bestimmt werden. Dies nennt man auch zyklische oder periodische Steuerung. So, und nicht über den Heckrotor, werden auch Kurven geflogen.

The main rotor, in its function as the central assembly of the helicopter, does more than generate lift; it is also a decisive control element. Unlike normal aircraft, which possess a basic flight stability, helicopters achieve their unique maneuverability at the price of an instability which cannot be solved aerodynamically. For this reason, the helicopter must be "coerced" into flying; to stay on course, the helicopter pilot must constantly correct various parameters.

Unlike a normal aircraft, a helicopter has a total of three controls, which the pilot uses to steer the craft. By using the stick and push rods, the pilot can incline the swash plate in all directions and thus determine the direction of motion of the helicopter. Another name for this kind of control is cyclic or periodic control. This is also the way the pilot flies into curves (not via the tail rotor).

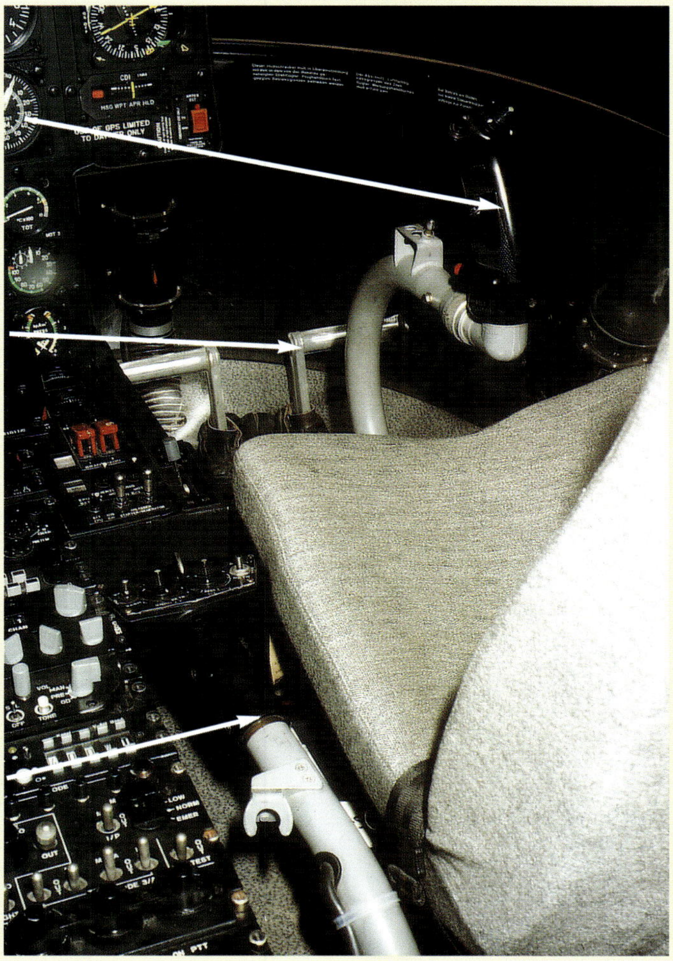

Steuerknüppel
stick

Pedale
pedals

Blattverstellhebel
pitch

Mit dem linken Arm bedient der Pilot den Blattverstellhebel (engl.: pitch). Dieser verstellt durch Heben oder Senken der Taumelscheibe, die am Rotormast gleitet, den Anstellwinkel der Hauptrotorblätter. Durch diese Veränderung des Auftriebs steigt oder sinkt der Hubschrauber. Man nennt dies auch kollektive Blattverstellung.

Dies reicht aber noch nicht für einen kontrollierten Flug aus. Der Hauptrotor der BO 105 dreht sich entgegen dem Uhrzeigersinn. Durch seinen Antrieb wird im Hauptgetriebe ein Drehmoment erzeugt, das den Rumpf des Hubschraubers entgegengesetzt zum Hauptrotor drehen ließe, wenn man keine Gegenmaßnahme ergreifen würde. Diese Gegenmaßnahme heißt Heckrotor. Er gleicht durch seinen Schub das Drehmoment aus und ermöglicht die Drehung des Hubschraubers um die Hochachse. Die dazu notwendigen Steuerorgane sind die Pedale (engl.: pedals), über die der Pilot den Schub des Heckrotors dem Drehmoment des Hauptrotors anpasst.

With his or her left arm, the pilot operates the pitch lever. This lever adjusts the pitch of the main rotor blades by raising or lowering the swash plate which slides on the rotor mast. The helicopter ascends or descends as a result of these changes in lift. This type of control is also referred to as collective pitch.

However, the above adjustments alone are not sufficient for controlled helicopter flight. The main rotor of the BO 105 rotates in a counterclockwise direction. The drive of this rotor generates a torque in the main gear box; if no countermeasures were taken, this torque would cause the fuselage of the helicopter to turn in a direction opposite to the main rotor. This countermeasure is provided by the tail rotor. The thrust produced by the tail rotor offsets the torque and allows the helicopter to turn around its vertical axis. The controls required for this turning are the pedals, which the pilot uses to adjust the thrust of the tail rotor to the torque of the main rotor.

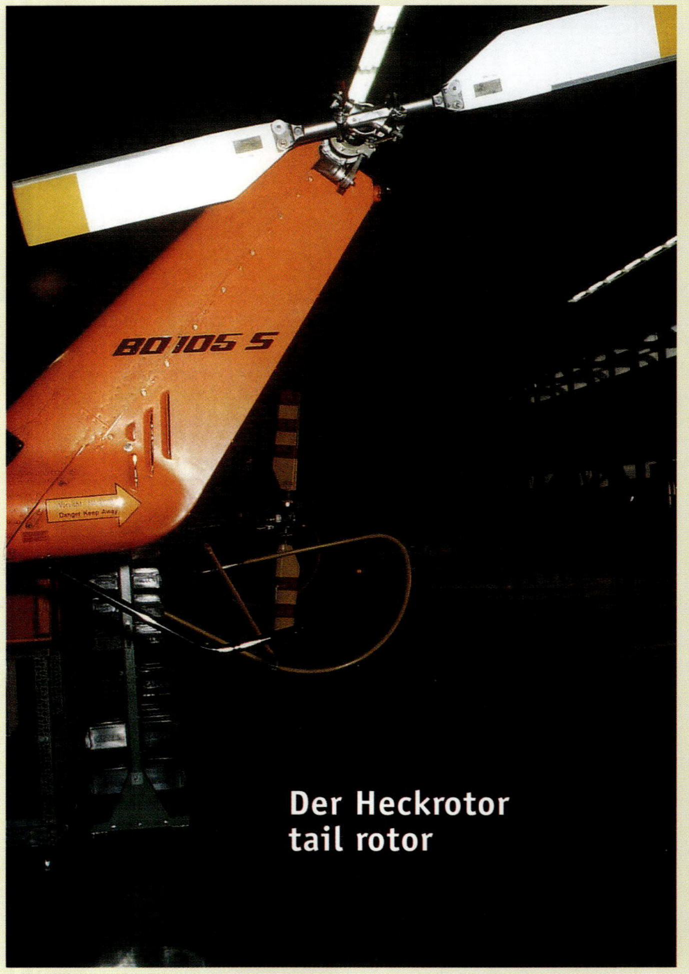

Der Heckrotor
tail rotor

Die Flugzustände werden hauptsächlich über die Abstimmung von periodischer und kollektiver Blattverstellung gesteuert. Der Heckrotor gewährleistet dabei die Beibehaltung der Fluglage bei sich ändernden Drehmomentverhältnissen.

So hält der Pilot im Schwebeflug mit dem „pitch“ die gleichmäßige Höhe über dem Boden. Mit dem „stick“ hält er die Position und korrigiert mögliche Windeinflüsse. Mit den Pedalen hält er die Schwebeflugrichtung oder dreht den Hubschrauber um die Hochachse. Will er nun aus dem Schwebeflug in den Vorwärts- und Steigflug übergehen, zieht er am „pitch“ und erhöht durch den höheren Anstellwinkel den Auftrieb, aber auch den Luftwiderstand des Rotors. Damit die Rotordrehzahl konstant bleibt und nicht zusammenbricht, werden über das Ziehen des „pitch“ auch die Kraftstoffregler der Triebwerke angesteuert und die eingespritzte Kraftstoffmenge erhöht.

Dieser Vorgang ist quasi mit dem Gasgeben beim Autofahren vergleichbar, wobei sich aber, im Unterschied zum Automotor, die Drehzahlen nicht verändern.

Da sich damit auch das Drehmoment erhöht hat, muss dieses über die Pedale korrigiert werden, um eine Drehung um die Hochachse zu verhindern. Zeitgleich hat der Pilot auch den „stick“ nach vorne bewegt und damit Vorwärtsfahrt aufgenommen.

Im Ergebnis müssen alle Steuereingaben gleichzeitig und gleichmäßig erfolgen und je nach Intensität der Steuereingabe dosiert werden. Diese ständige Koordination ist das eigentliche „Geheimnis“ des Hubschrauberfliegens.

Flight maneuvers are controlled mainly by coordinating the cyclic and collective pitch adjustment systems. The tail rotor allows the pilot to hold a flight position despite changes in torque.

When hovering, for example, the pilot keeps the helicopter at a constant height above ground by adjusting the pitch. He or she uses the stick to hold the aircraft steady and to offset the effects of any wind. With the pedals, he or she holds the direction of hovering flight or turns the helicopter around its vertical axis. If the pilot wants to make the transition from hovering to forward or ascending flight, he or she pulls the pitch lever; this higher pitch increases both lift and the air resistance of the rotors. To ensure that the rotor speed remains constant and does not drop precipitously, the pitch lever is also used to direct the fuel control system to inject more fuel into the engines.

This procedure can be roughly compared to the act of pressing the accelerator in a motor vehicle. In contrast to the automobile engine, however, the helicopter engine does not change its speed.

Since this step has also increased the torque, however, the pilot has to intervene with the pedals to prevent the helicopter from turning around its vertical axis. At the same time, the pilot moves the stick toward the front, thus initiating forward flight.

To achieve the desired result, all control measures must be carried out uniformly and simultaneously; in addition, they must be metered to reflect the desired intensity. The constant coordination is the real "secret" of flying a helicopter.

Einsatz für den Rettungshubschrauber
Mission for the Rescue Helicopter

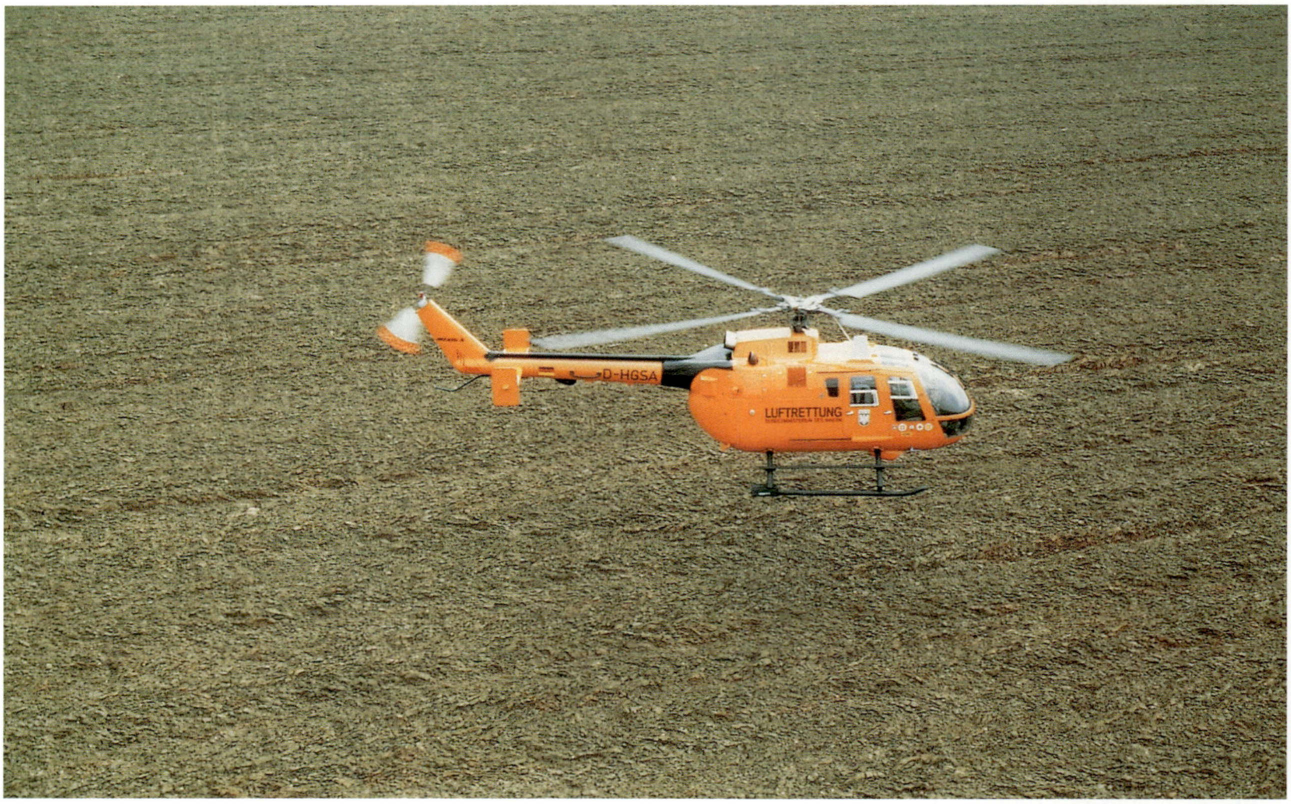

Ein Segelflugzeug soll abgestürzt sein: Der Rettungshubschrauber wird zur Suche eingesetzt.

A glider has reportedly crashed. A rescue helicopter is sent out on an SAR mission.

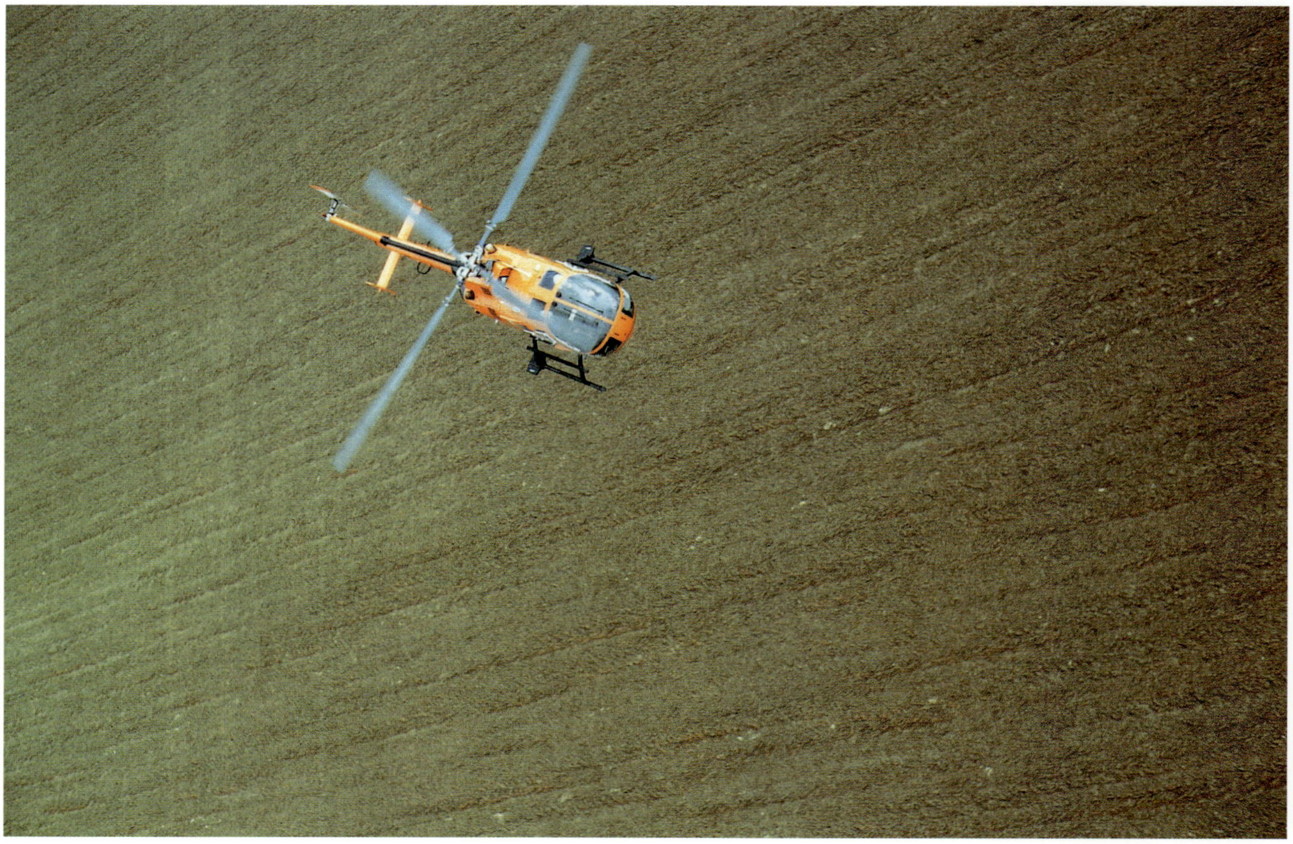

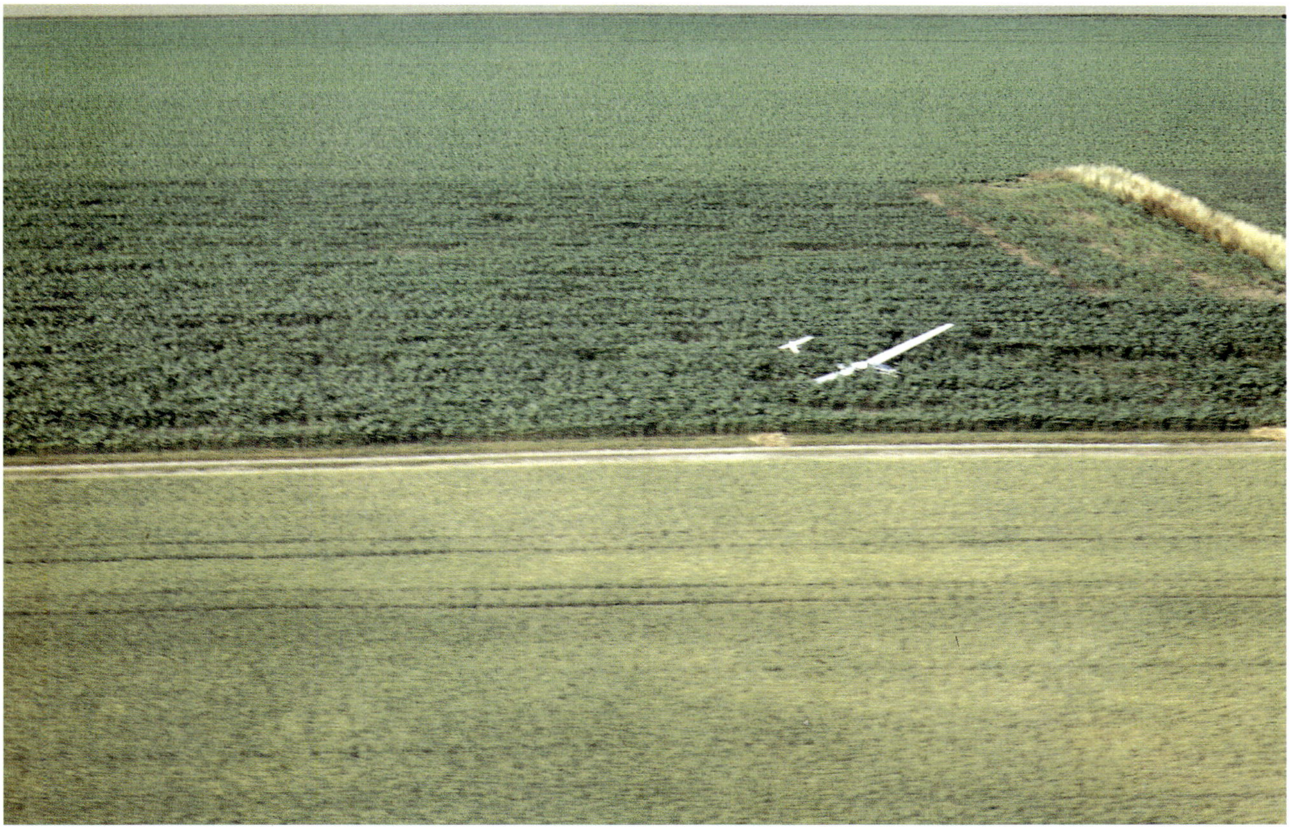

Beim Anflug erkennt die Besatzung des Rettungshubschraubers, dass der Pilot nicht im Cockpit des Segelflugzeugs sitzt. Der Rettungshubschrauber führt die bodengebundenen Einsatzkräfte an den Ort heran und beginnt mit der Suche nach dem Piloten.

During the approach to land, the rescue helicopter crew notices that the pilot is not inside the glider. In this situation, the rescue helicopter crew leads the rescue workers on the ground to the emergency site and commences a search for the pilot.

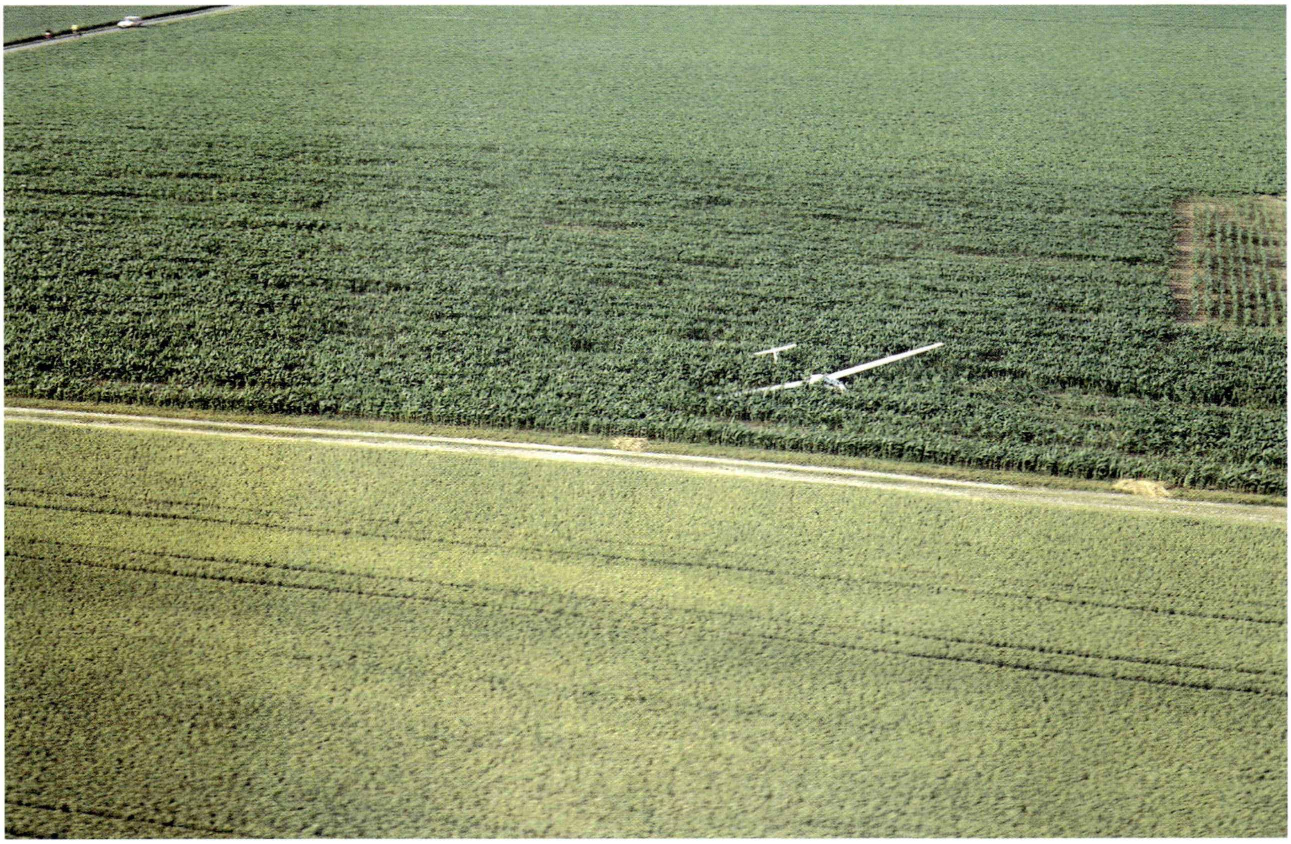

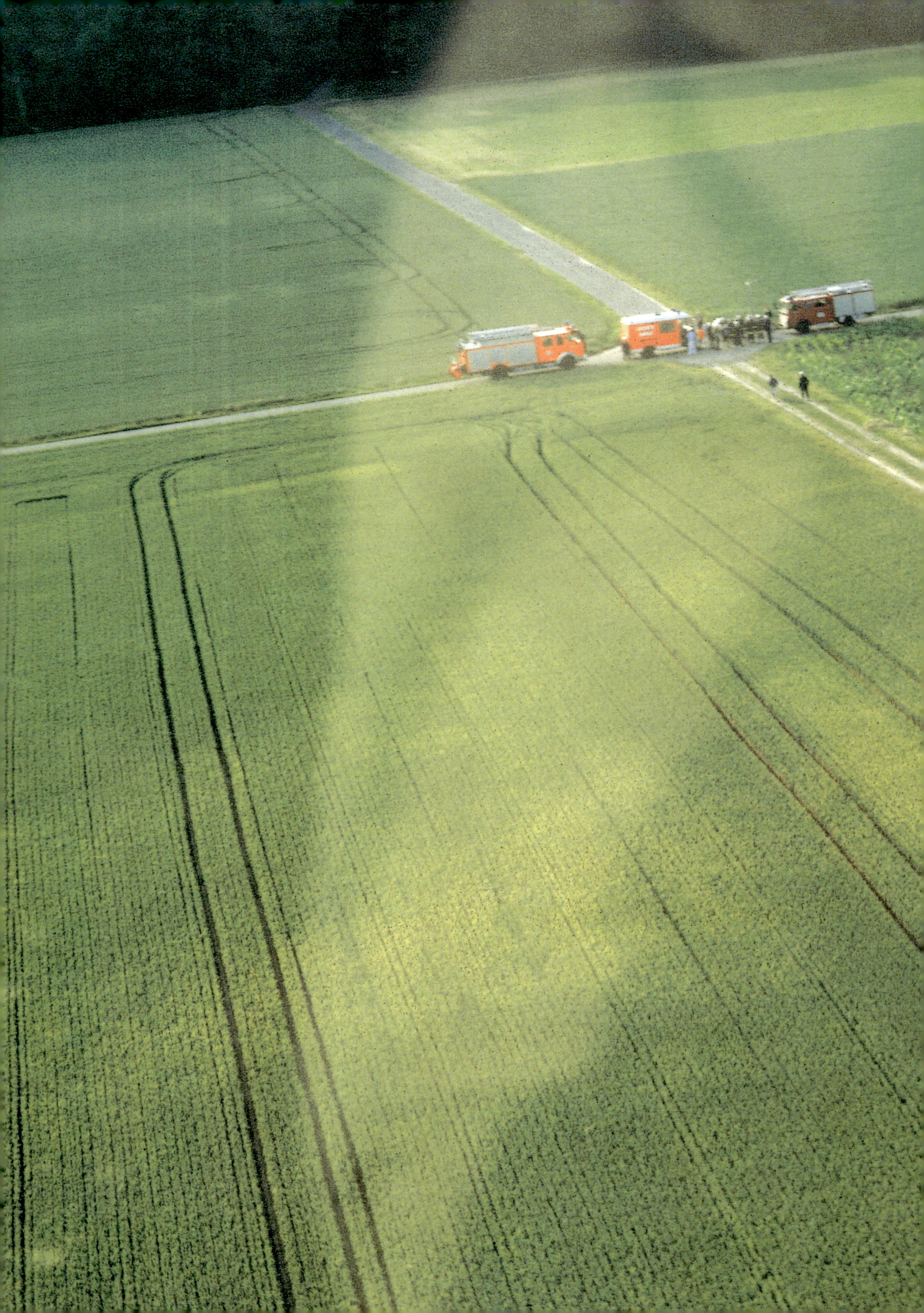

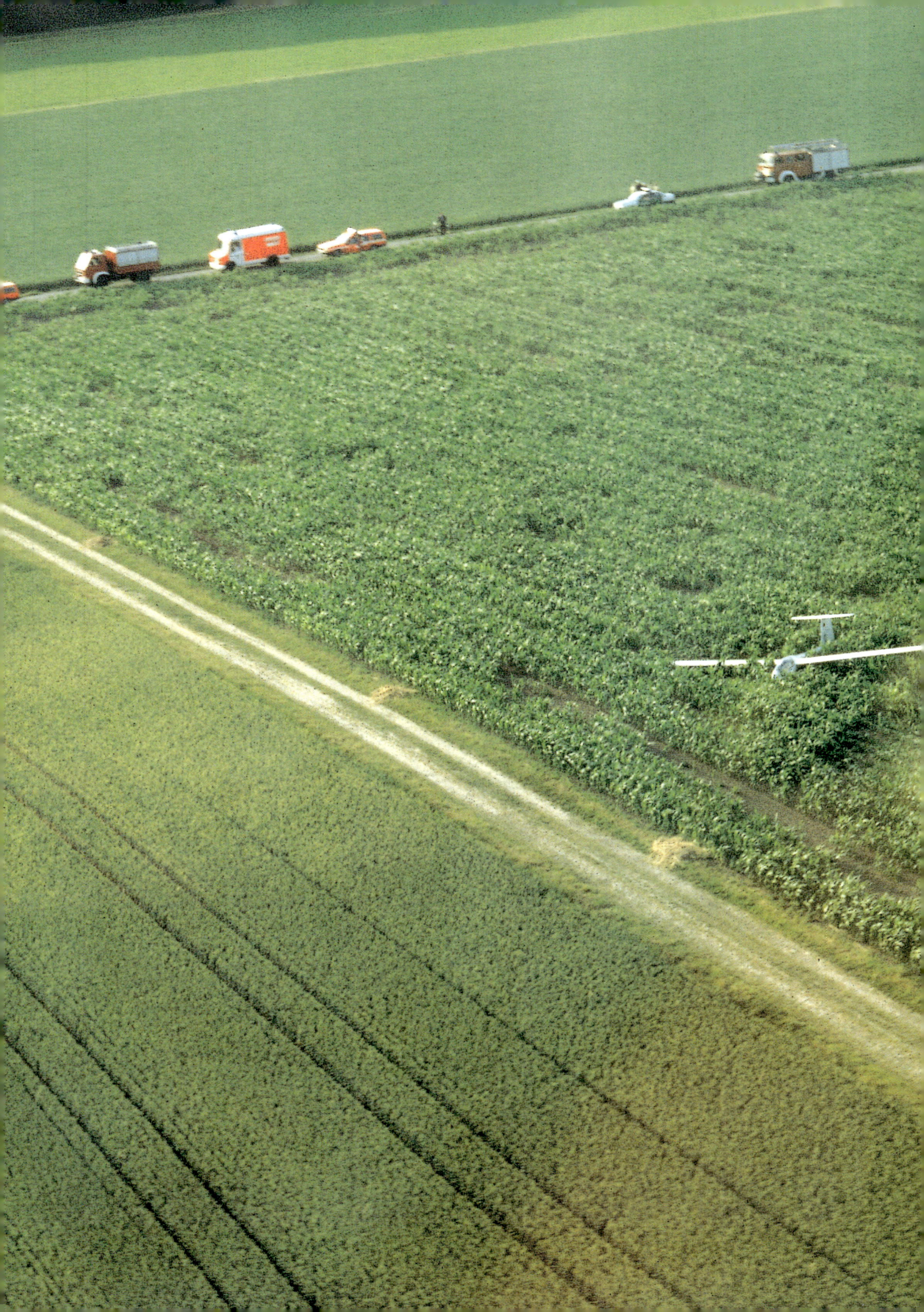

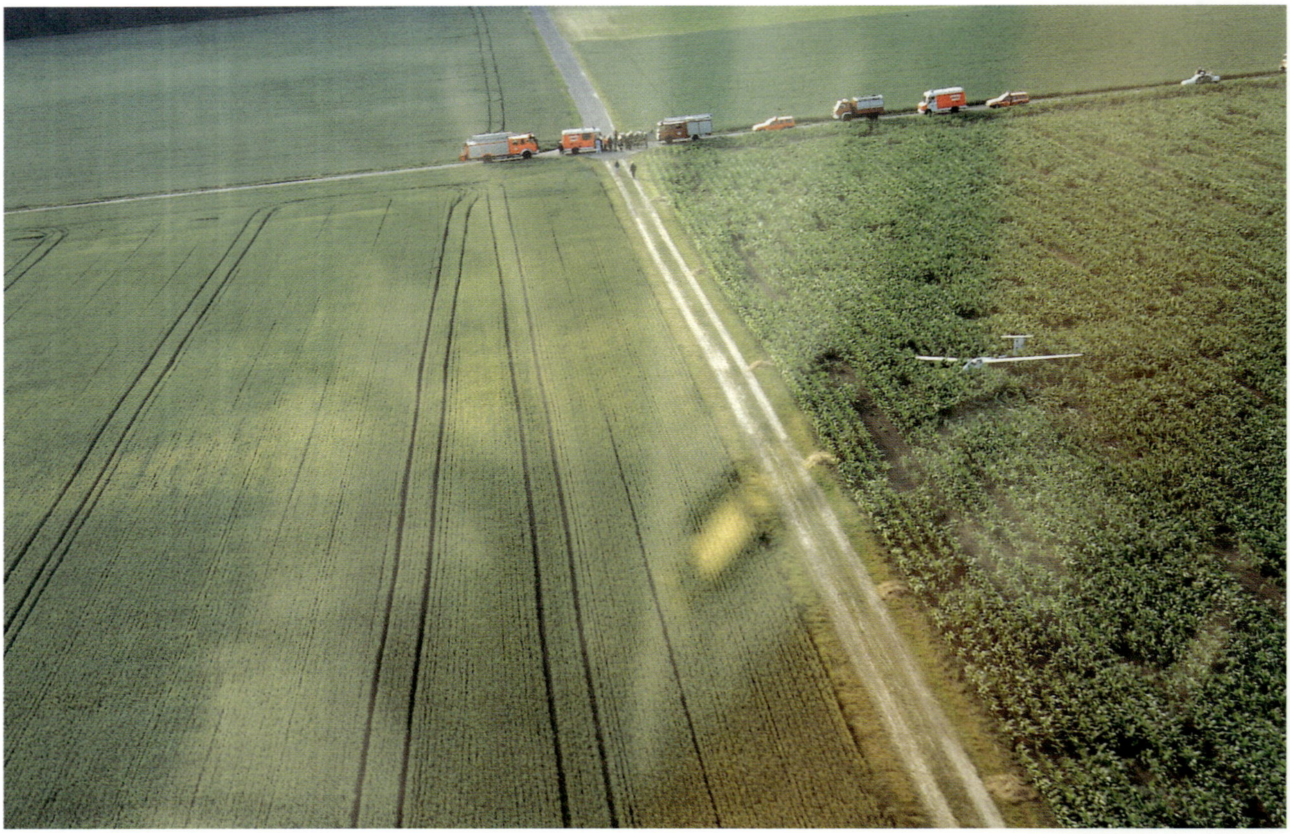

Entwarnung: Es war nur eine Notlandung. Der Pilot sitzt in einer Gaststätte und trinkt einen Kaffee.

False alarm: it was only an emergency landing. The pilot is sitting comfortably in a nearby restaurant drinking a cup of coffee.

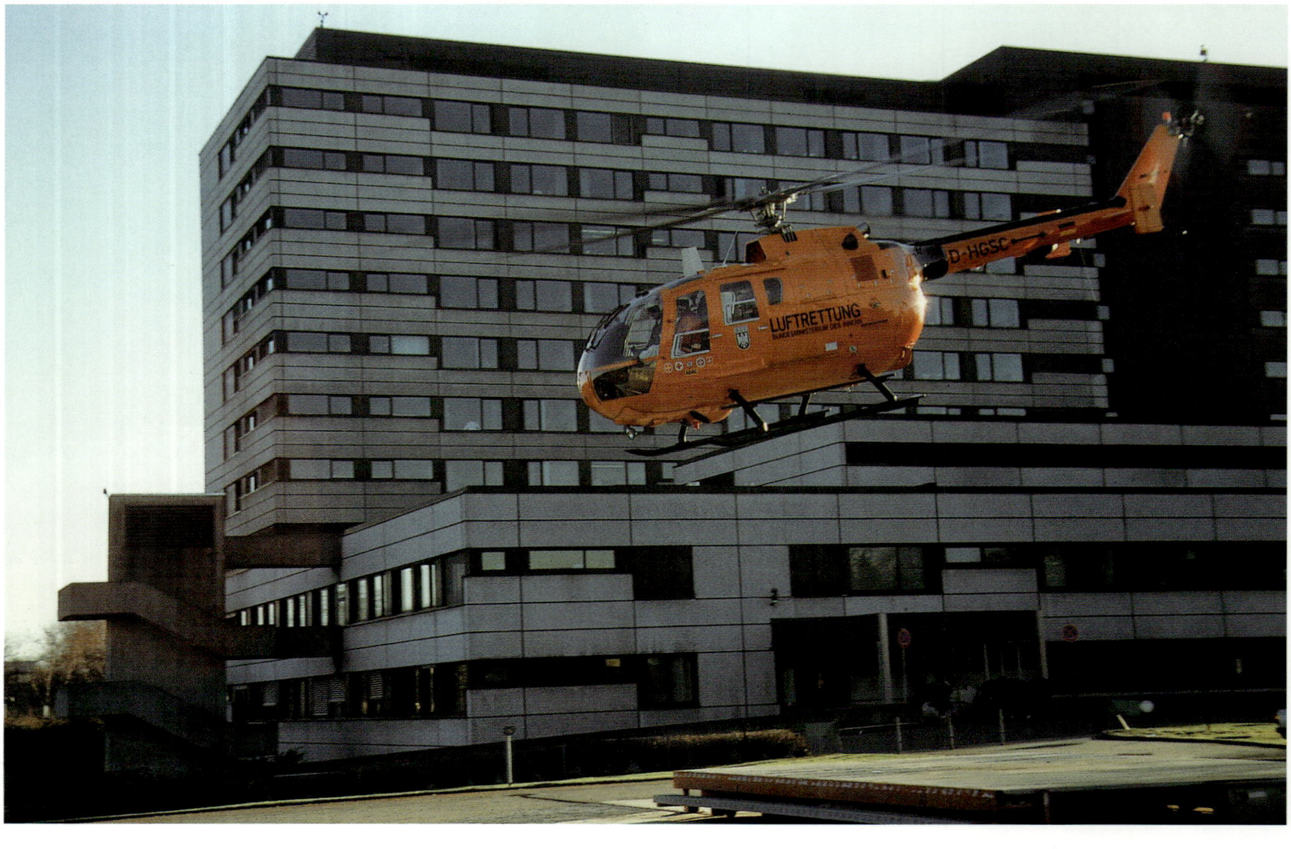

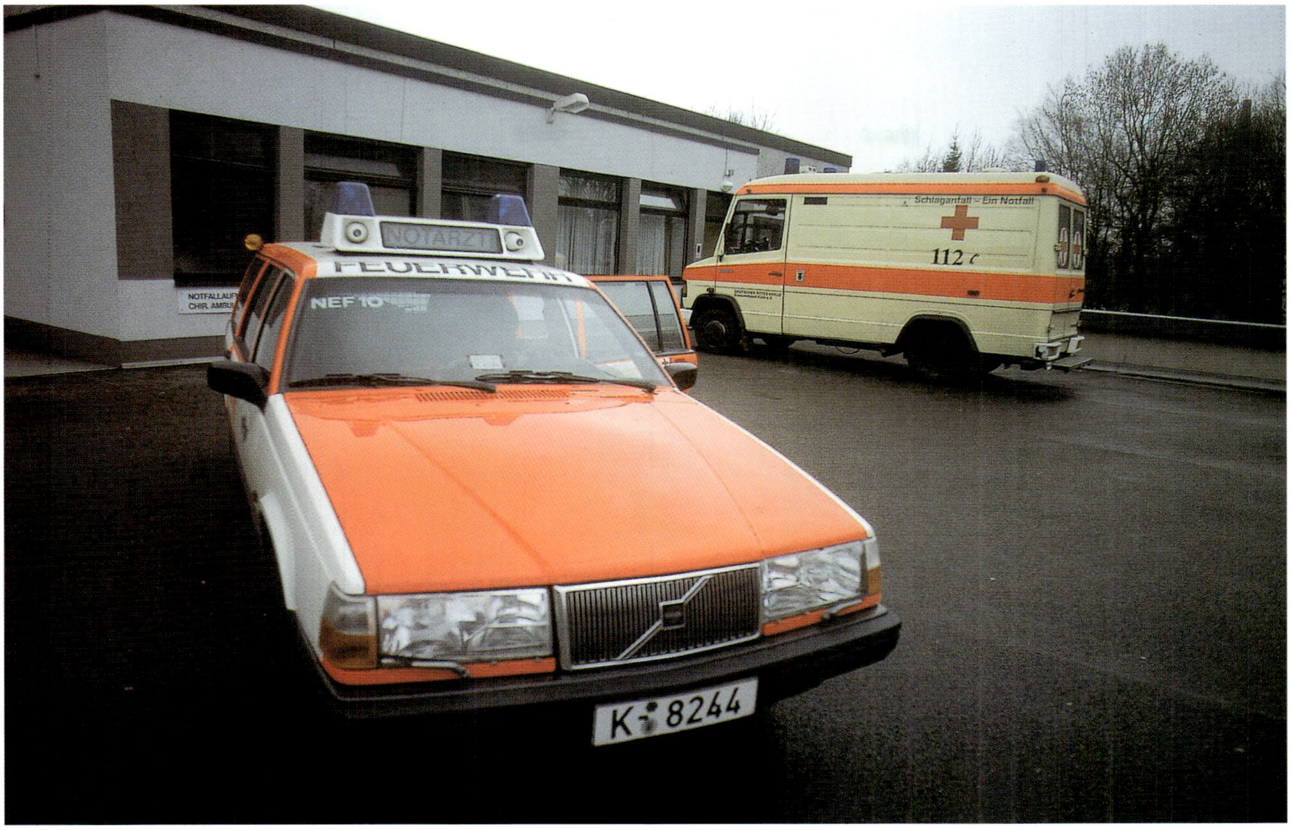

NEF und RTW im Rendez-Vous-System.

The emergency physician car (NEF), rescue ambulance and rescue helicopter all work within the framework of a rendez-vous system.

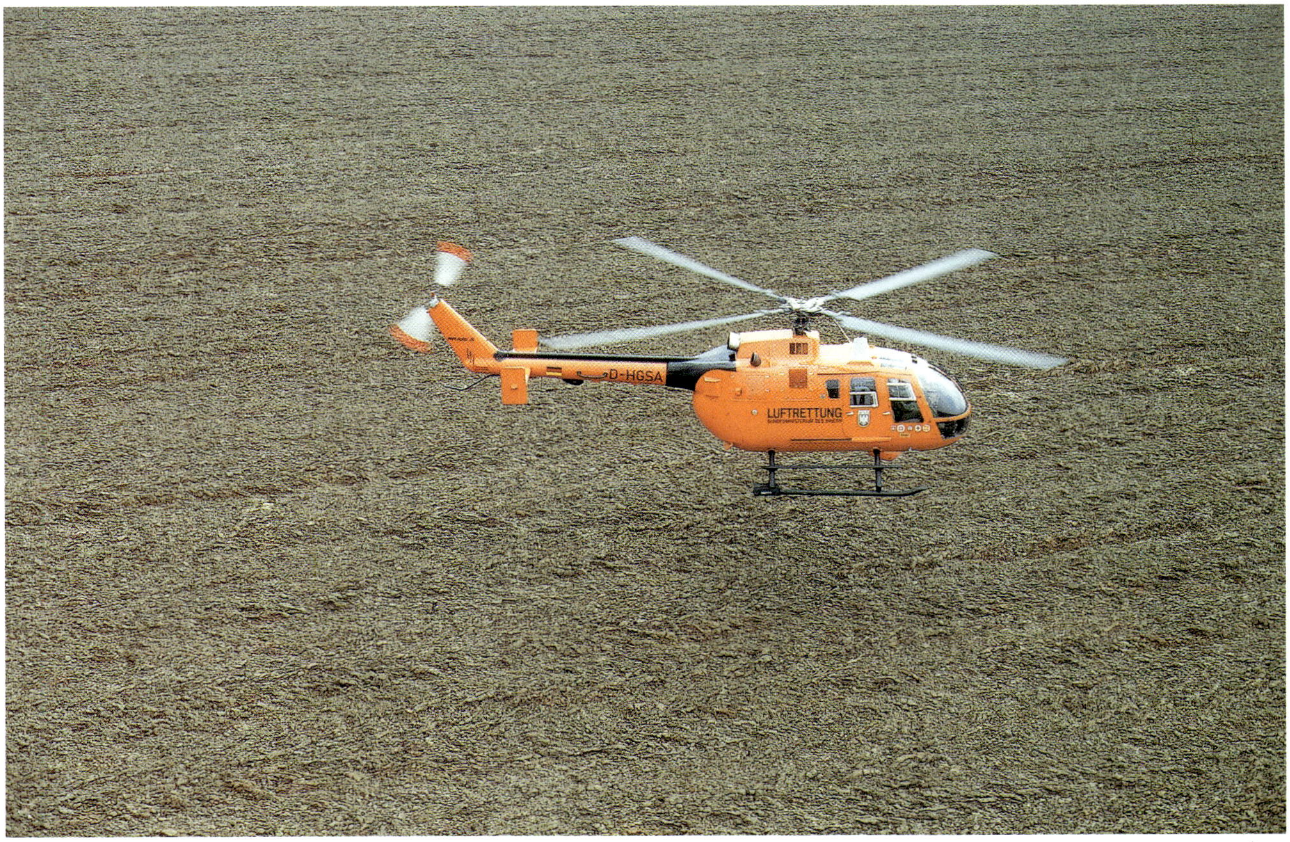

Einsatz für den Rettungshubschrauber
Mission for the Rescue Helicopter

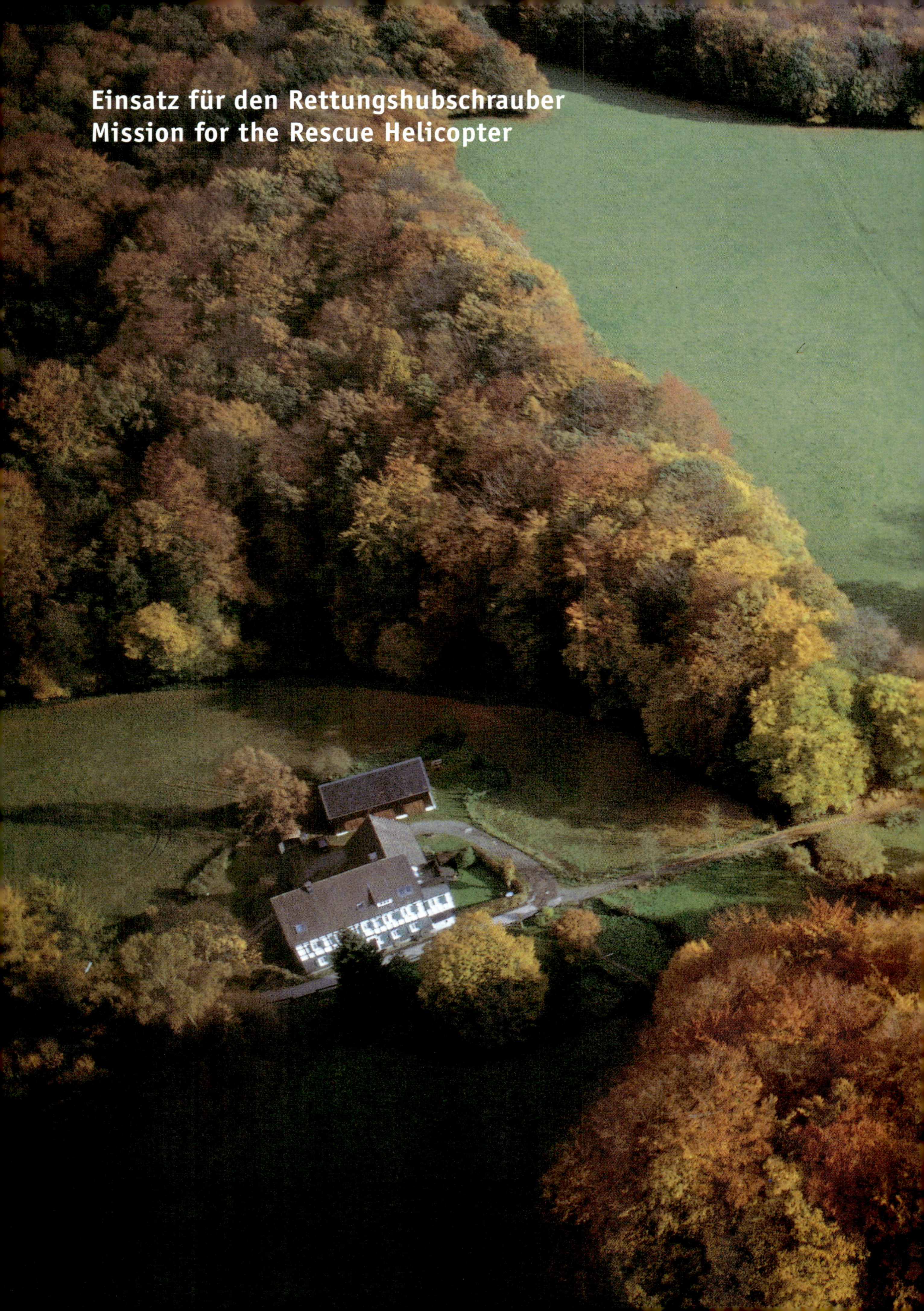

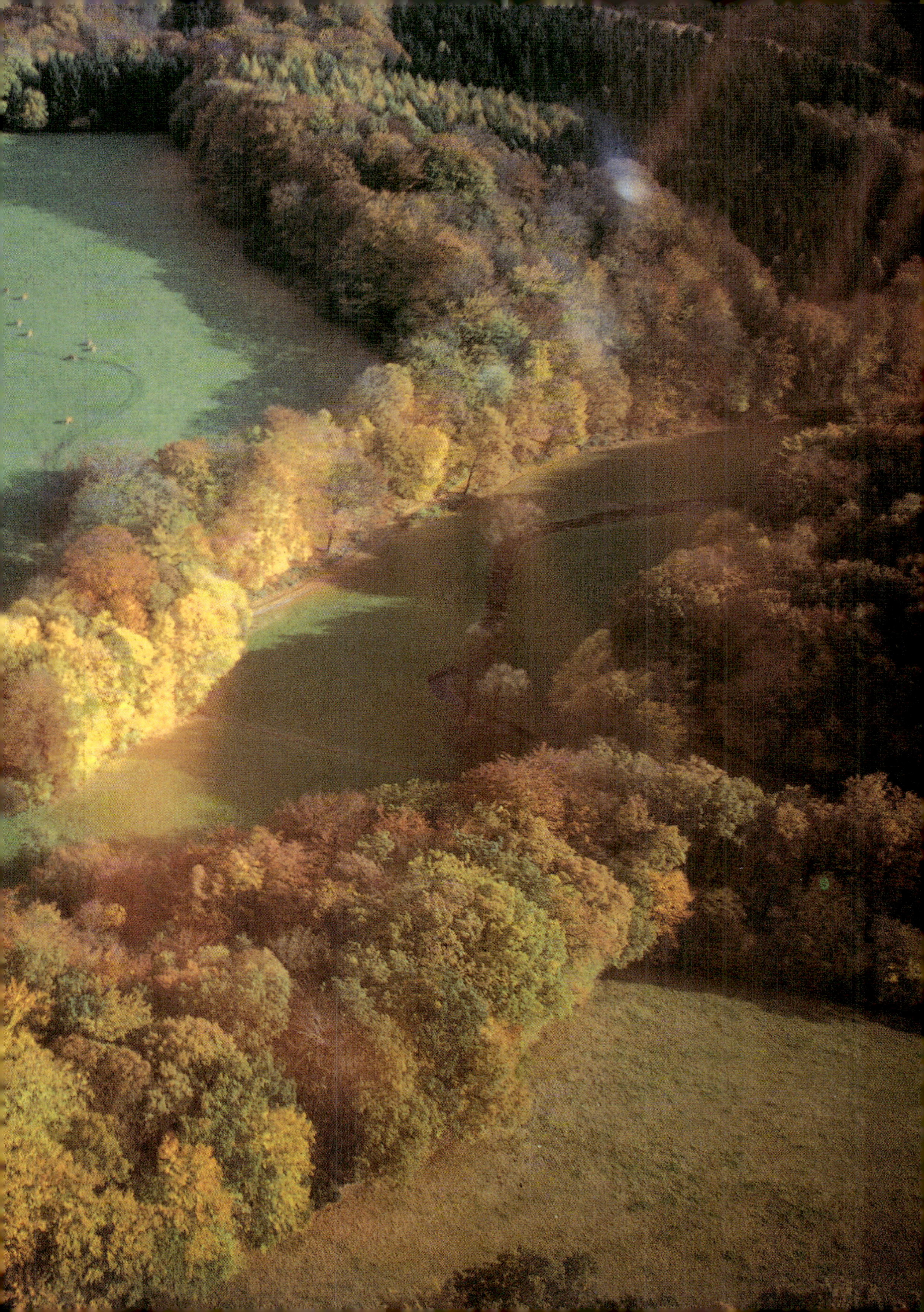

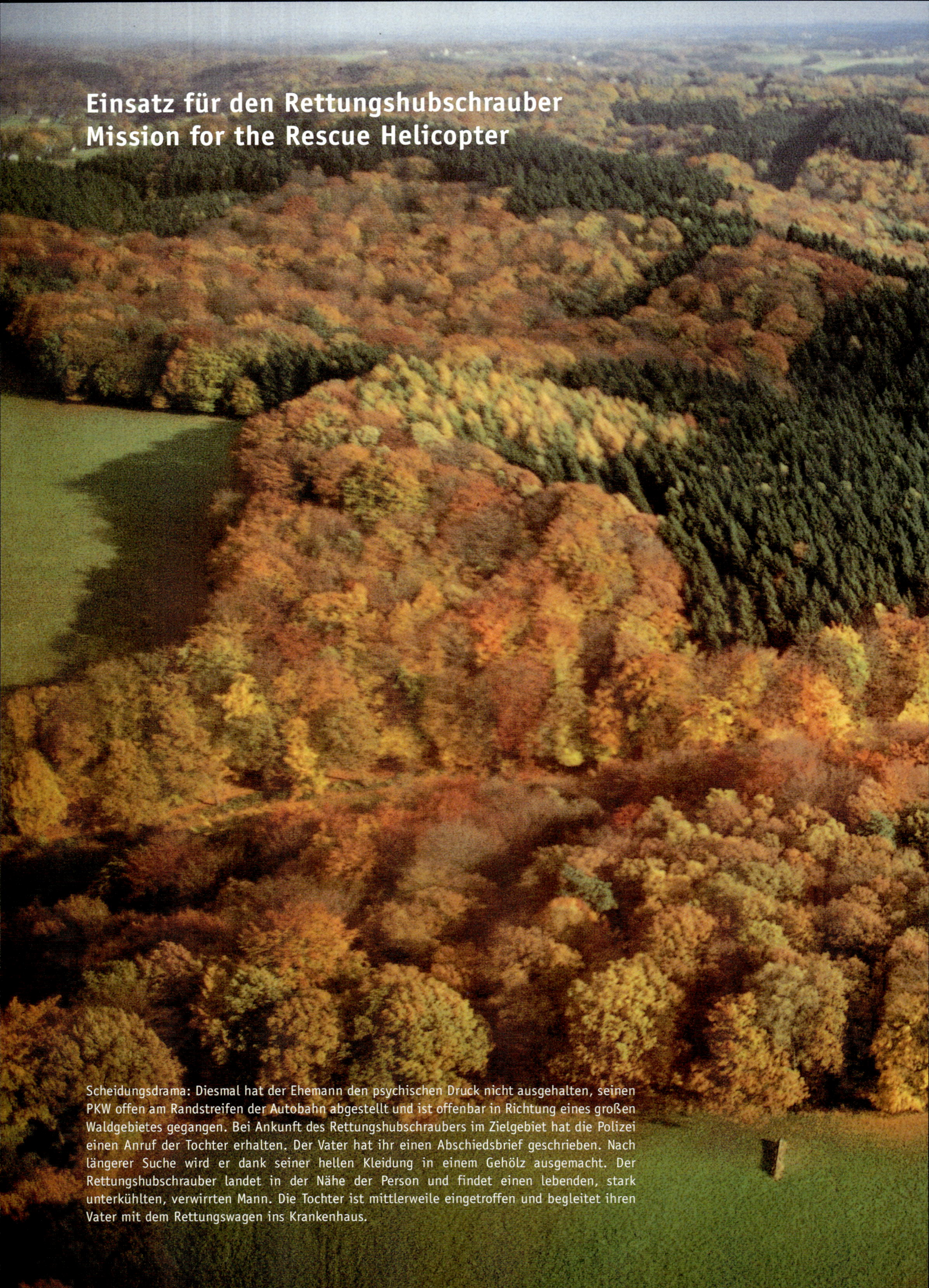

Einsatz für den Rettungshubschrauber
Mission for the Rescue Helicopter
Scheidungsdrama: Diesmal hat der Ehemann den psychischen Druck nicht ausgehalten, seinen PKW offen am Randstreifen der Autobahn abgestellt und ist offenbar in Richtung eines großen Waldgebietes gegangen. Bei Ankunft des Rettungshubschraubers im Zielgebiet hat die Polizei einen Anruf der Tochter erhalten. Der Vater hat ihr einen Abschiedsbrief geschrieben. Nach längerer Suche wird er dank seiner hellen Kleidung in einem Gehölz ausgemacht. Der Rettungshubschrauber landet in der Nähe der Person und findet einen lebenden, stark unterkühlten, verwirrten Mann. Die Tochter ist mittlerweile eingetroffen und begleitet ihren Vater mit dem Rettungswagen ins Krankenhaus.

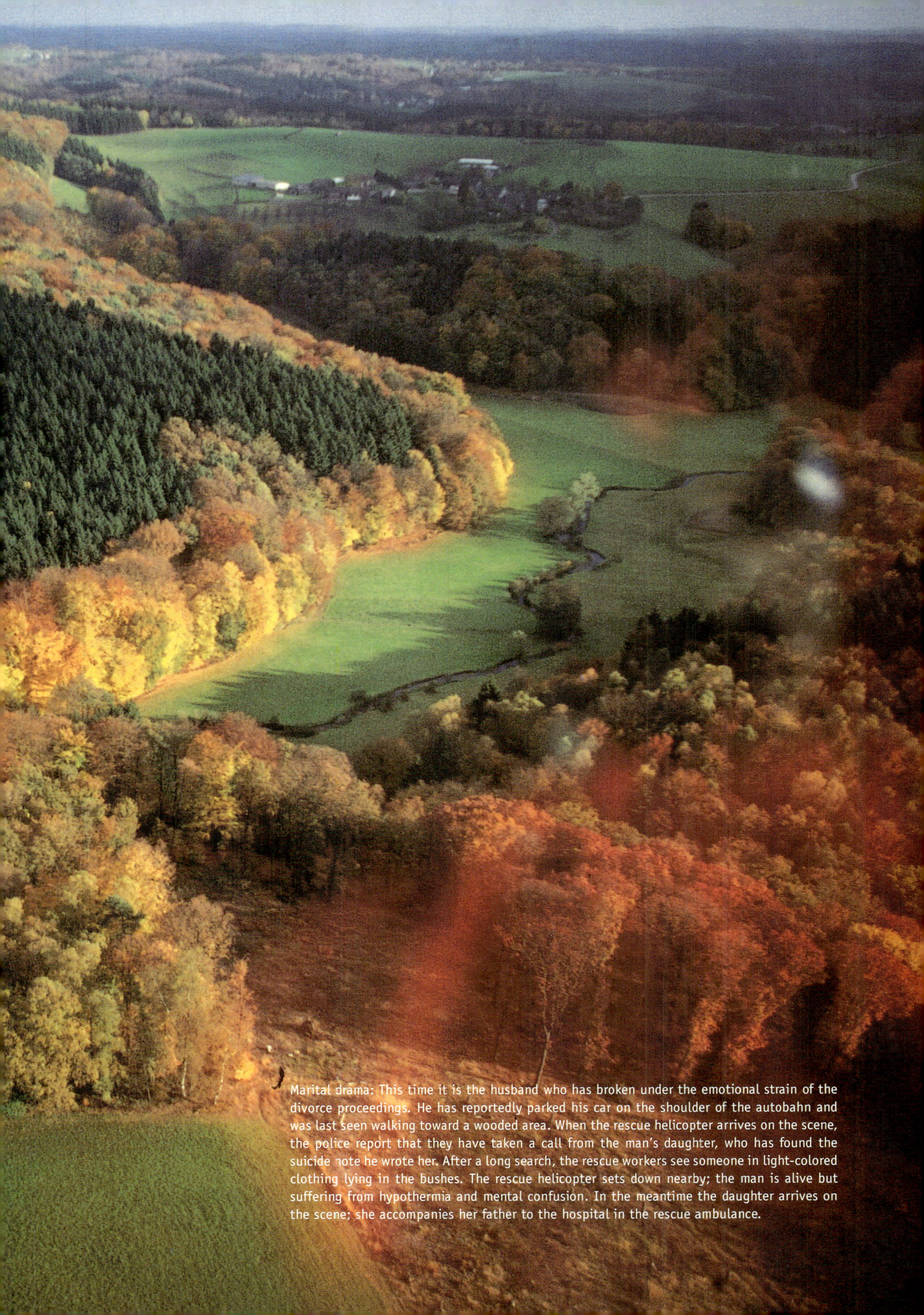

Marital drama: This time it is the husband who has broken under the emotional strain of the divorce proceedings. He has reportedly parked his car on the shoulder of the autobahn and was last seen walking toward a wooded area. When the rescue helicopter arrives on the scene, the police report that they have taken a call from the man's daughter, who has found the suicide note he wrote her. After a long search, the rescue workers see someone in light-colored clothing lying in the bushes. The rescue helicopter sets down nearby; the man is alive but suffering from hypothermia and mental confusion. In the meantime the daughter arrives on the scene; she accompanies her father to the hospital in the rescue ambulance.

Die häufigsten Fragen an der Einsatzstelle
Frequently Asked Questions

Wie wird man Pilotin oder Pilot auf einem vom Bundesgrenzschutz betriebenen Rettungshubschrauber?

Dazu muss man zunächst einmal die Ausbildung zum Polizeibeamten im BGS absolvieren. Der Bundesgrenzschutz stellt grundsätzlich nur Bewerberinnen und Bewerber mit mittlerem Bildungsabschluss (Realschule) für den mittleren Polizeivollzugsdienst oder Fachhochschüler und Abiturienten für den gehobenen Polizeivollzugsdienst ein.

Nach einer zweieinhalb bzw. dreijährigen Ausbildung, die für den gehobenen Polizeivollzugsdienst mit der Erlangung des Grades eines Diplomverwaltungswirtes (FH) endet, besteht die Möglichkeit sich im Rahmen einer BGS-internen Ausschreibung zum Eignungsauswahlverfahren für Piloten zu bewerben.

Dieses ca. einwöchige Auswahlverfahren findet an der Luftfahrerschule der BGS-Fliegergruppe in Sankt Augustin statt und beinhaltet auch die Feststellung der fliegerärztlichen Tauglichkeit beim Deutschen Zentrum für Luft- und Raumfahrt (DLR) in Köln.

Hat man dies „überstanden", beginnt die im Augenblick noch ca. zweijährige Ausbildung zur Berufshubschrauberpilotin bzw. zum - piloten. Dabei absolviert der Flugschüler etwa 260 Flugstunden und mehr als 900 Stunden Unterricht in über 15 Fächern von der Meteorologie über Navigation und Funknavigation bis hin zur Triebwerktechnik. Nach der Prüfung durch das Luftfahrtbundesamt besitzt er dann die zivile Berufspilotenlizenz und die Musterberechtigung für den auch im Einsatzbetrieb des BGS noch verwendeten Verbindungs- und Beobachtungshubschraubers SA 318 C „Alouette". In Zukunft wird dies übrigens der Eurocopter EC 135 sein.

Die Berufspilotenlizenz ist absolut vergleichbar mit der des Piloten bei einem Luftfahrtunternehmen. Wie diese auch, betreiben der Bundesgrenzschutz und alle Polizeihubschrauberstaffeln der Länder, deren Piloten teilweise ebenfalls beim BGS ausgebildet werden, zivil zugelassene Luftfahrzeuge, deren Wartung und Betrieb auf der Basis des Luftverkehrsgesetzes und nicht auf der Grundlage militärischer Vorschriften erfolgen. Fachaufsichtsbehörde ist deshalb auch das Luftfahrtbundesamt.

How can a man or woman become a pilot on a rescue helicopter operated by the German Border Police?

The first step is to complete training as a police officer in the Federal Border Police. The FBP only accepts applicants who have completed secondary modern school or commercial high school [Realschule] for the intermediate police service class and applicants with qualifications enabling them to study at a university ("A levels") or university of applied sciences [Fachhochschulreife] for the higher intermediate police service class.

After completing a period of training of two to three years culminating – for candidates aspiring to admission to the higher intermediate police service class – with the granting of a degree equivalent to a diploma in public administration from a university of applied sciences, the candidate can apply for pilot's training within the framework of an internal selection process conducted by the Federal Border Police.

The one-week selection process is carried out at the Aviation School run by the Aviation Group of the Federal Border Police in St. Augustin-Hangelar. It includes evaluation of medical suitability at the German Research Institute for Aeronautical and Aerospace Engineering (DLR).

If a candidate "survives" these hurdles, he or she can start training to become a professional helicopter pilot; at present this training takes approx. two years. During this training the student has to put about 260 hours of flying time under his or her belt and attend more than 900 hours of instruction in more than 15 subjects, ranging from meteorology over navigation and radio navigation to engine technology. After passing the examination conducted by the Federal Aviation Office, the student is granted a professional pilot's license and the type rating required to fly the liaison and observation helicopter type SA 318 C "Alouette" which is still used by the Federal Border Police. In the future, this role will be taken over by the Eurocopter EC 135.

This professional pilot's license is entirely comparable with the license possessed by pilots working for commercial airlines. Like the airlines, the Federal Border Police and all of the police flying squadrons in the various German states, which send their pilots to the German Border Police for training in some cases, operate aircrafts approved for civil aviation. These aircraft are serviced and operated on the basis of the civil aviation legislation and not according to military regulations. For this reason, the applicable supervisory authority is the Federal Office of Civil Aviation.

Rettungshubschrauber nicht mehr einsatzbereit
The Rescue Helicopter is no longer operational.

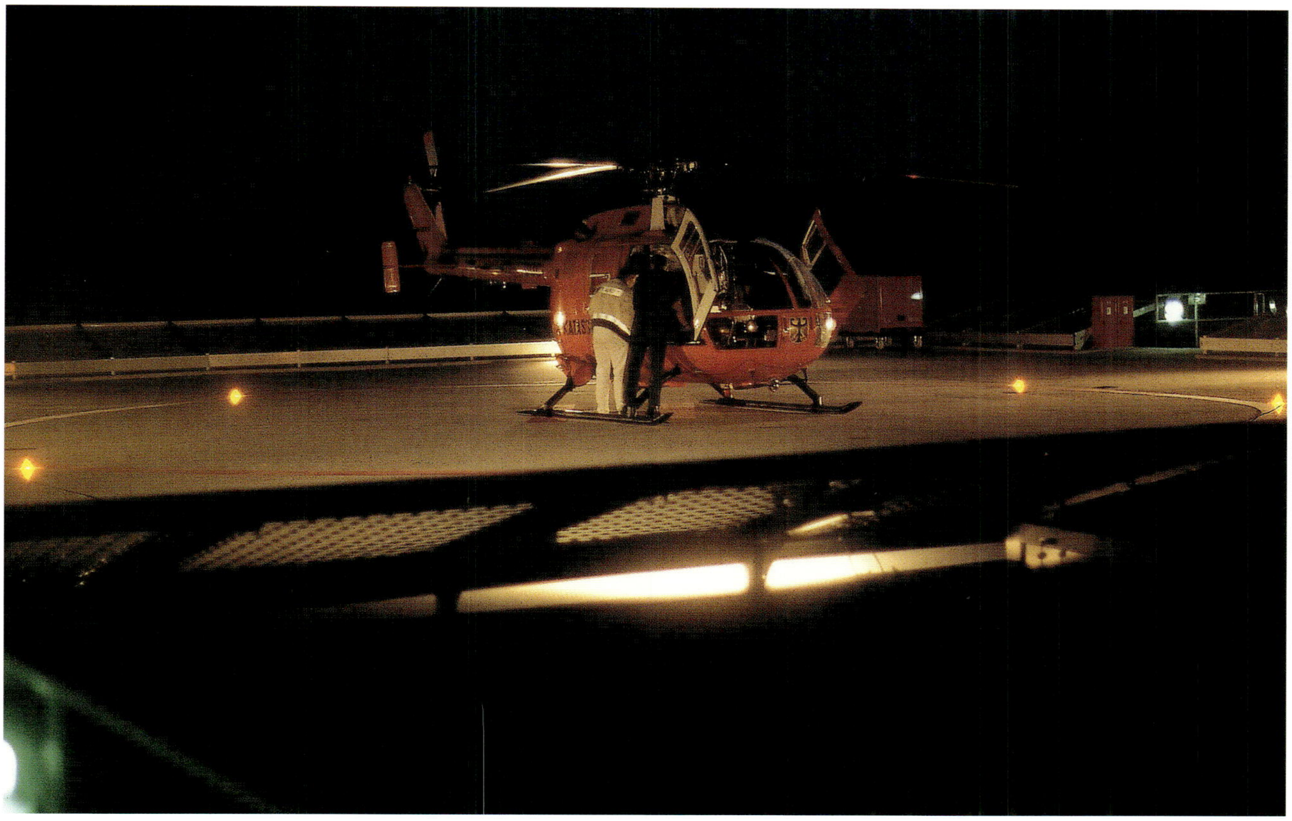

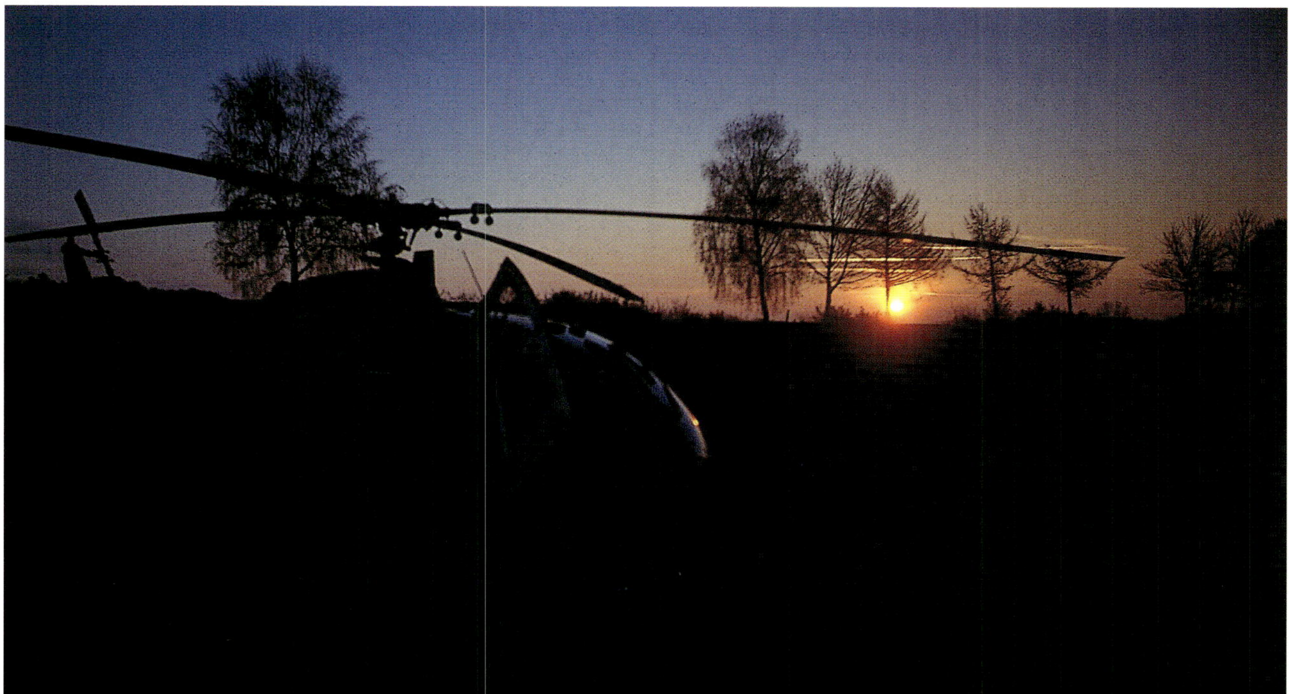

Nicht selten startet man kurz vor Sonnenuntergang noch zu einem Einsatz oder die länger andauernde Versorgung von Patienten lässt den Abend hereinbrechen. In solchen Fällen ist der Rettungshubschrauber wegen der Dunkelheit nicht mehr einsatzbereit, fliegt jedoch den bekannten Weg zum beleuchteten Landeplatz der Station zurück.

Frequently, the rescue helicopter starts out on a mission during daylight but is caught by darkness while the crew is administering emergency medical care. Once night falls, the helicopter is no longer operational; in such cases, it takes a familiar route back to the well-lighted helicopter landing site at its base.

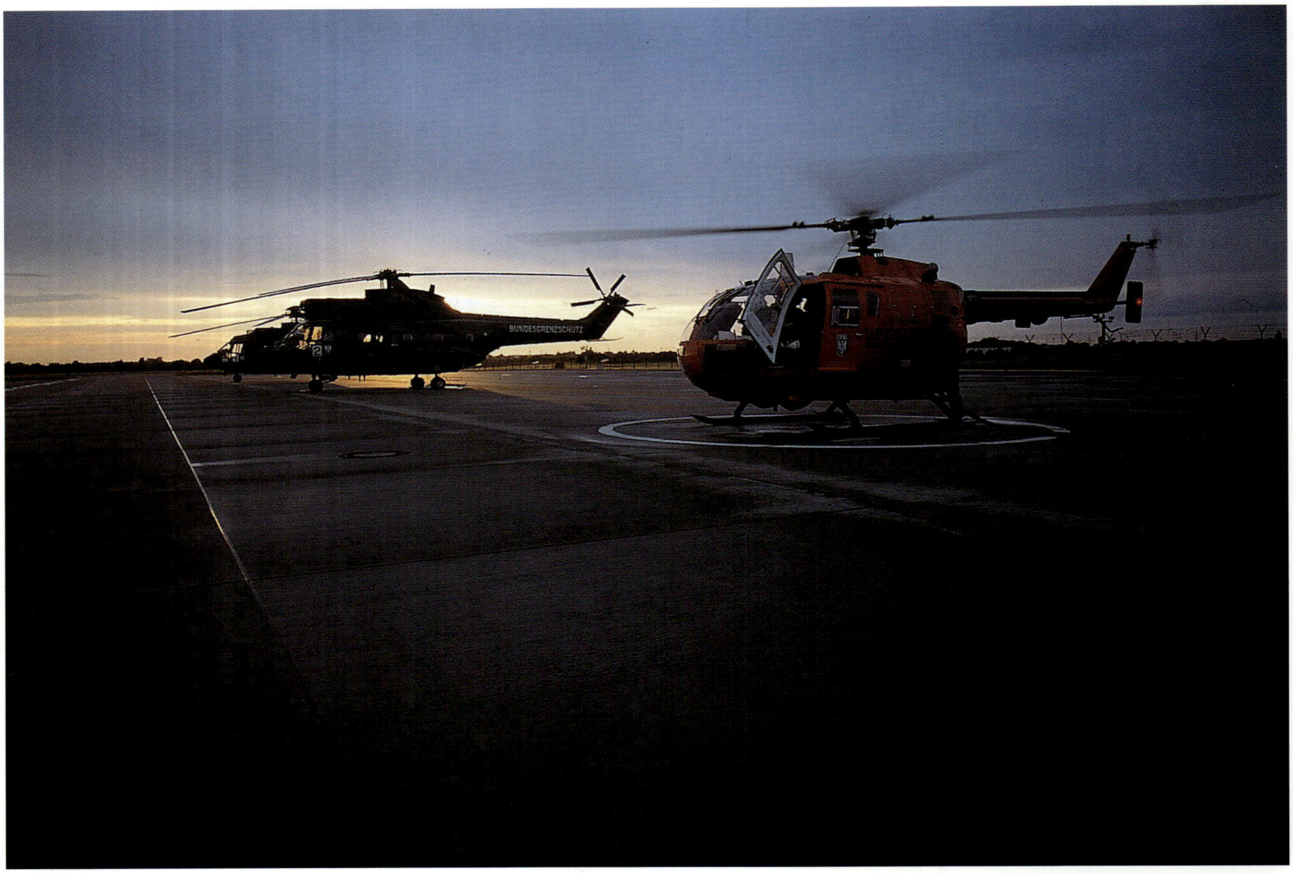

Die häufigsten Fragen an der Einsatzstelle
Frequently Asked Questions

Wieso haben manche Hubschrauber Kufen, andere jedoch Räder?

Besonders für Rettungshubschrauber sind Kufen von großem Vorteil, weil sie auf unbefestigtem Untergrund unempfindlicher gegen Beschädigung sind und in nassem Gelände weniger stark einsinken als Räder.

Ab einer bestimmten Größe (ca. 4 – 5 t Höchstabfluggewicht) sind jedoch die meisten Hubschrauber mit einem Radfahrwerk ausgestattet, da es die Manövrierfähigkeit am Boden erhöht und auf Landeplätzen der Schwebeflug (Abstrahl!) in Grenzen gehalten und gerollt werden kann.

An die Kufen einer BO 105 können Räder adaptiert werden, um den Hubschrauber im Falle eines Falles auch schieben zu können.

Why do some helicopters have skids and other wheels?

For rescue helicopters, in particular, skids are very advantageous because they are resistant to damage on unpaved landing sites and do not sink as far into the ground on muddy terrain.

Starting at a certain size (approx. 4 – 5 tons max. takeoff weight), however, most helicopters are equipped with landing gear which increase the maneuverability of the aircraft on the ground and ensure that hovering (downwash) is kept within limits at landing sites. In addition, helicopters with wheels can be rolled into the hangar.

The skids of the BO 105 can be fitted with wheels allowing the helicopter to be pushed in an emergency.

Einsatz für den Rettungshubschrauber
Mission for the Rescue Helicopter

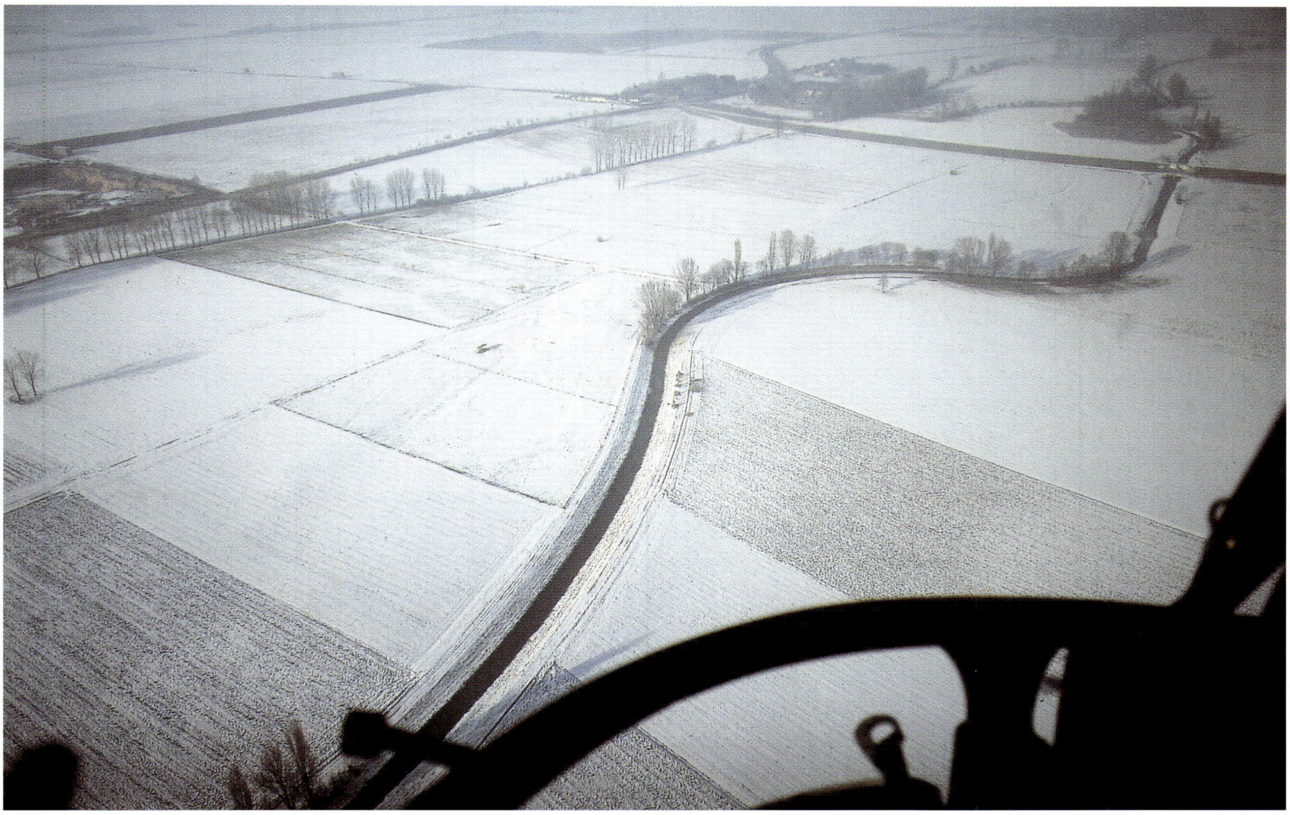

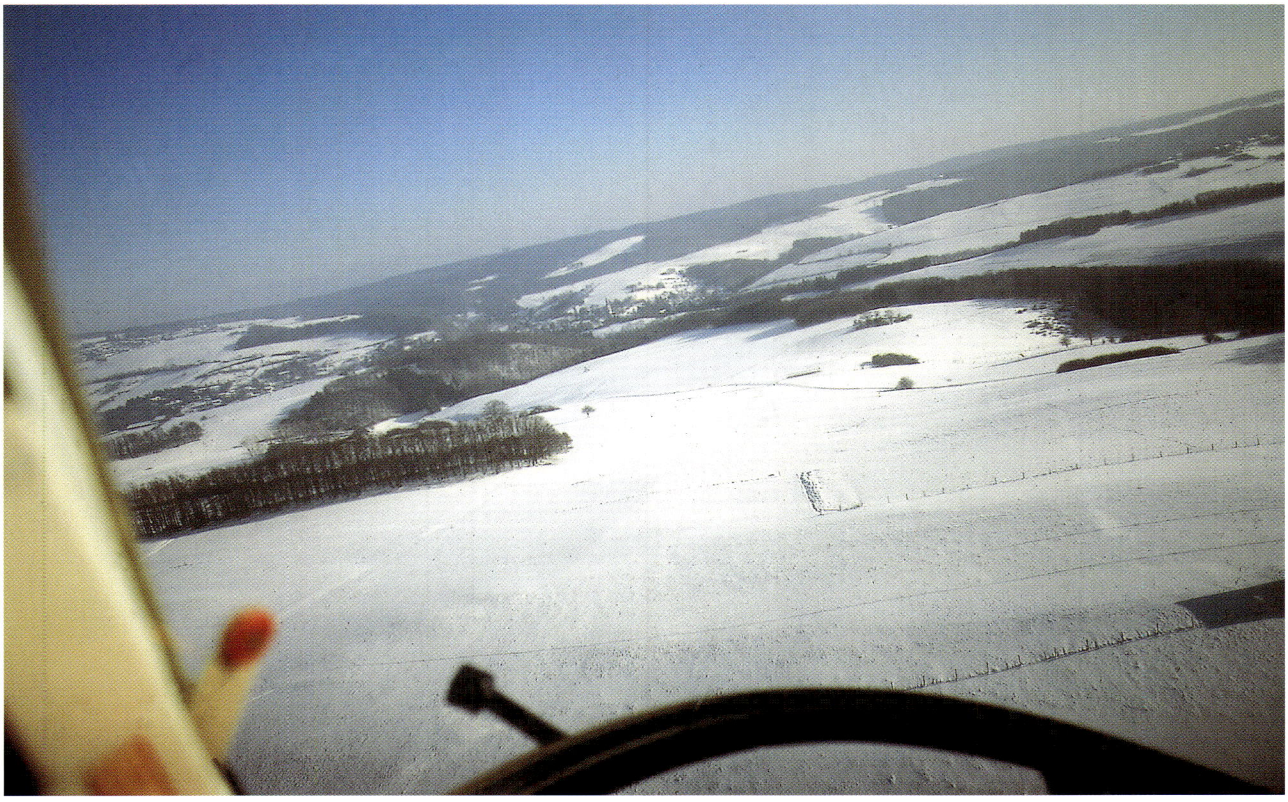

Ein Notarzt vor Ort hat den Rettungshubschrauber für seinen Patienten zum Transport in eine Spezialklinik angefordert.

A physician with emergency & rescue certification on the ground has requested a rescue helicopter to transport a patient to a specialized medical center.

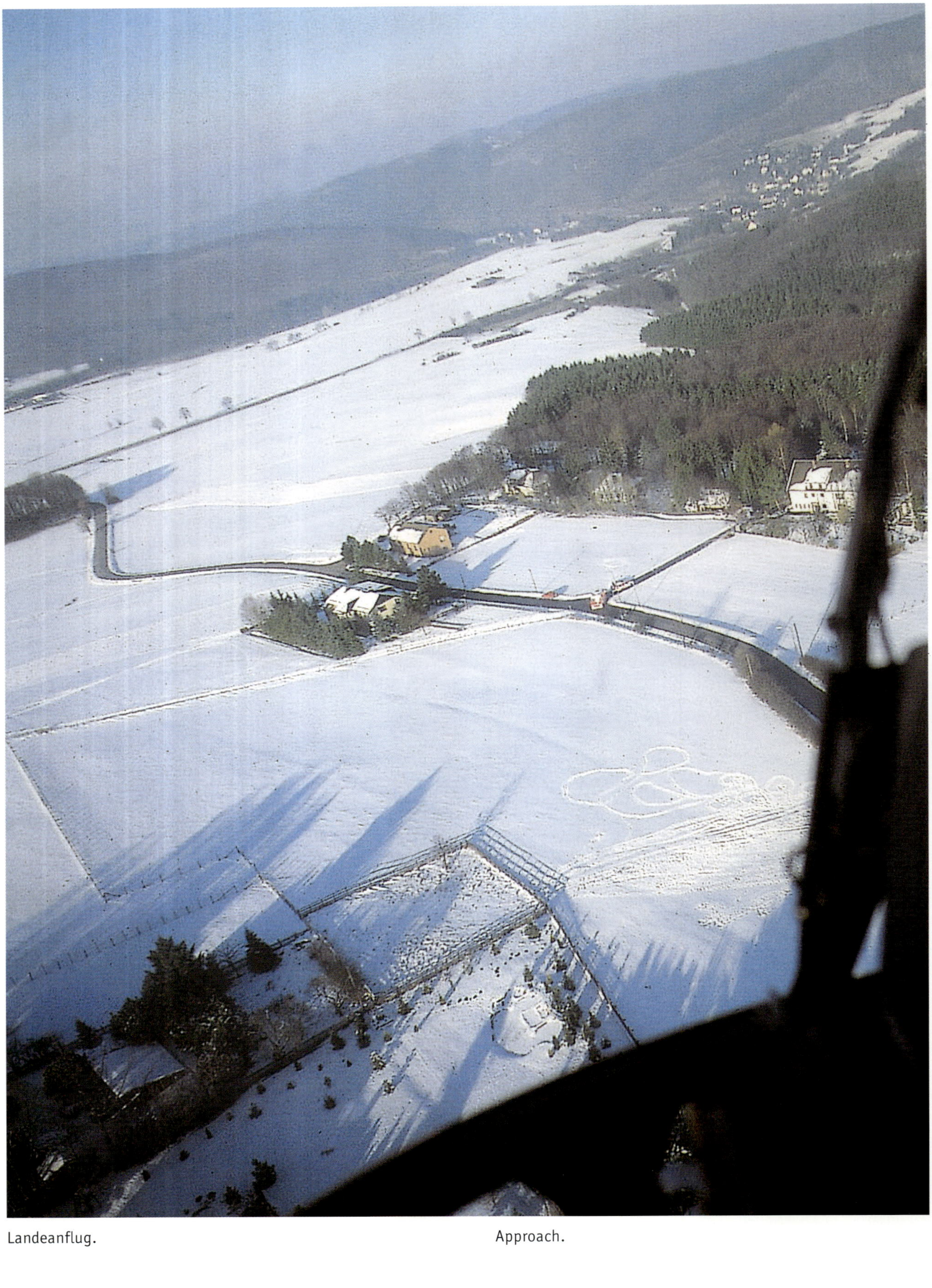

Landeanflug.

Approach.

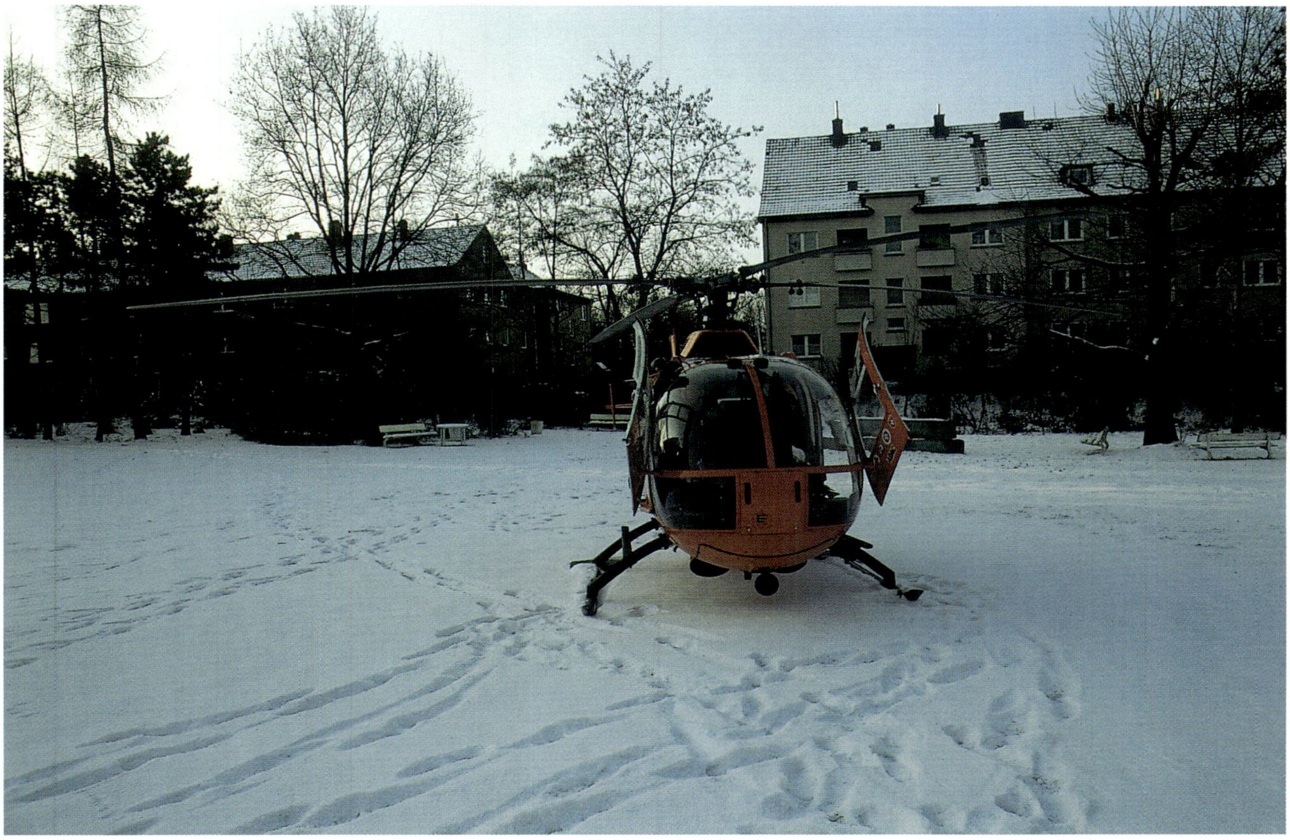

Im Winter verkürzt sich der Einsatztag von etwa 8.30 Uhr bis etwa 16 Uhr, bedingt durch den geänderten Sonnenauf- und untergang.

In winter the helicopter's operational day is shorter: it lasts from around 8.30 a.m. to about 4.00 p.m. depending on when the sun comes up and goes down.

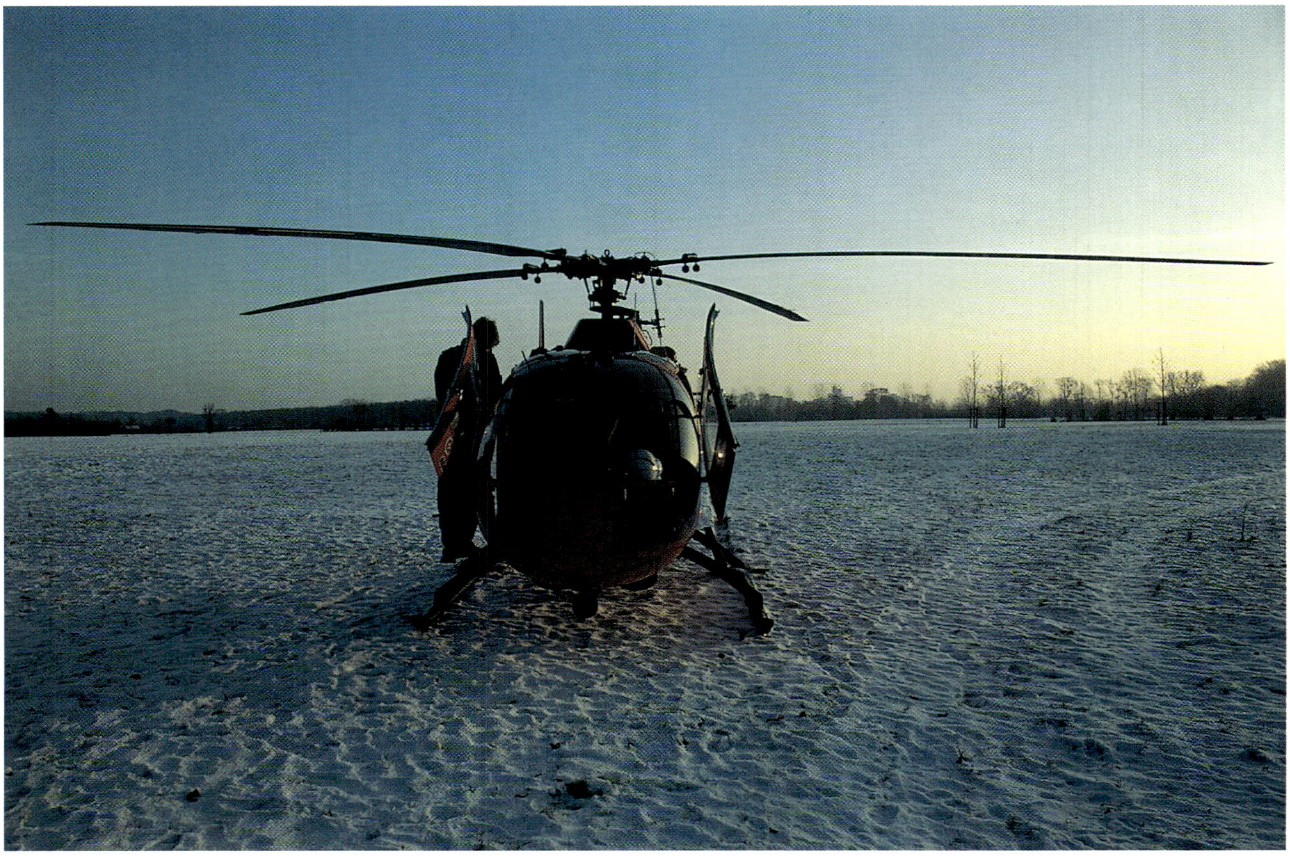

Der Christoph 3 im Internet
Christoph 3 in the Internet

von/by Erik Gladich

Am 12. September 1998 präsentierte sich der Christoph 3 als erster Rettungshubschrauber mit einer offiziellen Homepage im Internet. Dem vorausgegangenen war ein weiter Weg der Genehmigungen beim Bundesamt für Zivilschutz, beim Bundesgrenzschutz, bei der Berufsfeuerwehr Köln, bei dem Malteser-Hilfsdienst e.V. und dem leitenden Notarzt des RTH, PD Dr. med. Bertil Boullion.

Bei den vielen Gesprächen, die wir mit den einzelnen Vertretern führten, begegnete man uns mit einer überaus positiven Haltung gegenüber der neuen Möglichkeit der Darstellung des Rettungshubschraubers Christoph 3.

Auch im Internet wurde eben diese Darstellung weit über die Grenzen von Köln hinweg dankbar angenommen.

Im Monat besuchen etwa dreihundert Gäste die Homepage und nutzen dabei fleißig die Möglichkeit per eMail Kontakt mit uns aufzunehmen. Von Anfragen für Filmaufnahmen über den Wunsch, der Luftrettung eine Spende zukommen zu lassen, bis hin zu Patienten, die uns einfach nur Danke für die Hilfe sagen wollten, erreichten uns.

Die Homepage soll Interessierten einen Einblick in die Tätigkeit von dem Rettungshubschrauber Christoph 3 geben und dabei insbesondere über Neuerung informieren. Die Unterhaltung der Homepage wird ausschließlich auf Eigeninitiative von einigen Besatzungsmitgliedern betrieben.

Internetadresse:
http://www.christoph3.de
eMail: christoph.3@gmx.de

On 12 September 1998 Christoph 3 became the first rescue helicopter to have an official website This Internet debut was preceded by a long permit-gathering period during which crew members of the Christoph 3 applied to the Federal Office of Civil Defense, the German Border Police, the Cologne Professional Fire Service, Malteser-Hilfsdienst e.V. and PD Dr. med. Bertil Boullion, the stuff physician with emergency & rescue certification in the rescue helicopter service.

During the numerous conversations we had with the individual representatives of the above organizations, we met with an entirely positive response to this new possibility for presenting the rescue helicopter Christoph 3. In the Internet itself, this presentation has been viewed with great interest by Internet users far beyond the boundaries of Cologne.

About 300 people visit the site every month; many of them take advantage of the opportunity offered on the website to contact us by email. These emails have covered a wide range of topics ranging from a request for video films of the rescue helicopter over the wish to make a donation to the air rescue service straight through to a simple "thank you" from a former patient.

The website was set up to give interested members of the public an impression of the work of the rescue helicopter Christoph 3 and, in particular, to keep them abreast of new developments. The creation of the website is due solely to the initiative of several crew members.

URL:
http://www.christoph3.de
eMail: christoph.3@gmx.de

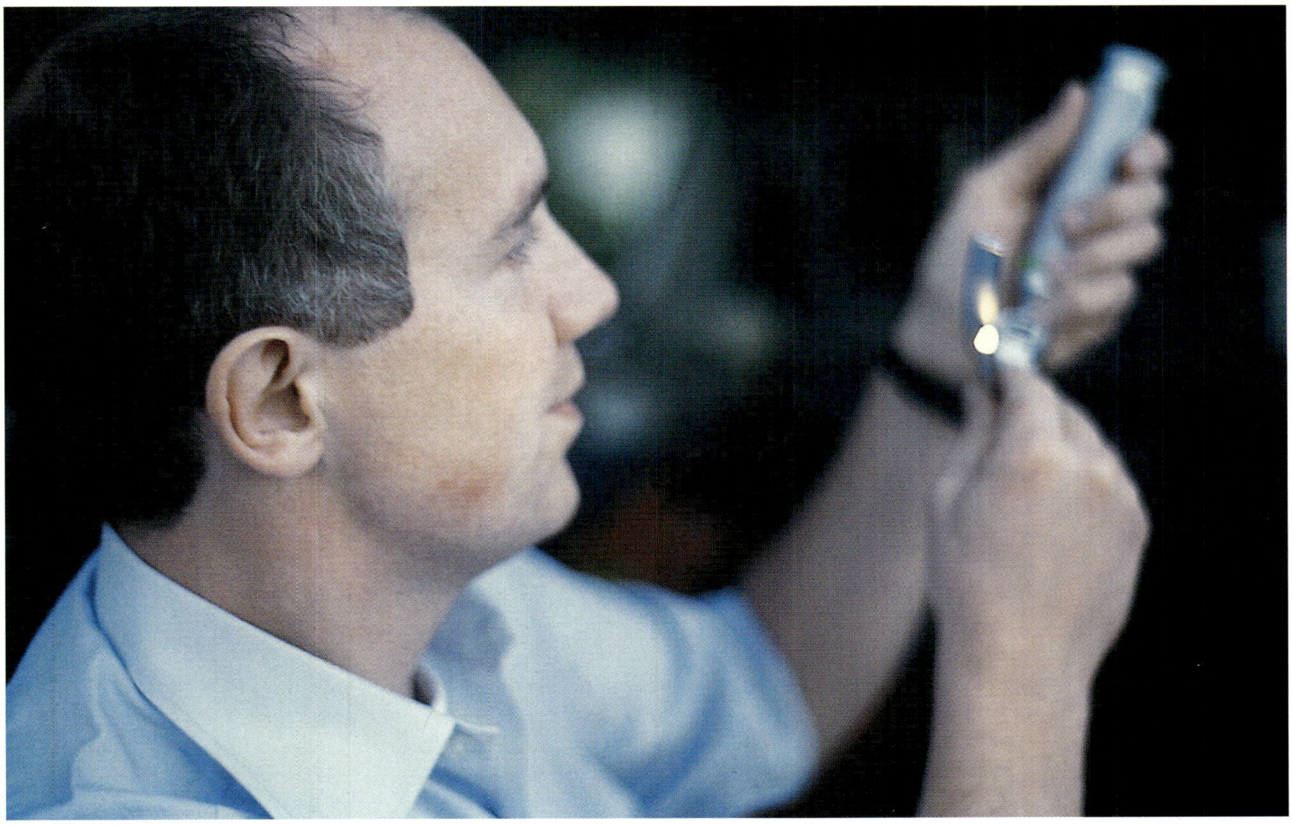

Der Luftrettungsassistent prüft die Funktion des Laryngoskops.

The air rescue paramedic checks the function of the laryngoscope.

Einsatz für den Rettungshubschrauber
Mission for the Rescue Helicopter

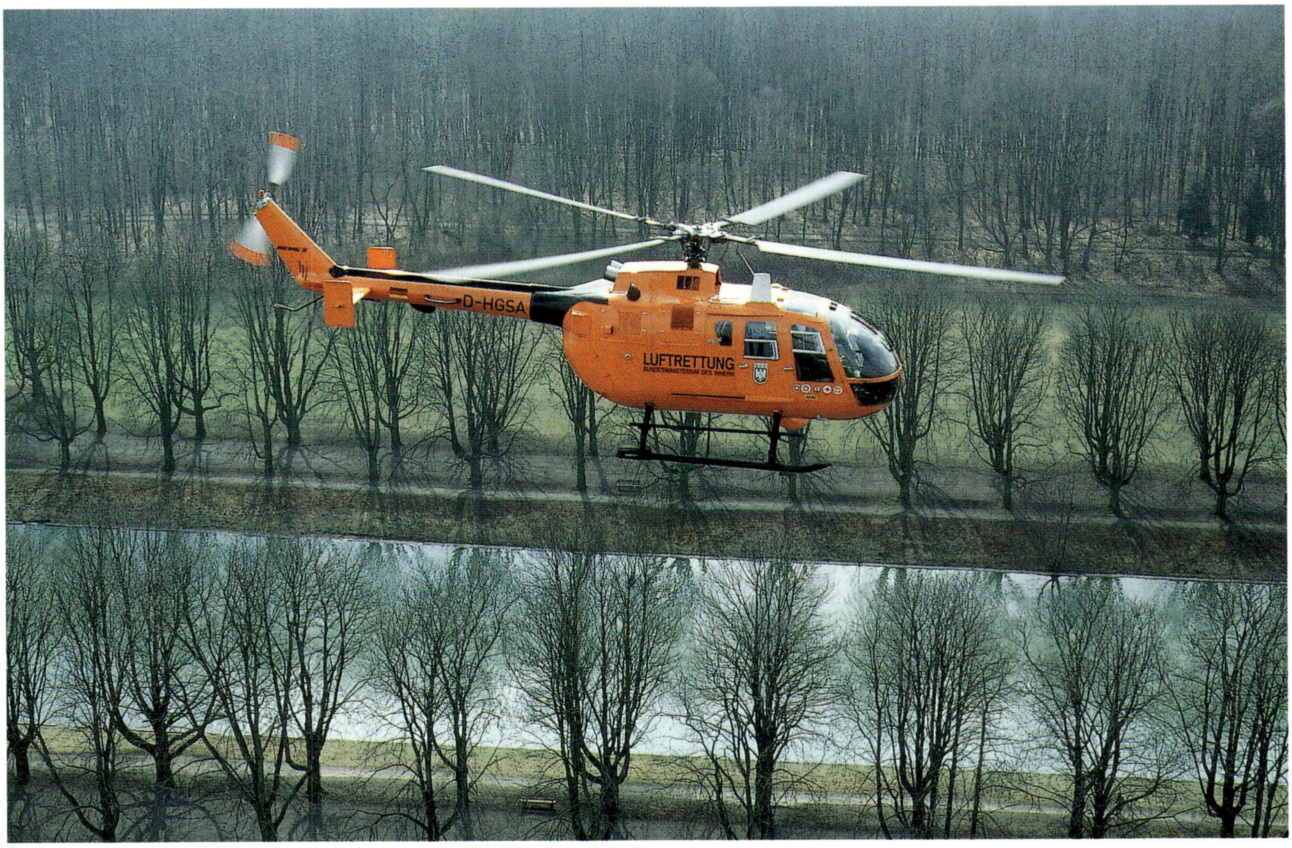

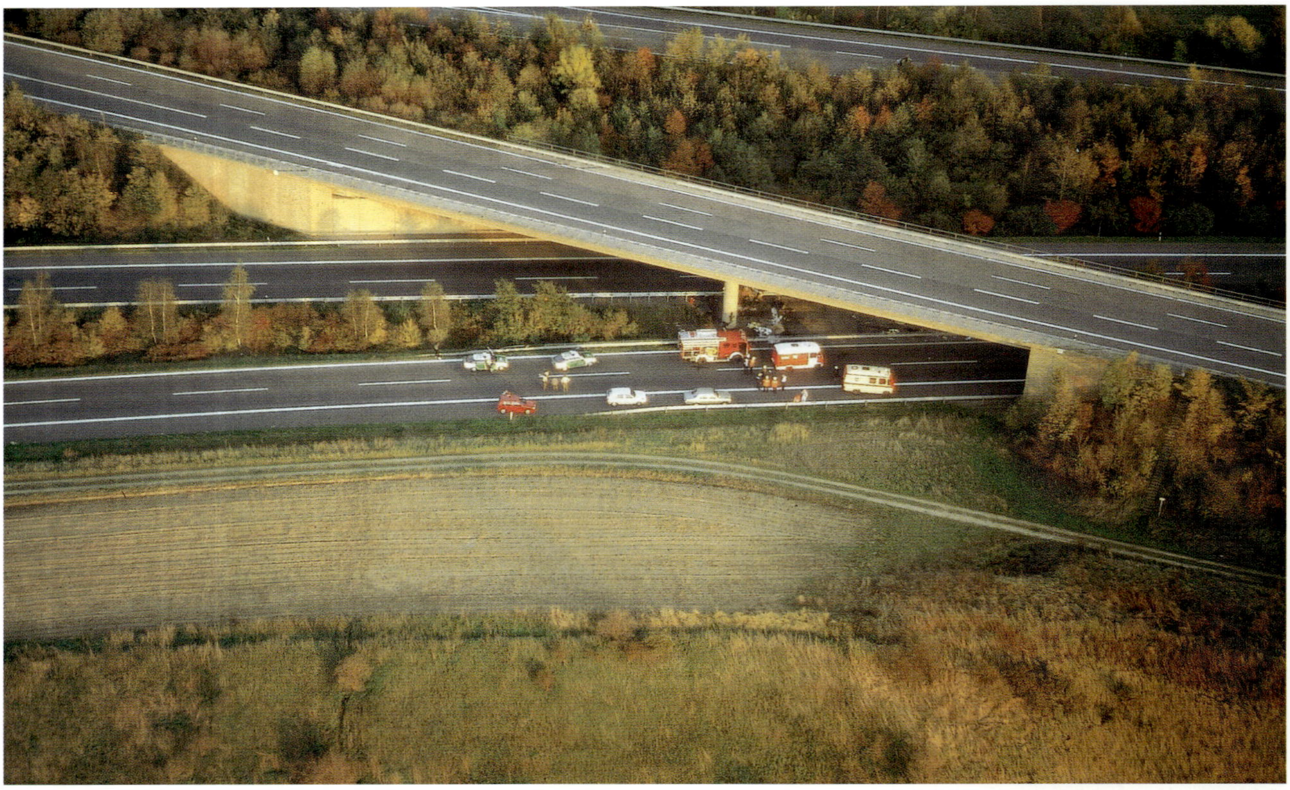

Ein streunender Hund rennt auf die Autobahn. Der Fahrer eines mit drei Insassen besetzten PKW macht eine reflexartige Lenkbewegung. Alle Insassen sind tot. Der Hund ist weitergelaufen.

A stray dog runs onto the autobahn. The driver of an automobile with two passengers instinctively grabs the steering wheel and swerves into the path of an oncoming car. Three people die in the accident. The dog runs away.

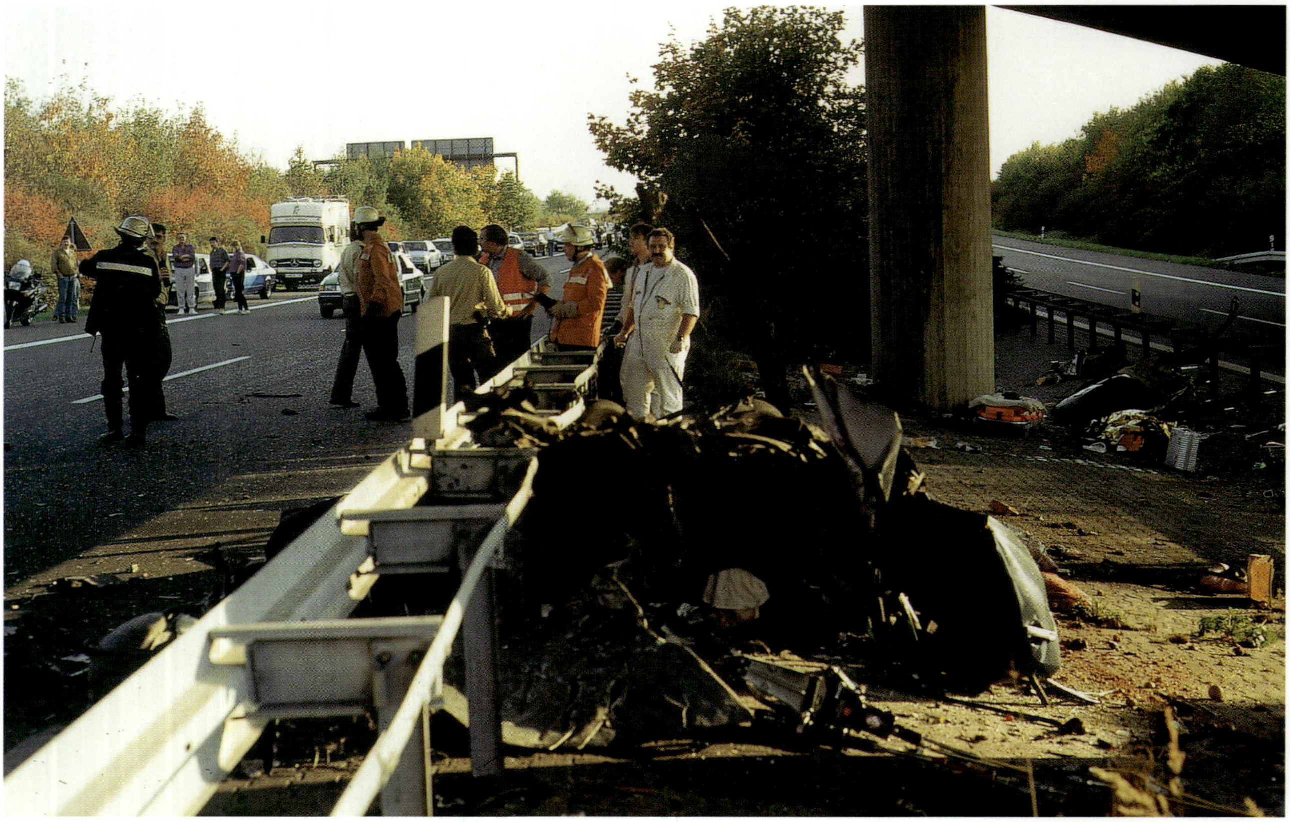

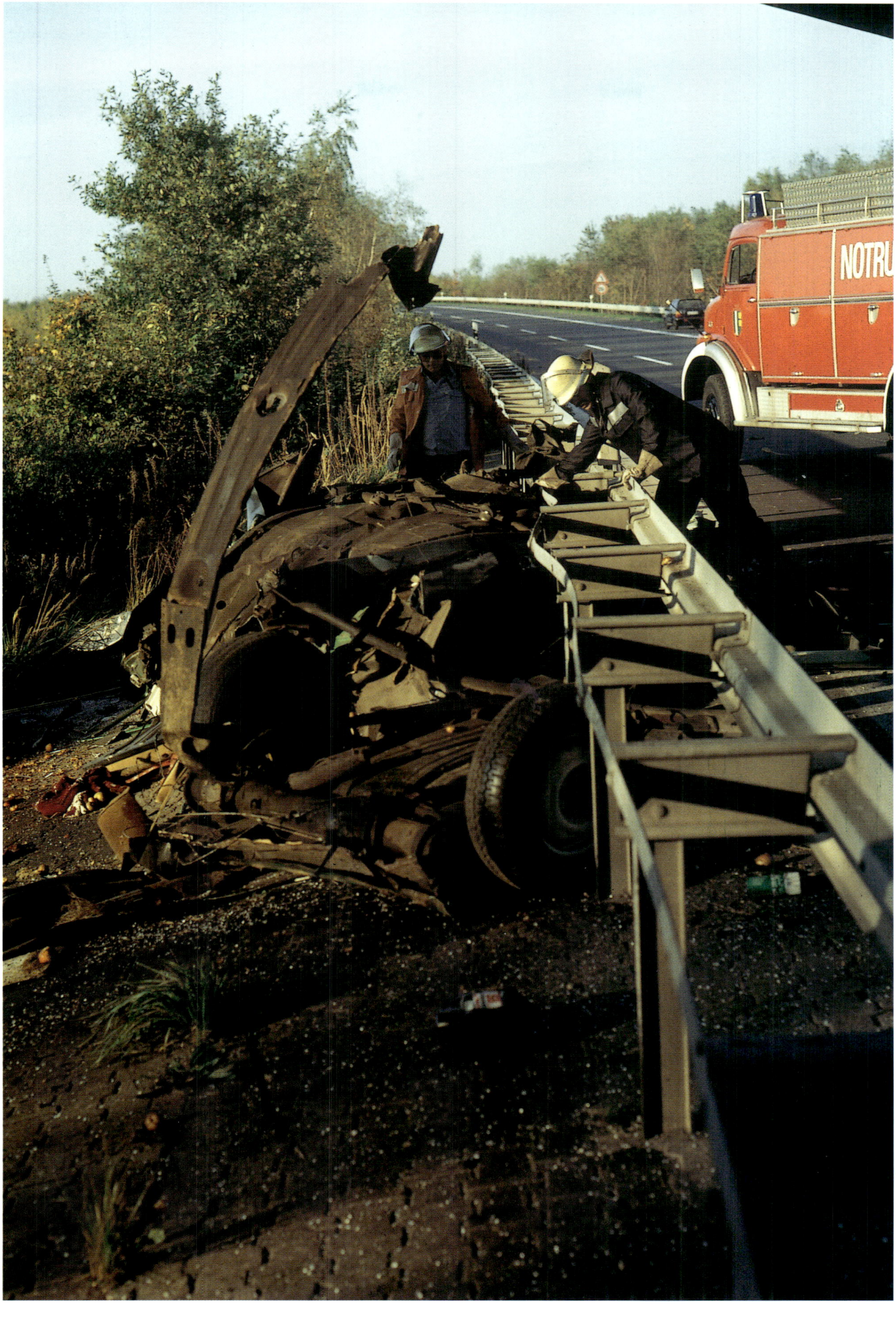

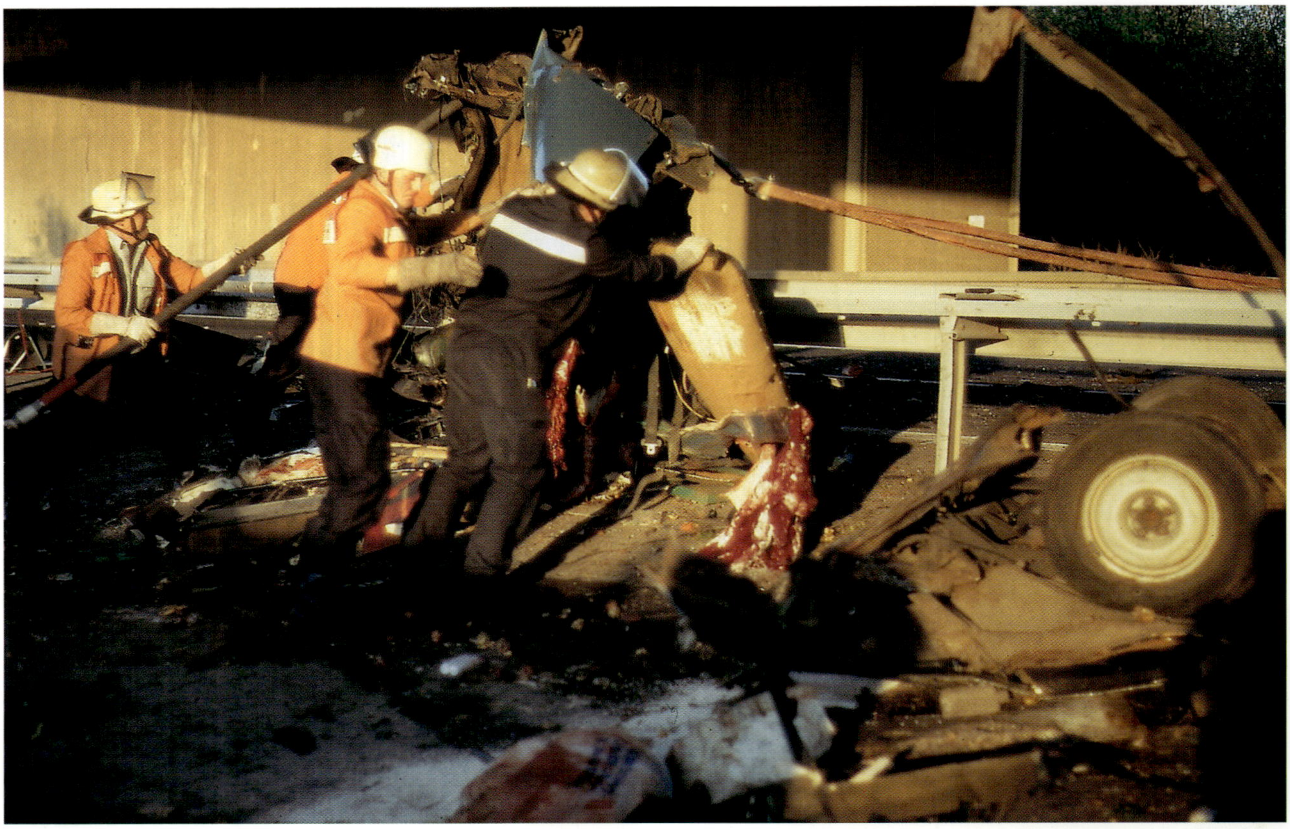

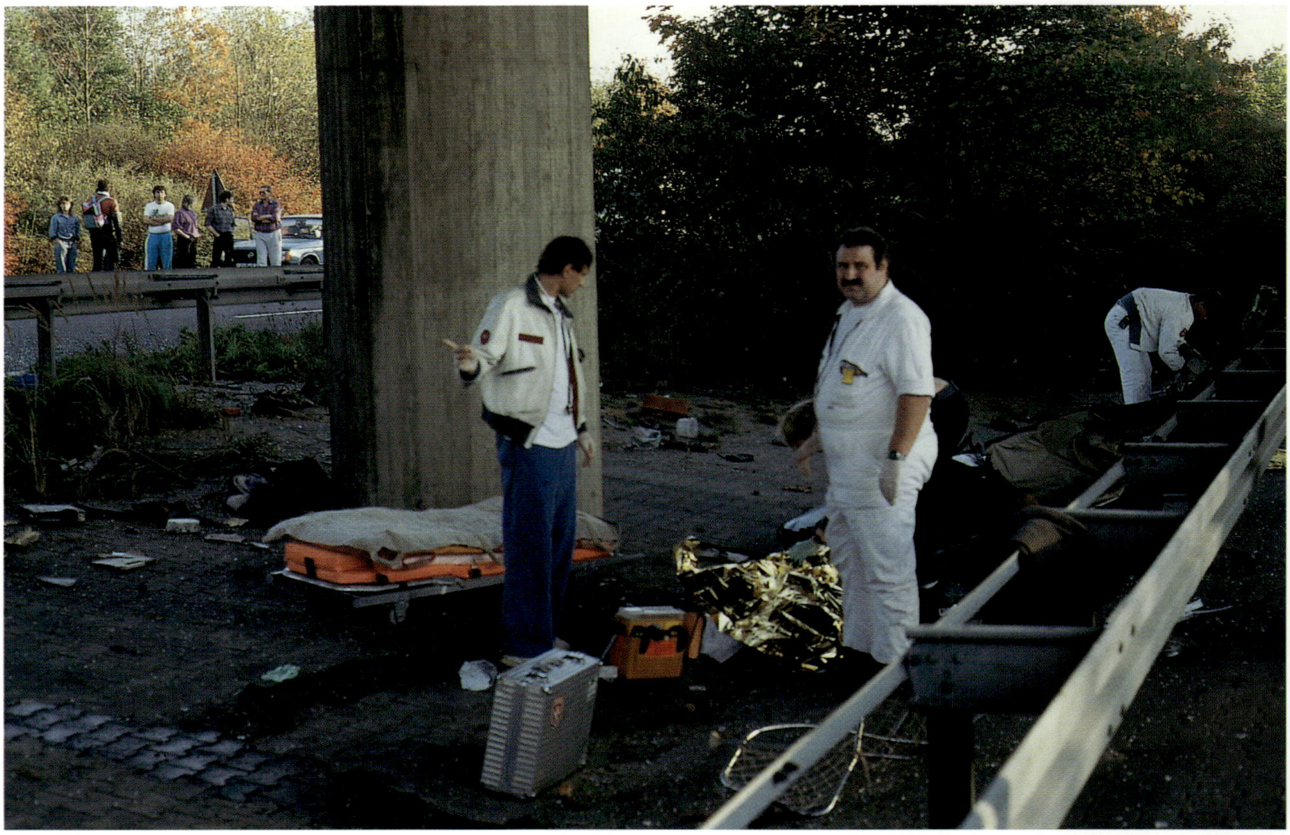

Einsatz für den Rettungshubschrauber
Mission for the Rescue Helicopter

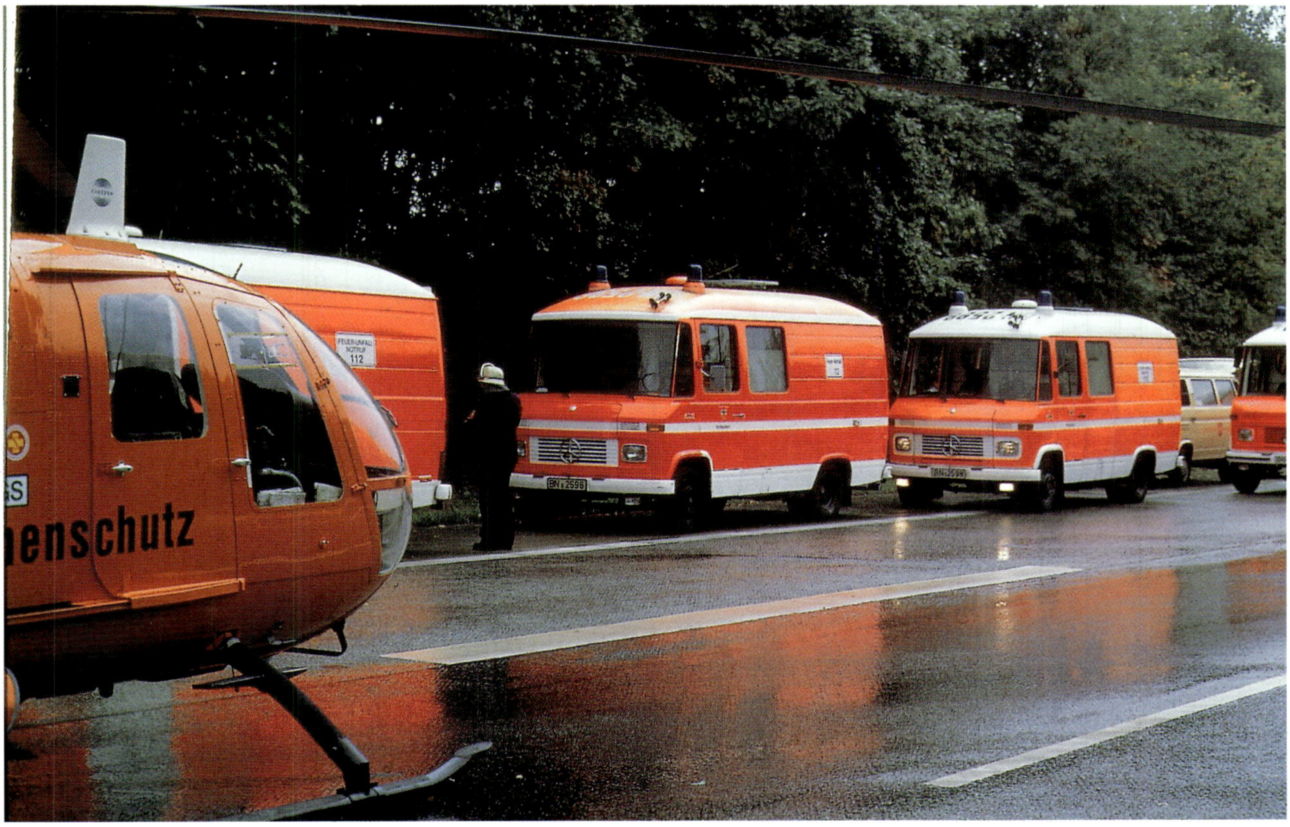

Massenanfall von Verletzten: ManV. Ein Reisebus ist umgekippt.

MassI: Accident with a large number of injured persons. A touring bus has turned over.

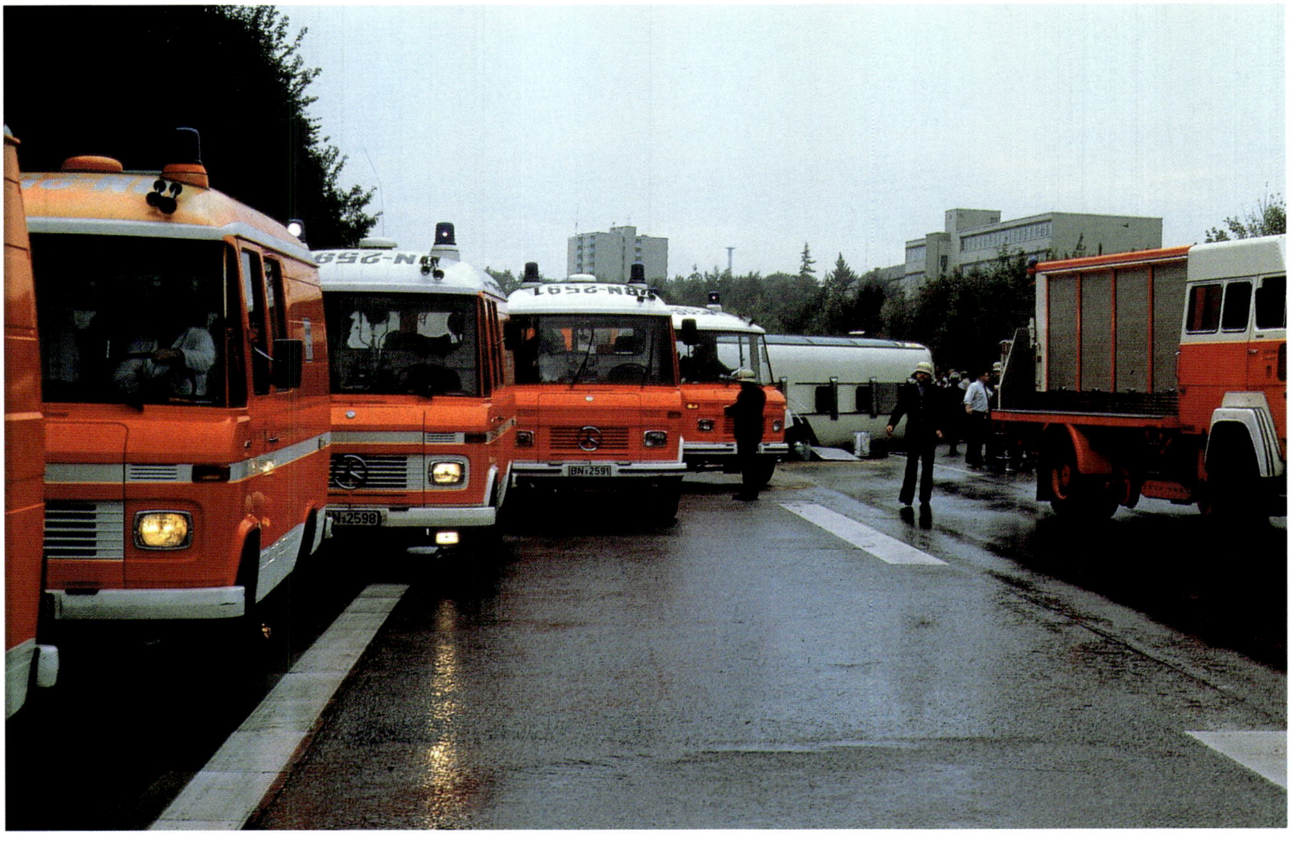

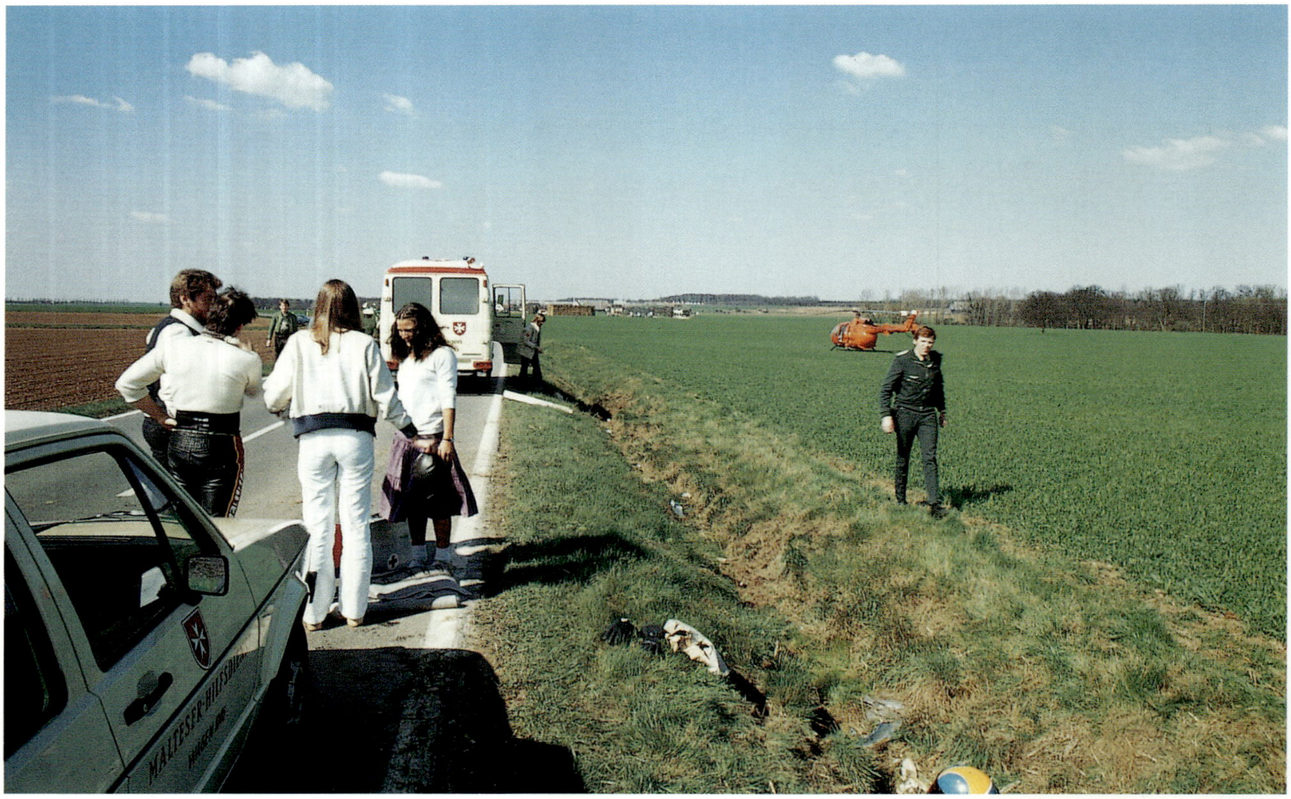

Einsatz für den Rettungshubschrauber
Mission for the Rescue Helicopter

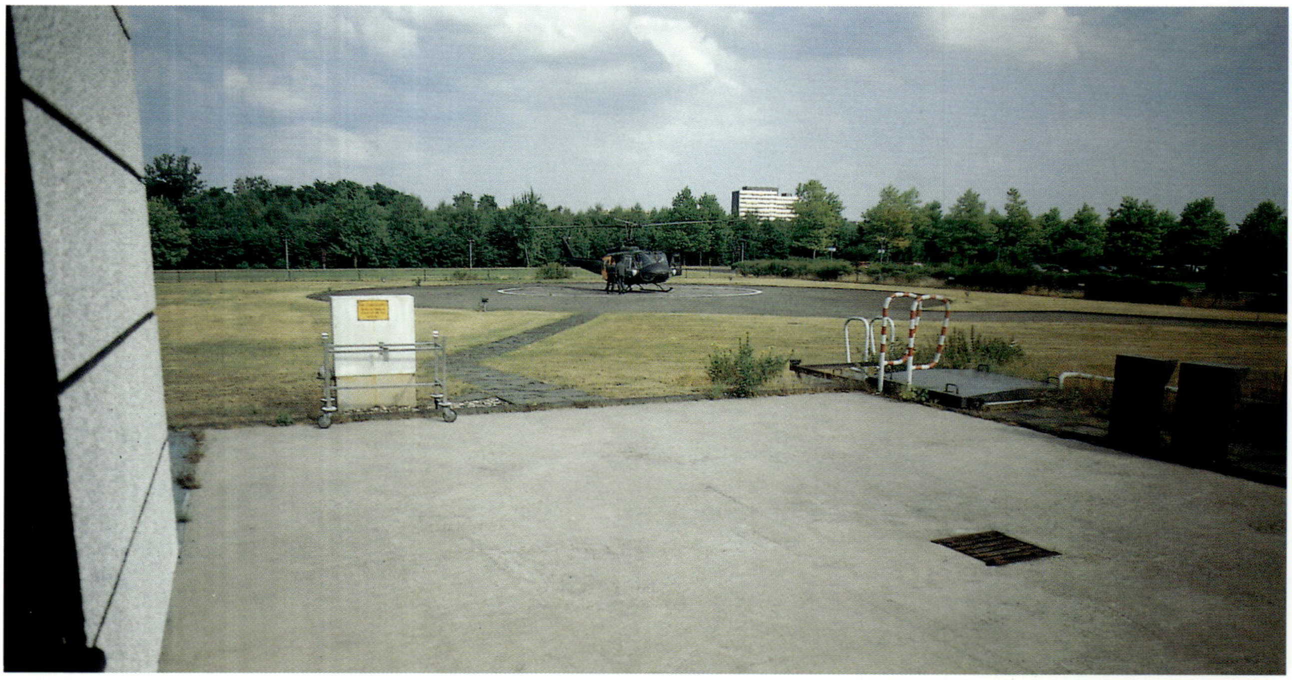

Christoph 3 ist durch einen technischen Defekt nicht einsatzbereit. Gleichzeitig läuft eine Einsatzanforderung zu einem Unfall mit drei verletzten Kindern ein. Der Leitstellendisponent hat Kenntnis, dass ein SAR-Hubschrauber zu einem Tag der offenen Tür auf einer Feuerwache steht. Ein kurzer Anruf genügt.

Owing to a technical defect, Christoph 3 is grounded. At the same time, an emergency call comes in: an accident with three injured children. The dispatcher at the Coordination Center knows that an SAR helicopter is on exhibit at a Fire Department "open house". A phone call is enough to mobilize the crew of the SAR.

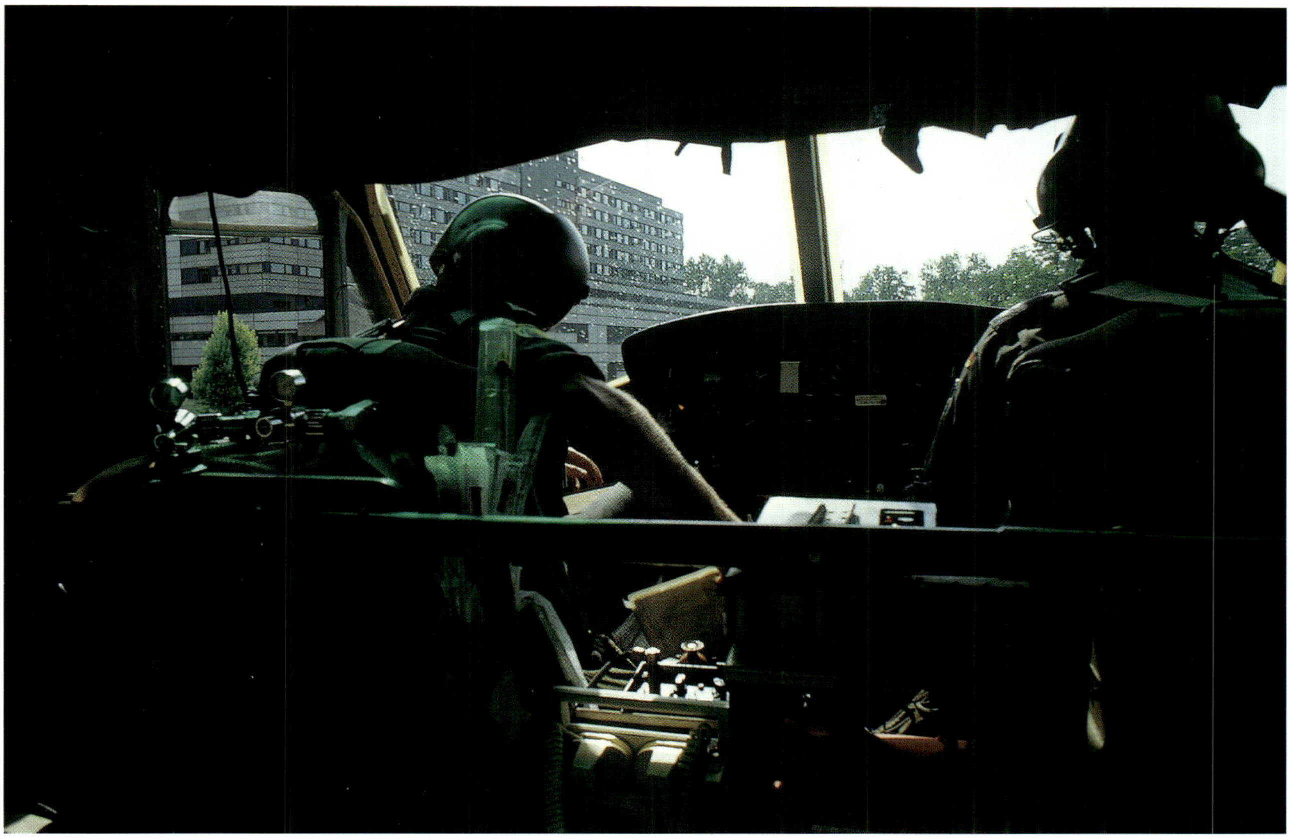

Innerhalb von Minuten ist der SAR-Hubschrauber auf dem Landeplatz von Christoph 3. Notarzt und Rettungsassistent steigen in den Hubschrauber ein. Drei Kinder werden versorgt.

Within minutes, the SAR helicopter touches down at the heliport usually used by Christoph 3. The physician with emergency & rescue certification and the air rescue paramedic board the SAR. Shortly afterwards, three children receive emergency medical attention.

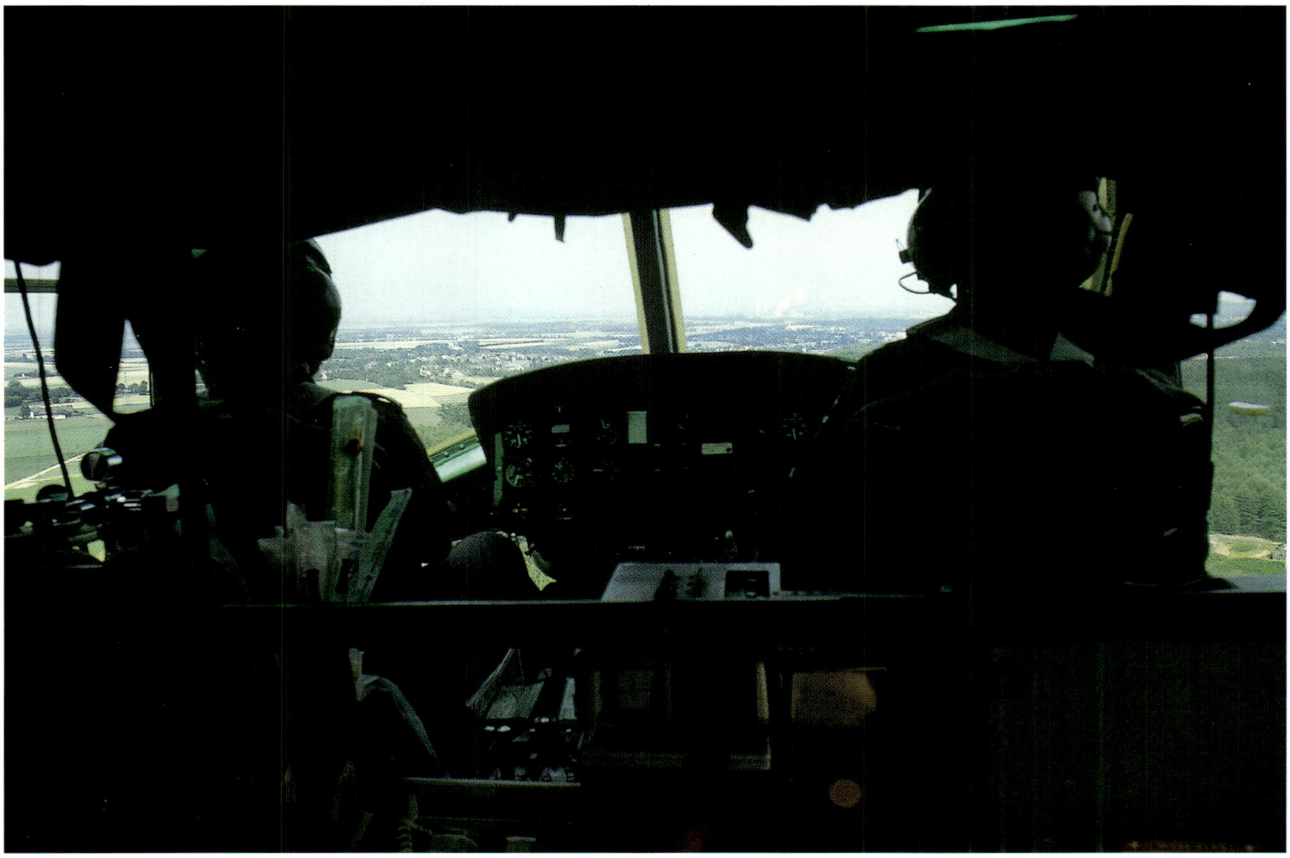

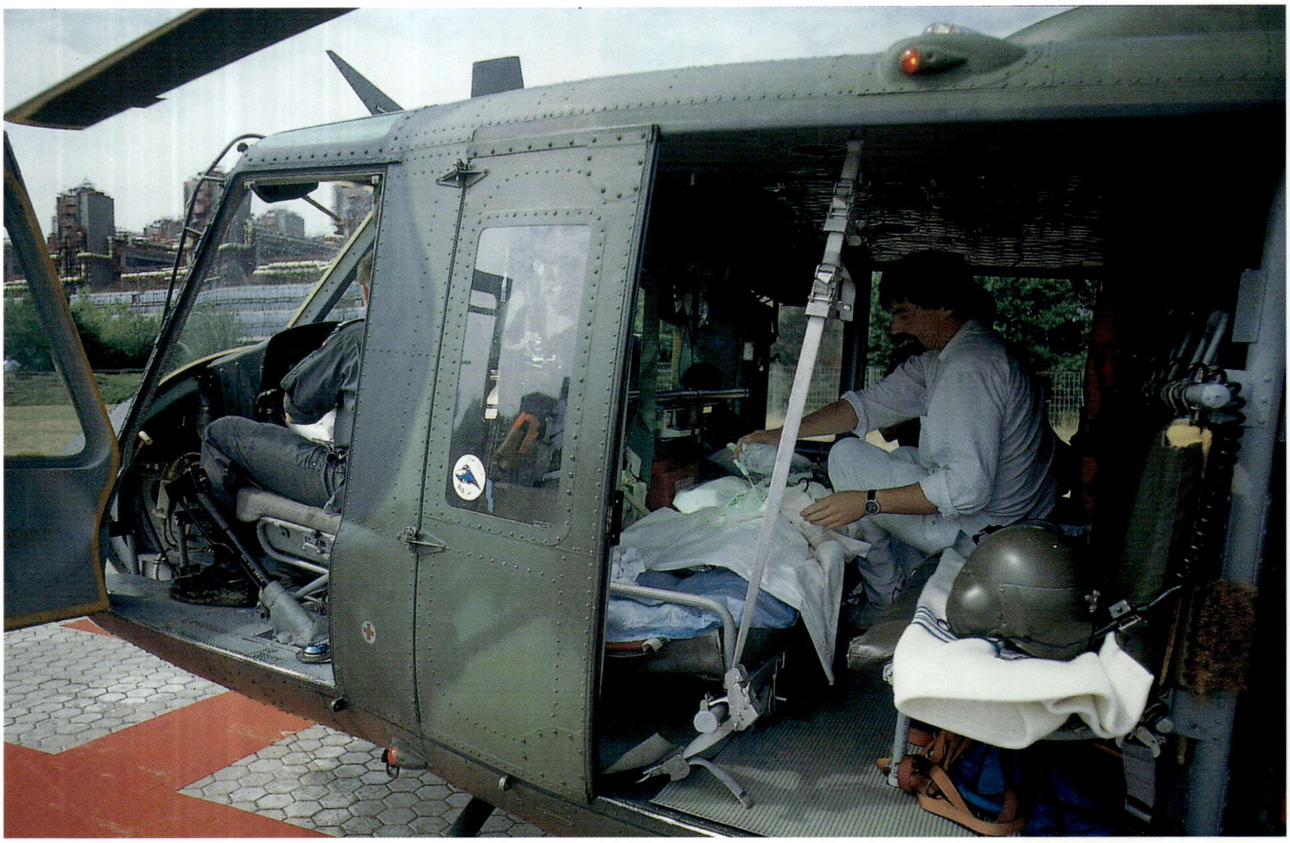

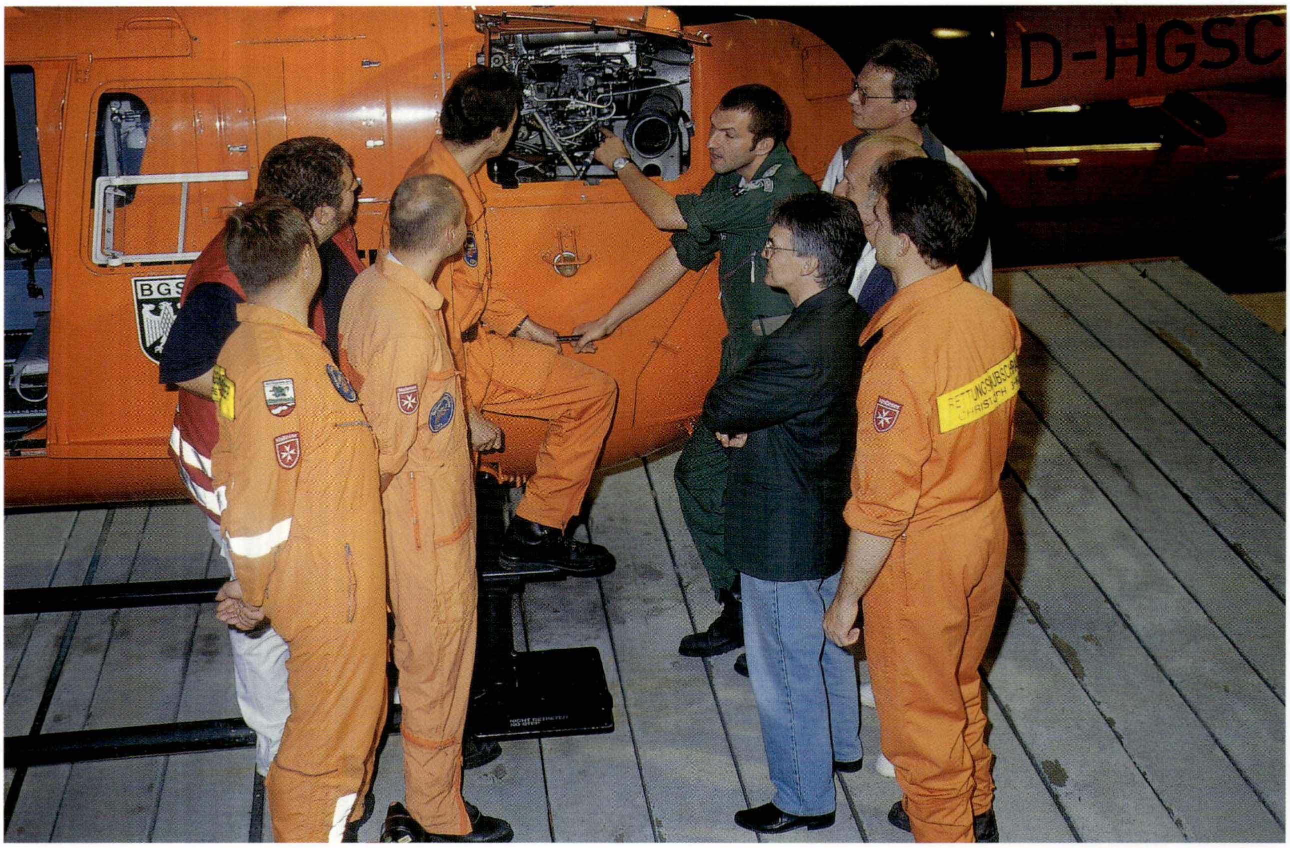

Piloten bilden die Luftrettungsassistenten auch vor Ort fort.

The pilot provides continued on-the-job training for air rescue paramedics.

Luftrettungsstationen in Deutschland
Air Rescue Stations in Germany

Stand: 03.2001
Last rerised:
March 2001

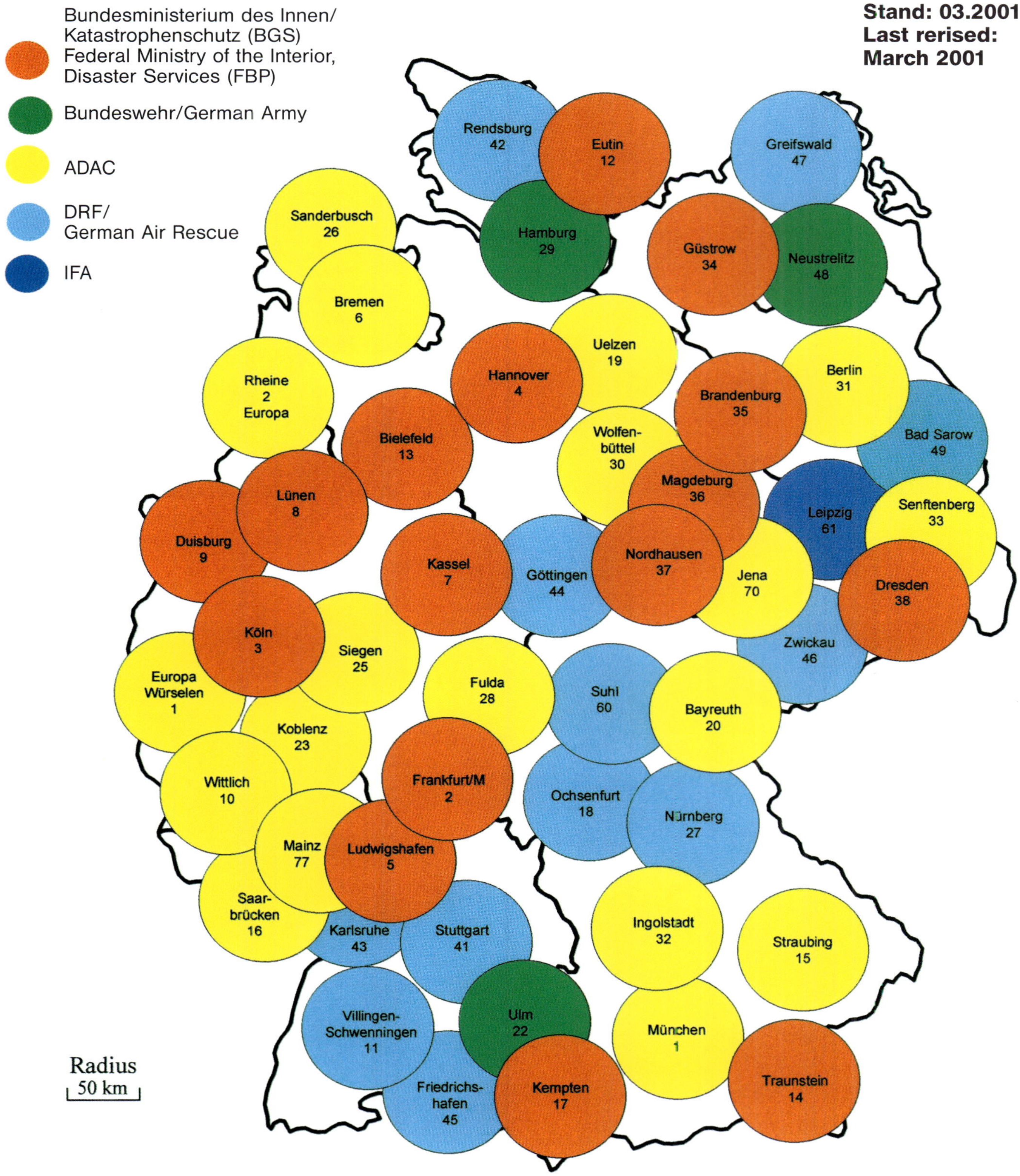

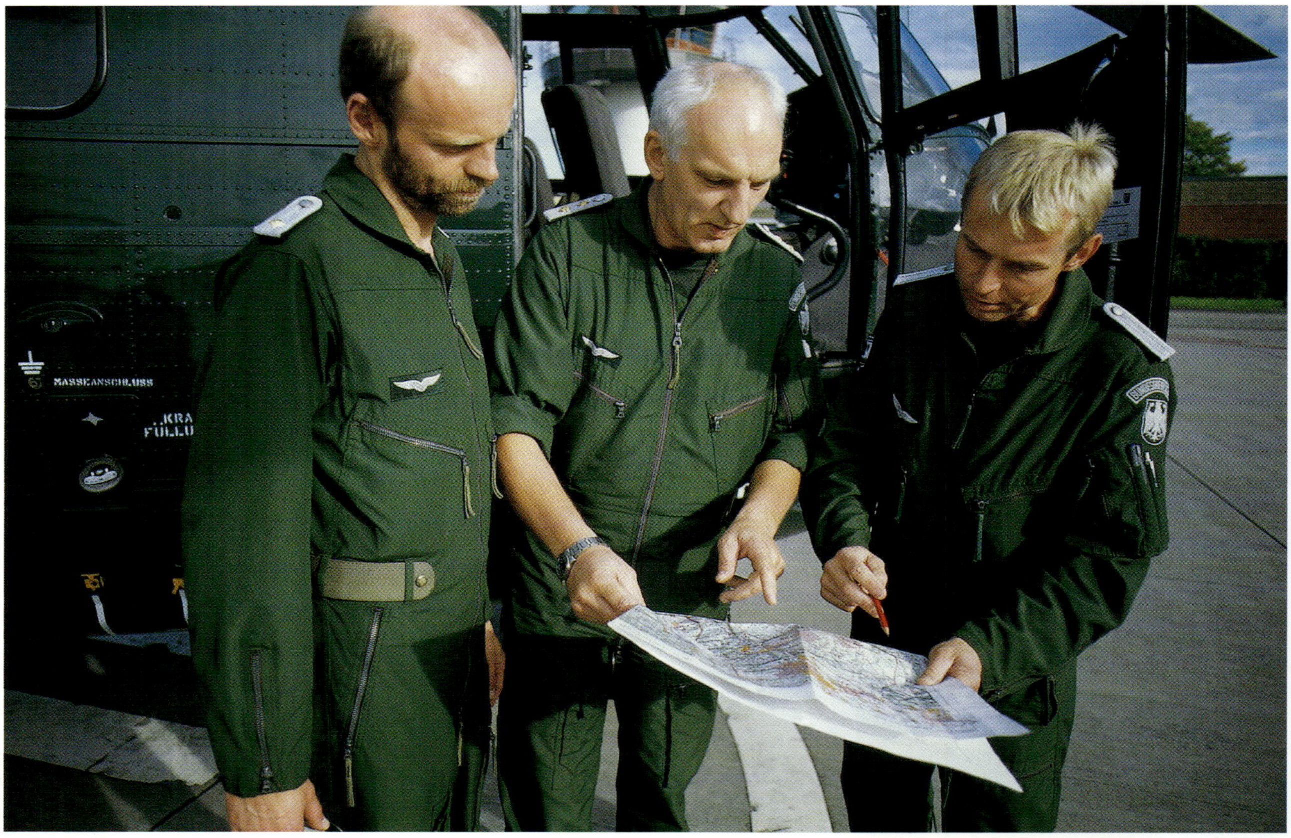

BGS-Rettungspiloten haben vielfältige Aufgaben. Hier bereiten drei Piloten einen Flug mit einem Staatsgast vor.

A rescue helicopter pilot's job within the FBP is highly diversified. In this photo three pilots prepare to transport a visiting dignitary – a very unusual kind of "secondary transport".

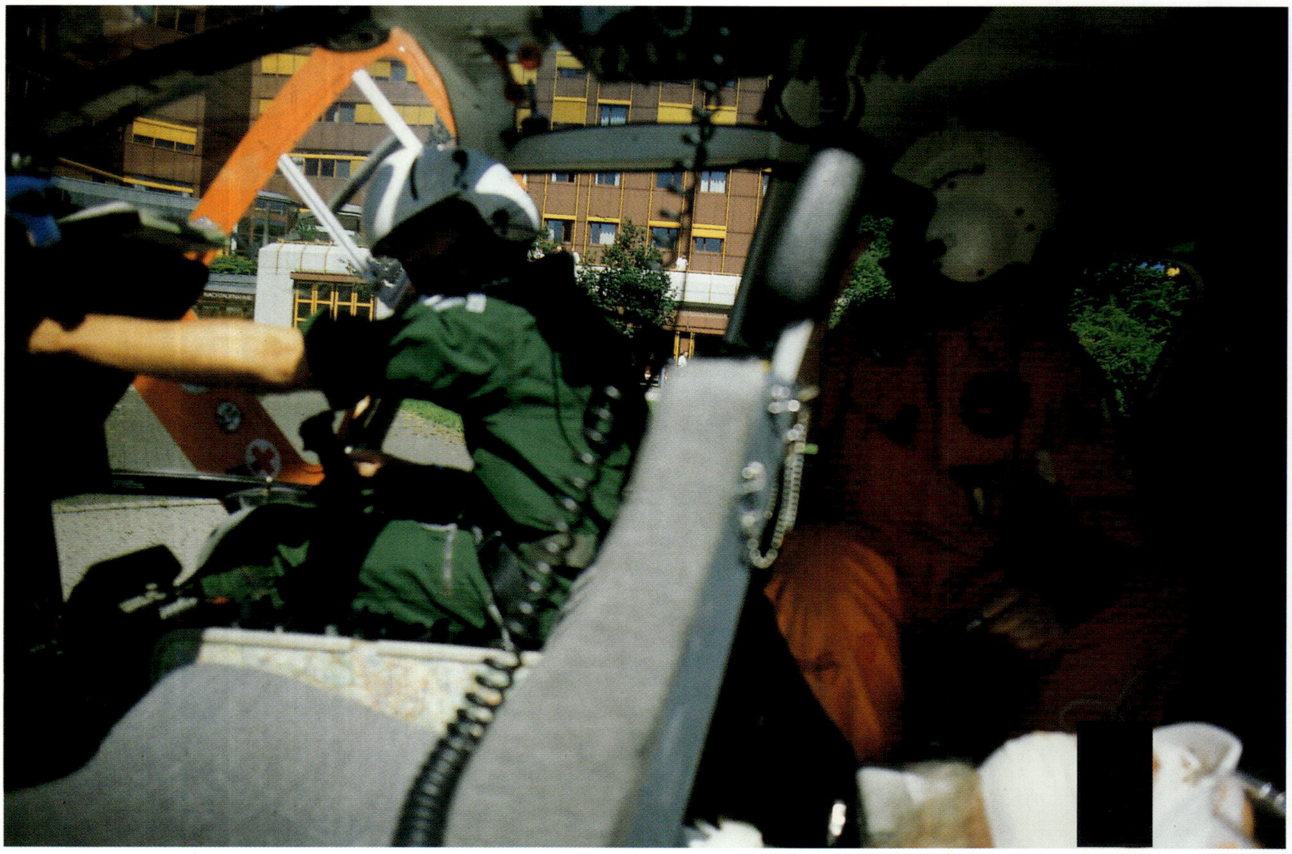

Interhospitaltransfer

Interhospital transfer

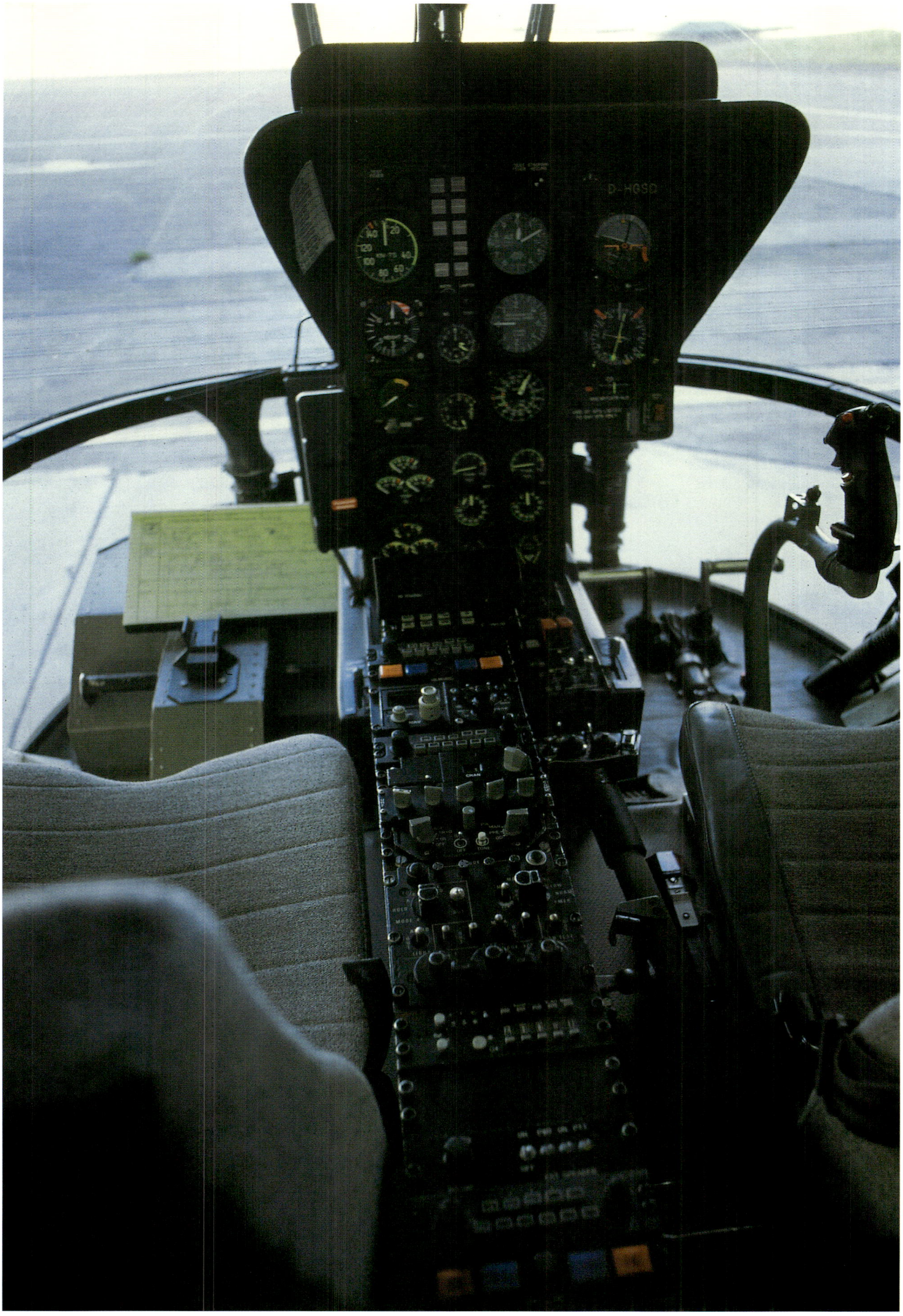
D-HGSD

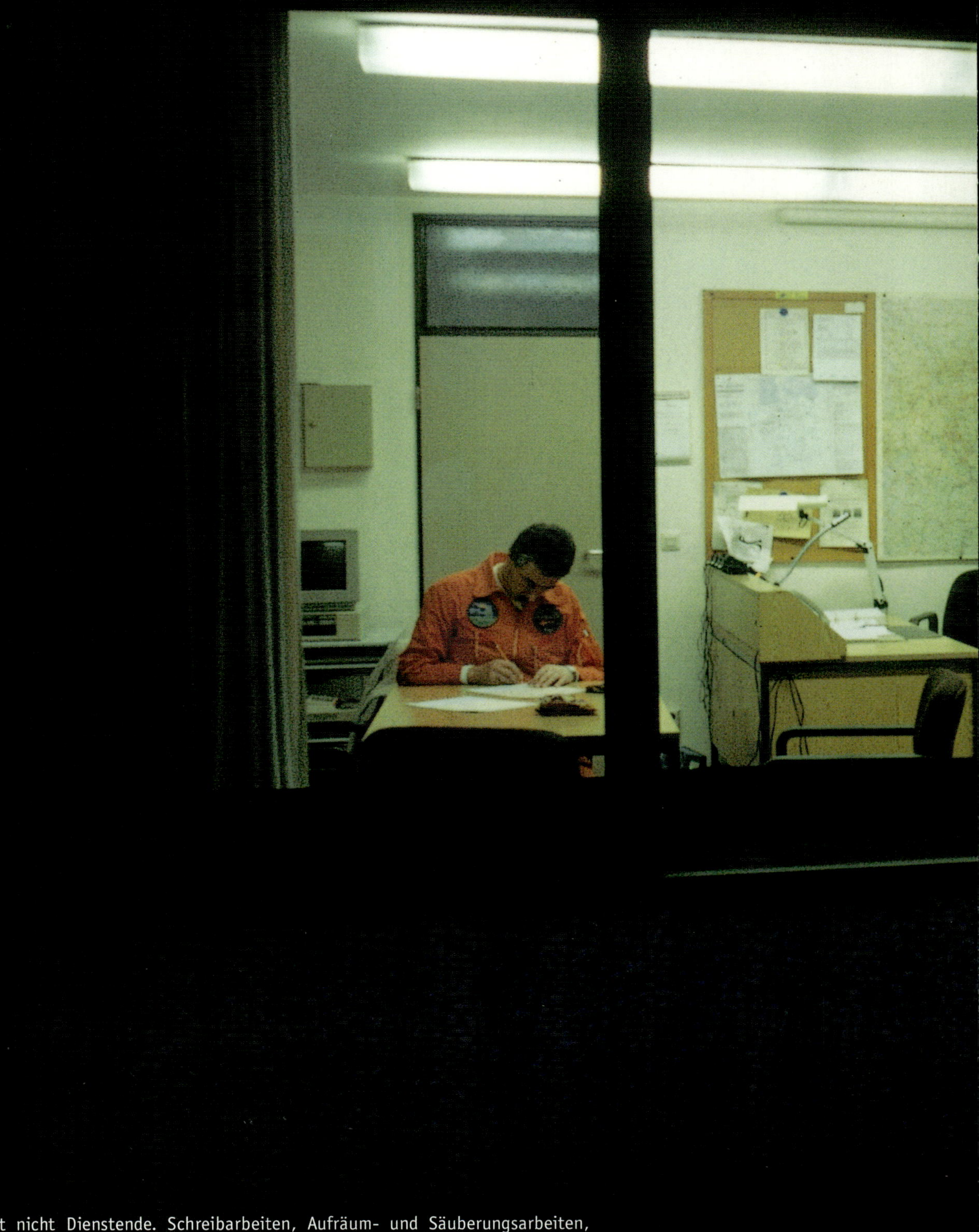

t nicht Dienstende. Schreibarbeiten, Aufräum- und Säuberungsarbeiten, ung,dringende Rückrufe und Anfragen, Nachflugkontrollen können das hinauszögern.

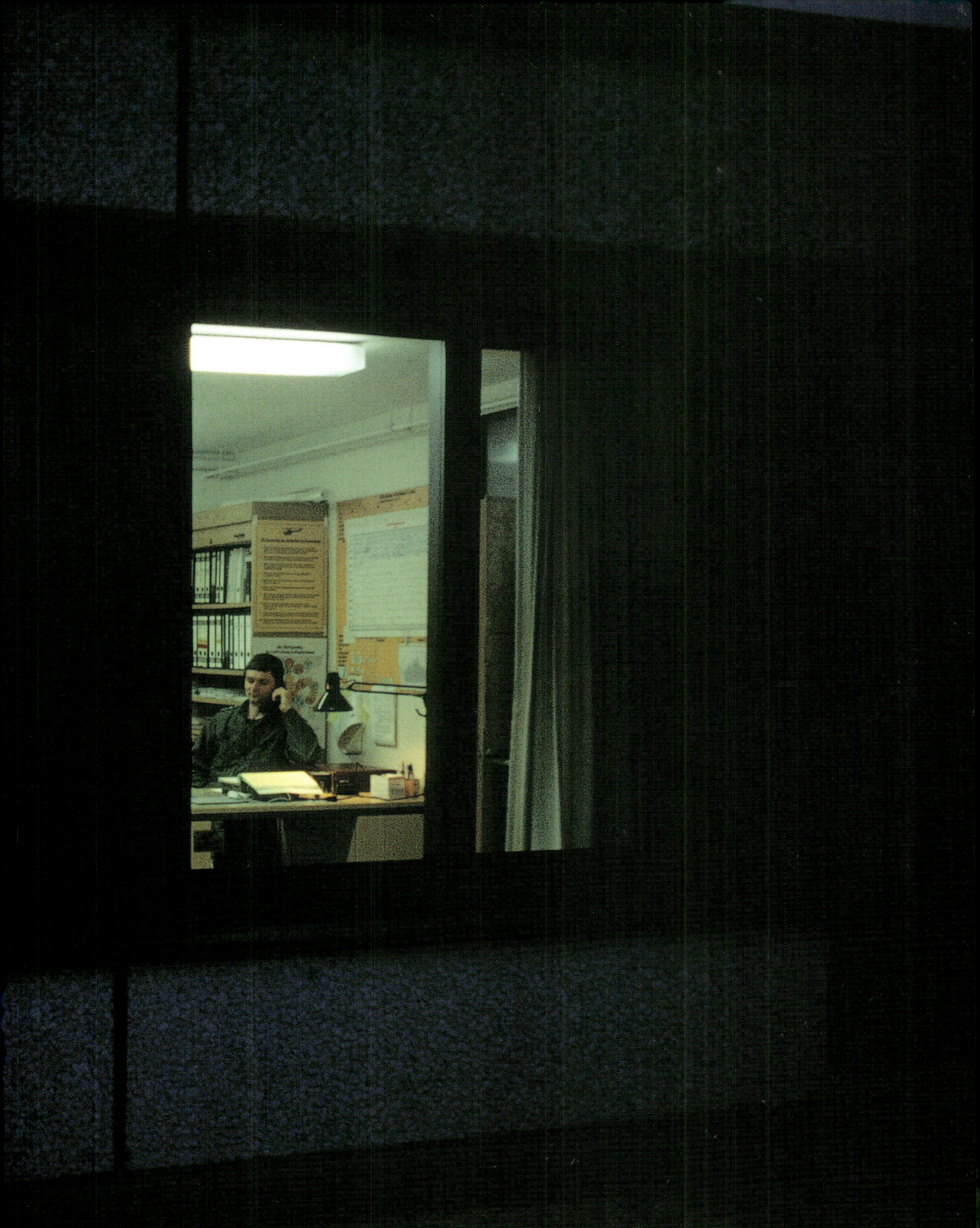

End of the mission but not of the working day. Paper work, phone calls, cleaning and straightening up. Personal data to be recorded and sometimes verified. Not to mention the requisite post-flight inspection.

Europäisierung der Luftrettung – HEMS! HEMS-proposals? – HEMS!

von/by Gunter Carloff

Als ich im November 1991 einen Telefonanruf von dem mir unbekannten Peter Curwen, Home Office Police Department, Vereinigtes Königreich, erhielt, und er mich fragte, ob ich der zuständige Beamte des BGS für die Luftrettung sei, war ich elektrisiert über das, was ich anschließend zu hören bekam. Die Arbeitsgemeinschaft der europäischen Luftfahrtbehörden (Joint Aviation Authorities; JAA) hätte im Oktober 91 einen Entwurf einer Betriebsvorschrift für die Luftrettung mit Hubschraubern veröffentlicht, die erhebliche Auswirkungen haben werde.

Einzelheiten sollten auf einem Treffen am 18.12.1991 im Airport Conference Center in Frankfurt mit Teilnehmern aus allen betroffenen europäischen Staaten diskutiert werden.

Neben den Chefpiloten des ADAC, der Deutschen Rettungsflugwacht (DRF) und meiner Person waren Vertreter aus Frankreich, Italien, Norwegen, Österreich, Schweden, der Schweiz und dem Vereinigten Königreich anwesend. Es wurde festgestellt, dass der vorliegende Entwurf der Betriebsvorschrift den meisten Betreibern der Luftrettung nicht bekannt war.

Forderungen nach Flugbetrieb mit 2 Piloten, leistungsstarken zweimotorigen Hubschraubern und sonstige erschwerenden Forderungen hätten auf die Luftrettung in der Bundesrepublik Deutschland verheerende Auswirkungen gehabt. Die Forderungen orientierten sich an theoretischen Forderungen der Flugsicherheit, die in der Praxis kurzfristig nicht erfüllbar waren. Hiermit begann eine intensive europäische Diskussion die in Deutschland mehrfach zu Schriftwechseln auf Ministerebene und Schlagzeilen in der Boulevardpresse führten. Auf der Arbeitsebene wurden die Regelungen praktikabler und Übergangsfristen immer wieder gestreckt. Die Betriebsvorschrift JAR-OPS 3 (Joint Aviation Requirements – Commercial Operations, Helicopters) ist mit seinem Teil HEMS (Helicopter Emergency Medical Service) seit 1998 in Deutschland in Kraft und mit der zweiten Änderung dieser Vorschrift, die in 2001 veröffentlicht wird, hat sich die langwierige und häufig mühselige Arbeit in internationalen Arbeitsgruppen offenkundig gelohnt. Der

In November 1991 I received a phone call from a Peter Curwen at the Home Office Police Department in the UK asking if I was the German Federal Border Police Officer in charge of air rescue. I had never met Peter Curwen before, but what he had to tell me was electrifying: the Joint Aviation Authorities (JAA) had published Draft Operating Regulations for Air Rescue with Helicopters in October 1991 which would have enormous implications for rescue activities.

Details of the new regulations were to be discussed at a meeting, to be attended by representatives of all the European nations concerned, scheduled for 18 December 1991 at the Airport Conference Center in Frankfurt/Main.

The German delegation consisted of the Head Pilot of the ADAC, a representative of the German Air Rescue Service (DRF) and myself. The other participants came from Austria, France, Italy, Norway, Sweden, Switzerland and the UK. It soon became evident that most of the operators of air rescue services did not know about the new Draft Operating Regulations.

The draft contained requirements – e.g. flight operations with 2 pilots, high-powered two-engine helicopters and other stipulations making life difficult for the rescue service operators – which would if enacted have had devastating effects on air rescue in the Federal Republic of Germany. The requirements were based on theoretical flight safety criteria which could not be satisfied in actual practice within the short term.

This draft triggered an intensive European discussion which repeatedly led to official correspondence between various ministries in the German government and made headlines in the boulevard press. On the operative level the regulations were made easier to implement and the transitional periods repeatedly extended. The Joint Aviation Requirements – Commercial Operations, Helicopters (JAR-OPS 3) – including a section on the Helicopter Emergency Medical Service (HEMS) – have been in force in Germany since 1998. A perusal of the Second Revision of the Regulations, to be published in 2001, shows that the protracted and sometimes tedious work carried out in the international working parties

Standard der Flugsicherheit ist in Europa nach vielen Jahrzehnten unterschiedlicher nationaler Lösungen erhöht und harmonisiert worden. Ein fortschrittliches Luftrecht ist entstanden, das sich mit dem bisher dominierenden US-Luftrecht unter dem Dach der Internationalen Zivilluftfahrtorganisation (JCAO) messen lassen kann.

Im Rettungshubschrauber hat sich ein Besatzungsmitglied bei medizinischen Hubschraubernoteinsätzen neben dem Piloten etabliert. Dieses „HEMS Crew Member" wird nach einem einheitlichen Plan, den die deutschen Luftretter 1998 gemeinsam erarbeitet haben, in seine besonderen Aufgaben zur Unterstützung des Piloten eingewiesen. Die nächste Generation von leistungsgesteigerten Rettungshubschraubern hat Einzug gehalten und Mängel an Landeplätzen werden Hindernis für Hindernis abgetragen.

Trotz aller Probleme, die bekanntlich im Detail stecken, ist mit JAR-OPS 3 zwischenzeitlich eine europäische Erfolgsstory geschrieben worden.

has obviously paid off. Following decades of non-uniform national solutions, the standard of flight safety in Europe has now been raised and harmonized. Progressive aviation legislation has been enacted which can stand up to any comparison with the dominant US aviation legislation under the umbrella of the International Civil Aviation Organization (ICAO).

For emergency medical missions with rescue helicopters, the "HEMS Crew Member" has become firmly established, in addition to the pilot and the physician with emergency & rescue certification, as a crew member who carries out both medical and aviation functions. In 1998 the German air rescue services drew up a uniform plan for instructing the HEMS Crew Members on the particular aviation tasks they are expected to perform as the pilot's right hand. The next generation of performance-enhanced rescue helicopters has already arrived; at the same time, the deficiencies noted at helicopter landing sites are being removed, obstacle by obstacle.

Despite the mass of problems that have had to be ironed out, the JAR OPS 3 is now a European aviation success story.

Über den Autoren • About the Author

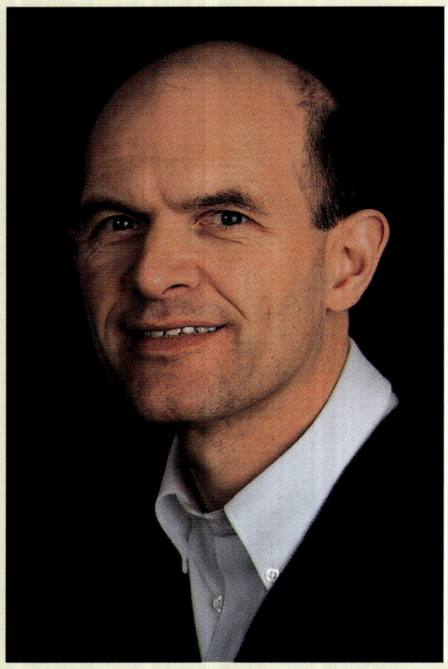

Privat-Dozent Dr.med. Bertil Bouillon,

geboren 1958, ist Oberarzt am II.Chirurgischen Lehrstuhl der Universität Köln im Klinikum Köln-Merheim. Nach seinem Wehrdienst, den er als Schiffsarzt bei der Marine absolviert,wurde er Assistenzarzt in Köln-Merheim. Heute ist er dort Facharzt für Chirurgie und besitzt ebenfalls die Teilgebietsbezeichnung für Unfallchirurgie. Als Notarzt war er im Rettungsdienst der Stadt Köln eingesetzt,war dann koordinierender Notarzt am Klinikum Merhein, ärztlicher Leiter des Rettungsdienstes der Stadt Köln und ist seit 1987 leitender Hubschrauberarzt für den Rettungshubschrauber Christoph 3. Er ist Mitglied in wichtigen medizinischen Fachgesellschaften und hat über 140 Publikationen in nationalen und internationalen Zeitschriften und Büchern veröffentlicht, sowie über 150 Vorträge auf nationalen und internationalen Kongressen und Symposien gehalten.

born in 1958, is Staff Physician attached to the Second Department of Surgery at the University Hospital Cologne in Cologne-Merheim. After completing his military service as a ship's doctor in the German Navy, he started his surgical residency at the Second Surgical Professorship in Cologne-Merheim. Today he is a specialist for surgery with the subspecialty traumatology. As a physician with emergency & rescue certification, he was sent on missions by the Rescue Service of the City of Cologne. He subsequently became Emergency Physician Coordinator at the University Hospital Cologne in Cologne-Merheim and then Medical Director of the Rescue Service of the City of Cologne. Since 1987 he has been the head physician with emergency & rescue certification working on the rescue helicopter Christoph 3. He is a member of important professional medical societies and has published more than 140 articles in national and international journals and books. In addition, he has presented upwards of 150 papers at national and international congresses and symposia.

Über den Autoren • About the Author

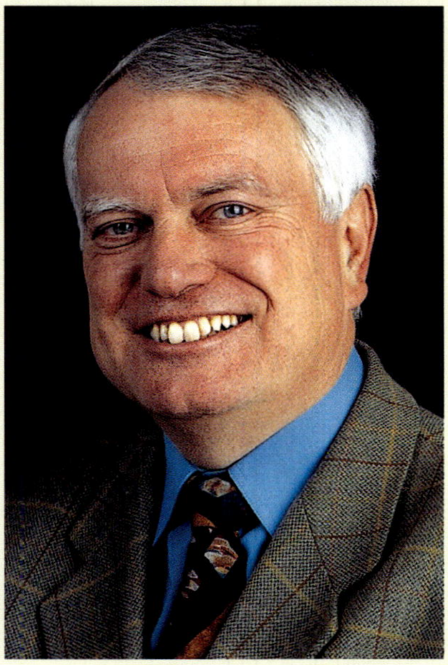

Ernst Brück,

geboren 1941, war als Geschäftsführer des Malteser-Hilfsdienstes in der Anfangszeit des Kölner Rettungshubschraubers für Einsatz, Leitstelle, personelle Besetzung des medizinischen Rettungspersonals und der Notärzte zuständig. Er war zudem für die gesamte rettungsdienstliche Ablauforganisation in der Phase des 1. Modellversuchs des Bundesministerium des Innern im Grossraum Köln-Düsseldorf „Hubschrauber im Katastrophenschutz und Rettungsdienst" verantwortlich. Nach Ende des Modellversuchs und Überleitung des Christoph 3 an den Kernträger, die Stadt Köln, und die angeschlossene Trägergemeinschaft bestehend aus Kreisen und kreisfreien Städten des Einsatzbereichs war er für die personelle Besetzung mit ehren- und hauptamtlichen Rettungsassisten zuständig. Im Juli 1997 wechselte er in die Bundesgeschäftsstelle des MHD.

born in 1941, now holds an executive position at the NRW State Office of the Maltester-Hilfsdienst. As Managing Director of the Malteser-Hilfsdienst at the beginning of the rescue helicopter era, he was responsible for helicopter missions, the Coordination Center, the medical personnel aboard the rescue helicopter, and the physicians with emergency & rescue certification. In addition, he was responsible for the entire workflow organization of rescue service operations during the first Model Program – "The Role of Helicopters in Disaster Relief and Rescue Services" – conducted by the Federal Minister of the Interior in the Cologne-Düsseldorf metropolitan area. At the end of the Model Program – when the responsibility for Christoph 3 was turned over to the core sponsor, the City of Cologne, and the affiliated sponsors' group (consisting of districts and cities which do not belong to any district) in the operational area of the helicopter – he was responsible for providing professional and volunteer paramedics for the rescue helicopter. In July 1997 he transferred to the National Office of the Malteser-Hilfsdienst.

Über den Autoren

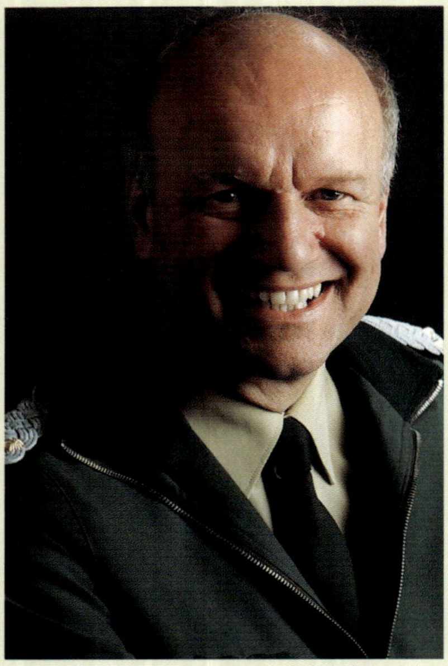

Gunter Carloff

geboren 1947, aufgewachsen in Hamburg,heute Polizeidirektor im BGS, begann nach dem Abitur seine Laufbahn beim Bundesgrenzschutz. Seiner Ausbildung zum Berufshubschrauberführer folgten Berufungen zum stellvertretenden Staffelführer der BGS-Fliegerstaffeln Mitte und Nord, fliegerische Fortbildungen zum Fluglehrer für die Hubschraubermuster SA 318 C, BO 105, Bell UH-1D und Bell 212. Nach einem zweijährigen Studium für den höheren Polizeivollzugsdienst wurde er Einsatzstabsoffizier und Leiter Luftrettungsdienst im Stab der BGS-Fliegergruppe. In dieser Funktion war ihm die Fachaufsicht über bis zu 22 Luftrettungsstationen übertragen. Zugleich war er Führer der Stabs- und Ausbildungsstaffel in Sankt Augustin-Hangelar. Seit 1996 ist er Leiter der Aus- und Fortbildung der BGS-Fliegergruppe. Seine wesentlichen Aufgaben der letzten Jahre waren die Erarbeitung einer Untersuchung über Flugunfälle durch Freileitungen, die Entwicklung eines Crew Coordination Concepts, die Konzeption für ein Crew Resource Management-Training, die Erprobung eines Hindernis – Warnsystems für Hubschrauber. Als gefragter Experte und Autor hat er zahlreiche Artikel über den Flugbetrieb mit Hubschraubern, die Luftrettung, über Landeplätze und über die Entwicklung des europäischen Luftrechts für Hubschrauber veröffentlicht. Gunter Carloff ist Fachberater des Luftfahrt-Bundesamtes und in folgenden Gremien tätig: Normung von Rettungshubschraubern (DIN/CEN), Ausbildung von Hubschrauberpiloten in Europa (JAR-FCL 2), Anforderungen an Flugsimulation in Europa (JAR-STD 1 H) und für Hubschrauberflugbetrieb in Europa (JAR-OPS 3). Er ist unverändert aktiver Pilot (ATPL-H) auf verschiedenen Hubschraubern u.a. AS 332 L1 Super Puma. Auch heute schlägt sein Herz für alle Belange der Luftrettung, die er als Rettungspilot seit den ersten Tagen der Christoph Luftrettung kennt.

About the Author

Gunter Carloff

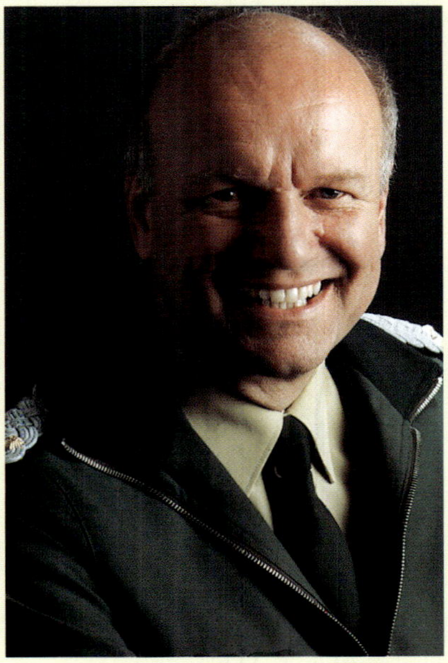

born in 1947, is now Police Director of the German Federal Border Police. Carloff jointed the FBP after graduating from college-track high school ("A levels") in his native Hamburg. After completing his training as a professional helicopter pilot, Carloff was named Deputy Squadron Leader of the Aviation Squadrons Central and North of the Federal Border Police. After undergoing further training in aviation, he became a flight instructor for the helicopter classes SA 318 C, BO 105, Bell UH-1D and Bell 212. After completing two years of further study to qualify for the higher police service, Carloff was appointed Head of Operations on the Staff of the FBP Aviation Group and Head of the Helicopter Emergency Medical Service (HEMS). In the latter capacity, he was responsible for all matters related to aviation at the 22 HEMS stations. At the same time, he was Head of the Staff and Training Squadron in St. Augustin-Hangelar. Since 1996 he has headed the Basic and Continued Training Program of the FBP Aviation Group.

In recent years Carloff has successfully undertaken several major projects; these include the design of a study on flight accidents caused by power lines, the development of a Crew Coordination Concept, the design of Crew Resource Management Training and the testing of an obstacle-warning system. He is also a sought-after expert and author who has published numerous articles on flight operations with helicopters, the helicopter emergency medical service, heliports and the development of European aviation law for helicopters. In addition, he is a consultant to the German Federal Office of Civil Aviation and a member of the following committees: Standards for Rescue Helicopters (DIN/CEN), Training of Helicopter Pilots in Europe (JAR-FCL 2), Requirements for Flight Simulation in Europe (JAR-STD 1 H) and for Helicopter Flight Operations in Europe (JAR-OPS 3). He is still an active pilot (ATPL-H) on various helicopters, including the AS 332 L1 Super Puma. He is still intensively involved in all aspects of HEMS operations, which he has followed closely as a rescue helicopter pilot since the first days of Christoph air rescue.

Über den Autoren • About the Author

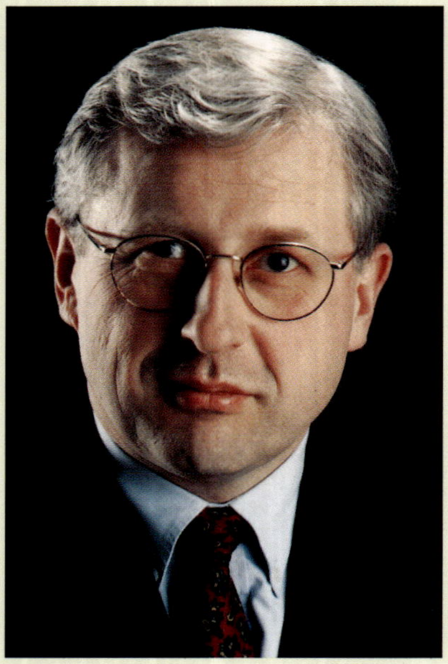

Bernd Falk,

geboren 1956 in Bonn. Nach kaufmännischer und medizinischer Ausbildung war er 12 Jahre lang Leiter der Rettungs- und Fahrdienste des Malteser-Hilfsdienstes auf Bundesebene. Er hatte die operative Leitung des boden- und luftgebundenen Malteser Rückholdienstes. Er ist Mitinitiator der „Ständigen Konferenz für den Rettungsdienst". Unter seiner Leitung gelang eine erfolgreiche Implementierung eines Qualitätsmanagementsystems an allen 150 Rettungswachen der Malteser mit Zertifizierung nach ISO 9001. Von 1979 bis 1999 war er ehrenamtlich als LRA auf dem Rettungshubschrauber „Christoph 3" in Köln eingesetzt. Seit 1999 ist er im Projektmanagement / Unternehmensentwicklung bei der gemeinnützigen ADAC-Luftrettung GmbH München tätig. Dort ist er unter anderem Leiter des Projektes EUCREW – Europäisches Schulungszentrum für Luftrettung und bodengebundenen Rettungsdienst.

born 1956 in Bonn. After completing commercial and medical training, he served as National Director of the Rescue and Transport Services of the Malteser-Hilfsdienst. He was Operative director of the airborne and land-bound Malteser Medical Repatriation Service. He was also Co-initiator of the „Standing Conference for the Rescue Service". Successful implementation of a quality management system at all 150 rescue stations of the Malteser-Hilfsdienst with certification in conformance with ISO 9001 was one of his jobs. From 1979 to 1999 he did volunteer service as an ARP on the rescue helicopter „Christoph 3" in Cologne. Since 1999 he is project management and corporate development for the non-profit organization ADAC-Luftrettung GmbH in Munich. Among other responsibilities at this organization, he serves as Director of the project EUCREW – European Training Center for Air Rescue and Land-Bound Rescue Service.

Über den Autoren • About the Author

Erik Gladich

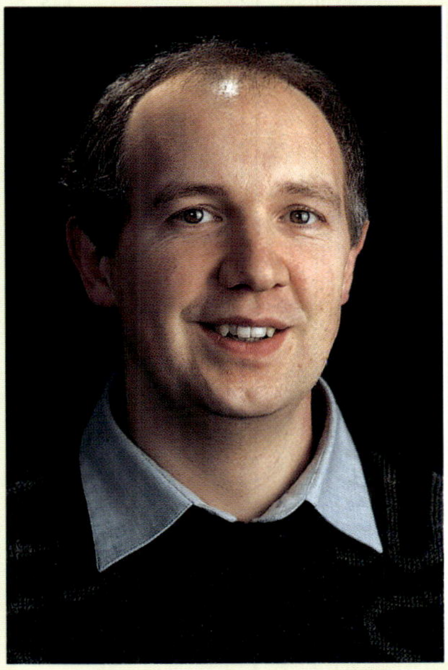

geboren 1963, ist seit dem Jahr 2000 Dienstgruppenleiter für den RTH und das NEF 5. Für beide ist er Qualitätsbeauftragter. Im Malteser-Hilfsdienst ist er hauptamtlich seit 1982, seit dieser Zeit ist er auch auf dem NEF eingesetzt. 1983 wurde er in die RTH-Crew berufen. Zuvor war er Zugführer, Ausbilder und im Stab Hauptverwaltungsbeamter als Sachbearbeiter für den Sanitätsdienst zuständig. In Köln gehört er wie alle anderen Luftrettungsassistenten auch zur ersten Generation der HEMS-Crew Member. Er hat die erste offizielle Homepage eines RTH konzipiert und ins Internet gestellt.

born in 1963, has been Head of the Paramedic Group for the rescue helicopters (RH) and the emergency physicians' car (NEF) since 2000. He is a quality assurance representative for both types of vehicles. Gladich has been employed by the Malteser-Hilfsdienst since 1982 and has worked aboard the NEF during this period. In l983 he was asked to join the rescue helicopter crew. Before this he worked as a platoon leader, trainer and administrative assistant concerned with the paramedic service on the staff of the chief executive officer. Like all the other air rescue paramedics in Cologne, he is a "first-generation" HEMS Crew Member. Furthermore, he designed the first official rescue helicopter website and placed it in the Internet.

Über den Autoren • About the Author

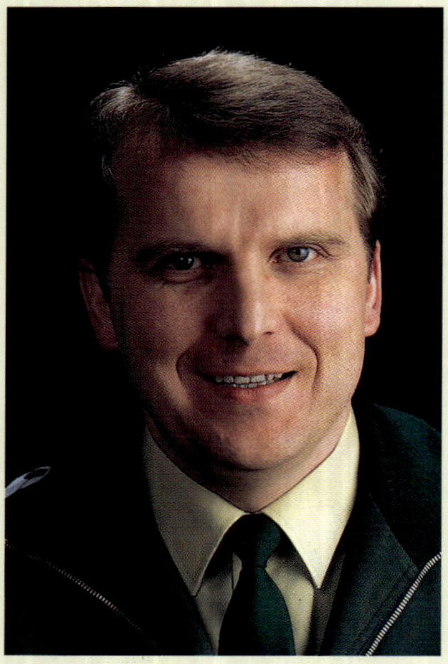

Thomas Helbig

geboren 1959, heute Polizeioberrat im BGS, begann seine Laufbahn nach dem Abitur. Mit dem Eintritt in den BGS studierte er an der Fachhochschule des Bundes für öffentliche Verwaltung und schloss dieses Studium als Diplomverwaltungswirt ab. Seiner Ausbildung zum Berufshubschrauberführer folgten die Tätigkeit als Flugeinsatzleiter in der BGS-Fliegerstaffel Süd sowie neben anderen Tätigkeiten die stellvertretende Staffelführung der BGS-Fliegerstaffel Nord. Nach einem zweijährigen Studium u.a. an der Polizei-Führungsakademie wurde er zunächst Leiter der Stabs- und Ausbildungsstaffel der BGS-Fliegergruppe und ist heute Leiter der daraus hervorgegangenen BGS-Fliegerstaffel West in Sankt Augustin-Hangelar.

born in 1959, today a senior police officer in the Federal Border Police, entered the FBP after graduating from college-track high school ("A levels"). He then completed the degree program in public administration at the College of Public Administration run by the German government. After undergoing training to become a professional helicopter pilot, Helbig served in various capacities at the Federal Border Police, including the positions of Head of Operations at the Aviation Squadron South and Deputy Squadron Leader of the FBP Aviation Squadron North. Following two years of further study at the Police Administration Academy and other educational institutions, he was appointed Leader of the Staff and Training Squadron of the FBP Aviation Group. Today he is Squadron Leader of the Aviation Squadron West – the successor to the Staff and Education Squadron – at St. Augustin-Hangelar.

Über den Autoren • About the Author

Dr. med. Dr. rer. nat. Alex Lechleuthner

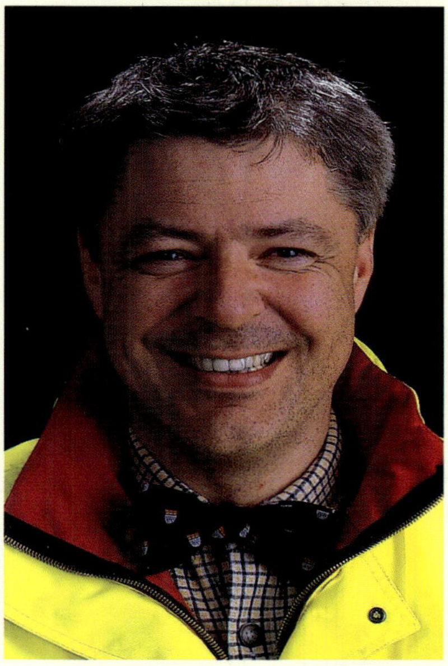

geboren 1959, studierte nach dem Abitur Humanmedizin und Chemie/Biologie in München und Freiburg. 1986 promovierte er zum Dr.med. in München und wurde approbiert, 1987 promovierte er zum Dr.rer.nat. in München. An der Universität in München und am Klinikum Köln-Merheim war er Assistenzarzt, hatte dann in Pittsburgh/USA einen Forschungsaufenthalt bevor er 1994 Facharzt für Chirurgie wurde.

Seit 1994 ist er Ärztlicher Leiter Rettungsdienst der Stadt Köln bei der Berufsfeuerwehr Köln. 1995 gründete er das Institut für Notfallmedizin der Berufsfeuerwehr Köln und leitet es seither. Im Jahr 2001 initiierte er den internationalen Studiengang „Rescue Engineering" an der Fachhochschule Köln. Seit vielen Jahren ist er auch aktiv im Notarztdienst auf dem NEF und dem Rettungshubschrauber Christoph 3 tätig.

was born in 1959. After studying medicine, chemistry and biology at universities in Munich and Freiburg, he received his "Dr. med" title and his medical license in Munich in 1986. In 1987 he went on do a doctorate in natural sciences, the "Dr.rer.nat." in Munich. He completed his residency at the University of Munich and University Hospital Cologne-Merheim before going to Pittsburgh, Pennsylvania (USA) on a research grant. Lechleuthner was awarded the title of "Specialist in Surgery" in 1994. Since 1994 he has been Medical Director of the Rescue Service at the Professional Fire Service of the City of Cologne. In 1995 he founded the Institute of Emergency Medicine at the Cologne Professional Fire Service and has headed this institute since then. In 2001 he initiated the founding of an international academic program in "Rescue Engineering" at the Cologne University of Applied Sciences. He has worked as a physician with emergency & rescue certification aboard the emergency physician car (NEF) and the rescue helicopter Christoph 3 for many years.

Über den Autoren • About the Author

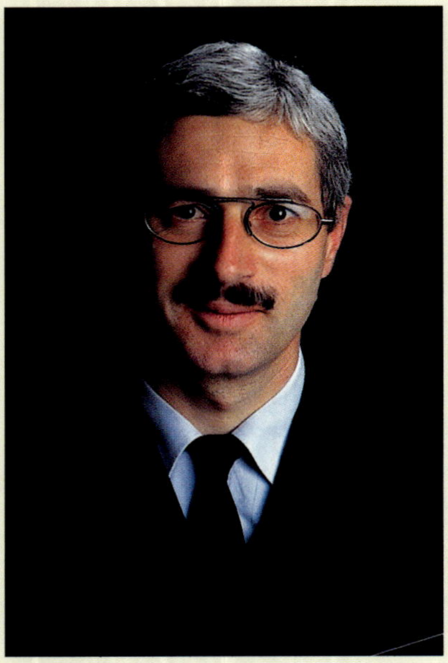

Klaus Maurer

geboren 1958, ist heute als Branddirektor stellvertretender Leiter der Berufsfeuerwehr Köln und dort zuständig für die zentrale Einsatzorganisation und leitet die Abteilung Gefahrenabwehr I. Nach dem Abitur studierte er an der Universität im Fachbereich Bauingenieurswesen mit der Fachrichtung Konstruktiver Ingenieurbau. Bevor er als Referendar in den Feuerwehrdienst eintrat, war er einige Jahre als wissenschaftlicher Angestellter am Lehrstuhl für Baumechanik der Universität tätig. Nach seiner Ernennung zum Brandrat war er als stellvertretender Leiter der Abteilung Einsatzdienst eingesetzt, dann war er Leiter der Abteilung Brandschutz, Hilfeleistung und Rettungsdienst der Berufsfeuerwehr Köln und nicht nur in dieser Funktion mit dem Rettungshubschrauber eng verbunden.

born in 1958, senior fire service officer, is now Deputy Chief of the Cologne Professional Fire Service, where he is in charge of Central Operations and heads the Department for Hazard Avoidance I. After graduating from college-track high school ("A levels"), he studied at the University of Wuppertal, where he had a major in civil engineering and a minor in structural engineering. Before entering the fire service as an administrative trainee, he worked for several years as an assistant lecturer in the Department of Building Mechanics. Following his promotion to the civil service grade of Brandrat in the higher intermediate fire service, Maurer was appointed Deputy Head of Operations and then Head of Fire Protection, Auxiliary Services and Emergency Medical Services at the Cologne Professional Fire Department. In this capacity – but not only in this capacity – he has been intensely involved in rescue helicopter activities.

Über den Autoren • About the Author

Wolfgang Nowak

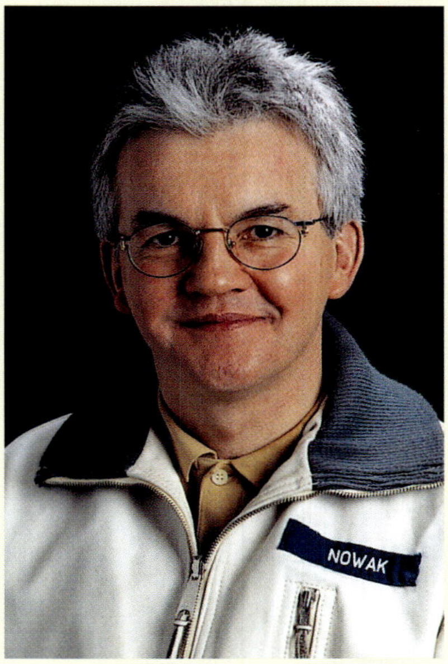

geboren 1951, war bereits als Fünfzehnjähriger ehrenamtlicher Helfer im Malteser-Hilfsdienst. Seine Ausbilderberechtigung für Erste Hilfe Kurse erwarb er kurz darauf. Nach dem Abitur absolvierte er einen der ersten Rettungssanitäterlehrgänge des Malteser Hilfsdienstes, arbeitete im Krankenhaus und sammelte Erfahrungen im bodengebundenen Rettungsdienst. Er zählt zu den Rettungssanitätern der ersten Jahre von Christoph 3. In dieser Zeit gelang es neben Anderen auch ihm, das neue Rettungsmittel RTH bei Polizeien und Rettungsdiensten bekannt zu machen und die Scheu vor einer Anforderung des RTH abzubauen. Die Vermittlung von neuen Einsatz- und Rettungsstrategien wurde ihm übertragen, und zwar zunächst an der zentralen Schulungsstätte des Malteser-Hilfsdienstes in Köln als Ausbildungsreferent, dann in gleicher Funktion und als Dozent im Rettungsdienst an der staatlichen Rettungsassistentenschule in Bonn.

born in 1951, joined the Malteser-Hilfsdienst as a volunteer at the age of 15. Shortly afterwards, he qualified to be a First Aid Trainer. After graduating from college-track high school, Nowak completed one of the first training programs for emergency medical technicians held by the Malteser-Hilfsdienst, worked as an EMT at various hospitals, and gained experience as a member of the rescue service on the ground. He is one of the "EMT pioneers" who worked aboard Christoph 3 in the early days of air rescue in Germany. During this period, he was also one of the "PR pioneers" who mounted information campaigns to explain the rescue helicopter to police and rescue services in an attempt to overcome their initial reticence to call in the new air ambulance. He was subsequently entrusted with the task of teaching new mission and rescue strategies. In this role, he first worked as an instructor at the Central Educational Facility of the Malteser- Hilfsdienst in Cologne and later as a lecturer on rescue service topics at the State School for Paramedics in Bonn.

Über den Autoren

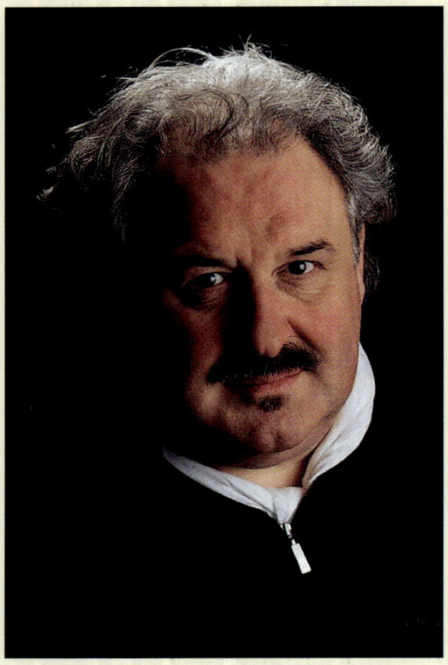

Karl Neno

geboren 1952, heute Gymnasiallehrer für Musik und Deutsch, hat seit Jugendtagen zwei große Interessen: die Musik und die Fotografie, die er immer parallel betrieb. Nach dem Abitur folgten ein Musikstudium an der Musikhochschule mit dem künstlerischen Hauptinstrument Trompete, Tonsatz und Kompositionsfächern, sowie ein Studium an der Universität in Germanistik, Philosophie und Pädagogik (Philosophikum). Zeitgleich begann seine Zeit im Ersatzdienst. Früh sammelte er Erfahrungen, zunächst im Krankentransport, dann im Rettungs- und Notarztdienst. Nach Abschluss seines Rettungssanitäterlehrgangs, bei dem er alle schriftlichen, mündlichen und praktischen Prüfungsteile mit der Bestnote sehr gut abschloss, bot man ihm an, im Luftrettungsdienst mitzuwirken. 22 Jahre war er dort ehrenamtlich tätig, zunächst als Rettungssanitäter, mit Einführung des Berufsbildes dann als Rettungsassistent und in Köln in der ersten Generation der HEMS-Crew Member.

Seine Portraitphotographien hat Karl Neno in mehreren Ausstellung vorgestellt und ist darüberhinaus als künstlerischer Fotograf anerkannt. Er wird in kontinuierlichen Abständen exklusiv im Kisterkall-Verlag weitere Fotobücher und Bildbände präsentieren. Neben seinen fotografischen Arbeiten hat Karl Neno in unterschiedlichen Formationen als Trompeter, sowie als Komponist und Arrangeur gearbeitet. Seine Kenntnisse hat er als Big Band Leader seinen Schülern weitergegeben. Die von ihm gegründete Band existiert seit über 20 Jahren. Einem Absolventen der Paul Mc Cartney's School of Music gefielen Neno's Pop-Songs so gut, dass Karl Neno weitere aus der Schublade holte und sie aufnahm. Für ihn ist das Musizieren eine Möglichkeit, sich in der Zeit auszudrücken, die Fotografie eine Möglichkeit, Zeitüberdauerndes zu schaffen. Auf der Foto – CD zum Buch finden sich neben Fotos aus dem Buch „Einsatz für den Rettungshubschrauber" auch einige seiner Pop-Songs und einige Titel seiner Instrumentalmusik.

About the Author

Karl Neno

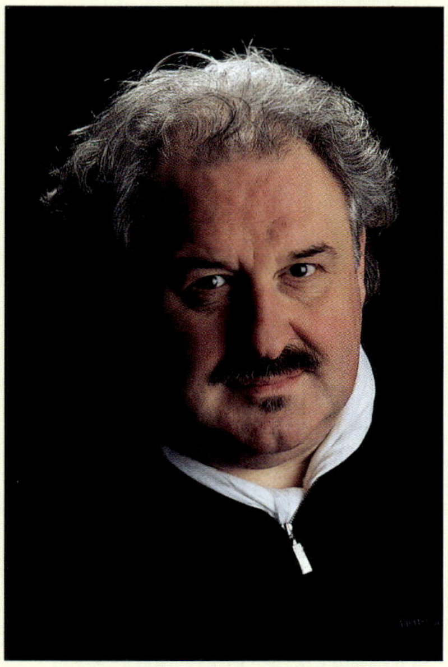

born in 1952, now a teacher of music and German at a college-track high school (Gymnasium), has had two parallel passions since childhood: music and photography. After completing his A levels, Neno was admitted to the Cologne Conservatory of Music (Staatliche Musikhochschule), where he studied the trumpet (his main instrument), music theory and composition. During this period of his life, he also studied German, philosophy and education at the University of Cologne. Neno's career in the emergency medical service started at about the same time, during his alternative service with the Malteser-Hilfsdienst. Here Neno gained valuable experience – first in patient transport, later in the emergency medical service and emergency physician service. After passing his examinations as an emergency medical technician with the top mark of "very good" in the written, oral and practical parts, he was offered a job in the helicopter emergency medical service (HEMS). He worked in the HEMS – first as an EMT and later in the new profession of "air rescue paramedic" – for 22 years. He is one of the "first generation" HEMS Crew Members in Cologne.

Portrait photography has always fascinated Karl Neno and his studio portraits have already been exhibited in several shows. However, he is also well known in photographic circles for his art photography. As part of an exclusive arrangement with Kisterkall Publishers, Neno plans to successively produce additional photo books – classical "coffee table books" as well as books explaining some aspect of photography – at regular intervals.

Over the years Karl Neno has continued to pursue his twin passions. Next to his photography, he has found time to play the trumpet – and work as a composer and arranger – for various bands and groups. Twenty years ago he founded a high school big band as a way of sharing his musical know-how with the younger generation. This "Big Band" has survived to the present day. On one occasion a graduate of Paul McCartney's School of Music liked one of Karl Neno's pop songs so much that Karl Neno took more songs out of his desk drawer and recorded them.

For Neno, making music is a way to express yourself in time, while photography is a possibility for creating something that lasts. The Photo-CD accompanying this book contains several of his pop songs and instrumental arrangements in addition to photos from the book "Mission for the Rescue Helicopter".

Über den Autoren • About the Author

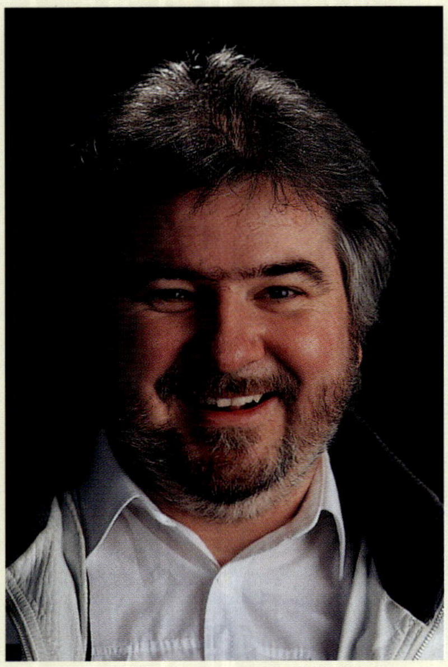

Peter Simon

geboren 1958, ist seit 1979 Luftrettungsassistent auf dem Kölner Rettungshubschrauber. Er besitzt eine weitere medizinische Berufsausbildung als Fachkrankenpfleger für Anästhesie und Intensivmedizin. 1980 wurde er zum leitenden Luftrettungsassistenten berufen und hat dieses Amt 20 Jahre lang ausgeübt. Als leitender Luftrettungsassistent war er für die Fortbildung der Luftrettungsassistenten und deren Einweisung in die Handhabung der medizinischen Geräte zuständig. Er gehört zur ersten Generation der Kölner Rettungsassistenten, die die Ausbildung zum HEMS Crew Member erfolgreich absolviert hat. Seit dem Jahr 2000 ist er wegen seines hohen fachlichen Könnens als Qualitätsbeauftragter für den Malteser-Rettungsdienst in der Region Nordrhein-Westfalen tätig, und ist Malteser Vertreter in den DIN-Normenausschüssen für Luftrettungsmittel, Krankenkraftwagen und Behindertentransportwagen.

born in 1958, has worked on the Cologne rescue helicopter as an air rescue paramedic since 1979. He has also completed nursing training in anesthesia and intensive care medicine. In 1980 he was appointed Head Air Rescue Paramedic and served in this capacity for 20 years. In this position he was responsible for organizing the continued education of air rescue paramedics and providing instruction on the handling of medical machines and devices. He is a member of the first generation of air rescue paramedics in Cologne who successfully completed their training as HEMS Crew Members. Owing to his extensive professional know-how, he has been appointed Quality Management Officer for the Maltese Rescue Service in North Rhine-Westphalia in 2000. He also represents the Malteser-Hilfsdienst on the DIN Standards Committees for air rescue resources, rescue vehicles and disabled-person transport vehicles.

Über die Übersetzerin • About the translator

Shawn Christoph

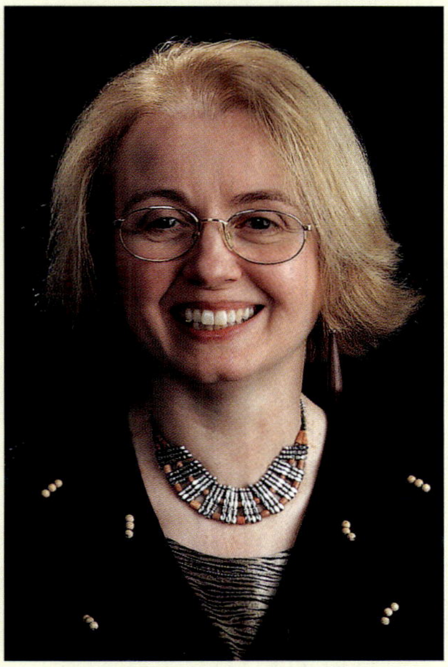

wurde 1946 in Washington, D.C. geboren. Sie studierte Mikrobiologie an der Universität Maryland und Publizistik an der Columbia-Universität in New York. Nach Ihrer Übersiedlung nach Essen im Jahre 1968 arbeitete sie als Journalistin, Dozentin und Übersetzerin. Seit 1986 ist sie als freiberufliche Übersetzerin tätig. Zu ihrem Kundenstamm zählen grössere, mittlere und kleinere Unternehmen, Werbeagenturen, Universitäten, Wissenschaftler, Ärzte, die Justizbehörden, Rechtsanwälte und Privatpersonen. Seit einigen Jahren spezialisiert sie sich zunehmend auf die Übersetzung medizinischer, pharmazeutischer und biotechnologischer Fachtexte.

was born in Washington, D.C. in 1946. After studying microbiology at the University of Maryland and journalism at Columbia University in New York City, she moved to Essen, Germany, in 1968. During her first 20 years in Germany, she worked as a journalist, teacher and translator. She has been a free-lance translator for the last 15 years; her customers include large companies, SMEs, advertising agencies, universities, scientists, doctors, the judicial system, lawyers and private individuals. In recent years, she has increasingly specialized in medical, pharmaceutical and biotechnology texts.

Vorankündigung

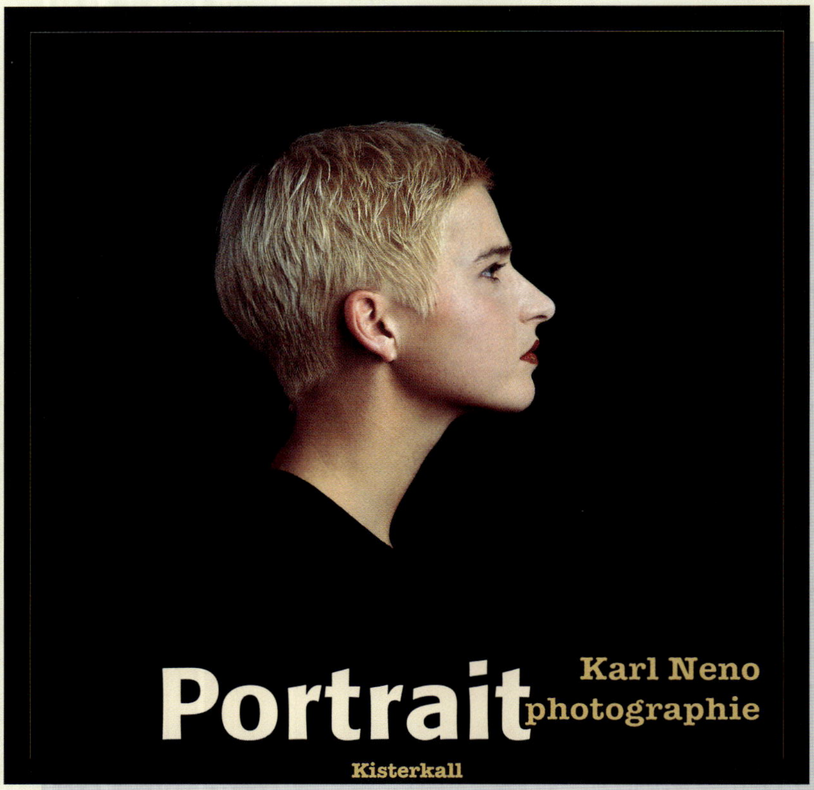

ISBN
3-935604-01-7

Der Kisterkall Verlag wird weitere Ratgeber und Kunstbände herausgeben.

In aktueller Vorbereitung ist ein Foto-Ratgeber von Karl Neno über künstlerische Portraitfotografie. Neno's Geschick, komplizierte Vorgänge einfach und anschaulich zu erklären, machen die Tipps des Buches für Anfänger wie Fortgeschrittene nachvollziehbar.Das Buch ist in Form eines großangelegten Workshops mit nur zwei Modellen, Sandra und Stephanie, fotografiert, um so zu zeigen, wie unterschiedliche Gestaltungen das Bild eines Menschen verändern können.

Weitere Bücher über Neno's Fotografien von Menschen werden folgen.

Informationen dazu erhalten Sie unter der Verlagsadresse, per Fax oder auf unserer Internet – homepage **www.kisterkall.de.**

Alle Fotos des Buches: Einsatz für den Rettungshubschrauber sind auch als Posterprints erhältlich.

Anfragen dazu richten Sie bitte an den Kisterkall Verlag!

Kisterkall will be publishing additional practical guides and art books within the near future. At present the publishing house is working on a guide to portrait photography by Karl Neno explaining the secrets of artistic photographic portraits. Owing to Neno's ability to explain complicated subjects clearly and understandably, his tips are easy to follow for experienced and novice photographers alike. The book has been designed as a photographic workshop; by working with only two models, Sandra and Stepahnie, the author shows how a multitude of different effects can be achieved by changing a few basic parameters.

This will be followed by other photo books containing Neno's photographs of people.

To obtain further information, contact us by mail, fax, or email – or visit our website at **www.kisterkall.de.**

All photos of the book: Mission for the Rescue Helicopter are also available as poster prints.

Please send any inquiries directly to Kisterkall Publishers.